# An Osteopathic Approach to Diagnosis and Treatment

## THIRD EDITION

# An Osteopathic Approach to Diagnosis and Treatment

## THIRD EDITION

**Eileen L. DiGiovanna, DO, FAAO, Senior Editor**
Professor Emerita
Former Chairperson
The Stanley Schiowitz, DO, FAAO Department of Osteopathic Manipulative Medicine
New York College of Osteopathic Medicine
New York Institute of Technology
Old Westbury, New York
Fellow of the American Academy of Osteopathy

**Stanley Schiowitz, DO, FAAO, Senior Editor**
Dean Emeritus
Former Distinguished Professor and Former Chairperson
The Stanley Schiowitz, DO, FAAO Department of Osteopathic Manipulative Medicine
New York College of Osteopathic Medicine
New York Institute of Technology
Old Westbury, New York
Fellow of the American Academy of Osteopathy

**Dennis J. Dowling, DO, FAAO, Editor and Illustrator**
Private Practice
Attending Physician & Director of Manipulation
Physical Medicine and Rehabilitation Department
Nassau University Medical Center
East Meadow, New York
Former Professor and Chairperson
The Stanley Schiowitz, DO, FAAO Department of Osteopathic Manipulative Medicine
New York College of Osteopathic Medicine
New York Institute of Technology
Old Westbury, New York
Fellow of the American Academy of Osteopathy

*With 20 Contributors*

ILLUSTRATED BY **Dennis J. Dowling, DO, FAAO**

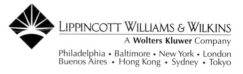

**LIPPINCOTT WILLIAMS & WILKINS**
A **Wolters Kluwer** Company
Philadelphia • Baltimore • New York • London
Buenos Aires • Hong Kong • Sydney • Tokyo

Acquisition Editor: Danette Somers
Developmental Editor: Keith Donnellan and Nancy Winter
Marketing Manager: Kathy Neely
Project Manager: Bridgett Dougherty
Typesetter: Maryland Composition, Inc.
Printer: Edwards Brothers, Inc.

530 Walnut Street
Philadelphia, Pennsylvania 19106

351 West Camden Sreet
Baltimore, Maryland 21201-2436 USA

Printed in the United States of America

**Library of Congress Cataloging-in-Publication Data**

An osteopathic approach to diagnosis and treatment / [edited by] Eileen L. DiGiovanna,
Stanley Schiowitz, and Dennis Dowling.—3rd ed.
     p. ; cm.
  Includes bibliographical references and index.
   ISBN 0-7817-4293-5
  1. Osteopathic medicine. I. DiGiovanna, Eileen L. II. Schiowitz, Stanley. III. Dowling,
Dennis J.
   [DNLM: 1. Osteopathic Medicine. WB 940 084 2004]
RZ341.0696 2004
615.5'33—dc22
                                      2004015188

# Dedication

*We dedicate this book:*

*To osteopathic students and physicians who share our belief that our hands are channels of healing;*

*To colleagues and mentors who have expanded our understanding of osteopathic manipulative medicine;*

*To our patients, who have taught us so much about the functioning of the human body, mind, and spirit;*

*To our families, who give us the support that allows us to continue.*

# Preface to First and Second Editions

The instruction of students in the concepts and principles of osteopathic medicine, as well as in the skills of manipulative medicine, began in a tiny frame building in Kirksville, Missouri, almost 100 years ago today. Andrew Taylor Still was the founder and professor of that school. He wrote down many of his thoughts and ideas, which were later collected into the first books of this profession.

Since that time, only a few books have been published on osteopathy, with most of the educational process relying on personal instruction and demonstration. To add to this, much of the information is scattered in obscure journals not available to everyone. Those texts which are available are generally limited to one or a few types of techniques.

Our goal here has been to prepare a text that organizes currently taught concepts and techniques into one comprehensive volume which might then serve as a reference for osteopathic medical students, as well as practicing physicians. The result is a book, which presents an integrated method for both the diagnosis and treatment of somatic and visceral problems manifesting in the soma. We have also added an extensive section on practical applications to serve as a demonstration of examples of osteopathic concepts integrated into the management of some commonly encountered conditions.

The osteopathic approach to diagnosis and treatment is unique. We hope this text will make it more readily available to all osteopathic medical students.

Eileen L. DiGiovanna, DO, FAAO
Stanley Schiowitz, DO, FAAO

# Preface to Third Edition

The osteopathic profession has continued to grow, both in numbers of physicians and students and in the understanding of osteopathic manipulative medicine, since the first publication of this text. The subject matter taught in the osteopathic collegesß¥ departments of osteopathic manipulative medicine has expanded to meet the needs of the students as they prepare for practice. The methods of testing the students has evolved with heavier emphasis on case histories.

The editors have revised this edition to meet the needs of both teachers and students of osteopathic manipulative medicine. Many more practical applications have been added to the text along with many of the newly developed techniques. Each section on a region of the body has been enhanced with case histories illustrative of situations where osteopathic manipulative medicine is applicable to the patientsß¥ needs.

We have retained the material we feel is essential for practicing osteopathic physicians to understand in order to best serve their patientsß¥ treatment needs.

Eileen L. DiGiovanna, DO, FAAO
Stanley Schiowitz, DO, FAAO
Dennis J. Dowling, DO, FAAO

# Acknowledgments

We wish to acknowledge the able assistance given us in preparing this book by the editorial staff at Lippincott William & Wilkins. And of course, thanks to our spouses, Joseph DiGiovanna, DO, Lillian Schiowitz, and Fran Dowling for their support and allowing us the time to complete this project.

# Contents

## SECTION III   CERVICAL SPINE

## SECTION VI   PELVIS AND SACRUM

## SECTION VII   THORACIC CAGE

## SECTION VIII   UPPER EXTREMITIES

# SECTION X CRANIAL OSTEOPATHY

# SECTION XI SYSTEMIC CONSIDERATIONS

# SECTION XII OSTEOPATHIC MANAGEMENT

# Contributors

**NANCY BROUS, DO**

Assistant Professor
Director of Islip Clinic
New York College of Osteopathic Medicine
New York Institute of Technology
Old Westbury, New York

**JOHN CAPOBIANCO, DO, FAAO**

Former Clinical Associate Professor
The Stanley Schiowitz, DO, FAAO Department of
  Osteopathic Manipulative Medicine
New York College of Osteopathic Medicine
New York Institute of Technology
Old Westbury, New York

**LISA R. CHUN, DO**

Private Practice
Kaua'i Osteopathic Inc.
Koloa, HI

**WILLIAM THOMAS CROW, DO, FAAO**

Associate Professor
Department of Osteopathic Manipulative Medicine
Philadelphia College of Osteopathic Medicine
Philadelphia, Pennsylvania

**ALBERT R. DERUBERTIS, DO**

Private Practice
Physical Medicine and Rehabilitation
Suburban Heights Medical Center
Chicago Heights, Illinois

**EILEEN L. DIGIOVANNA, DO, FAAO**

Professor Emerita and Former Chairperson
The Stanley Schiowitz, DO, FAAO Department of
  Osteopathic Manipulative Medicine
New York College of Osteopathic Medicine
New York Institute of Technology
Old Westbury, New York

**JOSEPH A. DIGIOVANNA, D.O.**

Former Acting Chairman and Associate Professor of
  Family Practice
Former Associate Professor of Osteopathic
  Manipulative Medicine
Smithtown, New York

**DENNIS J. DOWLING, DO, FAAO**

Attending Physician & Director of Manipulation
Physical Medicine and Rehabilitation Department
Nassau University Medical Center
East Meadow, New York
Former Professor and Chairperson
The Stanley Schiowitz, DO, FAAO Department of
  Osteopathic Manipulative Medicine
New York College of Osteopathic Medicine
New York Institute of Technology
Old Westbury, New York
Private Practice
Osteopathic Manipulative Medicine Associates
Syosset, NY

**BARRY S. ERNER, DO**

Private Practice
Cos Cob, Connecticut

**HUGH ETTLINGER, DO, FAAO**

Associate Professor
The Stanley Schiowitz, DO, FAAO Department of
  Osteopathic Manipulative Medicine
Director of Residency Program in Osteopathic
  Manipulative Medicine
New York College of Osteopathic Medicine
New York Institute of Technology
Old Westbury, New York

**JONATHAN F. FENTON, DO**

Private Practice
Essex Junction, Vermont

**MARY-THERESA FERRIS, DO**

Private Practice
Mechanicsville, VA

## BONNIE GINTIS, DO

Private Practice
Soquel, California

## MARY HITCHCOCK, DO, FAAO

Former Associate Professor
Stanley Schiowitz Department of Osteopathic
　Manipulative Medicine
New York College of Osteopathic Medicine
New York Institute of Technology
Old Westbury, New York
Deceased

## DAVID J. MARTINKE, DO

Private Practice
Tonawanda, New York

## DONALD PHYKITT, DO

Private Practice
Athens, Pennsylvania

## SONIA RIVERA-MARTINEZ, DO

Family Practice Resident
Long Beach Medical Center
Long Beach, New York

## PAULA D. SCARIATI, DO

Private Practice
Fayetteville, New York

## STANLEY SCHIOWITZ, DO, FAAO

Dean Emeritus
Distinguished Professor and Former Chairperson
The Stanley Schiowitz, DO, FAAO Department of
　Osteopathic Manipulative Medicine
New York College of Osteopathic Medicine
New York Institute of Technology
Old Westbury, New York

## CHARLES J. SMUTNEY III, DO

Private Practice
Bethpage, New York

## LILLIAN SOMNER, DO

Private Practice
Bethesda, Maryland

## TONI SPINARIS, DO

Private Practice
Colden, New York

## SANDRA D. YALE, DO

Private Practice
Buffalo, New York

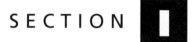

# Basics of Osteopathic Medicine

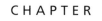

# Introduction

*Eileen L. DiGiovanna*

Osteopathic medicine represents one of two distinct schools of medicine in the United States. It is only in the United States that there are two groups of fully licensed physicians. Osteopathic medical institutions issue Doctor of Osteopathic Medicine or Doctor of Osteopathy (DO) degrees, and allopathic (nonosteopathic) medical institutions issue Medical Doctor (MD) degrees. The educational process is similar in both kinds of institutions, with distinctive differences in the osteopathic curriculum. Applicants to osteopathic medical schools have an undergraduate degree, and many have earned a master's or other postgraduate degree. They complete the Medical College Aptitude Test (MCAT), as do the applicants to the allopathic colleges.

The 4 years in osteopathic medical school are spent in the study of basic and clinical sciences, much as in nonosteopathic medical schools, but with an added focus on osteopathic principles and concepts and intensive study of osteopathic manipulative medicine. The third and fourth years allow rotations into clinic, office, and hospital settings with introductions to inner city, suburban, and rural types of practice.

After graduation, the DO may complete a rotating internship for 1 year and then enter a residency to specialize in any branch of medicine. The DO is qualified to write prescriptions, perform surgery, deliver babies, and undertake other medical services as needed for promoting good patient health. As of April 1985, DOs were certified in all specialties, including family practice. Subspecialization may be chosen in any field.

The uniqueness of osteopathic medicine lies in the application of osteopathic philosophy and concepts. Osteopathic medical practitioners follow accepted methods of physical and surgical diagnosis and treatment; they are also trained to expertly evaluate the neuromusculoskeletal system and seek to achieve normal body mechanics through the use of manual manipulative medicine. Osteopathic physicians recognize the body's ability to regulate itself and mount its own defenses against most pathologic conditions.

Osteopathic medicine thus recognizes the neuromusculoskeletal system as crucially important to the full expression of life. The viscera subserve the neuromusculoskeletal system by providing nourishment to it and by removing its wastes. As George Northup noted in *Osteopathic Medicine, An American Reformation:*

> The musculoskeletal system is intimately connected with all other systems of the body through both the voluntary and the involuntary nervous systems. . . . Thus, indications are that the musculoskeletal system is a mirror of both health and disease, responding as it does to inflammation and pain from disorder in other body systems.

Therefore, when assessing the patient, the osteopathic physician considers the body as an integrated unit comprising multiple complex functions and interrelated structures.

Another important principle in osteopathic medicine is that structure and function are intimately interrelated. An abnormality in the structure of any body part can lead to abnormal function, whether expressed locally or distantly from the deranged structure. To correct the mechanical disorders, the osteopathic physician undertakes therapeutic osteopathic manipulation. This

3

hands-on treatment is gentle and controlled; it may be directed toward joint motion or directed toward the muscles or fasciae. It is also used to affect circulation, body fluids, and nervous impulses.

The heart of osteopathy is the recognition of the body's ability to cure itself, with some external help, of many pathologic conditions. This tenet echoes the belief enunciated by Hippocrates more than 2,000 years ago: "Our natures are the physicians for our diseases."

Osteopathic medicine continues to grow even as it remains in a minority position in the health care system. From five schools in 1962, there are presently twenty schools, with more in the planning stages. The 2001 Annual Report on Osteopathic Medical Education numbers osteopathic physicians at 46,990 as of June 2001, with a total enrollment of students in the 19 osteopathic colleges of 10,817. Norman Gevitz, in *The D.O.s: Osteopathic Medicine in America*, published in 1982, estimated at that time that DO physicians and surgeons were providing health care services for more than twenty million Americans, or in excess of 10% of the population. He stated in a lecture recently that they now care for close to 20% of the population. More impor-

tantly, a large percentage of osteopathic physicians tend to go into the primary care specialties (64% as of 1999) and tend to practice in underserved areas.

The osteopathic profession has changed even as it has grown. It has achieved recognition as a significant part of the American health care system. It is now carefully defining its special contributions to medicine and is undertaking various kinds of research to prove the effectiveness of its manipulative techniques. With these and similar steps toward full realization of the potential of osteopathic medicine, the profession is securing its position in the modern medical climate.

## REFERENCES

DiGiovanna E, Schiowitz S. *An Osteopathic Approach to Diagnosis and Treatment*, 2nd ed. Philadelphia: Lippincott Raven, 1997.

Gevitz N. *The D.O.s, Osteopathic Medicine in America*. Baltimore: Johns Hopkins University Press, 1982.

Gevitz N. *From the Center to the Periphery*. Lecture for 2003 Convocation of the American Academy of Osteopathy. Ottawa, Canada, 2003.

Northup GW. *Osteopathic Medicine: An American Reformation*. Chicago: American Osteopathic Association, 1966.

Singer A. *AACOM 2001 Annual Report on Osteopathic Medical Education*. Chevy Chase, MD, 2001.

# History of Osteopathy

*Eileen L. DiGiovanna*

Andrew Taylor Still, the founder of osteopathy, was born August 6, 1828, in Jonesville (written as *Jonesboro* by one biographer, E. R. Booth), Lee County, Virginia, of English-Scottish-Irish-German descent. His father was a circuit-riding minister in the Methodist Episcopal Church, a physician, a farmer, and a millwright. His mother was a sturdy frontierswoman, Martha Poague Moore, who raised her children in a strongly religious home. It was from this background that Still developed a strong belief in God as the perfect Creator of all things. It was thus his belief that all of creation was perfect, including the human body. He proclaimed that a perfect body would be able to heal itself and would contain within it the means with which to do so.

As a young boy, Still experienced severe headaches. One day during such a headache, he went to sit in a rope swing his father had hung for him from a tree branch. Feeling ill, he removed the board from the swing and lay on the ground with the back of his neck resting against a blanket he threw over the rope. The pain eased, and he fell asleep. When he awoke, the headache was gone. He did this many times when a headache would occur and noted equal success. This observation contributed to later ideas relative to the involvement of the nervous system in body mechanics, eventually contributing to the development of osteopathy.

Being a hunter, as most men on the frontier were, Andrew Still would skin the animals he killed and developed a lifelong fascination with their muscles, bones, and joints. He never ceased his study of anatomy and always instructed his students in the significance of a strong background in anatomy as the basis for diagnosis and treatment.

He acquired his education in small school-houses as his father was moved ever further to the West. His informal education consisted of his incessant reading and information he learned as he followed his father on his rounds as minister-physician to the farms and small communities scattered around the countryside. Still gained his education in medicine primarily as an apprentice, although he claimed some formal training in Kansas City and was issued an MD degree by the state of Missouri.

Even as a youth, Still held strong opinions on many controversial subjects. One of these concerned slavery. He and his father were such strong abolitionists that his father, fearing for his family's safety, had to request a transfer from Missouri, a border state supporting slavery, to a Shawnee Indian Reservation in the Kansas Territory. Here, Andrew Taylor Still continued his fight against slavery. Here, also, he had access to Indian graves from which he exhumed and dissected bodies. As morbid as this may seem in today's enlightened times, this behavior was quite common for those studying medicine.

He joined the Kansas militia during the Civil War and rose from captain to the rank of major. It may have been during his service in the militia that he first learned about manipulation. European mercenaries who fought with the Union may have told him about "bonesetters," who were popular in England and other parts of Europe in the nineteenth century. There was undoubtedly some influence from this source because a card, distributed by Still from approximately 1883 to 1890, called him the "Lightning Bonesetter."

Later, as a member of the Kansas legislature, he assisted Kansas in becoming a state. While living with his family in Kansas, Andrew, his brothers, and father donated land and money for the building of Baker University in Baldwin, Kansas.

In the 1850s and 1860s, American medical practitioners were frequently poorly trained and had little understanding of the causes of disease. Very few had the advantage of a medical school education, and even those who did had received one that was extremely primitive compared to today's standards. Treatments were unsophisticated to the point of being dangerous. Some common remedies used in those years included laxatives, purgatives, bloodletting (sometimes to the point of unconsciousness), calomel (a mercury compound), narcotics, and drugs with alcohol bases. Dehydration, drug addiction, alcoholism, and mercury poisoning were among the results. Often the treatments were more dangerous than the illnesses. This time period occurred during the era known as the "Age of Heroic Medicine," not for the medical heroes that it produced but for the difficult and arduous interventions inflicted on the unfortunate patients.

Epidemics of typhoid, tuberculosis, influenza, yellow fever, "swamp fever" (malaria), measles, and meningitis, as well as other infectious diseases, often were rampant across the frontier. An epidemic of meningitis took the lives of three of Andrew's children; orthodox medicine was unable to save them. In his autobiography, Still reflected on this episode: "In sickness, had God left man in a world of guessing? Guess what is the matter? What to give and guess the result?" Still sought answers to these perplexing questions and began to develop a systematic method of treatment that would eliminate guesswork and bring health without the disastrous results of therapies current at that time. He worked largely with and through the musculoskeletal system and recognized the importance of the vascular and lymphatic systems. He believed in natural immunity, that the body had

its own "pharmacy" for healing itself. He developed a form of manipulation to help keep the body fit with unobstructed circulation and innervation.

Still broke with allopathy, as orthodox medicine was called, on June 22, 1874, when he "flung the banner of osteopathy to the breeze." "He moved about Kansas and Missouri as an itinerant physician, gaining a following of patients and finally settled in Kirksville, Missouri. He was later supported in letters and testimony by a fellow Missourian, Samuel Clemens (Mark Twain)."

Initially there were many difficulties. Prospective patients were suspicious and others practicing medicine were antagonistic. He was ostracized by the church that said he was trying to heal by the "laying on of hands." He was considered by many as a "quack." Even his brothers initially believed he was not in his right mind.

He began by treating people on outlying farms until the townsfolk recognized the seemingly miraculous results he was attaining. As his successes increased, his fame grew and huge crowds gathered for his new treatment. The small town was soon so overcrowded that a hotel had to be built by the railroad station to accommodate visiting patients. Eventually a sanitarium was built for use in treating patients and teaching.

Many requests came to Still to teach his new method of healing. He first attempted to teach the sons of a patient by preceptorship but failed when they could not understand his concepts. This led him to believe that osteopathy was something only he could do, but he was later successful in teaching his own sons. He then attempted to provide a course at Baker University in Baldwin, Kansas, the institution to which he and his brothers had contributed substantial land and financial support. He was not successful; osteopathy was considered quackery.

In 1892, Still purchased a small two-room building and started the American School of Osteopathy (ASO) in Kirksville, Missouri. The first class of twenty-two students graduated in 1893 and included five women, unusual at this time in history. Still quickly realized that 1 year was not enough and increased the curriculum to 2 years and then 3 years. In the first years, only anatomy and osteopathic manipulation were taught.

Dr. William Smith, a graduate of the prestigious Edinburgh University Medical School, was in America learning and selling surgical medical equipment. He was initially directed to Dr. Still by other physicians in an attempt to debunk the legendary osteopath; instead, he stayed on to become the first anatomy professor at the school in exchange for being taught manipulation. After he left, Jeanette (Nettie) Bolles, a member of the first class and a graduate of the American School of Osteopathy (ASO), became the anatomy professor.

Still trained his brothers, his children, some of his patients, and other MDs in his new profession. He never specifically wrote a technique book because he believed that his students should know anatomy exceptionally well and be able to devise their own techniques and adapt them based on that knowledge. He did write an autobiography and two concept books.

Still died in 1917 at the age of 89, 6 months after a statue in his honor was unveiled in the Kirksville courthouse square, where it stands today. He left behind a struggling profession and school. Many battles lay ahead for osteopathy to be accepted into the American health care system.

The American School of Osteopathy flourished and soon had to be moved to new quarters. By the turn of the century, there were more than seven hundred students enrolled in the school. One of the professional struggles occurred among the faculty of the ASO. Some wanted to develop a curriculum based on more scientific knowledge. Political dissention occurred as well among the faculty, and at one time a second school, The Andrew Taylor Still School of Osteopathy, was opened in Kirksville in 1922 with Still's son-in-law, George Laughlin, at its head. Eventually a truce was reached and the two schools merged. Many colleges of osteopathy had sprung up around the country. Some were providing adequate education in the principles and methods of osteopathy, whereas others were poorly run and some were merely diploma mills. Most closed for financial reasons or merged with another osteopathic school.

Another struggle occurred when all medical institutions were challenged regarding the quality of education. Abraham Flexner, a schoolteacher, was commissioned by the Rockefeller Institute to evaluate each of the medical school training programs in the United States, including osteopathic schools. Johns Hopkins University Medical School was used as the gold standard to which each was compared. Flexner's report was issued in 1910 and was scathing in its findings, with many of the institutions found sorely wanting and many institutions forced to close, including some of the poor-quality osteopathic schools. Legitimate osteopathic colleges chose to improve their medical curricula to meet the standards set for them. However, pharmacology was not included until 1929 because Still had so vehemently objected to doing so before his death.

Over the ensuing decades, DOs were concerned with developing places to practice, gaining hospital staff privileges, obtaining full licensure, and developing a mechanism for the accreditation of their colleges and hospitals. Many osteopathic hospitals sprung up to meet the needs of DOs who were not admitted to the staff of nonosteopathic hospitals. It was necessary to become aware of detrimental legislation and to lobby for inclusion in many of the medical laws and governmental medical programs. The American Medical Association's Code of Ethics forbade MDs from having any professional interaction with DOs

By the 1960s, there were six stable osteopathic schools located in Kirksville, Kansas City, Chicago, Philadelphia, Los Angeles, and Des Moines. In 1962, the profession suffered a major setback when the American Medical Association (AMA) changed its policy of fighting osteopathy and offered an alliance to DOs in California, urging them to join the California Medical Association. They had the cooperation of the California Osteopathic Association in the process. More than 2,000 DOs in the state accepted the offer. The school in Los Angeles was turned into an MD-granting institution that offered an MD degree to California DOs (and for a $65 fee to DOs all over the country). This college later became part of the California University System at Irvine. Legislation had been passed preventing the state from licensing DOs to practice in California. The profession lost a large number of DOs, the California Osteopathic Medical Society, more than 2,000 osteopathic physicians, one of its colleges, and approximately 60% of its residencies.

To the amazement of the AMA, some California DOs and most DOs in the rest of the country rejected the offer to become MDs and began a fight to reestablish osteopathy within the state, including a licensing board, a new Osteopathic Medical Society, and a new school located in Pomona (later named Western University College of Osteopathic Medicine). Legislation preventing DOs from becoming licensed was overturned in the early 1970s after a long court struggle.

As of 2004, there were 20 schools of osteopathic medicine, with two more to open in 2004. DOs are licensed in all 50 states; Vermont was the first (1896) and Mississippi was the last (1973) to license them with full practice rights. Licensure has been hard-won through many court battles, with many DOs spending time in jail for "practicing medicine without a license." As of 2001, all state licensing boards accepted the National Board of Osteopathic Medical Examiners (NBOME) College of Osteopathic Medicine Licensing Examination (COMLEX) as fulfilling the examination requirement for state licensure.

Osteopathic physicians continued for many years to fight for their rights—to join hospital staffs, to participate in health care insurance plans, and to be included in health care bills and laws, both state and federal. The American Osteopathic Association still maintains vigilance to protect the rights of its members, who are still threatened at times.

One of the rights that had to be established was the right to equal treatment with allopathic physicians by the military. As early as 1917, Theodore Roosevelt had written a letter to Congress requesting that DOs be admitted to the military as commissioned officers as MDs were. Congress did not act on his request. DOs were only able to join the military as regular recruits and often served as paramedics if they chose to join.

During World War II, MDs were drafted whereas DOs were not. When the MDs returned after the war, they found that they had lost many of their patients to the osteopathic physicians who had remained at home. After this, the American Medical Association (AMA) became an ally of the American Osteopathic Association (AOA) in lobbying for acceptance of DOs as commissioned officers in the military. In 1966, the military finally accepted osteopathic physicians as equal to allopathic physicians. There are now numerous osteopathic physicians in the military. The highest rank was achieved by Ronald Blanck, DO, who became commander of the Army Medical Corps and head of Walter Reed Army Hospital. He recently retired to enter academic medicine.

Many people have contributed to the growth of the profession. It would be impossible to name them all, but some outstanding contributors should be noted.

J. Martin Littlejohn, DO, MD, was a Scottish student of multiple professions, including theology and medicine. He came to the United States with his two physician brothers, and they found their way to Kirksville and attended the American School of Osteopathy. After graduation, he joined the faculty there. He encouraged the teaching of physiology and other "more scientific" subjects. He and his brothers moved to Chicago, where they founded the Chicago College of Osteopathy. J. Martin Littlejohn later moved to London and was instrumental in founding the British School of Osteopathy, one of the best-known and respected European schools, from which osteopathy spread throughout Europe.

William Garner Sutherland was another student of Still. When the grooves in the suture of a temporal bone caught his eye, he was led to believe that the cranial bones must be capable of motion. He likened them to the "gills of a fish." He thus began the study of cranial osteopathy and spent many years developing its theories and techniques, used today as a specialized form of osteopathy.

Harrison H. Fryette was a DO who studied the motion of the spine and of individual vertebrae through the use of fluoroscopy, and his work produced the *Physiologic Principles of Vertebral Motion*. This improved the knowledge of how the spine functions and is still used as a model today.

Fred Mitchell, Sr, performed extensive work with sacral motion and its relation to gait. He was a leader in the development of the Muscle Energy technique. He developed the technique based on some theories of a technique developed by T. J. Ruddy, an ophthalmologist. The technique was called Resistive Duction and had been used in the treatment of eye disorders. Tutorials were developed to teach Muscle Energy techniques to osteopathic college faculty and practicing osteopathic physicians.

Irwin Korr, PhD, a physiologist, spent years teaching in Kirksville, Michigan, and Texas at the osteopathic colleges. His strong commitment to osteopathy led him to perform research in the field of somatic dysfunction, and he published some of the finest work in this area, including *The Physiologic Basis of Osteopathy*. He contributed much knowledge regarding facilitation of the spinal cord and axonal transport of substances through the axons of nerves. He has been a vocal advocate of osteopathic medicine.

Lawrence Jones was a general practitioner in Oregon when he undertook the treatment of a patient with severe psoas spasm and, serendipitously, obtained information that led him to the development of the theories and techniques of strain/counterstrain. He first published this information in *The DO* in 1960 and later in a book, *Strain/Counterstrain*.

Stanley Schiowitz, Dean Emeritus of the New York College of Osteopathic Medicine, developed the technique known as facilitated positional release, one of the newest techniques to be introduced to the profession. He is also co-editor of this textbook and has devoted his life to improving the educational system within the profession, ensuring that osteopathic principles will be included in that system.

Richard Van Buskirk resurrected some of the practices of Dr. Still by studying some of the original writings as well as the book of one his earliest students, Charles Hazzard. These techniques were named the Still technique.

Louisa Burns was one of the earliest and most fastidious researchers in the profession. A graduate of the California school, she spent time at the Chicago school performing research and later moved to California to develop a research center where most of her research was performed. Her work contributed to the understanding of the development and treatment of somatic dysfunction. J. Stedman Denslow was another researcher who contributed to the literature of the profession. A large part of his work was performed at the Kirksville College of Osteopathy.

Many others contributed significantly to the development and growth of the profession, and for this we thank them.

## REFERENCES

Booth ER. *History of Osteopathy and Twentieth Century Medical Practice*. Cincinnati: Press of Jennings & Graham, 1905.

DiGiovanna EL. *An Encyclopedia of Osteopathy*. Indianapolis: American Academy of Osteopathy, 2002.

Gevitz N. *The D.O.s, Osteopathic Medicine in America*. Baltimore: Johns Hopkins University Press, 1982.

Hildreth AG. *The Lengthening Shadow of Dr. Andrew Taylor Still*. Kirksville, MO: The Journal Printing Co, 1938.

Jones BE. *The Difference a D.O. Makes*, millennium ed. Oklahoma City: Oklahoma Educational Foundation for Osteopathic Education, 2001.

Schiowitz S. *An Osteopathic Approach to Diagnosis and Treatment*, 2nd ed.. Philadelphia: Lippincott-Raven, 1997.

Still CE Jr. *Frontier Doctor Medical Pioneer*. Kirksville, MO: Thomas Jefferson University Press, 1991.

Trowbridge C. *Andrew Taylor Still 1828–1917*. Kirksville, MO: Thomas Jefferson University Press, 1991.

# The Philosophy of Osteopathic Medicine

*Dennis J. Dowling and David J. Martinke*

The precepts discussed in this section are ideals. Those who do incorporate them into their practice will have a more realistic view of health and disease from the perspective of osteopathic philosophy.

Osteopathic medicine is not merely a combination of traditional Western medicine and osteopathic manipulations. Rather, the principles and philosophy of osteopathic medicine apply not only to manipulative treatment but also to complete health care of the individual. This includes surgery, obstetrics, emergency medicine, internal medicine, pediatrics, geriatrics, and any other areas of care traditionally associated with conventional Western medicine. In fact, osteopathic principles and philosophy permeate all aspects of health maintenance and disease prevention and treatment.

*The American Heritage Dictionary* defines a philosophy as an "inquiry into the nature of things based on logical reasoning rather than empirical methods." By contrast, a principle is defined as a "rule or law concerning the functioning of natural phenomena or mechanical process." Unlike philosophies, these rules or laws can be proved by experimental design or laboratory analysis. With these definitions in mind, it will be clear that the descriptions outlined are properly termed philosophies, not principles, because for the most part they are based on logical reasoning rather than on experimental design.

The osteopathic faculty committee at Kirksville College of Osteopathic Medicine, Kirksville, Missouri, developed the first four of the following precepts in 1953. Sarah Sprafka, Robert C. Ward, and David Neff enumerated others in the *Journal of American Osteopathic Association*, September 1981, and others were added by common usage.

1. "The body is a unit."

    This is also sometimes noted as "The Person is a unit." The human body does not function as a collection of separate parts but rather as an integral whole. Obviously, the body does consist of parts—the heart, the lungs, the musculoskeletal system, and so forth—all working to benefit the organism in totality. However, the osteopathic physician refrains from selecting any part above the whole. The osteopathic physician regards the kidneys, of primary focus to a nephrologist, or the heart, of particular interest to a cardiologist, as components subservient to the greater interest of the body. Uniting the body's parts is the fascia, a deep fibrous tissue investing the muscles and organs and acting as a ground substance to support and unite the whole body from head to foot. Thus the fascia is a fluid mechanism of profound functional significance. Other systems such as the neurological and musculoskeletal system contribute communication and locomotion aspects that benefit and integrate the whole. The arteries carrying nutrition to structures and the veins and lymphatic vessels that are conduits leading away from various parts of the body act as the nutrition suppliers and waste removal systems of the body. In conjunction with the other organs and structures, the body is a functional unit. All of these would barely be functional without the direction, oversight, and modification from the central and peripheral nervous systems. Osteopathic medicine also relates that the person is a whole, consisting of mind, body, and spirit. The implications of the effect of the state of health of the mind on bodily functions and vice versa are a whole field of study, psychosomatics, in and of itself. These in conjunction with the spiritual side of the individual form a whole on which the life of as patient depends.

2. "Structure and function are interrelated."

Any body part performs a function dictated by its structure. As an example, lung structure dictates that gases, carried by and dissolved in the blood, pass through the pulmonary arteries to the small capillaries in close approximation to the alveoli, where gas exchange takes place. As structure governs function, similarly, abnormal structure brings about dysfunction. In the case of abnormal lung structure, as in pulmonary fibrosis or interstitial pneumonia, the gradient between the alveolar gases and blood gases is increased, resulting in decreased gas exchange. Function also modifies structure. As an example, certain bony protrusions, such as the mastoid process of the temporal bone, do not exist in the newborn infant. As the child develops, the sternocleidomastoid muscles maintain upright positioning of the head and allow for turning and side-bending of the neck. The chronic use of these muscles brings about enlargement and elongation of the bony attachments. It is almost intuitively understood that a muscle that is exercised becomes larger. Abnormal function also results in alteration of related structures. Constriction of blood vessels undergoing sympathetic nervous influence brings about

changes in these blood vessels as well as in other structures, such as the heart, kidneys, and eyes. Conversely, abnormal structure results in dysfunction. An enlarged heart, such as that occurring in cardiomyopathy, is inefficient and will be incompatible with health and perhaps with life.

3. "The body possesses self-regulatory mechanisms."

Many examples of this precept can be considered. First, neuronal reflex mechanisms are constantly monitoring body functions. For example, the carotid sinus and baroreceptors in the neck monitor blood pressure and adjust the heart rate and cardiac contractility in response to changes in blood pressure. Second, hormonal pathways are involved in self-regulation. The releasing hormones of the hypothalamus regulate the release of the stimulating hormones from the pituitary, which in turn causes release of end-organ products (such as hormones or steroids). These products in turn provide feedback and regulate the activity of the hypothalamic-pituitary axis. These hormonal pathways are part of the complex endocrine system that is involved in the self-regulation of the body. Third, many organs such as the heart and kidneys are able to regulate blood flow. This vascular auto-regulation allows the organ to maintain the appropriate blood flow in the setting of a changing vascular status. These examples represent only a few of the many ways in which the body can regulate its functions. The reconstructive nature of many of the systems, including the gastrointestinal allow for rebuilding of structures, exchange of toxic elements, and eventual elimination of waste products. All of this occurs without conscious control in a manner that also incorporates the body unity concept.

4. "The body has the inherent capacity to defend and repair itself."

It is amazing that illness does not occur more often given the environment of pathogens, irritants, and toxic substances in which we live. The first lines of defense commonly recognized are the skin and mucous membranes. Some pathogens and irritants enter through the portals of the respiratory system, the nose and mouth. Depending on the size, some are trapped in hairs and others may be soluble in mucous or saliva, swallowed and then denatured by the low-pH stomach milieu. Once these shields are violated, elements of the cellular and humoral immune system are called on to protect the body from present and future invaders. Defense mechanisms are constantly working to protect the body as it contacts thousands of microorganisms daily. Occasionally, the body walls-off a region to isolate an infection and in other instances reacts quickly to denature or eliminate the invader. The temperature, which is regulated by the central nervous system, can increase drastically in response to the presence of pathogens. A fever, a symptom that more traditional medicine took as the object of treatment in the past, is part of an attempt by the body to inhibit further replication of microorganisms. Maintaining a certain elevated temperature allows the body to exist while keeping the numbers or organisms limited and more susceptible to attack by other immune components. However, above a certain temperature, fever endangers the individual.

The body also has the ability to adapt and compensate for insults and injuries to the structure and function. The skin provides protection to the organs and structures deep to the surface, as well as an early warning system through the hairs and sensory organs embedded within. Temperature regulation, some waste removal, and communications are provided by the vessels and nerves. The skin, muscles, ligaments, bones, and other musculoskeletal structures can redistribute forces from activities or trauma. The body's ability to repair itself is easily substantiated by observing the healing of a laceration or a fracture. Granulation tissue and the regenerative properties of certain tissues allow healing to take place. Nature is the best healer. The physician may facilitate the process, but the inherent capacity of the body to repair itself brings about the actual healing. The physi-

cian's contribution is to remove obstacles to the body's performance.

There may be instances in which the body may find a part incapacitated or even destroyed. The redundancy of some systems allows for the complete loss of one of a pair of organs, compensation by the other in the set, and normal or near-normal functioning. A kidney damaged by disease or trauma often results in the one on the opposite side taking over the complete function. A significant portion of the intestines can be resected during surgery, with the remaining components maintaining function. The removal of the left lung will frequently result in the enlargement and increased efficiency of the right one. Even when there is only one of an organ, a fraction can be impaired while the remainder continues to function. The liver, which is responsible for a great deal of toxin removal, can still function despite significant damage. The compensation is not always to the level of previous functioning. The loss of a limb, an ear, or an eye will not necessarily result in a compensatory increase in the ability of the contralateral structure. The disability that occurs may severely hamper normal functioning.

The body goes through reconstructive processes constantly. Food, vitamins, and water are converted to energy sources and building blocks for the structures. Some surfaces, such as the covering of the tongue and the mucosal lining of the stomach and intestines, go through a rapid turnover. Other cellular processes go through replications and replacement that may take longer periods of time. Some, such as portions of the nervous system, only undergo growth and replication in the early years. All involve exchange of nutritive and other substances. The turnover in molecular and atomic substances is almost constant. Certain systems, including the visceral organs, are part of the maintenance and building process that assures further activity of the individual.

Defense mechanisms are also inborn for interacting with the environment on the visible level. Humans, as well as other animals, have a sympathetic nervous system that prepares and reacts to danger. The pupils enlarge, the hearing becomes more acute, blood is shunted to the arms and legs, perspiration increases, saliva and other fluids of the alimentary track reduce in production, energy conversion shifts, and the ability to mobilize is in readiness for an anticipated attack. This amounts to the ready state for a "flight" or "fight" response. The individual can defend himself and those under his protection by striking out at the danger, or he may use the same resources to attempt escape. These are reflexive reactions. Sometimes habits or training determine the actual outcome. A soldier trained in the use of weaponry may find herself using them to the fullest when trapped. At other times, escape may be the best response. At a lower threshold, the body responds to perceived threats. Students exhibit some of the same physiological responses without the manifest behaviors of fighting or escape. When faced with the threat of an important examination, the body prepares for the danger. Some mild activity is useful, because it heightens the senses. Persistent responses and those that are out of proportion to the situation can actually disrupt the thought processes and eventually even impact other systems.

5. "When normal adaptability is disrupted, or when environmental changes overcome the body's capacity for self-maintenance, disease may ensue."

Disease is an interaction of the person with the external and internal environments. It is caused by adverse environmental factors that overcome the body's defenses, or by the body's inability to adapt to a situation. In other words, the body can be overwhelmed or underprepared for what occurs. The cause may be the body's inability to adapt, as in the case of an abnormal structure or abnormal function. The body is susceptible to changes from within and without. These may be minute or of great consequence. Occasionally, a previously innocuous event may prove more deleterious. Bacteria and other pathogens surround us. Our systems typically handle small amounts quite effectively. It may take a certain exposure in time or number before sickness begins. At other times, the defense mechanisms may be deficient and allow disease to occur. This also happens when one illness follows another. The initial one debilitates the host and follow-up illness can find a more hospitable ground for disease growth. In other words, the innate adaptive, restorative, and defensive mechanisms are rendered ineffective by all insults. This was the case with certain epidemics. The Spanish flu pandemic of 1917 swept through the world. Although it was more virulent than previous versions, there apparently was a follow-up infecting agent that was responsible or contributed to millions of deaths.

6. "Rational treatment is based on the previous principles."

Osteopathic manipulative treatment was not mentioned in these precepts of osteopathic philosophy. When Still first announced his philosophy in 1874, he did not mention manipulation, and it was approximately 5 years later that he began using manipulation as a tool for diagnosis and treatment. Manipulation is not the only aspect of osteopathic philosophy, nor is it necessarily the most important. However, with recognition of the importance of the somatic component of disease, the value of manipulation will be correspondingly better appreciated.

Even though conventional osteopathy of the early 1900s did not incorporate the use of some other interventions, such as pharmacological ones, today many contemporary osteopathic physicians do use pharmacological interventions. This can be seen not in contrast or in abandonment of the principles, but rather in further analysis, as a further application of these principles. For example, medications such as antibiotics have bactericidal and bacteriostatic properties. In acting in this fashion, they may maintain or reduce the absolute load of bacteria to the point at which the individual's immunological mechanisms can recover and produce adequate defense against and removal of the invaders. In other words, they can be used to maximize the patients' potential and allow their innate abilities to manage the rest. Osteopathic manipulation would be directed at the same end. In totality, osteopathic physicians are "wholistic" in treating the whole patient and in their armamentarium in approaches. Typically, a physician who is presented with a symptom, dysfunction, or disease embarks on a search for the cause. A physician who only treats a disease is merely treating an effect and may have no great impact on the cause. The osteopathic physician who helps correct the cause by assisting the restoration of proper structure and function (at the organ, tissue, or cellular level) facilitates the natural processes. Once the cause is corrected, the body has the opportunity to heal itself through its inherent capacity for repair to the extent to which it is capable.

In addition to the basic principles of osteopathic philosophy, there are other corollary principles that help direct and govern the osteopathic physician's approach to a patient:

1. "Movement of body fluids is essential to the maintenance of health."

   The arteries and other tubular structures play a crucial role in carrying nutritive elements to their destination and carrying away waste materials to be expelled. Disturbances in the circulation will produce pathology, such as acute or chronic inflammation, atrophy, irritation, or trauma. If the vessels to these areas are compromised by intrinsic or extrinsic damage, then flow will be inadequate. Such an environment could delay or even stop the healing process. For example, if the compromised artery is a coronary artery, then angina or myocardial infarction might occur.

   The osteopathic physician focuses on areas of dysfunction that influence the circulation to an area involved by a pathologic process. If such dysfunction is corrected, then oxygen delivery by the arteries might increase, the venous congestion might be dispelled, and the healing process might be initiated. This process frees the body to make the repairs necessary for return of health.

2. "The nervous system plays a crucial part in controlling the body."

   The nervous system is a major factor controlling blood flow. Impaired autonomic nervous control of the upper thoracic spinal cord traveling to the cervical sympathetic ganglia can produce a vast array of vascular changes in the somatic dermatomes supplied by these nerves. The somatic changes possible when such a dysfunction occurs include increased temperature locally, moisture, tenderness, and edema. These signs, recognizable on palpation, are adaptive vascular responses to an abnormal autonomic nervous supply.

   Once dysfunction has been corrected, normal autonomic tone should resume, and vascular response and a higher level of health should occur. Therefore, thinking osteopathically requires knowledge of anatomy and the ability to reason from the region of pathologic manifestation to the site of autonomic control, not ignoring any of the tissues en route that may contribute to their dysfunction.

3. "There are somatic components to disease that not only are manifestations of disease but also are factors that contribute to maintenance of the diseased state."

   The somatic component of the disease process may be caused by a direct bodily injury (such as a blow to the skeletal structures), or it may represent the response of viscera to pathology.

   For example, in abdominal visceral pathology such as acute appendicitis or peritonitis, one may observe spasm or guarding of the abdominal musculature. Other musculoskeletal effects may develop at a segmentally related spinal region, creating osteopathic somatic dysfunctions. These somatic components of the visceral disease are major diagnostic clues. The mechanism of this somatic response is probably the segmentally integrated viscerosomatic reflex. The nervous system is the most important system connecting and integrating the visceral and skeletal organs.

In many instances, illness is an imbalance between the neuromuscular system and the visceral systems. This must be mitigated before the body can heal itself.

What is so "osteopathic" about these precepts? Dr. Still's purpose was not to violate or rewrite basic scientific principles of his time, but rather to elucidate them and position them centrally on a system of therapeutics that emphasized the promotion of the body's ability to regulate itself toward health, given an appropriate environment and adequate nutrition. Osteopathic medicine is generally applicable to all conditions; the osteopathic physician does not address one organ system or structure at the expense of another, but rather considers the person as an integral unit.

## REFERENCES

*American Heritage Dictionary*. W. Morris, ed. Boston: Houghton Mifflin, 1969.

Frymann VM. The philosophy of osteopathy. *Osteopath Ann* 1976;4:102–112.

Still AT. *Philosophy of Osteopathy*. Kirksville, MO: Published by author, 1899.

Still AT. *The Philosophy and Mechanical Principles of Osteopathy*. Kansas City, MO: Hudson Kimberly, 1920.

Sprafka S, Ward RC, Neff D. What characterizes an osteopathic principle? Selected responses to an open question. *J Am Osteopath Assoc* 1981;81:81–85.

# Somatic Dysfunction

*Eileen L. DiGiovanna*

The term *somatic dysfunction* has been adopted by the osteopathic profession as a substitute for the older designations, *osteopathic lesion* or *Still lesion*. Somatic dysfunction is a condition of the musculoskeletal system that is recognized solely by the osteopathic profession and was first defined by Ira Rumney, D.O. The accepted definition in the *Glossary of Osteopathic Terminology* is as follows:

> Somatic dysfunction is an impaired or altered function of related components of the somatic (body framework) system: skeletal, arthrodial, and myofascial structures, and related vascular, lymphatic, and neural elements.

Not all somatic lesions are somatic dysfunctions. Fractures, sprains, degenerative processes, and inflammatory processes are not somatic dysfunctions. Fred Mitchell, Sr has given a useful observation: "Implicit in the term 'somatic dysfunction' is the notion that manipulation is appropriate, effective, and sufficient treatment for it."

A somatic dysfunction is a change in the normal functioning of a joint and is diagnosed by using specific criteria. These criteria of diagnosis may be remembered as the mnemonic T-A-R-T.

1. *T* denotes *tissue texture changes*. The soft tissues around a joint in somatic dysfunction or regionally for a group of somatic dysfunctions undergo palpable changes. These changes occur in the skin, fascia, or muscle and vary with the acuteness or chronicity of the dysfunction.
2. *A* denotes *asymmetry*. The position of the vertebrae or other bones is asymmetrical. Deviations, atrophy, or hypertrophy are some asymmetrical findings that may be appreciated on palpation. This is a static, positional finding.
3. *R* denotes *restriction of motion* within the bounds of physiologic motion. The involved joint does not have a full, free range of motion. The restriction involves one or more planes; it most frequently involves the minor motions of any given joint. This restriction is found by motion-testing the joint in all planes.
4. *T* denotes *tenderness*. Although not an objective finding, tenderness is produced during palpation of the tissues where it should not occur if there was no somatic dysfunction.

A second mnemonic has been proposed for the diagnostic criteria, *S-T-A-R*, by Dennis Dowling, DO. In this mnemonic, the S represents *sensitivity*. *Tenderness* is a response by the patient to palpation by the physician. This occurs in tissue that should normally not be tender to palpation. However, the sensitivity change may be experienced by the patient as numbness, paresthesia, or anesthesia, or other subjective sensation. The T still represents *tissue texture changes*, the A, *asymmetry,* the R, *restriction of motion,* as in TART. This may be used if the student or physician finds it more helpful.

## ■ TISSUE TEXTURE CHANGES

Tissue texture changes are a significant diagnostic tool. They occur in response to a variety of factors, including the following:

A. Neurologic factors
   1. Somatic manifestations
      a. Hyperresponsiveness of segmentally related functions
         (1) Hypertonic muscles
         (2) Muscle spindle overactivity
      b. Sudomotor activity (the production of perspiration) is altered, either increased or decreased
      c. Neurologically induced vasomotor activity, either constriction or dilation of vessels
      d. Soft tissue tenderness or other sensitivity
   2. Reflex manifestations
      a. Pain referred to other than local site (somato-somatic reflex)
      b. Rigidity of tissues at reflex site
      c. Sudomotor activity may increase or decrease
      d. Changes in pulse rate (increase or decrease)
      e. Changes in skin temperature
B. Circulatory factors
   1. Macroscopic changes
      a. Temperature changes
      b. Erythema or blanching
      c. Edema (swelling)
      d. Changes in pulse and cardiac rate
   2. Microscopic changes
      a. Hyperemia of soft tissues
      b. Congestion and dilation
      c. Edema (swelling)
      d. Minute hemorrhages
      e. Fibrosis
      f. Local ischemia
      g. Atrophy

## ■ CRITERIA FOR EVALUATION OF SOFT TISSUES

Tissue texture changes vary somewhat between acute and chronic somatic dysfunctions. In the spinal area, the changes tend to occur at the articulations of the vertebrae, over the transverse processes, and over the spinous process. (Table 1)

### Asymmetry

On palpation of a joint involved in somatic dysfunction, the bony structure involved with the related joint will be found to lie in an asymmetric position with respect to its normal position and to the position of bones contiguous to it. For example, the spinous process of a vertebra involved by somatic dysfunction may lie to one side of the line formed by the spinous processes of other vertebrae (which should lie in the midline), or one transverse process may be more posterior than the ones superior and inferior to it and the contralateral one of the same vertebra. There may be an approximation of one transverse process to the vertebra below while the opposite transverse process is separated from the one below it. A spinous process may be found

## TABLE 4-1 FINDINGS IN ACUTE AND CHRONIC SOMATIC DYSFUNCTIONS

|  | ACUTE | CHRONIC |
| --- | --- | --- |
| Temperature | Increased | Slight increases or decreases (coolness) |
| Texture | Boggy, more rough | Thin, smooth |
| Moisture | Increased | Dry |
| Tension | Rigid, board-like | Slight increase, ropy, stringy |
| Tenderness | Greatest | Present, but less |
| Edema | Yes | No |
| Blood vessels | Venous congestion | Neovascularization |
| Erythema test | Redness lasts | Redness fades quickly or blanching occurs (Red reflex) |

Definitions of some of these terms from the *Glossary of Osteopathic Terminology* are as follows:
   **Bogginess.** A tissue texture abnormality characterized by a palpable sense of sponginess in the tissue, interpreted as resulting from congestion caused by increased fluid content. **Ropiness.** A tissue texture change characterized by a cord- or rope-like feeling. **Stringiness.** A palpable tissue texture abnormality characterized by fine or string-like myofascial structures.

closer or further than expected to the position of the next spinous process.

## Restriction of Motion

A joint involved by somatic dysfunction has a restricted range of motion. It is said to meet an abnormal "barrier" to motion. In the normally functioning joint, there are two barriers to motion (Fig. 4-1):

1. The *physiologic barrier* is that point to which the patient may actively move any given joint; it represents a functional limit within the anatomic range of motion. Some further passive motion is still possible past this point toward the anatomic barrier (Fig. 4-2A).
2. The *anatomic barrier* is that point to which the joint may be passively moved beyond the physiologic barrier (Fig. 4-2B). Restriction at this point occurs because of bone, ligament,

or tendons. To pass the anatomic barrier, a disruption of tissue (ligament, tendon, capsule, or bone) has to occur (Fig. 4-2C).

A *pathologic barrier* may also occur as the result of disease or trauma. An example is joint fusion caused by spondylitis or the joining of osteophytes in an arthritic joint. Inflammation or joint effusion will restrict normal motion. The osteopathic restrictive barrier is one that lies within the physiologic range of motion and that prevents a joint from moving symmetrically within the physiologic range of motion (Fig. 4-3).

In somatic dysfunction, a joint is restricted, or meets a *restrictive barrier*, in one or more planes of motion. Motion in the opposite direction will appear normal or relatively free. For example, a vertebra may move more freely into flexion but not be able to move all the way to the physiologic motion barrier of extension. Because

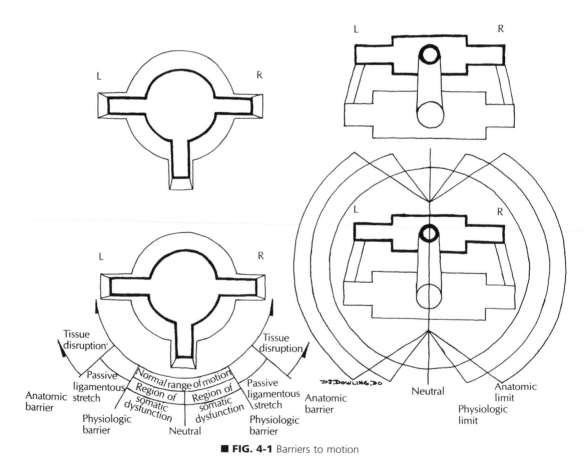

■ **FIG. 4-1** Barriers to motion

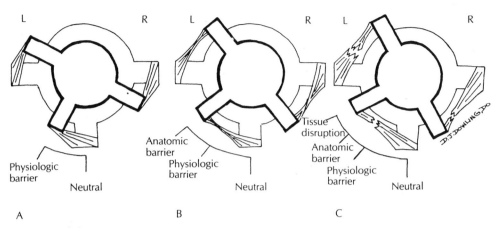

■ **FIG. 4-2 (A)** Physiologic barrier engaged by the patient. **(B)** Anatomic barrier engaged passively, with ligaments stretched. **(C)** Anatomic barrier has been passed, causing tissue disruption.

motion in one direction of the joint is affected, the motions in other cardinal directions of the joint are similarly affected. Often, restriction will be apparent in all three planes of vertebral motion, most noticeably in the minor motions of that joint. In vertebral somatic dysfunction, a

hypermobility, or increase in motion, may be found in the contiguous vertebrae. These apparent increases in motion may be compensations or the result of persistent regional restrictions.

It is important to understand that motion may be restricted as a result of "tethering" by a tight

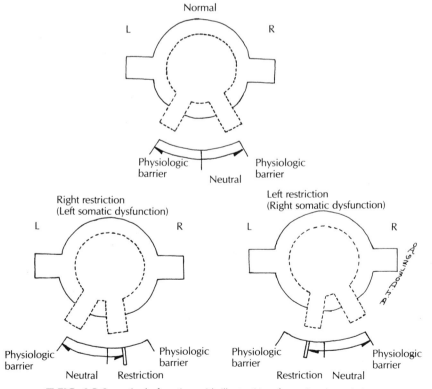

■ **FIG. 4-3** Somatic dysfunction with illustration of rotational restrictions.

muscle rather than from hitting against an obstacle. This is probably more often the case than not.

## Tenderness (Sensitivity Alterations)

Tenderness is the subjective sensation of pain or soreness that is reported by the patient in response to palpation of tissues by the physician. Tenderness is the most likely subjective finding. This sensation is almost always present in tissues surrounding a somatic dysfunction when the physician exerts no more than normal pressure. Pressing too firmly on soft tissues will almost always cause pain or tenderness. Pressure that should not normally cause pain will do so in tissues around a dysfunctional joint.

It is important to be aware that because tenderness is a subjective finding, not all patients report it as such at the site of somatic dysfunction. Some other subjective sensation may be reported, or none at all may be reported. If the other criteria are present, they are sufficient for the diagnosis to be made. Tenderness and other subjective sensations indicate the likelihood of a problem but are not a diagnosis in and of themselves. The physician must use these findings as part of a larger picture when making the diagnosis of somatic dysfunction.

## Diagnosing Viscerosomatic Reflex Dysfunctions

A tenet of osteopathic medicine is that visceral reflexes to the soma are an important cause of somatic dysfunction and are of major diagnostic significance. Dysfunctions caused by these reflexes may be either acute or chronic.

Acute viscerosomatic reflex dysfunctions are probably indistinguishable from any other acute somatic dysfunction. Chronic viscerosomatic dysfunctions have a few characteristics that may aid in differentiating them from somatic dysfunctions of other causes.

1. The skin tends to be more atrophic over the involved area.
2. The tissues display a firm, dry sponginess, as opposed to the bogginess of an acute dysfunction. The texture is very firm.

3. Joint motion is more restricted and seems more fixed than the usual dysfunction. Attempts to elicit motion in the involved joint produce a sluggish, rigid movement. The end feel at the barrier tends to be more "rubbery."
4. When such a dysfunction is corrected, it will tend to return to a dysfunctional state within 24 hours until the cause of the reflex is corrected.

It is important to know the location of sympathetic innervation in relation to the thoracic and upper lumbar vertebrae so that viscerosomatic reflex dysfunctions may be used for diagnostic purposes. The patterns appear to follow these autonomic nerve distributions.

## Naming Somatic Dysfunctions

A standard terminology has been devised for the purpose of recording somatic dysfunctions. In the case of vertebrae, it is traditional to refer to a functional vertebral unit, consisting of two vertebrae and the intervening disc, with the upper of the vertebrae being the one exhibiting the restricted motion. The somatic dysfunction is always named for the diagnosed relative freedom of motion, that is, the directions in which the vertebra can move most easily. For example, if the C3 vertebra is restricted in the motions of extension, side-bending to the right, and rotation to the right, then C3 is said to be flexed, side-bent to the left, and rotated to the left on C4. This is denoted as $C3FS_LR_L$. This may also be written $C_3FSR_L$.

The terminology reflects the fact that the vertebra assumes the position of its freedom of motion. T7 $ES_RR_R$ indicates that the seventh thoracic vertebra is extended, side-bent to the right, and rotated right on T8. In this case, the seventh thoracic vertebra is restricted in the motions of flexion, side-bending to the left, and rotation to the left.

Spinal somatic dysfunctions are classified as type I or type II dysfunctions. Type I dysfunctions follow Fryette's first principle of physiologic motion, which states that when the vertebrae are side-bent from a neutral position, rotation will occur in the opposite direction from the side-bending. These are group curves in the thoracic or lumbar regions involving more than one vertebra. When rotation and side-bending are involved, the rotation is opposite to the side-bending. Although type I dysfunctions are group curves, they are distinct from idiopathic scoliosis. Although type I somatic dysfunctions tend to occur with habitual posture and activity, they can result from trauma.

Type II dysfunctions follow Fryette's second principle of physiologic motion, which states that when side-bending occurs from a hyperflexed or hyperextended (non-neutral) position, rotation and side-bending of one segment are in the same direction. These are single vertebral dysfunctions and are often pathologic in nature. The involved vertebra will be found to be either flexed or extended on the vertebra below it and side-bent and rotated to the same side. Type II dysfunctions are more often traumatic in origin.

Type I and type II dysfunctions refer only to somatic dysfunctions in the thoracic and lumbar vertebrae because Fryette's principles only apply to these areas. However, in common usage, somatic dysfunctions in the typical cervical spine are often referred to as type II. Motion characteristics of the cervical region dictate that the typical cervical vertebrae side-bend and rotate toward the same side regardless of dysfunction or normal functioning. The distinction is the involvement of a flexion or extension component in the dysfunctional unit.

Somatic dysfunctions in other areas of the body, such as the extremities, are still named for their freedom of motion. For example, the radial head may move anteriorly or posteriorly. If it moves freely posteriorly and is restricted in anterior motion, it is named a "posterior radial head." Likewise, when it moves freely in an anterior direction and is restricted in posterior motion, it is named an "anterior radial head."

Because of some difficulty in standardization, some osteopathic physicians still use terminology that indicates barriers to free motion. In this case, in the interest of clarity, the term *restriction* should be used.

## Predisposing Factors

There are undoubtedly many factors that create conditions that predispose muscles and joint surfaces to be especially susceptible to the development of somatic dysfunction. Eventually a *facilitation* of the segmental spinal cord level maintains the somatic dysfunction for an extended period of time.

Certain factors that predispose to the development of a somatic dysfunction are as follows:

1. Posture
   a. Habitual
   b. Occupational
   c. Active (e.g., sports-related)
2. Gravity
   a. Body habitus
      (1) Obesity
      (2) Pregnancy
   b. Weight-bearing
3. Anomalies
   a. Abnormal size or shape of vertebra
   b. Abnormal facets
   c. Fusion or lack of fusion
      (1) Lumbarization
      (2) Sacralization
      (3) Spina bifida
4. Transitional areas (areas are especially prone to the development of somatic dysfunction)
   a. Occipitoatlantal (O-A)
   b. C7–T1
   c. T12–L1
   d. L5–S1
5. Muscle hyperirritability
   a. Emotional stress
   b. Infection
   c. Reflex from another somatic or visceral area
   d. Muscle stress
      (1) Overuse
      (2) Overstretch
      (3) Underpreparation
      (4) Accumulation of waste products
6. Physiologic locking of a joint, "close-pack position"
7. Adaptation to stressors—spontaneously reversible
8. Compensation for other structural deficits—stable

Type I somatic dysfunctions may be caused by any of the following:

1. Muscle imbalance
2. Short leg

3. Occupation
4. Trauma
5. Visceral reflexes
6. Disease or infection

## Etiology

The exact cause of somatic dysfunction is often debated. Some feel there is a true facet "locking." Most believe that muscle dysfunction is the major factor operating in the creation and/or maintenance of joint restrictions. Abnormal neural impulses, probably arising as a result of nociceptive activity and muscle spindle stretch responses, to the muscle, mediated through the muscle spindle, are probably the most significant cause of joint restriction and pain. Trauma (pain and force) is probably the major factor triggering an abnormal neural impulse.

Some other theories postulated in support of the facet locking include the following:

1. Meniscoid entrapment—based on the theory that vertebral facet joints have small menisci that may become trapped within the joint.
2. Meniscoid extrapment—based on the theory that the menisci may become trapped outside the joint.
3. Capsular compression.

The meniscoid theory was proposed by Kos and Wolf (Bogdvk and Jull) as a mechanism of "acute locked back" and was elaborated by Bogdvk and Jull. This theory is based on the premise that there are wedge-shaped menisci in the lumbar zygapophyseal joints. It is speculated that the apex of the wedge may become trapped between the articular surfaces or, on flexion, outside the joint cavity (Figs. 4-4 and 4-5).

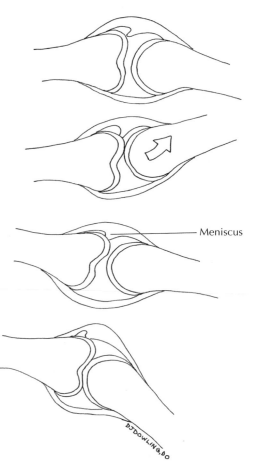

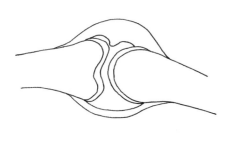

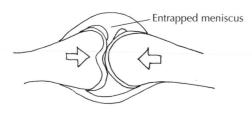

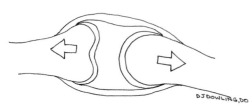

■ **FIG. 4-4** Meniscus entrapment theory. With joint motion, the meniscus is trapped between the joint surfaces. Traction is required to free the meniscus.

■ **FIG. 4-5** Meniscus extrapment theory. As the joint is flexed, the meniscus moves above the articular surface and occasionally is trapped there as the joint begins to extend. With further extension the meniscus bends, causing pain.

## REFERENCES

Bogdvk N, Jull G. The theoretical pathology of acute locked back: A basis for manipulative therapy. *Manual Medicine* 1985;1:78–82.

Burns L. Viscero-somatic and somato-visceral spinal reflexes. *J Am Osteopath Assoc* 1907:60.

DiGiovanna EL. *An Encyclopedia of Osteopathy*. American Academy of Osteopathy. Columbus, OH: Greydon Press, 2002.

Educational Council on Osteopathic Principles. *Glossary of Osteo Terminology*. American Osteopathic Association Directory, 1995.

Fryette HH. *Principles of Osteopathic Technique*. Kirksville, MO: Journal Printing Co, 1954:9.

Greenman P. *Principles of Manual Medicine*. Baltimore: Williams & Wilkins, 1991.

Mitchell F, Jr. Towards a definition of "somatic dysfunction." *Osteopath Manual: Medicine*. 1979.

Rumney I. The relevance of somatic dysfunction. *Yearbook of the American Academy of Osteopathy*. Colorado Springs: American Academy of Osteopathy, 1976.

Schiowitz S. *An Osteopathic Approach to Diagnosis and Treatment*, 2nd ed. Philadelphia: Lippincott-Raven, 1997.

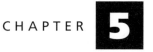

CHAPTER 5

# General Anatomic Considerations

*Stanley Schiowitz, Eileen L. DiGiovanna, and Nancy Brous*

The skin is the largest organ in the body. It is in constant contact with the environment, and many of its important functions have to do with protecting the body from environmental insults or with regulating the internal milieu as the external environment changes. The skin safeguards the internal structures from chemical and mechanical irritants and seals in bodily fluids to maintain a fluid internal environment. Salt and waste products are excreted through the skin. Dilation and constriction of blood vessels in the skin and evaporation of sweat from the surface of the skin aid in regulating body temperature. Finally, the skin acts as a sensory organ, relaying information about the environment to the central nervous system.

The skin consists of three layers. From exterior to interior, there are the epidermis, the dermis, and the fascia. The outer, epidermal layer is made up of dead and dying cornified cells. It has no vasculature and very few nerve endings. The middle and most important dermal layer is the least dense, consisting of approximately five layers of cells. It contains capillaries, small vessels, and most nerve endings. Hair and nails, specialized protective structures of the skin, are derived from dermal tissue. The deep, fascial layer of skin connects to the subcutaneous tissues. More vessels and nerve endings lie in this layer.

The circulatory elements of the skin have two functions: to conduct heat and to carry nutrition to the skin. Heat conduction is performed by venous plexi and arteriovenous anastomoses. The arteries and capillaries carry nutritive components. Other structures in the skin include two types of glands, *sudiferous*, or sweat-producing glands, and *sebaceous*, or oil-producing glands.

## ■ INNERVATION AND SENSATION

The skin is innervated by the autonomic (sympathetic) nervous system and the peripheral (sensory) nervous system. Sympathetic innervation affects the blood vessels, the muscles of the hair follicles, and the glands in the skin. Sympathetic innervation of the blood vessels in the skin contributes to vasoconstriction and vasodilation. The ends of the vasoconstrictor fibers apparently secrete norepinephrine, and it is believed vasodilation results from the secretion of acetylcholine at some of the endings. Vasodilation raises the temperature and causes a reddening of the skin. Vasoconstriction results in cooling of the skin and a blue color caused by the increase in deoxygenated blood. With severe or prolonged vasoconstriction, the skin hue pales as blood is squeezed out of the vessels. Sympathetic stimulation also causes sweating. These effects of sympathetic stimulation contribute to osteopathic diagnosis. Increased or decreased temperature, sweating, and changes in skin texture are associated with somatic dysfunctions in the involved area.

The skin is responsive to four types of sensation—touch (pressure), heat, cold, and pain. These sensations are detected by mechanoreceptors that are expanded nerve endings in the skin. Also present are some unmyelinated, or free, nerve endings. All four sensations are elicited in skin where only free nerve endings exist; thus, the free nerve endings apparently respond to all types of stimuli. The mechanoreceptors or expanded nerve endings (Merkel's disks and Ruffini endings) and encapsulated endings (Pacini corpuscles, Meissner's corpuscles, and Krause's end bulbs) (Fig. 5-1) appear to be sensation-specific. Merkel's disks are sensitive to touch (two-point discrimination). Meissner's corpuscles are sensitive to touch, and Pacini corpuscles to vibration and deep pressure. It has been postulated that Ruffini endings are sensitive to heat and Krause's end bulbs to cold.

## The Physician's Skin

Mechanoreceptors and other neural elements in the skin of the palpating physician's hand convey information about the patient. Because the dorsum of the hand is thinner-skinned than the palm, temperature is best palpated with the dorsum. Merkel's disks are most numerous in the palm and especially in the finger pads, which makes the finger pads most sensitive to touch. Thickening of the skin, as in calluses, decreases sensitivity. Because the receptors fatigue, the physician may find it necessary to rest or change fingers during palpation to ensure maximum sensitivity.

## ■ FASCIA

Anatomists define fascia as a dissectable mass of fibroelastic connective tissue. The osteopathic physician defines fascia as all the connective tissue of the body that has a supportive function, including ligaments, tendons, dural membranes, and the linings of body cavities.

Fascia is very extensive. If all other tissues and organs were removed from the body, with the fascia kept intact, then one would still have a replica of human anatomy. Fascia surrounds every muscle and compartmentalizes muscle masses. It surrounds and compartmentalizes organs in the face, neck, and mediastinum. Fascia forms sheaths around nerves and vessels. It envelops the thoracic and abdominopelvic organs. It forms the pleura, pericardium, and peritoneum. Fascia connects bone to bone, muscle to bone, and forms tendinous bands and pulleys.

Fascia is continuous throughout the body. The majority of the fascial planes are arranged in a longitudinal direction. Areas of hypertonicity or muscular imbalance can impose functional restriction on the natural longitudinal glide of the body's fascial sheets. Therefore, one area of restriction can influence adjacent and distal areas.

Several functional transverse diaphragms exist in the body. Restrictions of these dia-

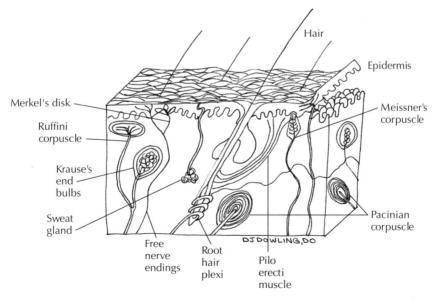

■ **FIG. 5-1** Mechanoreceptors in the skin.

phragms can cause major alterations in the function of surrounding structures. The respiratory diaphragm permits passage of the aorta, esophagus, vena cava, azygous veins, thoracic duct, vagus, and phrenic nerves. The urogenital diaphragm supports the pelvic viscera, allows sacrococcygeal mobility, and transmits the anal canal, urethra, vagina, lymphatics, and neurovascular bundles. The cranial base and dura transmit the jugular veins and cranial nerves IX, X, and XI through the jugular foramen. Any restrictions in these major transverse diaphragms will inhibit longitudinal fascial motion above and below and thus affect function of those structures it encompasses.

## Functions

The fascia has varied functions. It acts to stabilize and maintain upright posture through the lumbodorsal fascia, the iliotibial band, the gluteal fascia, and the cervical fascia. Fascia also protects enclosing muscle groups while defining their motion. This delimiting function channels muscle energy into specific action while simultaneously preventing muscles from rupturing and tearing. Therefore, fascia coordinates the action of muscle and muscle groups for smoother coordination and supports organs, muscles, neurovascular bundles, and lymphatic channels. It restrains and binds motion.

Fascia aids the circulation of body fluids. It keeps veins open and widens them as it is tensed during muscle contraction. Fascia is inherently contractile and elastic. As it contracts along the muscle, it compresses the veins within it, increasing venous return. Any contraction, tension, or imbalance in the fascia can impede or inhibit this dynamic contractile-elastic activity and result in decreased venous return and congestion.

The distribution of arterial blood to any part of the body requires adequate blood pressure and unobstructed arterial channels. The heart must be able to contract freely in the thorax without fascial or bony restrictions. Innervation to the heart must be free from mechanical irritation along its distribution. Adequate venous return is needed. Again, any restrictions in fascial sheaths housing the neurovascular bundles or even in neighboring fascial planes can decrease blood flow to an area.

The lymphatic vessels are arranged in a superficial and a deep set. Both pierce the fascia and accompany the veins. Therefore, lymphatic drainage can also be affected by restrictions in the fascial planes.

As the immediate external environment of every living cell, fascia directly or indirectly influences the metabolism of these cells. Abnormal pressure or tension will alter the diffusion of nutrients and the elimination of wastes, resulting in alterations in cell function. A cell needs proper maintenance of osmotic pressure and tissue tension of the surrounding interstitial fluid and ground substance for proper metabolism.

## Cellular Composition

The most abundant cellular component of fascia is the fibroblast. The fibroblast is under control of the endocrine system. Fibroblasts are responsible for the production of collagen and ground substance, and their response to physicochemical changes is important. Under pressure, fibroblasts produce collagen organized along the same stress lines as the direction of force. Therefore, fascia can adapt to external stresses by cross-linking of collagen. This increase in strength can also decrease fascial flexibility and can cause restrictions and potential compression of vessels and nerves.

## Circulatory Effects

Fascia directly or indirectly influences the health of the body by being coordinated with the musculoskeletal system, by cooperating in the circulation of body fluids, and by allowing generous passageway for nerves. Derangement in the fascial planes can result in venous congestion, abnormal reflexes, and a decreased range of motion. It is important that the osteopathic physician evaluate the fascia as a part of the structural examination and treat any tensions or restrictions found within it.

## ■ MUSCLES

It is interesting to note that muscles are the only tissues found in the body that have the ability to shorten. It is this contractile characteristic of muscle that allows them to shorten and thus move bones at their articulations.

## Muscle Action on Joints

Joint motion is created by the action of the skeletal muscles. These muscles create motion by contracting. A muscle can contract in three different ways:

1. *Isotonic contraction*, in which a muscle shortens.
2. *Isometric contraction*, in which a muscle maintains the same length.
3. *Isolytic contraction*, in which a muscle contracts while being lengthened.

## Muscle Contraction Definitions

1. **Concentric contraction.** The muscle shortens, using the property of contractility to perform the task.
2. **Eccentric contraction.** The muscle lengthens, using extensibility to perform the task.
3. **Static contraction.** The muscle is in partial or complete contraction without changing its length. There is no rotary joint motion.

## Example of Forward Bending of the Head

1. In the upright position, the eccentric contraction (lengthening) of the extensor muscles controls the speed of forward bending. These muscles are exercised.
2. In the supine position, the concentric (shortening) contraction of the flexor muscles lifts the head off the floor. These muscles are exercised.
3. In the prone position, the patient may try to bend forward, but the floor will prevent the motion. This will create static contraction of the neck flexors, which are exercised.

## Classification

The manner in which muscles are constructed determines how far a muscle can shorten, relative to its strength. This is classified according

to the arrangements of its muscle fibers. In a *fusiform* muscle, the fibers are parallel to each other along the long axis of the muscle and its tendons. This type of arrangement allows for the greatest amount of shortening. In *unipennate* and *multipennate* muscles, the fibers run obliquely to the tendons. These fibers when enervated will contract maximally, but because of their oblique orientation, their action does not result in the same amount of shortening of the muscle as found in a parallel muscle.

## Moment of Force

Muscle power is used to move one part of the skeletal system around another part, with their articulation acting as a fulcrum. This creates a torque or *moment of force*. The torque around any point equals the product of the amount of force and its perpendicular distance from the direction of force to the axis of rotation (*moment arm*). If one were to hold a 5-pound weight in the palm, with the elbow flexed at a 90-degree angle, and if the distance from the elbow joint to the weight were 1 foot, then 5 foot-pounds of flexor muscle effort would be needed to maintain this position. If the elbow were flexed at a 45-degree angle, the force, the 5-pound weight, would stay the same but the moment arm would be reduced. Less than 5 foot-pounds of flexor muscle effort would be needed to maintain this position.

## Lever Action

The use of the joint as a fulcrum brings into play Newton's laws of levers.

1. A first-class lever has the fulcrum placed between the point of effort and resistance.
2. A second-class lever has the resistance placed between the fulcrum and the point of effort.
3. A third-class lever has the point of effort between the fulcrum and resistance.

Of the three levers, the second-class lever is most efficient with regard to minimizing effort needed to move a resistance. A wheelbarrow is an example of such a lever. Most of our long muscles act as third-class levers. The biceps muscle's flexion effort in moving the forearm is an example of such a lever action. The triceps' action causing forearm extension is an example of a first-class lever. First-class lever action usually requires less effort for motion than third-class lever action.

An interesting demonstration of lever action is afforded by the brachialis muscle in flexion. Simple forearm flexion represents a third-class lever action; however, with a weight in the palm, lowering the forearm from a position of flexion to one of extension reverses the designations, in that gravity becomes the effort or moving force, while the insertion of the brachialis becomes the resistant force. This creates a second-class lever action.

## Spurt-and-Shunt Action

MacConaill and Basmajian define the spurt-and-shunt action of muscles as follows: when a muscle contracts, it creates two vector forces with regard to the articulation. One is a swing (rotation) force around its axis (spurt action). The second is transarticular motion into the joint in relation to its axis (shunt action). Both of these motions are present simultaneously, but in different proportions in all muscles. A large spurt-to-shunt ratio permits greater rotary motion with diminished joint stability. The reverse is true with an increased shunt-to-spurt ratio.

The biceps flexion motion of the forearm is primarily a spurt action at the elbow, but contraction of the long head of the biceps is a stabilizing, shunt action at the glenohumeral articulation.

A third motion is created by muscle contraction—spin motion. The amount of spin will depend on the difference in the planes of the origin and insertion of the muscle. Spin motion plays a part in the second law of myokinematics.

## Laws of Myokinematics

The first law of *myokinematics* (MacConaill and Basmajian, 1977), the law of *approximation*, states that "when a muscle contracts it tends to bring its attachments (origin and insertion) closer together." In most activities, the effect of this law is modified by using other muscle activity or resistant force to stabilize either the insertion or the origin end of the muscle. This creates motion at one end of the muscle only.

The second law, the law of *detorsion*, states that "when a muscle contracts, it tends to bring its line of origin and its line of insertion into one and the same plane." A simple example is sternocleidomastoid action. Unilateral contraction creates ipsilateral side-bending, flexion, and contralateral rotation of the head.

A less commonly recognized application of this principle is in hip extension. Pure gluteus maximus contraction tightens the hip joint and raises the femur somewhat toward the ilium in the frontal plane. To achieve hip extension, the pelvis rotates anteriorly in the sagittal plane. This rotation changes the planar relationships of the origin and insertion of the muscle. The law of detorsion is activated, and the insertion will try to match the plane of muscle origin. The more the pelvis is rotated, the greater the hip extension.

## Gravity

Gravitational force is the attraction of each mass-particle in the universe for every other mass-particle. Gravitational force has three unique characteristics:

1. It is applied constantly.
2. It is applied in one direction only.
3. It acts on each mass-particle of the body.

This force is constantly exerted on all parts of the musculoskeletal system. Its effects, however, can be modified by body position. In the upright anatomic position, gravity assists in stabilizing the hip, knee, and ankle joints. At the same time, it creates instability of the glenohumeral articulation. In the supine position, gravitational force on all these joints is markedly different. The physician must be aware of the action of gravity when using exercise treatment. Bending the head forward in the upright position does not exercise the cervical flexor muscles. Gravity is the primary force involved. Extensor muscles are brought into play if control of the speed of forward bending is desired. In the supine position, forward bending or bringing the chin to the chest would necessitate use of the neck flexors.

# ■ THE JOINTS

All bones that have freedom of movement will move on other bones at their respective joints. Several factors influence these motions. Knowledge of why, when, and how joint motion is induced is essential for the understanding of functional anatomy and for the diagnosis and treatment of osteopathic somatic dysfunctions.

## Classifications

Joints are usually divided into three classifications by composition: fibrous, cartilaginous, and synovial joints. *Fibrous joints (synarthroses)* are connected by dense fibrous tissue. Their motions are greatly limited. Commonly, they are found in the skull. The cranial articular surfaces are irregular, yet they form specific suture match and interlock. They are joined together by fibrous tissue, which is very firm and practically fills the joint space. This type of articulation allows greater motion in infants, with gradual reduced motility with aging.

*Cartilaginous joints (amphiarthroses)* are characterized by the presence of fibrocartilaginous disks between the two contiguous surfaces. Very firm and strong ligaments, contiguous to the discs, hold the joint together. A small amount of rocking and sliding motion is permitted. The best examples are the intervertebral discs and the symphysis pubis.

*Synovial joints (diarthroses)* are the most common joints found in the body and the ones with which the practitioner is usually most familiar. The following characteristics are shared by all of these joints: their articular surfaces are covered by hyaline cartilage and the articulation is enclosed by a joint capsule creating a closed joint, which contains synovial fluid that lubricates the hyaline cartilage. Some joints contain intra-articular discs or menisci, such as the knee. These menisci separate the articular surfaces of the bones and aid in creating better-matching articular surfaces.

The structure of the articular surfaces further classify joints into *plane, spheroid, condylar, ellipsoid, trochoid, sellar,* and *ginglymus* joints.

A *plane joint* has two almost flat surfaces and is usually limited to a sliding motion. An example of this surface type is the triquetral-pisiform articulation.

A *spheroid joint (ball and socket)* has a round convex head that articulates with a concave surface. This articulation has the greatest amount of motion, with freedom of motion in all three planes. An example of this type is the hip joint.

A *condylar joint* is a modified ball and socket, with partial flattening of both articular surfaces. This flattening limits the motions available as compared to a spheroid joint. An example of this is the metacarpal-phalangeal articulation.

The *ellipsoid joint* modifies the spheroid joint by a head shaped as an ellipsoid (football-shaped). It has greater motion than the condylar joint but less than the spheroid joint. An example of that is the radiocarpal articulation.

The *trochoid joint* is composed of a ball shape that is surrounded by a circle composed of bone and ligaments. Its motion is primarily rotation. An example of this is the articulation between the atlas and axis.

The *sellar joint* is composed of two bones whose articular surfaces are saddle-shaped, with one surface convex and one concave. This allows for greater motion in all planes. An example of this is the trapezium–metacarpal (thumb) articulation.

The *ginglymus joint* is a hinge joint. Its articular surfaces fit one another in such a way that it allows for an especially large freedom of motion in one plane, an action similar to a hinge. An example of this is the humerus–ulna articulation.

## Biomechanics of Joint Motion

None of the articular surfaces of the body is truly flat. They are ovoid or sellar (saddle-shaped) (Fig. 5-2). The joints that have evolved are an attempt at a mating of these forms: sella to sella and ovoid convex to ovoid concave. The articulations thus formed are not truly congruent, permitting greater freedom of joint movement and

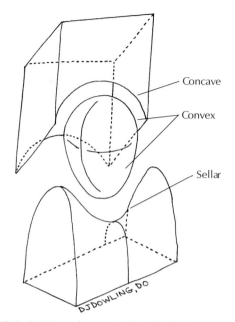

■ **FIG. 5-2** Bony shapes. At this articulation, an ovoid shape sits in a sellar shape. Convex and concave surfaces are shown.

geometrically created coupled and accessory motions.

Individual joint motions can be described in terms of spin, roll, and slide. *Spin* is defined as one bone rotating on its mechanical axis, in place, on another bone. *Roll* is defined as movement resulting from an increase or decrease in angle between the two articulating bones. *Slide* (glide) is a translatory motion of one bone sliding over the surface of another bone (Fig. 5-3).

The curved articular surfaces, moving one on another, develop complex patterns of motions. The coupled motions created by convex–concave mating articulations follow specific patterns. When a concave surface moves on a convex surface, the roll and slide motions are in the same direction. However, when a convex surface moves on a concave surface, the roll and slide motions are in opposite directions.

Femoral extension on the tibia follows these patterns of motion. As the stance leg extends in gait, the femur rolls anteriorly with posterior slide on a fixed tibia (Fig. 5-4). However, the swing leg on extending creates tibial roll and slide anteriorly (in the same direction) on the distal femur (Fig. 5-5). Full femoral extension can be described as an anterior femoral roll with a posterior slide, accompanied at full extension by a medial femoral spin on the tibia.

The fully extended knee undergoes another prescribed motion in its final stage of extension. This is a conjunct rotation created by the geometry of the articulating surfaces (see Chapter 92, Anatomic Considerations of the Knee Joint).

Articular stability is a combined function of the shape of the joint, its ligamentous and muscular attachments, the strength of its capsule, and the balance of joint pressure to atmospheric pressure. Variation in any of these factors may contribute to somatic dysfunctions.

It is usual to describe motion as occurring in cardinal planes about fixed axes. Shoulder abduction would be described as motion in a fron-

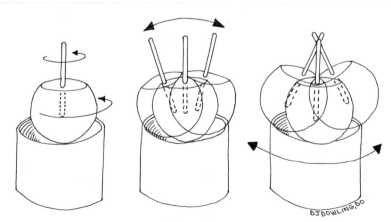

■ **FIG. 5-3 (A)** Spin. **(B)** Roll. **(C)** Slide.

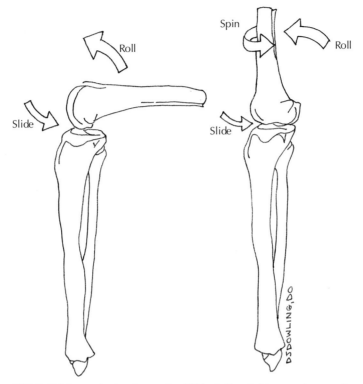

■ **FIG. 5-4** Femoral extension on fixed tibia. Roll and slide occur in opposite directions.

tal plane about an anteroposterior axis. However, we know that the head of the humerus, a convex surface, moves on the concave glenoid fossa with an upward roll and downward slide. Because this is a coupled, continuous motion, it cannot be about a fixed axis. This type of motion is said to be about an *instantaneous axis of rotation*. This axis defines multiple motions, rotary and translatory, that occur simultaneously in the same plane. The abduction motion would require continuous determinations of its instantaneous axis as it moved. This would give a true pathway of the joint motion. This motion is still typically only in one plane.

In full extension the femur rolls, slides, and spins. The motion is multiplanar and involves more than one axis; it is said to occur on a *helical axis*. The helical axis completely defines a three-dimensional motion between two rigid bodies. Active functional motions, appendicular as well as vertebral, are usually motions about helical axes.

The addition of force to joint motions may bring into play accessory motions. Accessory motions cannot be performed voluntarily; they can only be activated against resistance or by an outside force. An example is long-axis traction on the phalangeal articulations. The restriction of small accessory motions is a major factor in the creation of somatic dysfunctions, especially in the articulations of appendages.

Motion is affected by ligamentous relationships. A *"close-packed" joint* position is one in which the ligaments have twisted, bringing the bones together into maximum congruence. The bones cannot be separated without first loosening the ligaments. Joint motion is lost, and forces are more easily transmitted through this joint into the next one. Tangential force will more likely cause fracture than sprain.

In weight-bearing joints, the close-packed position replaces muscle activity for maintenance of support. In the spine, motion is transmitted through the bodies of close-packed verte-

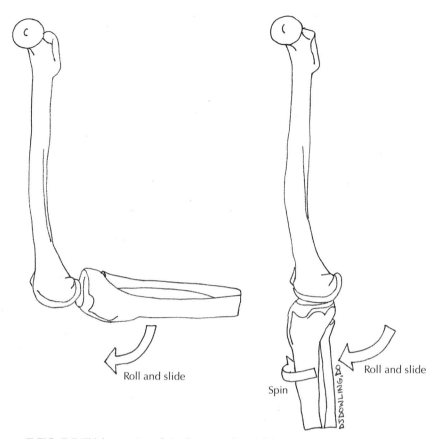

■ **FIG. 5-5** Tibial extension of the femur. Roll and slide occur in the same direction.

brae into the first movable zygapophyseal articulation. Somatic dysfunction can result.

## Biomechanics of Intervertebral Joint Motion

The general principles of motion discussed with regard to appendicular articulations also pertain to spinal synovial articulations. The vertebral articulations, however, have a tripod arrangement, which further complicates their motions. This tripod consists of an anterior synarthrosis, the vertebral bodies with intervertebral disks, and a pair of matched posterior synovial articulations. These three articulations are involved simultaneously in every vertebral motion.

Common factors that influence segmental motion include the design and spatial relationships of the individual facets; the vertebral ligamentous and muscular attachments and their function; the size and health of the intervertebral disks; the osteology of the vertebra; and the age, sex, and health of the patient. In addition, preload, gravity, tone, and the amount and direction of applied load and stress must be taken into account.

## ■ SPINAL COLUMN

### Vertebral Osteology

The various shapes and structures of the vertebrae may also affect their motions. The cervical vertebral bodies are sella-shaped, which encourages freedom of motion. The joints of Luschka modify the translatory lateral motion of the cervical vertebral bodies. The shingle effect created by the thoracic spinous processes can restrict extension. A similar restriction can occur in the lumbar region if the spinous processes are elongated. The ribcage restricts lateral flexion and unilateral joint rotation.

The fifth lumbar vertebra is subject to a

greater number of congenital abnormalities than any other bone. These abnormalities affect motion and create the tendency for dysfunction. A very common abnormality of this region, usually not reported radiologically, entails a change in the fifth lumbar vertebra-sacral base articular facet relations. It is common to find atypical bilateral horizontal articulations or one horizontal and one vertical facet articulation in this region. This creates an imbalance that develops into low back dysfunction.

A functional unit of the vertebral column is composed of two segments: an anterior segment that consists of two neighboring vertebral bodies separated by an intervertebral disk, and a posterior segment consisting of the two neural arches, their pedicles, laminae, superior and inferior articulations, transverse processes, and a spinous process (Fig. 5-6).

The main functions of the anterior segment are supportive, weight-bearing, shock-absorbing, and, in combination with the posterior segment, protective of the spinal cord. The posterior segment primarily effects directional guidance of joint motion. In the upright position, it is almost nonweight-bearing.

## Facets

The facets of the typical cervical vertebrae, C3 through C7, are flat and oval. Their average spatial orientation is a 45-degree angle between the horizontal and frontal planes. The superior facets face backward and upward (Fig. 5-7). They therefore have great freedom of motion in all planes. Because of the 45-degree spatial planar relationship, the coupled motions of rotation and lateral flexion always occur in the same direction.

The thoracic articular facets are flat, with the superior facets facing backward, upward, and laterally. The spatial orientation is a 60-degree angle from the horizontal to the frontal plane, and a 20-degree rotation from the frontal to the sagittal plane in a medial direction (Fig. 5-8). Without the rib attachments, the coupled motions of lateral flexion and rotation would be excellent. Flexion is greatly reduced by the 60-degree angle toward the frontal plane. Combined lateral flexion with rotation can be in the same or opposite directions.

The lumbar facets have curved surfaces. The superior facets are concave and face backward and medially. The inferior facets mirror them by being convex, facing forward and laterally. The rules of concave–convex relationship are evident with joint motion. Lateral flexion is a coupled roll-and-slide motion. This creates a slight rotary movement. As in the thoracic region, lateral flexion and rotation can be in the same or opposite directions.

The average lumbar facet spatial orientation is a 45-degree angle from the frontal to the sagittal plane, turning in the lateral direction (Fig. 5-9). The greatest motion is found in flexion–extension; some lateral flexion is present with slight rotation. The described typical motion patterns may vary segmentally if other factors intervene.

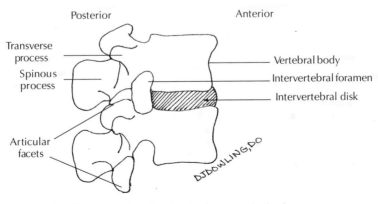

■ **FIG. 5-6** Functional unit of the vertebral column.

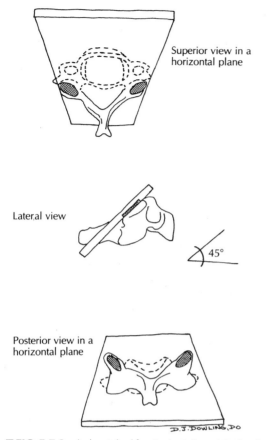

**FIG. 5-7** Cervical vertebral facet orientation at the level of C4.

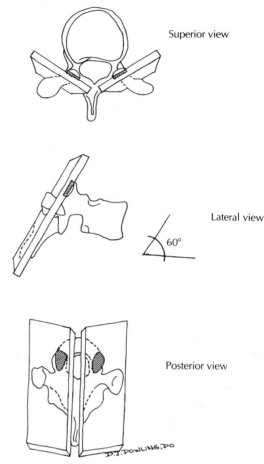

**FIG. 5-8** Thoracic vertebral facet orientation at the level of T6.

The motion found at transitional intervertebral segmental levels is unpredictable. The additional stress created by changes in curve directions and the osseous shape variations create a climate for the development of somatic dysfunctions.

## Vertebral Ligaments

The anterior and posterior longitudinal ligaments limit extension and flexion, respectively. Posteriorly, they are joined by the interspinous and supraspinous ligaments and the ligamentum flavum. Collectively, they create a firm connection, linking all the vertebrae together. This supports and limits excessive motion. Dysfunction can develop when degenerative disks allow a loosening of the supportive ligaments, and posterior or anterior spondylolisthesis occurs.

## Vertebral Muscular Attachments

The muscular attachments are commonly described as bilaterally symmetric. Unfortunately, this is not the case. Everyone has asymmetric development. This causes unstable hypotonic or hypertonic muscular development. Even simple spinal motions would become imbalanced if not for the synergistic or stabilizing assistance of other groups of muscles. All motions are susceptible to dysfunction because of these factors. The greater the imbalance, the greater the tendency for the development of somatic dysfunction.

When evaluating muscle function or using muscle contractive force therapeutically, the clinician must be cognizant of the differences in strength and action between the superficial, powerful muscles and the deep, weaker muscles.

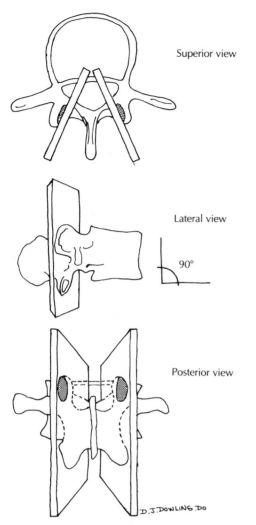

Superior view

Lateral view

90°

Posterior view

D.J.DOWLING.DO

**■ FIG. 5-9** Lumbar vertebral facet orientation at the level of L3.

The deep muscles, because of their vertebral attachments, create localized intervertebral balancing movements. The clinician uses the localized but lesser strength of the deep muscles in muscle energy treatment.

## Intervertebral Disks

The intervertebral disks influence vertebral joint motion in a number of ways. The annulus consists of layers of fibroelastic fibers that are attached to the superior and inferior vertebral endplates. These fibers intertwine in oblique patterns that permit rolling, rotation, and translation of one vertebra on another. The relative size of the disk with reference to its attached vertebrae is proportional to the motion allowed.

Disk degeneration, with a reduction in height, creates an imbalance of the articular facet relationship. The possible ligamentous effect was discussed previously.

## Preload and Gravity

Normally, the effects of preload (gravity, weight, and muscle tone) are greater at the fifth lumbar vertebra than at the fifth cervical vertebra in the upright subject. However, the cervical muscles of a patient who has been living with constant stress may be chronically contracted, with a marked increase in tone. The disks would be subjected to a constant increased preload. Slight force can create great dysfunctions. The effect of scoliosis at any level creates an imbalance in muscle tone, with increased preload on one side of the disk. One-sided muscular overdevelopment, a common occurrence over time in most humans, can produce dysfunction in this manner.

Normal gravitational force directly affects the functional spinal unit. A gravitational force that is not directed toward the center of gravity of an object creates a secondary rotary force vector. None of the functional spinal units is completely horizontal to the earth. There are normal or abnormal lateral physiologic spinal curvatures and multiple compensatory scoliotic patterns. Thus, spinal muscles are in a constant state of hypertonicity, trying to maintain an upright stature against gravity's rotary force. All of these factors affect articular motion and function.

## Vertebral Motion at the Functional Spinal Unit

Coupled motions are normally present in a functional spinal unit. **Flexion** is the rotary motion of anterior vertebral approximation coupled with ventral translatory slide. **Extension** is the rotary motion of anterior vertebral separation coupled with dorsal translatory slide.

**Rotation right** is the turning of the anterior aspect of the body of the vertebra toward the right, coupled with a diminution of interverte-

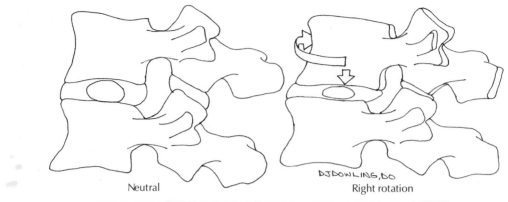

Neutral

Right rotation

DJDOWLING,DO

■ **FIG. 5-10** Coupled rotation and translatory motion in the horizontal plane.

bral disk height, described as vertical translatory compression (Fig. 5-10).

**Rotation left** is the turning of the anterior aspect of the body of the vertebra toward the left, coupled with the previously described vertical translatory compression. As the vertebra turns back toward the midline, either from right or from left rotation, the intervertebral disk returns to its usual height.

**Lateral flexion right or left** is a rotary motion that causes the side of upper vertebral body to approximate the one below it, right or left, accompanied by a contralateral translatory slide (Fig. 5-11).

Each of these described coupled motions occurs in a single plane and on an instantaneous axis of rotation. If two of these coupled motions occur simultaneously, i.e., lateral flexion accompanying rotation, then multiple planes are involved, and the combined motions occur on a helical axis of rotation.

A diagnosis of somatic dysfunction, $T_4ES_RR_R$, indicates that the motion of the fourth thoracic vertebra on the fifth thoracic vertebra is greater in the directions of extension, right lateral flexion, and right rotation. These three coupled motions occur in three planes simultaneously on a helical axis of rotation (Fig. 5-12). The barriers to freedom of the described motion would all be in the opposite directions, but on a similar helical axis of rotation.

Many osteopathic diagnostic and therapeutic

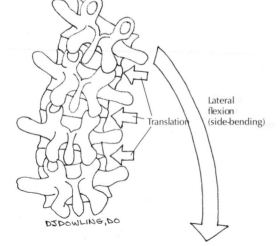

Lateral
flexion
(side-bending)

Translation

DJDOWLING,DO

■ **FIG. 5-11** Coupled rotator and contralateral translator motions in the frontal plane that occur during side-bending.

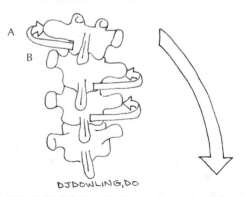

A

B

DJDOWLING,DO

■ **FIG. 5-12 (A)** Type II side-bending and rotation in same direction. **(B)** Type I side-bending and rotation in opposite directions.

approaches can be explained by combining the laws of physiologic motion, vertebral biomechanics, and the kinetic principle of the effect of resistance to linear motion. The effect of resistance to linear motion can be described as follows. If an object in linear motion encounters an obstacle or resistance, then it will turn about its point of contact with the interfering factor.

For example, on palpation, the transverse process of the fourth thoracic vertebra is more prominent posteriorly on the right. Is it part of a somatic dysfunction complex involving three planes and six motions on a helical axis? The vertebra is placed into a position of flexion. The right transverse process becomes more prominent posteriorly. It is assumed that this has happened because there is a barrier present to the motion of flexion, and the vertebra is responding according to the rule of the effect of resistance on linear motion. That is, on meeting this flexion barrier, the vertebra turns away from and around it in the direction of allowable freedom of motion, or right rotation.

Two parts of the diagnosis are now available. Freedom of motion in extension (flexion barrier) and right rotation. According to the laws of physiologic motion, if flexion or extension is involved in the motion diagnosis, then lateral flexion is in the same direction as the motion of rotation. Therefore, the diagnosis is $T_4ES_RR_R$, moving on a helical axis.

## REFERNCES

Basmajian JV. *Muscles Alive*, 4th ed. Baltimore: Williams & Wilkins, 1978.

Becker FR. The meaning of fascia and continuity. *Osteopath Ann* 1975;3:8–32.

DiGiovanna E, Schiowitz S. *An Osteopathic Approach to Diagnosis and Treatment*, 2nd ed. Philadelphia: Lippincott-Raven, 1997.

Ealton WJ. *Textbook of Osteopathic Diagnosis and Technique Procedures*, 2nd ed. Colorado Springs, CO: American Academy of Osteopathy, 1970.

Educational Council on Osteopathic Principles. *Glossary of Osteopathic Terminology*. Chicago: American Osteopathic Association, 1995.

Fujiwara M, Basmajian JV. Electromyographic study of two joint muscles. *Am J Phys Med* 1975;54:234–242.

Hoag JM, Kosok M, Moser JR. Kinematic analysis and classification of vertebral motion. *J Am Osteopath Assoc* 1960; 54:899–908, 982–986.

Kapandji IA. *The Physiology of the Joints*, 2nd ed. Edinburgh: Churchill Livingstone, 1974.

MacConaill MA. The movements of bones and joints. *J Bone Joint Surg [Am]* 1949;(31B)1:100–104.

Basmajian JV. *Muscles and Movements*. Huntington, New York: Robert E. Krieger Publishing, 1977.

Moore KL. *Clinically Oriented Anatomy*. Baltimore: Williams & Wilkins, 1980.

Pratt NE. *Clinical Musculoskeletal Anatomy*. Philadelphia: J.B. Lippincott Company

Rasch PJ, Burke RK. *Kinesiology and Applied Anatomy*, 6th ed. Philadelphia: Lea & Febiger, 1978.

Sauer GC. *Manual of Skin Diseases*, 4th ed. Philadelphia: J.B. Lippincott, 1980.

Warwick R, Williams P. *Gray's Anatomy*, 35th British ed. Philadelphia: W.B. Saunders, 1973.

Wells KF, Luttgens K. *Kinesiology*, 6th ed. Philadelphia: W.B. Saunders, 1976.

White AA, Panjabi MM. *Clinical Biomechanics of the Spine*. Philadelphia: J.B. Lippincott, 1978.

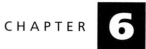

# General Physiologic Considerations

*Dennis J. Dowling and Paula D. Scariati*

In essence, osteopathy is based on the concepts of structure and function. At its simplest interpretation, structure is anatomy and function is physiology. An understanding of physiology and neurophysiology in particular is essential to understanding the mechanisms of somatic dysfunction and the logical application of osteopathic manipulation. Some basic terminology needs to be clarified:

**Afferent nerve.** A nerve carrying impulses toward the central nervous system (CNS).

**Efferent nerve.** A nerve carrying impulses from the CNS.

**Ventral horn.** The anterior portion of the gray matter in the spinal cord where efferent motor neurons leave the spinal cord.

**Dorsal horn.** The posterior portion of the gray matter of the spinal cord where afferent sensory nerves enter the spinal cord.

**Contraction.** Physiologic shortening of muscle length from its usual resting length.

**Contracture.** Abnormal, fixed shortening of muscle length.

**Agonist.** Muscle or muscle groups primarily responsible for performing some motion (i.e., flexion).

**Antagonist.** Muscle or muscle groups that oppose the motion of the agonist and produce an opposite motion (i.e., extension).

Sensory nerves carry impulses from sense organs to the spinal cord or brain. Those that enter the spinal cord do so through the dorsal horn. Those destined to terminate locally end in the gray matter of the spinal cord, where they pro- duce local segmental responses such as excitation, facilitation, and reflex actions. They may directly affect a motor or sympathetic nerve or do so through an intermediary interneuron. These interneurons may be either excitatory or inhibitory. Those with distant terminations or other intermediaries travel to integrative areas higher in the spinal cord, the brain stem, or the cerebral cortex.

The body is artificially divided into groups of structures identified as organs, glands, ligaments, muscles, neural tissue, vessels, bone, and skin. This differentiation is anatomically correct but functionally misleading. The somatic and visceral components act synergistically to fulfill the body's needs and functions. However, this interaction is often visualized as a strictly mechanistic process in which one part of the body causes the action to be initiated, either automatically or volitionally, and the rest of the body simply performed orders. By contrast, osteopathic medicine holds that each part of the body is in some manner responsible for and responsive to every other part.

The spinal cord is the organizer of information, which is processed from the brain to other regions. Feedback from these areas to the brain helps maintain normal function. A difficult concept to grasp is that parts of the body may communicate directly with one another without the brain's intervention. In these communications, the nervous system is less like a two-way intercom system in a large apartment house than like a fully interactive telephone system with the brain acting as the operator. A common example is *the knee-jerk reflex*, which occurs automatically in response to appropriate stimuli without direct intervention from the brain. Modification can be produced centrally in the brain or sometimes by other factors. Conscious attention to a hammer striking the patellar tendon can blunt or eliminate the reflexive effect of knee extension. It is often necessary to use techniques of distraction such as closing one's eyes, sticking out the tongue, or performing an isometric exercise with the hands. The use of caffeine, thyroid medication, stimulants, alcohol, and the effect of stress and anxiety can all modify reflexes.

Some reflexes serve an apparent survival benefit early in life but apparently fade quickly in infancy. The *Babinski reflex* appears to change significantly. Initially the toes curl about a stroking stimulus and later the toes curl upward and there is withdrawal of the foot. The *Moro reflex* consists of arm abduction and neck flexion in response to a sudden backward fall. The asymmetric tonic reflex, also known as either the fencer's reflex or the bowman's reflex, results in contraction of the triceps, psoas, and hamstrings with relaxation of the biceps brachii on the side of the head and neck rotation, with the exact opposite effect on the contralateral side. There is an agonist contraction with antagonist relaxation throughout. Each of these reflexes may be considered survival mediators and apparently fade in preparation for coordinated motion. In truth, there is an inhibitory effect centrally, and these reflexes are suppressed throughout most of life. Unfortunately, they recur in response to damage of the central nervous system.

## ■ THE AUTONOMIC NERVOUS SYSTEM

The autonomic nervous system can be thought of as an involuntary manager, indicating that modification occurs without conscious effort. It is divided into sympathetic and parasympathetic nervous systems. The autonomic nervous system controls the moment-by-moment activity of the viscera. Its components, often described as antagonistic, are more realistically understood as cooperative or complementary.

The somatic component is often discussed as a totally independent, voluntary system responsible for the musculoskeletal system. It is not customarily thought of as interacting with the autonomic nervous system. However, the somatic component has undeniable effects on the autonomic nervous system, and vice versa.

## ■ THE SYMPATHETIC NERVOUS SYSTEM

The sympathetic chains of ganglia are bilaterally oriented in a cephalad–caudad direction at the levels of the first thoracic segment to approximately the second lumbar segment. The fibers exit the cord along with the somatic motor axons as the ventral roots via the intervertebral foramina. These preganglionic fibers exit the root along the white ramus and into the ganglia. They synapse with postganglionic nerves at various levels of the chain. The postganglionic axons return to the spinal nerve via the gray ramus. For much of their course, the sympathetic nerves travel intimately with the somatic axons (Fig. 6-1).

Another important anatomic feature of the sympathetic chains is their relationship to the ribs. The ganglia lie anterior to the junction be-

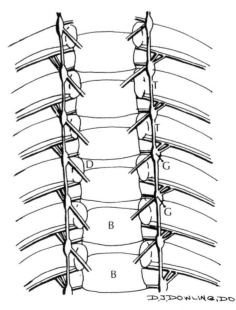

■ **FIG. 6-1** Sympathetic chain. B, vertebral body; G, sympathetic trunk ganglion; T, sympathetic trunk; D, intervertebral disc.

tween the head and neck of the ribs but posterior to the pleura. The range of influence is further extended superiorly as far as the sympathetic plexi to the head and upper extremity by the cervical ganglia and to the lower extremities by the lumbar splanchnic nerves.

The sympathetic nervous system assists the body in managing the stresses and requirements of the external environment. It is responsible for the *"flight or fight" response*. Reactions are constantly moderated and adjusted in response to information received by higher centers. Visceral function is fine-tuned. Circulation, metabolism, smooth muscle tone, intestinal motility, cardiac function, and pulmonary response are regulated.

## ■ THE PARASYMPATHETIC SYSTEM

The parasympathetic system is also known as the craniosacral portion of the autonomic nervous system because of the sites of origin of the preganglionic fibers. The cranial portion has ganglia associated with the third, seventh, ninth, and tenth cranial nerves. Spinal cord segments S2, S3, and S4 comprise the sacral portion.

The parasympathetic ganglia are located close to the innervated organ. Fibers from the oculomotor, facial, and glossopharyngeal nerves supply ganglia for organs found in the head, whereas the remainder of the visceral organs receive their innervation from the vagus and the sacral axis. The vagus alone supplies the heart, lungs, trachea, liver, gallbladder, esophagus, stomach, pancreas, spleen, kidneys, small intestine, and the ascending and transverse colons. The nervi erigentes, constituting the pelvic nerve, send fibers to sex organs, external genitalia, and the bladder and its sphincters. There is no parasympathetic innervation of the extremities.

Despite the fact that the parasympathetic nerve fibers innervate various organs, there are regions of the body where more than 50% of the fibers are actually sensory in nature. The visceral organs are under dual control of the sympathetic and parasympathetic nervous systems. The process is a synergistic rather than a competitive one, with activation usually occurring reciprocally. The primary function of the parasympathetic system is internal maintenance, including

digestion and excretion. Among other functions, the cranial axis causes constriction of the pupil and decreases in heart rate. The parasympathetic division operates most effectively during times of recovery and rest.

## ■ SKELETAL MUSCLE SYSTEM

The skeletal or somatic nervous system is under voluntary control, although some processes can be performed automatically. A joining of the ventral and dorsal roots inside the vertebral canal forms the typical spinal nerve. Sensory fibers have their cell bodies in the dorsal root ganglion and then synapse in the dorsal horn. The ventral root contains the motor neurons. The rami of the 31 pairs of spinal nerves split into a dorsal and ventral ramus. These in turn are subdivided into other branches. The structure is fairly consistent but is best represented by the thoracic nerves. All of the skeletal muscle nerves arise or terminate in common origins in the spinal cord and exit via the vertebral foramina. The sympathetic pathways are shown in Figure 6-2.

### Neuromuscular Reflexes

Ventral motor neurons give rise primarily to two types of nerves that exit the anterior horn to innervate skeletal muscle, alpha motor neurons and gamma motor neurons. Alpha motor neurons transmit impulses via nerve fibers to innervate large skeletal muscle fibers. A single alpha motor neuron excites a few to several hundred skeletal muscle fibers known as the *motor unit*. Gamma motor neurons transmit impulses via nerve fibers to innervate small skeletal muscle fibers called *intrafusal fibers*. These fibers contribute to the muscle spindle apparatus (Fig. 6-3).

Two primary and separate muscular reflex systems, each with its own apparatus, function, and response, play major roles in stabilizing and modulating muscular activity. The muscle spindle reflex sends information to the nervous system about muscle length or the rate of change in muscle length. The Golgi tendon reflex sends information to the nervous system about muscle tension or the rate of change in tension. Both

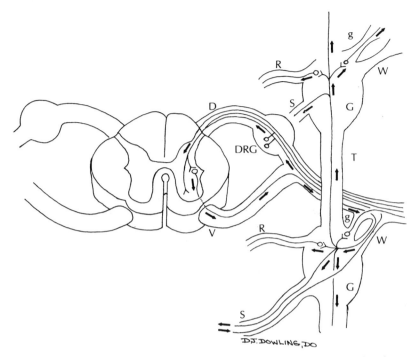

■ **FIG. 6-2** Sympathetic pathways (D, dorsal root; V, ventral root; DRG dorsal root ganglion; S, splanchnic; R, recurrent meningeal; g, gray rami communicantes; W, white rami communicantes; G, sympathetic trunk ganglion; T, sympathetic trunk).

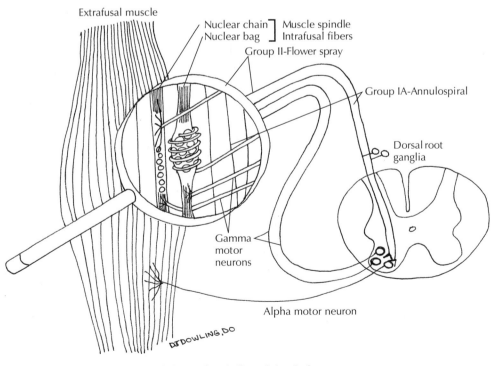

■ **FIG. 6-3** Muscle spindle and detail of components.

can be thought of as protective to the stability of the muscle. Overstretching of the central portion results in muscle spindle activity and reflex tension and shortening as a means of splinting. Golgi tendon activation protects the attachment portion of the muscles, and increased tension results in reflexive muscle relation.

# ■ MUSCLE SPINDLE REFLEX

Muscle spindles are intrafusal mechanoreceptors that are widely distributed within skeletal muscle fibers in the belly of the muscle. They exist in parallel with the much larger extrafusal skeletal muscle fibers, and the connective tissue around the muscle spindles is continuous with the connective tissue around the other muscle fibers. The muscle spindles mediate a response to a load placed on the muscle; this is known as the *load reflex*. Muscle spindles have a dampening function, as well. They prevent some types of oscillation and jerkiness in body movement. In fact, tremors noted, especially during times of extreme anxiety or stimulation, represent a failure to dampen this response smoothly. In addition to serving at a subconscious level, the muscle spindle reflex is invoked in voluntary motor activity.

Muscle spindles are composed of two types of intrafusal muscle fibers: nuclear bag fibers and nuclear chain fibers. The nuclear bag fibers have nuclei that appear to be bunched in the center of the cell, and the nuclear chain fibers have their nuclei aligned single-file in the center as in a series. There are two to five nuclear bag fibers and six to ten nuclear chain fibers in a typical muscle spindle. The central portions of either type of fiber have very poor contractile ability, whereas the ends that are attached have greater contractility. The components of an intrafusal muscle spindle are diagrammed in Figure 6-3.

The sensory afferents of the muscle spindle comprise group Ia fibers (primary endings), which send branches to every intrafusal fiber in the muscle spindle, and group II fibers (secondary endings), which innervate the nuclear chain endings only. The larger primary endings (Ia) surround the center of the muscle spindle much like a coil, whereas the smaller secondary endings (II) terminate on either side of the primary endings in a branch-like fashion. The Ia fibers are known as *annulospiral endings*, and the type II fibers are called *flower-spray endings*. Although both respond to length changes, the nuclear bag/annulospiral complex responds primarily to rate of change and the nuclear chain/flower-spray complex reacts more to absolute length change. They both react somewhat to both conditions.

Stimulation of the muscle spindle occurs either with lengthening of the whole muscle, which stretches the midpoint and excites the receptors, or with contraction of the endpoints of the intrafusal fibers, which also stretches the midpoint and excites the fiber. Stretching the muscle spindle increases the rate of firing, whereas shortening the muscle spindle decreases the rate of firing. In the so-called neutral position, a baseline background of firing occurs (Fig. 6-4A). However, in a compacted or hypershortened position, theoretically, cessation of the firing may occur. Thus, the musculoskeletal system can send a positive signal or no signal to the spinal cord to indicate the status of the muscle.

The nerve fiber from the type Ia or II group passes through the dorsal horn into the ventral region of the spinal cord. The effect there is stimulation of the alpha motor neuron. Stimulation of this fiber results in activation and contraction of the larger extrafusal muscle component. This results in shortening of the whole muscle unit. The submerged and smaller muscle spindle is then shortened, resulting in a decrease or elimination of the firing in the sensory fibers.

A simple example of the muscle spindle reflex is the patellar tendon reflex. The knee, when flexed to 90 degrees, places the quadriceps muscle into a relatively stretched position. The sudden strike of a hammer against the tendon results in a dynamic stretch of the spindle and firing of the Ia (and possibly II) fiber; the alpha motor neuron is then stimulated and in turn induces quadriceps contraction and knee extension (Fig. 6-4B).

Slow stretch of the length of the receptor portion of the muscle spindle produces the static stretch reflex. The number of impulses transmitted from the primary and secondary endings increase in proportion to the amount of stretch,

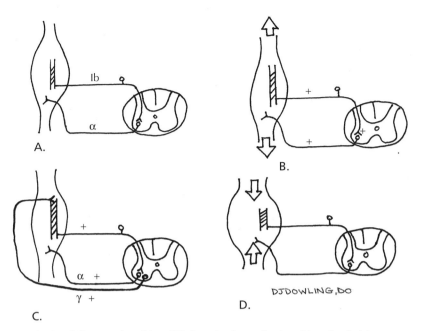

■ **FIG. 6-4 (A)** Neutral position. **(B)** Stretch of extrafusal and intrafusal alpha motor neuron stimulated to reflexively initiate extrafusal muscle contraction. **(C)** Gamma motor neuron innervation of muscle spindle. Contraction of ends stretches spindle, activating Ib fibers. Ib sensory fiber activates alpha motor neuron to cause extrafusal muscle contraction. **(D)** Compression of whole muscle or contraction of extrafusal muscle results in shortening of muscle spindle and deactivation of sensory fiber firing.

and signals are transmitted as long as the muscle is stretched. The static stretch reflex is thought to be mediated primarily by nuclear chain fibers, because these are the only fibers innervated by both primary and secondary endings. The static gamma fibers, which mainly excite the nuclear chain fibers, enhance the static reflex but contribute little to the dynamic reflex.

Motor efferents of the muscle spindle consist of static and dynamic gamma fibers, which make different contributions to the stretch reflex mediated by the muscle spindle. Static gamma fibers primarily innervate nuclear chain fibers, producing tonic activity in Ia afferent fibers. Dynamic gamma fibers primarily innervate nuclear bag fibers, generating phasic activity in Ia afferent fibers. Overall, the gamma motor neurons serve two functions: (1) they cause the intrafusal fibers to contract, thereby stretching the central portion of the muscle spindle and causing activity of the sensory endings (this is theorized to be the mechanism for maintaining postural

tone); and (2) they cause the intrafusal fibers to contract sufficiently to stretch the muscle spindle toward threshold, thereby increasing the sensitivity of the muscle spindle apparatus (Fig. 6-4C).

The gamma motor neurons are very numerous and in some regions may actually constitute 70% of the motor neurons exiting the spinal cord. The effect of establishing or maintaining a steady state of the spindle also leaves the system vulnerable to over-regulation. The resultant contraction of the end portions of the spindle results in greater susceptibility to further stretch (Fig. 6-4D). Too constant, rapid, or frequent firing or maintenance of firing past the time required results in a high gain set. Sudden stretching of muscular tissue that has not been prepared with concomitant gamma stimulation results in an even more powerful response. Inappropriate maintenance of the gamma motor neuron stimulation may result in a stretch reflex, despite the fact that the muscle is actually in the neutral or a relatively shortened position.

Analogous to the muscle spindle but without tensile ability are the stretch receptors in other soft neuromusculoskeletal tissue. The Pacinian corpuscles are present in fascial and ligamentous tissue and may respond to sudden or over-whelming stretch by "signaling" the spinal cord. Even though the ligaments have no true intrinsic contractile ability, the afferent signal may inter-act at the segmental level with the elements of the muscle spindle. Efferent signals may actually travel to the extrafusal muscles of the immediate region and initiate a cascade of stretch and mus-cle contraction. This may serve a protective func-tion by using structures other than the ligaments and fascia themselves, namely the muscle, to ef-fect regional contraction and limited range of motion of the regional joints.

### Neuronal Circuitry of Muscle Spindle Reflexes

The monosynaptic pathway, in which sensory input fibers synapse directly with motor output fibers, governs the primary endings (Ia) that me-diate the dynamic stretch reflex. The type II fi-bers may occasionally terminate monosynapti-cally, but most terminate on multiple interneurons in the gray matter of the spinal cord. Type II fibers transmit more delayed sig-nals to the anterior motor horn.

### ■ GOLGI TENDON REFLEX

*Golgi tendon organs*, sometimes called tendon spindles, are encapsulated sensory mechanore-ceptors located in mammalian tendons between the muscle and the tendon insertions. There is one tendon organ for every three to twenty-five muscle fibers. Tendons, because of their more fibrotic and less contractile nature, are subject to a stretching effect while there is contraction of the muscle belly. Golgi tendon organs detect the degree of skeletal muscle tension and convey this information to the CNS. The Golgi tendon organs are in series with the extrafusal fibers and are stretched whenever the muscle contracts.

Afferent neurons from the Golgi tendon mechanoreceptor are larger myelinated neurons of the Ib group. On entering the gray matter of the spinal cord, the afferent Ib neuron synapses with inhibitory interneurons. It also synapses with other interneurons that ascend to higher CNS levels. The inhibitory interneurons synapse with the large alpha motor neurons located in the anterior gray horn of the spinal cord. The alpha motor neurons that are inhibited are to the same muscle in which the Ib afferents origi-nate (Fig. 6-5). This results in reflex relaxation of the muscle.

Increased tension in a skeletal muscle distorts the Golgi tendon organ, producing a generator potential that initiates an action potential. The action potential travels over the Ib neurons to the spinal cord. Afferent action potentials acti-vate the interneurons, which inhibit the alpha motor neurons back to the skeletal muscle. The increased muscle tension that initiates the reflex can result from contraction of the skeletal muscle or from marked passive stretch of the muscle.

Interneurons, as the name implies, are bipolar neurons that connect two other neurons. They are located in all areas of the spinal cord, not just the anterior horn. Interneurons are small, highly excitable, and often spontaneously active. They can fire as rapidly as 1,500 times per second.

Certain interneurons located in the anterior horn in close association with the motor neurons constitute the *Renshaw inhibitory system*, which causes inhibition of neurons surrounding the motor neuron carrying a given excitatory im-pulse. This phenomenon is known as *recurrent inhibition*. The function of the Renshaw inhibi-tory system is to sharpen the signal of the motor unit. It prevents the signal from diffusing into adjacent nerve fibers, which would weaken the signal.

Because the basic Golgi tendon reflex results in reflexive inhibition of the muscle, the opposite effect of the stretch reflex produced by the mus-cle spindle, it is sometimes called the *inverse stretch reflex*. This autogenic inhibition is more commonly known as the *lengthening reaction* or the *clasp-knife reflex*. Like a pocketknife, in-creased muscular tension may result in sudden relaxation. An example is the sudden extension of the elbow in the loser of an arm-wrestling contest.

Both the muscle spindle and the Golgi tendon organ reflexes serve the same basic purpose: to

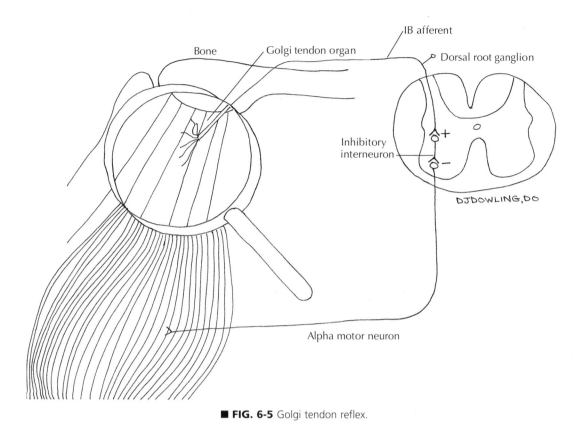

■ **FIG. 6-5** Golgi tendon reflex.

prevent disruption of the tissue. In the case of the muscle spindle, it is to dynamically prevent tearing or overstretching of the belly of the muscle. The Golgi apparatus protects the tendinous portion from tearing or even avulsion of the bony attachment. Both, when inappropriately set or activated, create or maintain abnormal muscle function.

## ■ FLEXOR REFLEXES

### Crossed Extensor Reflex

The crossed extensor reflex is the response elicited by stimulation of a given muscle (e.g., the biceps of the right arm, causing flexion) in the muscle of opposite function on the opposite side of the body (e.g., contraction of the triceps in the left arm, creating extension). The crossed extensor reflex is mediated via many sensory and motor interneurons in the spinal cord. Some act to inhibit the contralateral agonist and stimulate the contralateral antagonist. The reflex usually

occurs in response to prolonged stimulation (200–500 msec) after a painful stimulus and continues long after the provoking stimulus has been withdrawn (Fig. 6-6). The effect is necessary for coordinated balanced activity such as walking, crawling, climbing, and running. As one arm extends, the opposite flexes.

## ■ RECIPROCAL INNERVATION

Reciprocal innervation is the stretching of a given muscle, stimulating the contraction of that muscle via the muscle spindle. The antagonist muscle is inhibited.

### Segmentalization

Dermatome mapping of the cutaneous innervation is an established method of localizing a pathologic disease process to a particular segment. Although variations might exist in a given individual, the overall pattern is fairly consistent. A different type of segmentalization is not as well

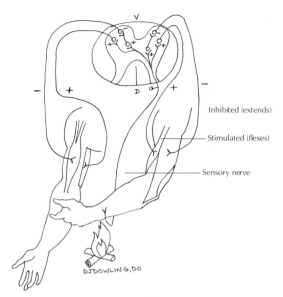

**■ FIG. 6-6** Crossed extensor reflex with reciprocal inhibition.

Inhibited (extends)

Stimulated (flexes)

Sensory nerve

known: the sympathetic system also shows segmental preference in regard to the visceral organs. According to *Gray's Anatomy*, the afferent fibers that accompany the preganglionic and postganglionic fibers of the sympathetic system occur in a segmental arrangement. Painful stimuli to the viscera are carried back to the cord via the sympathetics (Fig. 6-7). When all clues are combined, knowledge of this segmentalization can assist in the diagnosis of visceral disorder. For example, pain fibers from the heart pass to the first five thoracic spinal cord segments, mainly through the middle and inferior cardiac nerves. Ischemia of the heart muscle often produces pain substernally, with radiation to the chest, shoulder, neck, jaw, and abdomen.

Pain secondary to appendicitis is generally noted to be initially in the periumbilical region. Anatomically the appendix is not within this region of the abdomen. However, the innervation for the appendix is derived from the tenth thoracic segment, as is the area around the umbilicus. This segmental relationship demonstrates the intertwining of different regions anatomically. The typical progression of pain in the right lower quadrant of the abdomen only results when an inflamed appendix makes contact with

a sensitive peritoneum in that region. This represents direct mechanical and inflammatory impingement rather than a neurological pattern.

## Viscerosomatic Reflexes

A viscerosomatic reflex is one in which disruption, irritation, or disease of an internal organ or tissue results in reflex dysfunction of a segmentally related musculoskeletal region. In 1907, Louisa Burns, DO, attempted, through experiments on animals, to demonstrate the physiologic processes occurring in viscerosomatic and somatovisceral reflexes. By stimulating various visceral organs, she elicited contractions of segmentally related muscles. Irritation of the visceral pericardium and the heart muscle initiated contractions in the second through sixth intercostal and spinal muscles. Stimulation of abdominal organs similarly yielded results (Korr, Wilkinson, and Chornock, 1966, 1967; Korr, Chornock, Cole, and Wilkinson, 1967; Korr and Appeltauer, 1970). The importance of these findings has yet to be determined, but it is readily apparent that disruption by compression would limit or eliminate any benefits obtained from this nutrition. With complete separation of the axon, Wallerian degeneration occurs and innervated fibers are lost. Interestingly enough, Dr. Still wrote about the *"nerves of nourishment"* as important in the maintenance of normal functioning. An in-depth examination of his writings indicates that there was no confusion of vascular structures with nerves in regard to this observation.

## Facilitation

Facilitation indicates that an area of impairment or restriction develops a lower threshold for irritation and dysfunction when other structures are stimulated. Reflexes of either the somatosomatic or the viscerosomatic type may activate it. These low-threshold segments showed reflex hyperexcitability in response to pressure placed on the corresponding spinous processes, in response to pressure placed on the spinous processes of distant high-threshold segments, and in response to impulses from proprioceptors associated with positioning, from remote areas of skin, and from

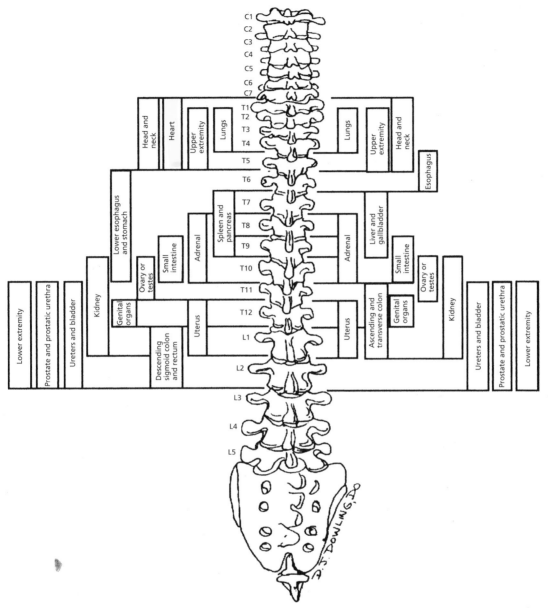

■ **FIG. 6-7** Segmentalization of sympathetic nervous system.

higher centers (Denslow et al., 1947) (Fig. 6-8). Facilitated segments are chronically hyperirritable and hyper-responsive. Muscles in the region are maintained in a hypertonic state, which constricts the available spinal motion. All of the supportive structures and their innervations may become afferent sources of facilitation. Reasonably, the neural controls would be expected to accommodate to the high level of activity, and this does occur in some cases. According to one theory, the muscle spindles, which monitor muscle length through gamma neuron control, are improperly set and therefore react inappropriately to stimuli. In comparison with messages sent from normally reactive neighboring neural tissue, messages sent from inappropriately reactive tissues are presented to the spinal cord and higher centers as confused. In other theories, the

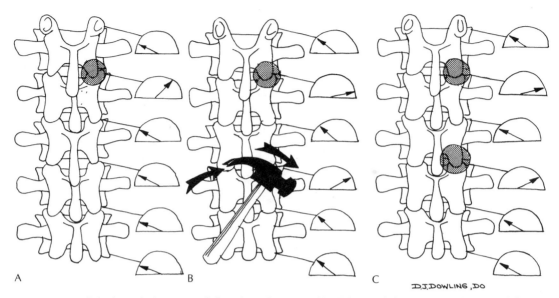

■ **FIG. 6-8** Facilitated vertebral segment. **(A)** Facilitated segment (shaded region) shows increased activity. **(B)** Force or stress applied some distance away from facilitated segment produces increased activity of all levels but especially of the facilitated segment and the struck segment. **(C)** Both the stressed segment and the facilitated segment exhibit hyper-reactivity.

spinal cord itself is considered able to adapt to the higher activity level and to channeling impulses to the affected region as if it were a "neurologic lens" (Korr, 1986).

## Nociception

At a local level, pain can be appreciated by several sensory endings that have a high concentration, especially in the skin. Local biochemical neuropeptides such as substance P, calcitonin gene-related peptide (CGRP), histamines, and interleukins mediate inflammatory changes and also increase local neural and tissue sensitivity. The fascia and adventitia of muscular blood vessels have numerous unmyelinated group IV and small group III myelinated fibers. Pressure, stretch, prolonged contractions, thermal and chemical changes, and ischemia may excite or sensitize these fibers. There is a high concentration of nociceptive-sensitive neurons in laminae I, II, IV, and X in the spinal cord. Some of these mediate local responses, and others project to the central nervous system via the spinothalamic, spinoreticular, and spinohypothalamic tracts. Higher center involvement of the hypothalamus, the locus coeruleus, and the pituitary lead to involvement of neuro-endocrine-immune as well as cortex responses. The cyclic nature of pain–inflammation–restriction of motion–contraction–histochemical changes–dysfunction is well known. The persistence of this recurring cycle depends on many factors, not the least of which is duration of the condition.

## Causes of Muscle Pain

Muscle spasms of diverse origin can cause pain. Prolonged muscle contractions irritate the splinting muscle and the associated ligaments and tendons, producing further spasm and initiating a pain cycle. The severity of the pain reflects the duration of a sustained contraction.

Ischemia, or localized anemia caused by obstruction of blood at a specific site, is a well-known cause of muscle pain, occipital tension headaches, and intermittent claudication. Retention of irritating metabolites and waste products also causes muscle pain. Blood flow to the area must be increased to remove these substances. Proper delivery of oxygen, glucose, and other nutritive substances cannot occur if impedances persist.

Pain caused by trauma or irritation (e.g., by an osteophyte) can be alleviated with the use of therapies that decrease muscle tension and improve local tissue circulation, affording subjective and objective relief from pain and spasm.

Some pain has been correlated to the existence of interleukin substances that have been described as necessary members of an inflammatory healing cascade. Substance P has been found in elevated levels, especially in people with chronic myofascial pain syndromes. Medications such as capsaicin are thought to contribute to analgesic control of pain by blocking the formation of substance P.

Failure of calcium to accumulate in the sarcoplasmic reticulum, abnormal interaction between the muscle fibril's actin and myosin, and anxiety may cause muscle pain.

## Manipulation

The goal of manipulation is to restore the whole body to maximal functioning. There is no standardized algorithm to be rigidly applied in all cases but rather is individually tailored to the patient. The discovery of somatic dysfunctions describes the regions to be treated. In the case of facilitated segments, whether one imagines resetting the gamma gain or re-establishing a coherent neural communication, the end goal is to bring about normal, comfortable motion.

Somatovisceral reflexes produce unmeasured changes on the internal organs. Sympathetic stimulation may promote or maintain a disease process. Relief of this source, if performed early enough, should alleviate the symptoms and the disease process. The viscerosomatic reflex is less amenable to cure. Manipulating the affected soma should have a beneficial effect in reducing symptoms, but the overall effect on the visceral component is indeterminable at this time. If we postulate a "tape loop" that promotes the whole process, then anything that breaks the cycle is of importance.

The changes created by osteopathic manipulative treatment are mediated at a local level but have the potential to be far-reaching and interactive. Proper control of muscle function depends on local excitation in conjunction with continuous feedback from the brain about muscle status.

## ■ PRACTICAL APPLICATIONS OF NEUROPHYSIOLOGY IN OSTEOPATHIC MANIPULATIVE TREATMENT

### Myofascial/Muscle Techniques

1. **Stretch reflex.** Quick stretch of a muscle excites the muscle spindle, causing reflex contraction. To prevent this reflex, myofascial therapy is performed slowly for correction of contracted or contractured muscles. A quick stretch can be used if the goal of therapy is to stimulate muscle tone.

2. **Moist heat** applied to muscle usually increases its **elastic** response to stretch. It also aids in increasing circulation. Dry heat is not as effective and does not penetrate as deeply as moist heat. The application of **ice** may seem to have a paradoxical effect, especially when one sees that heat increases local tissue relaxation and stretch. Cold has multiple effects. It is an analgesic and when applied to a region may even increase local circulation. The timing in the application of one of these modalities may affect the response significantly. Heat in the initial inflammatory stage may actually increase localized edema. Cold may produce or increase muscle contraction. Applications of 15 or 20 minutes with equivalent latency periods may be more effective than constant use. Some patients even respond to alternating heat and cold.

3. Connective tissue placed under prolonged **mild tension** shows plastic elongation.

4. **Servo-assist function of the muscle spindle reflex.** If the extrafusal fibers contract less than the intrafusal fibers, then the muscle spindles will maintain a stretch reflex to further excite the extrafusal fibers. This technique is used in active resistive myofascial therapy.

5. **Golgi tendon organ reflex.** When tension on the tendon becomes extreme, the inhibitory effect from the tendon organ can become so great that it causes a sudden relaxation of the entire muscle. This technique is used in active resistive myofascial therapy.

6. **Reciprocal innervation.** When a stretch reflex excites one muscle, it simultaneously inhibits the antagonist muscle. Reciprocal

innervation is of use in active indirect myofascial therapy, with or without resistance.

7. **Crossed extensor reflex.** When a stretch reflex excites one muscle, it simultaneously excites the contralateral antagonist muscle; the motion created crosses from one side of the spine to the other side in an X pattern. The crossed extensor reflex is helpful in active myofascial therapy, usually with isokinetic resistance.

# ■ COUNTERSTRAIN AND FACILITATED POSITIONAL RELEASE TREATMENTS

The theories of counterstrain and facilitated positional release treatments are discussed in detail in later chapters.

Prolonged shortening of a muscle allows shortening of the intrafusal (muscle spindle) and extrafusal fibers. The gamma motor neurons then increase their firing rate to maintain tone in the muscle, resulting in hypersensitive muscle spindle fibers in the shortened muscle. If the shortened, hypersensitive muscle is now lengthened rapidly (the muscle spindle responds to length and rate of change of length), a reflex overstimulation of the alpha motor neurons will occur and muscle spasm will ensue. The sensory signals also travel to the higher centers of the CNS, which are not capable of interpreting them properly and thus respond with excessive gamma motor stimulation, which maintains the spasm.

Reshortening the muscle allows the muscle spindle to shorten and resume normal firing. The CNS is now able to interpret the signals properly, so it resets its gamma motor neurons. This takes approximately 90 seconds to accomplish.

Adding a facilitating force along the axial spine with the addition of passive positioning in muscle shortening may compress the muscle spindle and reduce and eliminate the firing of annulospiral and flower-spray endings and reset the gamma motor neuron influence in a more immediate fashion.

# ■ MUSCLE ENERGY TECHNIQUES

Muscle energy treatment combines elements of the Golgi tendon reflex, reciprocal innervation, and elastic stretch. Muscle energy techniques that use the Golgi tendon reflex are much like active myofascial techniques in that extreme tension is used to create an inhibitory effect that will produce a sudden relaxation.

To engage the mechanism, the physician must resist the patient's efforts with an isometric force after placing the muscle group or joint into its pathologic barrier. The patient contracts for 3 to 5 seconds with sufficient minimal force to activate the local muscles. The Golgi organ initiates reflexive relaxation of the muscle by inhibiting the alpha motor neuron. After a brief period, the physician may slowly stretch the involved muscles and engage a new barrier.

Direct muscle pull causes an elastic stretch, such as occurs during periods of relaxation between active contractions and also at the passive stretch administered at the end of muscle energy treatment.

In reciprocal innervation when a stretch excites one muscle, it simultaneously inhibits its antagonist.

# ■ HIGH-VELOCITY LOW-AMPLITUDE THRUST

Although it is not necessarily thought of as a soft tissue technique, high-velocity low-amplitude thrust (HVLA) may result in regional changes in the musculature. Usually the surrounding soft tissues should be relaxed before the technique is used. The effect of the quick thrust of low amplitude, as long as it does not initiate a stretch reflex, may be to reduce local proprioceptive and nociceptive impulses from the joint. The sudden restoration of normal movement may help interrupt the cycle of pain–inflammation–restriction of motion–contraction–histochemical changes–dysfunction. The full mechanism is not well understood.

# ■ FASCIAL RELEASE (MYOFASCIAL RELEASE)

Fascia is a tissue that intimately covers all tissue, and the tension that results from spasm cannot separate the combination of fascia and muscle. As a substance that acts like a sheath and a colloid, fascia begins to show histochemical changes after trauma or prolonged stress. Resolution of somatic dysfunction must involve reversing such tensions.

# ■ INHIBITION/STIMULATION

The theories concerning the process of inhibition are not well documented. One of the oldest techniques of manipulation, its application is very similar to, and perhaps no different from, accupressure. The physician grasps or pushes a location, usually with one or two fingers; some practitioners use elbows and large surface areas such as the forearm or palm of the hand. The pressure engaged is firm and constant. After a period of time, the tissue appears to soften and the patient may describe that pain or sensitivity has diminished.

When this technique is applied to the thoracic or other spinal regions related to visceral innervation, the objective is to reduce stimulation, sympathetic or parasympathetic, to an organ or system. Some theories stress that the effect is simply muscular and may be caused by localized ischemia. Others state that painful stimuli or muscular contraction reduces because of accommodation. Accommodation occurs many times during the day. A person who wears eyeglasses becomes unaware of the stimuli of the frame resting on the bridge of the nose. We become less aware of our clothing as we proceed through the day. However, a collar or waistband that intermittently irritates may be more noticeable than one, however tight, that is constantly irritating.

Stimulation, also used for thousands of years, may be directed toward the muscle or the underlying structures. A flaccid muscle may be stimulated to activity by pressuring or kneading. This may activate some of the stretch receptors, such as the muscle spindle apparatus, and the body of the muscle contracts. When used to address visceral concerns, the effect may be stimulation of the parasympathetic or sympathetic underlying components. Stimulation in the suboccipital region or along the sacrum may initiate the former, whereas activity in the thoracolumbar spine may involve the latter.

With either of these techniques, the physician may intend to accomplish a certain goal, but it is the patient's response that is important. Changes in health may not occur so much because of a simple "knob turning" approach. As physicians using manipulative medicine, we facilitate the individual's own ability to reset his or her condition back to the more normal, functional state.

## REFERENCES

Barry G. *Lecture, Physiology.* Old Westbury, NY: New York College of Osteopathic Medicine; 1984.

Becker FR. The meaning of fascia and continuity. *Osteopath Ann* 1975;3:8–32.

Bullock J, Boyle J III, Wang MB, et al. The National Medical Series for Independent Study: Physiology. New York: John Wiley, 1984.

Cathie AG. *Manual of Osteopathic Principles and Practice—Second year, article C-17.* Philadelphia: Philadelphia College of Osteopathy, 1966.

Denslow JS, Korr IM, Krems AD. Quantitative studies of chronic facilitation in human motoneuron pools. *Am J Physiol* 1949;150:229–238.

Ettlinger H. Myofascial Release. *Osteopathic Principles and Practice.* Old Westbury, NY: NYCOM, 1987.

Ganong WF. *Review of Medical Physiology.* Palo Alto, CA: Lange Medical Publications, 1981.

Guyton AC. *Textbook of Medical Physiology,* 7th ed. Philadelphia: W.B. Saunders, 1986.

Hollinshead HW. *Textbook of Anatomy,* 3rd ed. Hagerstown, MD: Harper & Row, 1974.

Kandel E, Schwartz JH. *Principles of Neural Science.* New York: Science Publishing, 1985.

Korr IM. Somatic dysfunction, osteopathic manipulative treatment and the nervous system: A few facts, some theories, many questions. *J Am Osteopath Assoc* 1986; 86(2):109–114.

Appeltauer GSL. Continued studies on axonal transport of nerve proteins to muscle. *J Am Osteopath Assoc* 1970;69: 76–78.

Chornock FW, Cole WV, Wilkinson PN. Studies in trophic mechanisms: Does changing its nerve change a muscle? *J Am Osteopath Assoc* 1967;66:79–80.

Wilkinson PN, Chornock FW. Studies in neurotrophic mechanisms (abstr). *J Am Osteopath Assoc* 1966;65: 990–991.

Wilkinson PN, Chornock FW. Axonal delivery of neuroplasmic components to muscle cells. *J Am Osteopath Assoc* 1967;66:1057–1061.

Langley LL, Telford IR, Christenson JB. *Dynamic Anatomy and Physiology.* New York: McGraw-Hill, 1980.

Moritan T, Moramatsu S, Neuo M. Activity of the motor unit during concentric and eccentric contractions. *Am J Physiol* 1987;66:338–350.

Nicholas AS. Palpation in osteopathic medicine. *Osteopath Ann* 1978;67:36–42.

Patterson MM, Howell JN, eds. *The Central Connection: Somatovisceral/Viscerosomatic Interaction: 1989 Interna-*

*tional Symposium*. Athens, OH: University Classics, Ltd, 1992.

Sauer GC. *Manual of Skin Diseases*, 4th ed. Philadelphia: J.B. Lippincott, 1980.

Schiowitz S, DiGiovanna E, Ausman P. *An Osteopathic Approach to Diagnosis and Treatment*. Westbury, NY: NYCOM, 1981.

Smith PE, Copenhaver WM, eds. *Bailey's Textbook of Histology*. Baltimore: Williams & Wilkins, 1984.

Taber W. *Taber's Cyclopedic Medical Dictionary, 2nd ed*. Philadelphia: F.A. Davis, 1970.

Upledger JE, Vredevoogd JD. *Craniosacral Therapy*, chap. 5. Seattle: Eastland Press, 1983.

Willard FH, Patterson MM, eds. *Nociception and the Neuroendocrine-Immune Connection: 1992 International Symposium*. Athens, OH: University Classics, Ltd, 1994.

Williams PL, Warwick R, eds. *Gray's Anatomy*, 36th ed. Philadelphia: W.B. Saunders, 1980.

# Structural Examination and Documentation

*Stanley Schiowitz and Dennis J. Dowling*

## ■ STATIC SYMMETRY

Any observation of a patient that can be used to differentiate normal from abnormal function is an asset in determining a differential diagnosis. Changes in skin color, gait, or regional motion restrictions are used daily to this end. This chapter describes ideal and variant postures of an immobile, upright patient as seen in the sagittal, anterior, and posterior planes. The technique of structural examination and common causes of abnormal findings are described in the next section.

### Sagittal Plane Symmetry

In an ideal erect posture, a plumb line dropped from the ceiling along the body's midline would pass through the following points:

1. Slightly posterior to the apex of the coronal suture
2. Through the external auditory meatus
3. Through the bodies of most of the cervical vertebrae
4. Through the shoulder joint
5. Through the bodies of the lumbar vertebrae
6. Slightly posterior to the axis of the hip joint
7. Slightly anterior to the axis of the knee joint
8. Slightly anterior to the lateral malleolus

Any deviation from these relationships is considered a normal variant or an abnormal postural relationship.

## ■ PHYSIOLOGIC CURVES IN THE SAGITTAL PLAN

The adult has four normal sagittal curves, as follows:

1. In the cervical region, C1 to C7, convex forward, normal lordosis
2. In the thoracic region, Tl to T12, concave forward, normal kyphosis
3. In the lumbar region, Ll to L5, convex forward, normal lordosis
4. In the sacral region, the fused sacrum, concave forward

These curves are physiologic and biomechanical and were created by the body's functional development. At birth, the cervical, thoracic, and lumbar vertebrae form one continuous kyphotic (concave forward) curve. As the cervical extensor muscles develop, allowing the head to stay raised, the normal cervical (convex forward) lordosis develops. As the child begins to stand and walk, the back muscles strengthen and normal lumbar lordosis (convex forward) is achieved. This process begins at approximately age 3 years and is fully developed by the age 10 years. The thoracic spine retains its kyphotic posture, but the angle of the curve is usually decreased.

## ■ TRANSITIONAL ARTICULATIONS

The normal sagittal spinal curve changes from anterior convexity to anterior concavity and back at specific articulations: C7 on Tl, T12 on Ll, and L5 on the sacral base. These articulations have special osteologic constructions that assist in maintaining balance and reduce local mechanical stress. A transition in the curve at any other articulation causes local strain and dysfunction.

The sagittal spinal curves are interrelated in function. An increase in lumbar lordosis will result in increased thoracic kyphosis and increased cervical lordosis. In addition, the curves promote spinal flexibility and strength, allowing the spine to withstand stress. The spine has elastic properties under force, aiding the supporting function of the ligaments and muscles. A straight spine would transmit vector forces through the vertebral bodies, contributing to fracture.

## ■ SACRAL BASE RELATIONSHIP

The normal angle between the lumbar spine and the sacral base is 25 to 35 degrees (in the sagittal plane). A greater or lesser angle will affect the lumbar curve and cause compensatory changes in the curves higher in the spine. Flexion of the sacrum in the sagittal plane increases lumbar lordosis (anterior convexity). This will be accompanied by a similar increase in thoracic kyphosis and cervical lordosis. Extension of the sacrum reduces the lumbar anterior convexity, decreasing lumbar lordosis and providing a similar flattening of the thoracic and cervical curves.

## ■ COMMON VARIATIONS IN SAGITTAL POSTURES

Kypholordotic posture (Fig. 7-1A)

1. Head forward
2. Cervical spine lordotic
3. Thoracic spine kyphotic
4. Scapulae abducted
5. Lumbar spine lordotic
6. Anterior pelvic tilt
7. Hip joints slightly flexed
8. Knee joints extended
9. Plantar flexion of ankle joints in relation to angle of legs
10. Anterior bulging of abdomen

Swayback posture (Fig. 7-lB)

1. Head forward
2. Cervical spine lordotic, thoracic spine kyphotic
3. Decreased lordosis of lumbar spine

4. Posterior tilt of pelvis
5. Hip and knee joints hyperextended

Flat back posture (Fig. 7-1C)

1. Head forward
2. Cervical spine has slightly increased lordosis
3. Thoracic spine slightly kyphotic in upper portion, then flattens in lower segments
4. Lumbar lordosis flattened
5. Hips and knees extended.

Military-bearing posture (Fig. 7-1D)

1. Created by drilling in "chest out, stomach in" position
2. Head tilted slightly posteriorly
3. Cervical curve and thoracic curve normal
4. Chest elevated, creating anterior cervical and posterior thoracic deviation from plumb line
5. Increased lordosis of lumbar curve
6. Anterior pelvic tilt
7. Knees extended
8. Ankles plantar flexed

Anterior postural deviation (Fig. 7-lE)

1. Entire body leans forward, deviating anteriorly from the plumb line
2. Patient's weight supported by metatarsals

Posterior postural deviation (Fig. 7-1F)

1. Entire body leans backward, deviating posteriorly from plumb line
2. Balance maintained by anterior thrust of pelvis and hips
3. Marked lordosis from mid-thoracic spine down

Rotary posture (Fig. 7-1G)

1. Body rotated to right or left
2. Entire body may be involved, with rotation beginning from ankles and proceeding up
3. Lateral alignment appears completely different when viewed from right and left sides in scoliotic posture, rotation primarily of thorax, in direction of scoliotic convexity

Lumbar lordosis

1. Number of variations, described by increase in lumbar curve and height of curve
2. Simple lordosis: lordotic curve increased but contained within the lumbar region
3. High lordosis: lumbar lordotic curve passes into thoracic region, including half to two-thirds of thoracic spine in anterior convex-

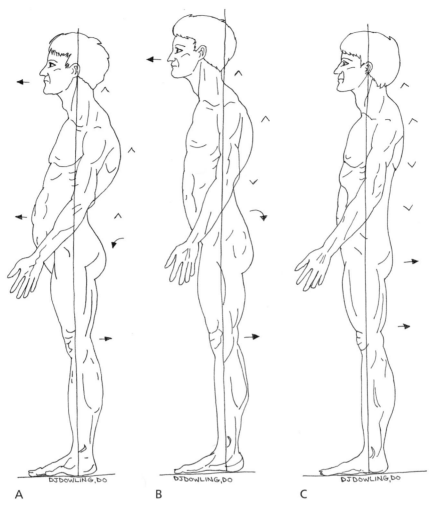

■ **FIG. 7-1 (A)** Kypholordotic posture. **(B)** Swayback posture. **(C)** Flat back posture.

ity; apex of curve moves upward toward first lumbar vertebra

4. These described variations of posture are commonly created by changes in pelvic, hip, and knee angles, or by multiple combinations of muscle hypotonicities and hypertonicities.

## Localized Thoracic Flattening

The examiner may find a localized area of thoracic spine, encompassing no more than three contiguous vertebrae, that exhibits severe flattening of the usual kyphotic pattern. This relationship can occur at an area of change of direction of a scoliotic curve, such as a right convexity becoming a left convexity. If rotation in both directions is severe, then the spinous processes of the vertebrae involved will be rotated off the midline. Failure of these processes to point directly posteriorly causes the flattened appearance.

Localized thoracic flattening may also be caused by chronic somatic dysfunction in two contiguous vertebrae. The examiner should look for a segmentally related visceral–somatic reflex pattern as the underlying cause. Chronic visceral pathology can cause this condition.

## ■ POSTERIOR PLANE SYMMETRY

In a completely symmetric posture (Fig. 7-2), a plumb line dropped from the ceiling to the floor would pass through the following points:

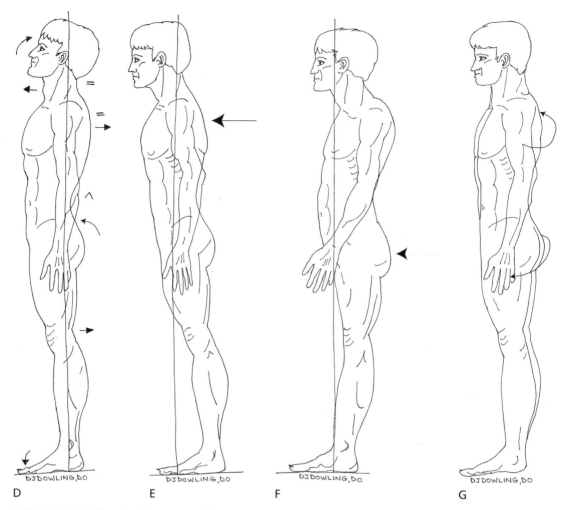

■ **FIG. 7-1 (D)** Military-bearing posture. **(E)** Anterior postural deviation. **(F)** Posterior postural deviation. **(G)** Rotary posture.

1. The inion
2. The midline of the vertebrae
3. The midline of the sacrum
4. The midline of the coccyx
5. A point midway between both medial malleoli

## Scoliosis

Muscles and ligaments balance the spine bilaterally. A second group of muscles maintains the position and alignment of the scapular girdle with respect to the spine. A difference in function between muscles and ligaments on the two sides of the spine will pull the spine out of alignment. The spine is not rigid but is made up of multiple maneuverable vertebral links. In response to asymmetric pull, one or more vertebrae will move from the position of symmetry. This vertebral motion can occur in three planes—the sagittal plane (flexion, extension), horizontal plane (rotation), or frontal plane (side-bending—and always represents a combination of multiple planar motions.

Scoliosis is defined as an appreciable deviation of a group of vertebrae from the normal straight vertical line of the spine, as viewed in the posterior plane. Scoliosis can be structural (organic) or functional. A structural curve is fixed when the patient side-bends into the convexity of the curve and it does not straighten

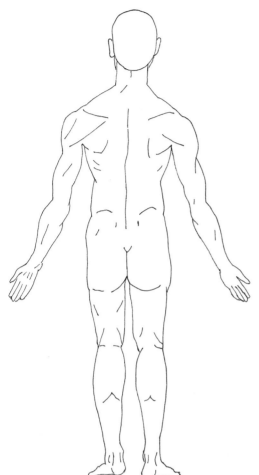

DJDOWLING,DO

■ **FIG. 7-2** Posterior view of the body. An ideal plumb line alignment is shown.

out. A functional scoliotic pattern will correct with side-bending. If an acute muscle contracture is causing a scoliotic appearance, placing the patient in the prone position will straighten the curve. A functional scoliotic curve that remains uncorrected for a number of years can give rise to musculoskeletal changes and become a fixed structural curve.

Harrison Fryette, in *Principles of Osteopathic Technique*, discussed specific coupled motion patterns. Of relevance here, when the spine is at rest, normal lateral flexion in one direction will cause the vertebral body to rotate in the opposite direction. (This rule applies only to the thoracic and lumbar regions.) If a group of vertebrae side-bend toward the right, the vertebral bodies will

rotate to the left. If this vertebral position is fixed, the patient would have a scoliotic curve. The scoliosis is said to have a left convexity. The spinous processes are deviated to the right of the midline and the left transverse processes are rotated posteriorly. If the thoracic region is involved, the rib cage will rotate and side-bend with the vertebrae. The ribs will be more posterior and separated on the left side. The scapular girdle may follow the rib cage in its displacement. Muscle imbalance, representing unilateral hypotonicity or hypertonicity, will create scoliotic patterns. The examiner must be aware of the line of force of the muscles involved, and of the complexity of multiple muscle actions at one region. The assignment of cause or effect to postural changes requires a thorough understanding of functional anatomy

What happens to the spine when the sacral base is not level? In the frontal plane, sacral base unleveling will cause a lumbar scoliotic pattern convex in the direction of the inferior sacral side, if the spine is flexible. The convexity may continue up through the thoracic region to create one thoracolumbar C-shaped scoliotic curve (Fig. 7-3). The body tries to compensate for the imbalance created by the C curve by creating a secondary, compensatory curve above the first lumbar curve. The side of convexity of the second curve is opposite that of the primary curve, producing an S-shaped curve (Fig. 7-4). Additional compensatory scoliotic curves can develop higher in the spine, into the cervical region, with alternating convexities. Because the body always attempts to maintain the eyes on a level plane, the last compensatory maneuver may be side-bending of the head. The body waist crease lines usually follow the pattern of the largest scoliotic asymmetry. The waist crease would have the most acute angle at the site and side of the greatest lateral flexion concave curve.

## Factors That Commonly Influence or Cause Scoliosis

(See also Chapter 45)

1. Structural or organic scoliosis—all causes
2. Bone deformities caused by congenital, traumatic, or disease conditions.

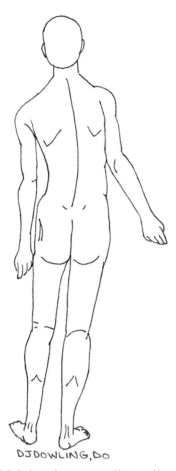

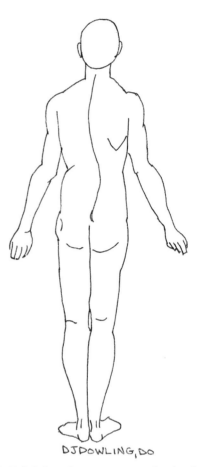

**FIG. 7-3** C-shaped curve caused by sacral base unleveling, posterior view.

**FIG. 7-4** S-shaped curve compensating for thoracolumbar scoliosis, posterior view.

3. Muscle tone changes caused by hypotonicity, hypertonicity, hypertrophy, or atrophy
4. Postural changes created by habits or occupation
5. Unilateral structural changes: short leg or unilateral flat foot or pronation; tibial torsion, knee deformity, or hip deformity; sacral torsion or pelvic torsion
6. Somatic dysfunctions
7. Compensatory and noncompensatory fascial patterns

## ■ COMMON VARIATIONS OF FRONTAL POSTURES

1. Right-handedness
   a. Upper thoracic scoliosis, concave to right
   b. Right shoulder lower than left
   c. Right buttock deviated away from midline

2. Left-handedness
   a. Upper thoracic scoliosis, concave to left
   b. Left shoulder lower than right
   c. Left buttock deviated away from midline
3. S-type compensated structural scoliosis
   a. The lumbar and thoracic scoliotic convexities are in opposite directions
   b. The rib cage will rotate posteriorly with the thoracic convexity
   c. The shoulders may be level
   d. The iliac crest heights may be level
   e. The buttocks are not deviated away from the midline
4. C-type compensated structural scoliosis
   a. Thoracic and lumbar scoliotic convexity form one continuous curve in same direction

    b. Rib cage rotated posteriorly with thoracic convexity

    c. Buttocks not deviated away from midline

    d. Iliac crest heights may be level

5. Lateral pelvic tilt functional curve, cephalad on right, C-type

    a. Thoracic and lumbar curves continuous and convex to left

    b. Scapula lower on right

    c. Rib cage rotated posteriorly on left

    d. Waist crease has more acute angle on right

    e. Neck laterally tilted to left

6. Lateral pelvic tilt functional curve, cephalad on right, S-type

    a. If compensated, should act as described in item three, except that iliac crest height is higher on right

7. Unilateral erector spinal muscle hypertonicity

    a. Side-bending of spine in direction of hypertonic muscle

    b. Scoliotic convexity in opposite direction

    c. Elevated iliac crest on side of hypertonicity

    d. Placing patient prone should change above findings

8. Unilateral upper trapezius muscle hypertonicity

    a. Head tilted toward side of hypertonic muscle

    b. Shoulder girdle elevated on affected side

    c. Scapula on hypertonic muscle side rotated upward and slightly adducted

The patterns of asymmetry described in this chapter are not all-inclusive. The body exhibits various biomechanical responses to all factors that influence the musculoskeletal system.

## ■ TECHNIQUE OF STATIC SYMMETRY EXAMINATION

A postural examination begins with the patient and physician in a fixed, reproducible position, so that observations may be correlated with observations made on future examinations. The patient stands on a level surface, without shoes. All extremities should be in full extension. The feet are placed 6 to 8 inches apart with the heels in the same frontal plane and the toes abducted approximately 15 degrees. The physician stands facing the aspect of the patient to be evaluated (front, back, or side) and at a sufficient distance to permit a complete body view. In the course of the examination, the physician will step closer to observe local areas of interest. The examiner's eyes should be at the level of the part being viewed, which may entail crouching or kneeling during evaluation of lower body portions. Light palpation may be used, too. Observations are highlighted in Figure 7-5.

## Posterior View

For posterior inspection, a good method is to observe the patient in the following sequence:

### Distant Evaluation, Posterior View

1. General observation of gross body symmetry and asymmetry
2. Achilles tendon
3. Medial malleoli
4. Popliteal lines
5. Gluteal creases
6. Greater trochanters
7. Posterior superior iliac spines
8. Heights of iliac crests
9. Thoracolumbar spines for deviations from midline symmetry, or flattening
10. Waist creases
11. Level of inferior angles of scapula, abduction-adduction
12. Rib cage rotation or scapular rotation
13. Level of shoulders
14. Level of fingertips
15. Deviation of cervical spine and skull from midline
16. Level of earlobes

Note the following factors:

    a. Head

    b. Earlobes

    c. Neck

    d. Shoulders

    e. Shoulder girdles

    f. Spine

    g. Rib cage

    h. Waist crease lines

    i. Iliac crests

    j. Gluteal creases

    k. Fingertips

    l. Popliteal creases

    m. Achilles tendons

    n. Heels

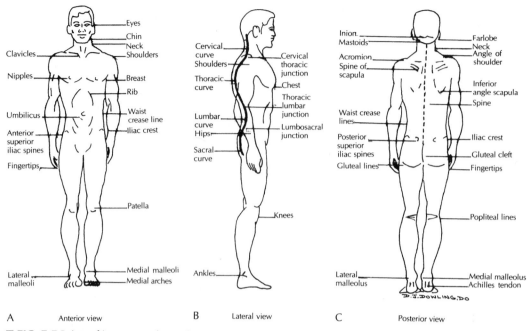

**■ FIG. 7-5** Points of interest on the static symmetry examination. **(A)** Anterior view. **(B)** Lateral view. **(C)** Posterior view.

After gaining an overall impression, the examiner steps within arm's length of the patient and adds palpation to confirm visual observation. The sequence of observations is repeated.

### Close Evaluation With Palpation—Posterior View

1. Is the head straight? Palpate the inion. Is it in the midline?
2. With one finger on the inion, place a finger of the other hand at the gluteal cleft. Are they in a line vertically to each other?
3. Touch the earlobes; measure their heights. Touch the tips of the mastoid bones. Are they level?
4. Are the neck and head tilted?
5. Put one finger of each hand on the right and left trapezius muscles where the neck meets the trunk. Are they level?
6. Slide those fingers laterally to the top of each acromium process. Are they level?
7. Place one finger at the inferior angle of each scapula, at approximately the level of the seventh thoracic vertebra. Are they level?
8. Move both fingers up the vertebral borders of the scapulae to the medial aspect of their spines. Are they level?
9. Place a palm flat on the posterior surface of each scapula, with your fingers resting on the superior scapular border. Are the scapulae rotated? Are they level?
10. Have the patient bend forward. Slide your palms over the angles of the ribs. Is there an exaggerated rib hump indicating scoliotic convexity?
11. Place one finger on the spinous process of the first thoracic vertebra. Slide it down the spine, one vertebra at a time, to the sacrum. Are the spinous processes symmetric with respect to each other in all three planes?

   a. Frontal plane—feel for deviation from the midline.
   b. Sagittal plane—feel for depression or prominence.
   c. Horizontal plane—feel the space between the tips of the spinous processes. Are they equal?
   d. Do areas of the spine seem flat?

12. Follow the waist crease lines. Are the angles equal? Does the more acute angle coincide with the concavity of a spinal scoliosis?

13. Measure the posterior superior iliac spines bilaterally. Place your thumb or index finger at each dimple in the lower back. Identify the most prominent (posterior) bony point. Bend down by flexing your knees, so that your eyes are at finger level. Note the following:

    a. Are they at the same height?
    b. Are they of the same depth?

14. Move these fingers up the iliac crest until they are resting on the uppermost portion of the ilium bilaterally. Are the crest heights level?

15. Place a finger of each hand at the gluteal lines. Move your eyes to that level. Are the lines level?

16. Bend down further and measure the heights of the popliteal lines. Are they level?

17. Measure the distance from the fingertips to the floor.

18. Trace each Achilles tendon to its insertion. Are they bowed or straight?

## Anterior View

The sequence for anterior observation is as follows:

### Distant Evaluation, Anterior View

1. General observation of gross body symmetry and asymmetry
2. Medial longitudinal arches
3. Medial malleoli
4. Patellae
5. Greater trochanters
6. Anterior superior iliac spines
7. Heights of iliac crests
8. Waist creases
9. Rib cage angle
10. Rib cage rotation
11. Nipple levels—males or children only
12. Level of shoulders
13. Level of fingertips
14. Deviation of cervical spine and skull from midline
15. Level of earlobes
16. Level of eyes

Note the following factors:

a. Head
b. Eyes
c. Neck
d. Chin
e. Shoulders
f. Clavicles
g. Chest wall
h. Rib angle
i. Nipples
j. Umbilicus
k. Iliac crests
l. Patellae
m. Fingertips
n. Medial malleoli
o. Medial arches

After completing the general evaluation, the examiner moves forward and adds palpation to confirm visual observations.

### Close Evaluation With Palpation—Anterior View

1. Is the head straight? Palpate the level of the earlobes.
2. Are eyes level?
3. Is the chin deviated from midline?
4. Palpate and measure the shoulder heights at the top of the acromium processes. Are they level?
5. Palpate and measure the clavicle heights. Are they level?
6. Note chest wall symmetry and rotation. If asymmetric, does it match the posterior view findings?
7. Note nipple heights (men and children only).
8. Measure the rib cage angle and the angle of the arm at the elbow.
9. Is the umbilicus at the midline? Are there scars on the abdomen?
10. Palpate the waist crease lines and note their length and angle.
11. Palpate the anterior superior iliac spines and note their heights and anterior posterior orientation (examiner's eyes at that level).
12. Follow the iliac crests to their greatest heights and measure them (examiner's eyes at that level). Are they equal?

13. Palpate the superior aspect of both patellae and measure their heights (examiner's eyes at that level). Are they level? Do they point anteriorly, medially, or laterally?
14. Measure the heights of the tips of the fingers from the floor. Are they equal? Are the hands internally rotated?
15. Measure the heights of the lowest aspect of each medial malleolus from the floor. Are they equal?
16. Measure the height of each medial arch. Are they equal?

### Sagittal Plane View: Distant Evaluation, Sagittal Viewv

1. Head
2. Cervical curve
3. Cervical–thoracic junction
4. Thoracic curve
5. Thoracolumbar junction
6. Lumbar curve
7. Lumbosacral junction
8. Sacral curve
9. Shoulders
10. Hips
11. Knees
12. Ankles
13. Anterior silhouette, chest to abdomen

With these observations in mind, the examiner moves forward and adds palpation to confirm visual observations, reproducing the sequence of evaluation.

### Close Evaluation With Palpation—Sagittal Plane View

1. Is the head displaced anteriorly?
2. Is the anteroposterior cervical curve exaggerated or flattened?
3. Is the transition from the cervical lordosis to thoracic kyphosis a smooth minimal curve?
4. Is the upper thoracic posterior convexity increased?
5. Is the thoracic posterior convexity a smooth curve? Is its kyphosis exaggerated? Do segments seem flattened?
6. Is the thoracolumbar junction at the articulation of the 12th thoracic and first lumbar vertebrae? Is the transitional curve smooth?
7. Is the lumbar anteroposterior curve smooth? Is it exaggerated or flattened?
8. Is the lumbosacral junction a smooth transitional curve? Does the lumbosacral angle appear normal?
9. Is there marked posterior angulation of the sacrum?
10. Look directly at the nearest shoulder. Is it forward, depressed, rotated? Can you see the other shoulder without moving your head?
11. Repeat the same examination with the scapulae and rib cage. Are they rotated?
12. Is the body rotated?
13. Bend down and look at the hips. Are they rotated? Are they fully extended?
14. Look at the knees. Are they rotated? Are they fully extended? Are they hyperextended?
15. Look at the ankles. Are they rotated?
16. Look at the anterior silhouette. What is the shape and position of the chest? What is the relationship of the chest to the abdomen in position and size?
17. Does the body seem displaced from the midline anteriorly or posteriorly?

## ■ FACTORS THAT COMMONLY INFLUENCE THE SAGITTAL CURVES

### Osseous-Muscular Factors

1. Bone deformities, of which the most common result from:
   a. Congenital deformities of the vertebrae
   b. Trauma creating fracture or dislocation
   c. Diseases such as tumors, infections, and osteopenia/osteoporosis
2. Ventral or dorsal muscle tone changes, commonly caused by:
   a. Muscle disuse or atrophy secondary to neurological disease, immobilization, or age
   b. Obesity or pregnancy, creating abdominal muscle stretch
   c. Contracture of muscles due to bumps, overdevelopment, injuries, or viscerosomatic reflexes

### Structural–Mechanical Factors

1. Change in location of transitional areas of the sagittal curves, commonly caused by:

  a. Congenital vertebral formation
  b. Sacral base imbalance in the sagittal or frontal plane
  c. Localized regional scoliotic patterns
  d. Organic kyphoscoliosis
  e. Wearing high-heel shoes
  f. Habit or occupation
2. Endomorphic characteristics (usually increase the lordotic curve)
3. Hereditary characteristics (increase lordotic curve)
4. Foot defects such as pronation or calcaneal valgus (increase lumbar lordosis)
5. Genu valgus or varus (influences lumbar curve)
6. Hip joint changes such as femoral ante/retroversion or femoral valgus/varus (influence lumbar curve)
7. Localized somatic dysfunctions (flattened thoracic kyphosis)

## ■ GENERAL CONSIDERATIONS

In all close examinations, the examiner should use palpation whenever it can help confirm visual observations. The eyes should be at the level of the body part observed during close examinations. Looking up or down can distort the findings. The examiner may bend down by flexing the knees or sit in a suitable chair.

The first observations should be from a distance. The examiner first develops a sense of body symmetry and then uses closer observation and palpation to confirm or rule out initial impressions.

## ■ DOCUMENTATION

As with other entries for medical record-keeping, details as to the structural findings should be recorded as pertinent positive and negative components relevant to the patient's condition. Documentation in a patient's chart is for the purpose of recording progress or changes over time and as a means of communicating to other osteopathic physicians and other health personnel. Specifics as to the deviation from normal, the side of asymmetrical findings and common references should be included. Occasionally, a pictorial representation may summarize the findings more easily than prolonged written descriptions.

When providing documentation on a patient's chart, common nomenclature and abbreviations should be used. For example, "R" indicating "right" and "L" indicating "left" is easily understood by anyone reading the chart; "HM" for "hypertonic muscles" would not be.

For the common abbreviations used for somatic dysfunctions, see Chapter 4.

### REFERENCES

Basmajian JV. *Muscles Alive.* 4th ed. Baltimore: Williams & Wilkins, 1978.

Calliet R. *Scoliosis.* Philadelphia: F.A. Davis, 1975.

Fryette HH. *Principles of Osteopathic Technique,* Carmel, CA: Academy of Applied Osteopathy, 1954.

Heilig D. Some basic considerations of spinal curves. *Osteopath Ana* 1978;311:318.

Kapandji IA. *Physiology of the Joints,* 2nd ed, vol 3. Edinburgh: Churchill Livingstone, 1974.

Kendall FP, McCreary EK. *Muscles: Testing and Function, 3rd ed.* Baltimore: Williams & Wilkins, 1983.

MacConaill MA, Basmajian JV. *Muscles and Movements, 2nd ed.* Huntington, NY: Robert E. Krieger, 1969.

Northup GW. Osteopathic lesions. *J Am Osteopathic Assoc* 1972;71:854–864.

Schiowitz S. Static symmetry and asymmetry. *Osteopath Ann* 1980;8:9.

# Palpation

*Eileen L. DiGiovanna*

**P**alpation is a particularly important means of uncovering information. Palpation can disclose subtle changes in the texture of the soft tissues of the body—the skin, fascia, muscles, ligaments, and tendons. Tissue changes that occur in response to the effects of sympathetic innervation may be manifested by an increase or decrease in skin temperature or moisture. Edema of the underlying soft tissues will produce a palpable bogginess. Changes in the quality of joint motion may be felt before they produce visible symptoms. Deeper palpation is used to search for masses, outline organ size and consistency, test muscle tone, and feel the impulse of the heart.

During palpation, the physician concentrates on the sensations received through the fingers and hands. The distribution and depth of receptor organs determine which part of the hand is most useful in specific tests. Because the heat receptors lie deep, the ulnar or dorsal aspect of the hand (where the skin is thinner than on the palms) should be used to test for temperature changes. Touch receptors such as Merkel's disks and Meissner's corpuscles are most numerous in the pads of the fingers, making these the most sensitive areas.

Observation is an important aid to palpation. The area being examined should be inspected for color changes (pallor) or erythema (redness). Increased erythema may indicate infection or inflammation and commonly occurs with acute somatic dysfunction. Pallor may occur with chronic somatic dysfunction. Areas of hyperpigmentation may be significant. The physician should also look for signs of trauma, such as scars, bruises, lacerations, abrasions, and swelling. Blemishes or masses on the skin's surface should be noted.

## ■ PALPATION OF THE SKIN AND SOFT TISSUES

The following is an organized approach to the development of palpatory skills. Practice each of these until you feel comfortable with your findings.

### Temperature Changes

1. Palpate lightly. Pressure or friction causes vasodilation, creating temperature changes.
2. See which area of the hand is most sensitive to temperature: the back or side of the hand, the fingertips, the wrist. (Thinner-skinned areas are most sensitive.)
3. Palpate various areas of the back to discriminate temperature differences. The thoracic area is usually warmer because of the underlying heart and great vessels. Compare the skin temperature of various body regions in several individuals.

### Evaluation of Skin Drag

1. Slide fingertips lightly across the surface of the skin to see if any drag can be felt on the fingertips.
2. Increased drag may be caused by a fine film of moisture.
3. A decrease in drag may be caused by exces-

sive moisture, oily skin, or abnormally atrophic skin.

## Evaluation of Skin Texture

1. Palpate for roughness or smoothness. Compare individual skin differences.
2. Feel for sebaceous activity (oiliness).
3. Try palpating through cloth to get the feel of its effect on reception of sensation by the hand.

## Palpation of Fluid in Tissues

1. Excess fluid in tissues is called *edema*. Edema results in a spongy or boggy feel to the tissues. Edema of significant proportions may accumulate over the sacrum or anterior aspect of the lower legs and ankles. It is also found in hives or welts.
2. Soft tissues involved in acute somatic dysfunction will have some edema. Try to palpate the bogginess of the tissues.

## Turgor (Elastic Rebound of the Skin)

1. Pick up the skin and then release it.
2. Observe how it returns to its former tautness. If the skin returns to its original state immediately, it has normal turgor. If the skin remains tented, it has poor turgor.
3. Lack of turgor is found in dehydration, aging, and certain metabolic diseases.

## Evaluation of Erythema (Red Reflex)

1. Rub the skin with the fingers in a firm stroke. Observe for blanching (whiteness) or erythema (redness). Note the length of time required for the skin color to return to normal.

*Note:* Are both sides equally red? Does the redness fade equally? Does one side remain red longer than the other? Areas of acute somatic dysfunction tend to remain red longer. Chronicity of the somatic dysfunction tends to lead to blanching of the skin that persists for a time.

## Tenderness

Tenderness is a subjective rather than an objective finding. Palpation of certain areas may cause the sensation of pain to the patient. This is known as tenderness. Because it is subjective, this finding is not as reliable as the objective findings of the physician.

## Layer-By-Layer Palpation

During palpation, it is helpful to mentally visualize the depth of the palpation. A gradually increasing pressure of the fingertips gives the sensations and textures of structures deeper and deeper in the body. Looking at an anatomical atlas while palpating a region assists in learning the feel of various structures of the body.

### Subcutaneous Tissues

Beneath the surface of the skin lie the subcutaneous tissues, consisting of various connective tissues, fascia, and fat. These tissues normally have a slightly spongy feel. Edema fluid may collect here and produce a "doughy" feel. Sometimes these tissues will "pit" with pressure. The pitting will remain for a time and is almost always indicative of edema. Pitting may be observed when pressure is applied to edematous ankles or sacrum.

In the subcutaneous tissues lie some of the superficial blood vessels. Palpate veins over the back of the hand or in the antecubital fossa. Occlusion with a tourniquet makes the veins more prominent. Note the springy feel. Palpate the radial and carotid arteries. Note that they are much firmer than unoccluded veins. Palpate the back for any abnormal tensions in the subcutaneous tissues. This may indicate contracture or fibrous changes of the fascia.

### Muscle

Muscle tissue consists of bundles of fibers arranged in parallel fashion.

1. Press more deeply into the tissues until you contact the firmer muscle tissues.
2. Select several large muscles (trapezius, biceps, sternocleidomastoid, deltoid) and follow the directions of their fibers to the muscle attachments.
3. Palpate the paraspinal muscles, feeling for the following:
   a. **Tone:** The normal feel of a resting muscle (if palpation is too rough, it may change the tone):

(1) *Hypertonic*—an increase in normal tone
(2) *Hypotonic*—a decrease in normal tone
(3) *Atonic*—no tone; a limp, flaccid muscle

b. **Contraction:** Normal tension built up in muscle as it shortens
c. **Contracture:** Abnormal fixing of a muscle in a shortened position with fibrous changes in the tissue
d. **Spasm:** Abnormal contraction maintained beyond physiologic need
e. **Bogginess:** Increased fluid in a hypertonic muscle; feels like a wet sponge
f. **Ropiness:** Cord-like or rope-like feel to a muscle that has been chronically contracted
g. **Stringiness:** A finer version of ropiness—the muscle feels as if it were made of tense strings

## Tendons

Tendons are fibroelastic strands of connective tissue attaching muscle to bone.

1. Palpate the Achilles tendon at the heel and the biceps tendon at the elbow.

Note the firmer feel of these tissues as compared to muscle.

## Ligaments

Ligaments are tough fibrous bands that connect bone to bone. Because they lie very deep, they are difficult to palpate. Some are not accessible to palpation.

1. The lateral collateral ligament of the knee may be palpated by asking the patient to cross his or her legs so that one ankle lies on the knee of the other leg. The knee should be flexed and the thigh externally rotated. The ligament may be palpated crossing the joint space laterally and slightly posteriorly.

**REFERENCES**

DiGiovanna E. *Encyclopedia of Osteopathy.* Indianapolis, IN: American Academy of Osteopaths: Indianapolis, IN, 2002.

DiGiovanna E, Schiowitz S. *An Osteopathic Approach to Diagnosis and Treatment, 2nd ed.* Philadelphia: Lippincott-Raven, 1997.

Educational Council on Osteopathic Principles. *Glossary of Osteopathic Terminology.* Chicago: American Osteopathic Association, 2001.

Nicholas AS. 1978. Palpation in osteopathic medicine. *Osteopath Ann* 1995;67:36–42.

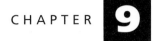

# CHAPTER 9

# The Role of Exercise in Osteopathic Management

*Stanley Schiowitz and Albert R. DeRubertis*

The average physician, before prescribing a specific drug, will have arrived at a working diagnosis and a therapeutic plan. The physician is expected to know the appropriate drug dosage, its side effects, its compatibilities with other drugs, and its effects on other clinical entities that the patient might have.

These minimal requirements of physician capability hold equally true in the prescription of exercise as a therapeutic modality. All physicians encounter patients who are voluntarily pursuing some form of exercise or for whom an exercise program should be prescribed. This chapter addresses the primary care physician's use and prescription of exercise therapy for musculoskeletal dysfunctions.

It is recommended that the reader review the discussion of the functional anatomy of muscle as described in General Anatomic Considerations, Section I, Chapter 5.

## Classification of Exercise

1. **Isotonic.** A dynamic exercise with a constant load. The resistance is the product of the load and the resistance arm (moment arm) and, therefore, is not constant.
2. **Isokinetic.** A dynamic exercise in which the speed of motion is controlled by varying the resistance.
3. **Isometric.** A static exercise in which the muscle contracts with little or no shortening (static contraction).

*Note:* The example of elbow flexion by contraction of the biceps with a weight held in the palm can be described as follows:

1. As flexion proceeds from a position of 90 degrees, the moment arm lessens; therefore, the resistance lessens. If the contraction force of the biceps is maintained constant, then the speed of flexion will correspondingly increase. This is an example of isotonic exercise.
2. If, as the moment arm lessens, the weight in the palm correspondingly is increased, then the resistance continually increases with flexion. The speed of flexion will remain constant. This is an example of isokinetic exercise, which can only be performed by using machines designed for this purpose.
3. If the weight in the palm were too heavy to be moved, then as the biceps contracted, flexion would not be created, the muscle would not change its length, and the moment arm and resistance would be constant. This is an example of isometric exercise.

*Isokinetic* exercise increases the work a muscle can do more rapidly than either isometric or isotonic exercise. It is more efficient. *Isometric* exercise should be used when motion of the joint is contraindicated or creates pain. For skill training, the best form of exercise is isotonic repetition of the motions needed in performing those skills.

## Indications for Exercise Therapy

1. To develop a sense of good postural alignment

2. To relax or lengthen contracted or shortened musculature
3. To achieve flexibility of joint motion within its normal range of motion
4. To increase muscle strength as needed to attain and maintain proper function.

Other chapters of this book describe methods for determining if these indications exist: static symmetry scan, regional motion testing, joint motion testing, palpation, and intersegmental motion testing. The only dysfunction testing not yet described is that used for muscle strength.

## Testing for Muscle Function (Strength–Contractility)

The general procedure for strength testing is to direct the patient to concentrically contract the muscle to be tested and then quantitatively measure the results and classify the findings.

1. Procedure for strength testing
   a. Place the segment in a completely relaxed position with minimal influence of gravity.
   b. Position the segment of the body involved so that the motion being tested can occur.
   c. Have the patient contract the involved muscle in an attempt to achieve concentric contraction and joint motion.
   d. Evaluate results.
2. Classification
   a. No contraction at all—grade 0.
   b. Contraction felt by examiner's fingers, but no motion—grade 1.
   c. Contraction with motion not against gravity—poor—grade 2.
   d. Contraction with motion against gravity but not resistance—fair—grade 3.
   e. Contraction against gravity but not fully against resistance—fair—grade 4.
   f. Full contraction against both gravity and resistance—excellent—grade 5.

## Inactivity and Hypokinetic Disease

Kraus and associates reported on studies performed to measure strength and flexibility of the trunk and leg muscles in children. Whereas only 8.7% of European children failed this test, 57.9% of American children failed. The poor American showing may be explained by the high degree of mechanization available.

In addition to mechanization, civilization has inhibited the "fight or flight" response. Urbanized humans live in an almost constant alert reaction phase. This imbalance in our lives—excessive unresolved stimulation—combined with insufficient exercise keeps us living in a potentially pathogenic environment.

The terms *tension neck, tension headache,* and *tension back pain* are common to the primary care physician. These syndromes are difficult to diagnose and even more difficult to treat. A multifactorial approach, incorporating behavior modification with relaxation and lengthening exercises, is advisable. Prevention by means of global relaxation and lengthening exercises and stress modification techniques should begin in childhood and continue throughout life.

## Kraus-Weber Test (Modified)

The modified Kraus-Weber test is a scanning procedure for evaluating groups of muscles acting together to perform specific body motions. Tests 1 through 5 primarily evaluate muscle strength. As the primary agonist muscles are contracted, the antagonist muscles are stretched. Contracture of these antagonist muscles might lead to a false interpretation of agonist muscle weakness. Tests 6 and 7 primarily test for muscle shortening (loss of extensibility).

Physicians treating musculoskeletal dysfunctions should use some form of screening to assist in prescribing effective exercise therapy. Numerous other tests are available, in addition to the ones described here.

**Test 1** tests upper abdominal–psoas muscle strength (Fig. 9-1):

1. **Patient position:** Supine, with hands folded across chest and legs fully extended.
2. **Physician position:** At foot of table holding patient's feet down.
3. Patient is instructed to curl head and body up, off the table. If the back is elevated 30 degrees or more off the table, then the upper abdominal muscles are functioning adequately. If the back is elevated more than 60 degrees to the fully upright position, psoas muscle strength is being used and tested.

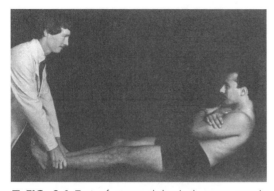

■ **FIG. 9-1** Test of upper abdominal, psoas muscle strength.

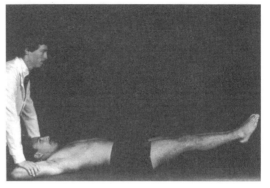

■ **FIG. 9-3** Test of lower abdominal muscle strength.

**Test 2** tests abdominal muscle strength without psoas involvement (Fig. 9-2):

1. **Patient position:** Supine, with hands folded across chest, hips and knees flexed, with feet flat on table.
2. **Physician position:** Holding patient's feet down flat on table.
3. Patient is instructed as before to curl the body up to a seated position.
4. Measure degree of compliance.

**Test 3** tests lower abdominal muscle strength (Fig.9-3):

1. **Patient position:** Supine with hands behind neck and both legs extended.
2. **Physician position:** At head of the table, holding patient's shoulders to the table.
3. Patient is instructed to lift both feet off the table, with legs extended, to a height of 10 inches, and to hold this position for 10 seconds.
4. Measure degree of compliance.

**Test 4** tests upper back muscle strength (Fig. 9-4):

1. **Patient position:** Prone, with pillow under abdomen, legs fully extended, hands clasped behind back.
2. **Physician position:** At foot of table, holding patient's hips and legs down to table.
3. Patient is instructed to raise his chest and abdomen off the table and hold this position for 10 seconds.
4. Measure degree of compliance.

**Test 5** tests lower back muscle strength (Fig. 9-5):

1. **Patient position:** Prone, with pillow under abdomen, legs fully extended, hands clasped behind neck.

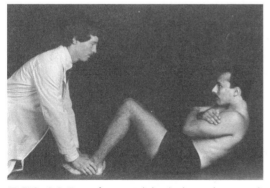

■ **FIG. 9-2** Test of upper abdominal muscle strength without psoas involvement.

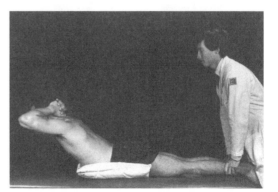

■ **FIG. 9-4** Test of upper back muscle strength.

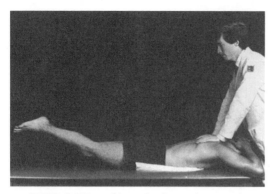

■ **FIG. 9-5** Test of lower back muscle strength.

2. **Physician position:** At head of table holding patient's shoulders down.
3. Patient is instructed to raise both legs off the table, without bending the knees, and to hold this position for 10 seconds.
4. Measure degree of compliance.

**Test 6** tests hamstring extensibility (Fig. 9-6):

1. **Patient position:** Upright, completely erect, feet together, hands at sides.
2. Patient is told to bend forward, trying to touch the floor, without bending the knees.
3. Physician measures the distance of the fingertips from the floor to determine degree of compliance.

**Test 7** tests hamstring extensibility (Fig. 9-7):

1. **Patient position:** Supine, both legs fully extended.

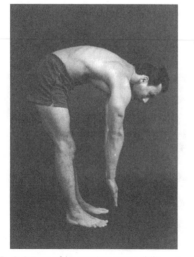

■ **FIG. 9-6** Test of hamstring extensibility, standing.

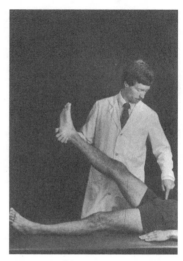

■ **FIG. 9-7** Test of hamstring extensibility, supine.

2. **Physician position:** At side of hamstrings to be tested.
3. Physician places one hand under the patient's heel. The physician's other hand is at the ipsilateral anterior superior iliac spine.
4. Physician passively raises the fully extended leg off the table until rotary motion is felt at the anterior superior iliac spine.
5. Measure the degree of hip flexion. Less than 60 degrees of flexion is considered loss of hamstring extensibility.
6. Flexion of 80 to 90 degrees indicates good extensibility of the gluteus maximus muscle. More than 90 degrees of flexion indicates good extensibility of the erector spinae muscle.

*Note:* The interpretation of this test can be invalidated by the presence of radiculitis or hip joint restriction.

## Planning an Exercise Program—General Principles

1. Do not perform if exercise causes pain.
2. Evaluate the gravitational force and patient's position.
3. Evaluate the effect of exercising two joint muscles on both joints.
4. Start with relaxing (postural) exercises, then add mild corrective exercise, gradually increase to more strenuous corrective exercises, specifically planned and to patient's tolerance.

5. Exercises should begin and end gradually with stretching and relaxing exercises used in warm up and cool down phases.
6. Instruct patient to relax between individual exercises.
7. Change position of patient and vary the exercises.
8. Multiple repetitions of identical movements should be avoided. Perform only two or three of the same exercise in one session.
9. All exercises are performed slowly and smoothly.
10. Avoid patient fatigue.
11. Perform regimen regularly.

## General Precautions

These precautions should be taken into account when writing exercise prescriptions.

1. Protect one body segment from strain while exercising another part.
2. Be aware of the needs, expectations, and limitations of the older patient.
3. Be aware of the needs, expectations, and limitations of debilitated patients.
4. Patients may have illness that may be worsened with active exercises.
5. Always prescribe specific therapy for specific purposes.
6. Avoid overdose of exercise therapy.
7. Do not cause pain by movement.
8. Prescribe supportive medications as indicated.
9. Prescribe follow-up treatments.
10. Prescribe home therapy and exercise as you would prescribe drug therapy.

## Relaxing Exercises

There are many variations and styles of relaxing exercises. The one described here uses static muscle contraction.

1. **Patient position:** Supine, legs extended, and arms at sides. Instruct patient as follows:
2. Bring your ankles and toes into full dorsiflexion; now, try to push the foot and toes into further dorsiflexion. Hold for a count of 4 seconds, relax.

3. Contract your calf muscles statically, hold for a count of 4 seconds, relax.
4. Contract your buttocks statically, hold for a count of 4 seconds, relax.
5. Bend your hips and knees and place your feet on the floor. Push your low back to the floor as firmly as possible, hold for a count of 4 seconds, relax.
6. Raise your back off the floor so that you are supported by your feet, upper spine, and shoulders. Push down on your upper spine and shoulders. Hold for a count of 4 seconds, relax.
7. Contract your hands, making a firm fist. Hold for a count of 4 seconds, relax.
8. Contract your forearm muscles statically. Hold for a count of 4 seconds, relax.
9. Contract your biceps muscles statically. Hold for a count of 4 seconds, relax.
10. Shrug your shoulders up toward your ears, as far as possible. Hold for a count of 4 seconds, relax.
11. Bring your shoulders forward, trying to meet in the midline. Hold for a count of 4 seconds, relax.
12. Tuck your chin in, then push your neck firmly backward toward the floor. Hold for a count of 4 seconds, relax.

## Writing an Exercise Prescription

The exercise prescription must do the following:
1. Be specific for musculoskeletal dysfunctions
2. Take into account the patient's physical and mental condition
3. Take into account the patient's muscle function:
   a. Ability to shorten—*contractility*
   b. Ability to lengthen—*extensibility*
   c. Ability to return to normal size—*elasticity*

Below is an example of an exercise prescription.

   **Patient's name: ____ Date: ____ Goals: ____**
   **Procedures to follow:**

1. Patient position: perform the following relaxing exercises:
   a. ____    time ____
   b. ____    time ____
   c. ____    time ____
   d. ____    time ____

2. Rest; change position; perform the following mild exercises (specific for goals):
   a. _____ time _____
   b. _____ time _____
   c. _____ time _____
3. Rest; change position; perform the following more difficult exercises, without pain (specific for goals):
   a. _____ time _____
   b. _____ time _____
   c. _____ time _____
4. Rest, repeat item two.
5. Rest, repeat item one.

You have completed this set of exercises. It should have taken _____ minutes to complete them.

Repeat this set of exercises _____ times daily.

You are to continue these exercises until your next appointment at this office on _____ (date).

*Warning: Do not perform any of the prescribed exercises if they create pain. Call my office for advice before continuing with this program.*

## REFERENCES

Ashmore EF. *Osteopathic Mechanics.* London: Tamor Pierston, 1981.

Bove AA, Lowenthal DT. *Exercise Medicine.* New York: Academic Press, 1983.

Cailliet R. *Soft Tissue Pain and Disability.* Philadelphia: F.A. Davis, 1977.

Carew TJ. The control of reflex action. In: Kandel ER, Schwartz JH, eds. *Principles of Neural Science, 2nd ed.* New York: Elsevier, 1985:464.

Daniels L, Worthingham C. *Muscle Testing, 3rd ed.* Philadelphia: W.B. Saunders, 1972.

Daniels L, Worthingham C. *Therapeutic Exercise, 2nd ed.* Philadelphia: W.B. Saunders, 1977.

De Lateur B, Lehmann J, Stonebridge J. Isotonic versus isometric exercise. *Arch Phys Med Rehabil* 1972;53:212–217.

DiGiovanna EL, Schiowitz S. *An Osteopathic Approach to Diagnosis and Treatment, 2nd ed.* Philadelphia: Lippincott-Raven, 1997.

Gowitzke BA, Milner M. *Understanding the Scientific Basis of Human Movement.* Baltimore: Williams & Wilkins, 1980.

Kendall FP, McCreary EB. *Muscles: Testing and Function, 3rd ed.* Baltimore: Williams & Wilkins, 1983.

Kraus H. *Clinical Treatment of Back and Neck Pain.* New York: McGraw-Hill Book Co.

Kraus H, Hirschland RP. Minimum muscular fitness tests in school children. *Res Q* 1954;25(2):178–188.

Kraus H, Prudden B, Hirschorn K. Role of inactivity in production of disease: A hypokinetic disease. *J Am Geriatr Soc* 1956;4(5):463-471.

Moffroid M, Whipple R, Hofkosh J, et al. A study of isokinetic exercise. *Phys Med Ther* 1969;49:735–746.

Thiistle, HG, Hislop HJ, Moffroid M. 1967. Isokinetic contraction: A new concept of resistive exercise. *Arch Phys Med Rehabil* 1967;48:279–282.

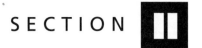

# Osteopathic Manipulation

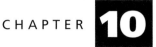

# History of Manual Medicine

*Eileen L. DiGiovanna*

The history of manual medicine is intermingled with that of medicine beginning in ancient times. Probably one of the earliest uses of the hands in medicine was for the treatment of dislocations and fractures. Massage was, likewise, practiced from early times and carried throughout the ages into modern times as a treatment for various soft tissue aches and pains. It flourished in Greek and Roman times. Aietaeus, a Greek physician, used massage for headaches, vertigo, and epilepsy, among other ailments. Hieroglyphics suggest that early Egyptians used their hands to treat injury and disease. Some early manuscripts by Hippocrates, the father of modern medicine, describe manual medicine techniques, frequently used to treat dislocations and spinal deformities. Writings of other historical physicians, such as Galen, describe various procedures using the hands in treating patients.

In the Orient, the Japanese and the Chinese used their hands to treat patients with dislocated shoulders, jaws, and other injuries. The *Kong-Fou,* describing Chinese massage, is considered to contain the earliest mention of massage as a medical treatment. Manually directed rollers were used on the abdomens of patients to treat constipation. Greenman reports in his text, *Principles of Manual Medicine,* evidence in the form of statuary more than 4,000 years old that indicates the use of manual medicine in Thailand.

In many religions and among many shaman, healers, and medicine men and women, ritualistic "laying on of the hands" was common. It was believed that a healing force or some form of energy passed from the healer to the patient that would effect a cure.

Various devices were used by Roman physicians and by physicians during Medieval times to assist in orthopedic treatments. Racks for stretching the spine, in some cases hanging the patient upside down, were devised, as were tables with attached pulleys and ropes that would put traction on a dislocated joint to assist in replacing it.

In nineteenth century England and throughout Europe, there arose a class of manipulators known as "bonesetters." These practitioners jealously guarded the "secrets" of manipulation passed down through families for generations. They served as a major source of medical care for the common people who could not afford the physicians of the day. Royalty also employed bonesetters when the care of the court physicians was insufficient or ineffective. In London, one famous bonesetter, Mrs. Mabb, sometimes referred to as Mrs. Mapp, became the bonesetter to the royal court and was soon driving around London in a coach with white horses because of her successes.

In the 1860s bonesetters attracted the attention of some well-known physicians. Sir James Paget noted that they were able to effectively treat some joint problems that had not responded to traditional medical care. He warned his colleagues that they should pay attention to what these bonesetters were doing because they were likely to be significant competition. A few years later, Dr. Wharton Hood wrote a book in which he described his own experiences as a bonesetter's apprentice.

In colonial times, bonesetters immigrated to

the United States. Most notable among them was the Sweet family who practiced in Rhode Island and Connecticut for almost 200 years. Andrew Taylor Still probably learned of bonesetters either from Hood's book or during his time in the military when he was in contact with soldiers from the East and mercenaries from Europe. From approximately 1883 until 1890, Still distributed cards identifying himself as the "Lightning Bone Setter." He did not attribute his knowledge to any instruction he received.

Medicine in the United States went through a time of turmoil in the nineteenth century. Samuel Thompson (1769–1843) was one of the first to challenge the practice of traditional medicine. He rejected all of the usual methods of treatment, believing that drugs should not be used as a treatment. Animal magnetism, as developed by Franz Mesmer, became popular for a time. This apparently had an effect on Still, who once advertised himself as a "magnetic healer." Samuel Hahnemann developed a method of treatment known as *Homeopathy*, which was quite popular at the time and is still practiced today in a modified form. These alternative treatments undoubtedly contributed to Still's belief that drugs were harmful and the use of manipulation was a safer choice for treating patients.

In the United States, the use of manipulation divided into two major movements. Andrew Taylor Still developed *Osteopathy,* which moved finally along the path of combining manipulation with traditional medicine in the twentieth century, and *Chiropractic*, still practiced today as a treatment aimed primarily at "adjustment" of the spine.

Chiropractic was developed by Daniel David Palmer (1845–1913), a Davenport, Iowa businessman turned "magnetic healer." Palmer is believed to have made contact with Still as early as 1893. He was reported to have arrived in Kirksville, Missouri with a student in the first class of osteopathy named Strothers. Arthur Hildreth reported that Blanche Still told him Palmer had been a dinner guest in the Still home. After approximately 1 week, he left and returned to Iowa, where he opened the first chiropractic college in 1896. D. D. Palmer died in an accident in which an automobile occupied by his son struck him during a parade. Chiropractic gained momentum when his son, Benjamin J. Palmer took over the school and began active promotion of the profession.

Although osteopathy and chiropractic have been the main sources of manipulation in the United States, other professions have developed an interest in manual medicine. Many physical therapists have integrated manipulation into their treatment regimens. Some medical doctors, especially orthopedists and physiatrists, have begun to use manipulative techniques. In England, James Mennell and Edgar Cyriax, both physicians, brought awareness of manipulation to the traditional medical community. Cyriax was aggressive in his promotion of manipulation as part of his orthopedic practice but denigrated the value of osteopathic manipulation, maintaining that osteopaths were quacks. However, many medical doctors in Europe were stimulated to use manipulation as part of their practice.

An organization of physicians using manipulation was formed, with membership including physicians from Europe, Canada, and the United States, known as the Federation International de Medicin Manuelle (FIMM), now also known as the International Federation of Manual/Manipulative Medicine. This organization conducts annual scientific seminars with presenters from the United States, Europe, and other countries.

## REFERENCES

DiGiovanna E. *Encyclopedia of Osteopathy.* Indianapolis, IN: American Academy of Osteopathy, 2000.

Gevitz, N. *The D.O.s, Osteopathic Medicine in America.* Baltimore: Johns Hopkins Univeristy Press, 1982.

Greenman PE. Models and mechanisms of osteopathic manipulative medicine. *Osteopath Med News* 1987;IV: 11–14, 20.

Greenman PE. *Principles of Manual Medicine, 2nd ed.* Baltimore: Williams & Wilkins, 1996.

Hildreth AG. *The Lengthening Shadow of Dr. Andrew Taylor Still.* Macon, MO: A.G. Hildreth, 1938.

Northup GW. *Osteopathic Medicine: An American Reformation.* Chicago: AOA, 1966.

Trowbridge C. *Andrew Taylor Still, 1828–1917.* Kirksville, MO: Thomas Jefferson University Press, 1990.

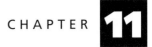

# Goals, Classifications, and Models of Osteopathic Manipulation

*Eileen L. DiGiovanna*

Osteopathic manipulative treatment (OMT) includes a variety of techniques using the hands in the diagnosis and treatment of patients by osteopathic physicians. It is a part of the overall treatment plan for many types of injuries and disease processes. This plan may include pharmacological agents, exercise, nutritional counseling, modalities, surgical procedures, and lifestyle counseling. OMT is directed specifically at the treatment of somatic dysfunctions, which involve the body framework—joints, muscles, fascia, tendons, and ligaments, as well as the blood vessels and nerves that are involved with these structures.

Palpation plays a major roll in the diagnosis of somatic dysfunction. The physician uses the hands to diagnose somatic dysfunction as well as other pathologies of the musculoskeletal system. Observation, motion testing, strength testing, and a variety of special tests are incorporated into the diagnostic evaluation of the patient.

The ability to perform OMT well requires a constant feedback to the physician's hands from the tissues of the patient. During the treatment, the physician must remain alert to palpatory sensations that indicate where the problem is located and how the tissues are responding to the treatment being performed. Compensatory mechanisms must be identified and the basic causes isolated.

The *Goals* of OMT include the following:

A. Relief of pain and reduction of other symptoms
B. Improvement of function
C. Increased functional movement
D. Improved blood supply and nutrition to the affected areas
E. Sufficient return flow of fluids via the lymphatic and venous systems
F. Removal of impediments to normal nerve transmission

The goals that are set for each individual must be realistic and placed within a reasonable time frame. Each patient (and physician) must realize that a "cure" may not be effected in all cases. Generally, the longer the patient has had a problem, the longer it will take to resolve it, if at all. A return to complete health may be an unrealistic goal. It needs to be understood, however, that although the problem may not be entirely resolved, it may often be expected that there will be some beneficial effects seen, such as decreased pain, some improvement in motion short of normal, or other improvement in quality of life.

Goals need to be re-evaluated at each visit and modified to reflect the true nature of the patient's condition. Sometimes an end goal cannot be set at the beginning of the treatment. The original goal may only be for the short-term, with long-term goals best set after the physician has become familiar with the response of the patient's body to treatment.

## Classifications of Manipulation

One classification of osteopathic techniques includes *direct* and *indirect* techniques.

1. **Direct:** Direct techniques are ones in which the restricted joint or tissue is initially taken in the direction of the restriction to motion. The restricted part is carried to the barrier at the beginning of the treatment. In some, an operator-generated force allows the joint or tissue to move beyond the restrictive barrier to motion. In others, the motion occurs gradually during the treatment.
2. **Indirect:** Indirect techniques are those that initially position the joint or tissue away from a barrier to motion and toward the relative ease or freedom of motion. Indirect techniques allow neural mechanisms or fascial tensions to be altered so as to permit improved motion of the joint or tissue.
3. **Combination:** There are a few techniques in which part of the technique is indirect and then a direct component is added or, conversely, a technique may begin as a direct technique then an indirect component added. Indirect to direct is most common.

Another classification system divides manipulative techniques into *passive* and *active*.

1. **Passive:** Passive techniques are those that are performed by the physician without any active participation by the patient.
2. **Active:** Active techniques require significant participation by the patient, guided by the physician. Voluntary muscle contraction and respiratory effort are two examples of active participation.

## Models of Manipulation

A system of *models of manipulation* is helpful in determining a plan for choosing types of techniques to be used as well as in goal-setting.

A. Postural, structural, or biomechanical model

This is probably the most commonly used model and is directed toward the treatment of the musculoskeletal system for the relief of pain and improvement of motion. The structure and the function of the affected area are evaluated and the OMT is geared toward returning dysfunctions to as near-normal a state as possible, being aware that structure and function are closely inter-related.

B. Neurological model

This model is chosen for treating by influencing the sensory, motor, or autonomic nervous systems or the reflexes associated with them. These may be affected at a variety of sites such as in the thoracic and upper lumbar spine, in the region of the cervical ganglia, or locally where a nerve pierces a muscle. Certain osteopathic techniques are directed specifically to the nervous system.

C. Respiratory/circulatory model

This model is chosen to influence the movement of fluid, such as lymph or blood, to improve respiratory capacity, or to reduce the work of breathing. Techniques may be directed to the thorax, diaphragm, ribs, and spine. This model is useful in the treatment of cardiac and respiratory problems or the removal of edema fluid.

D. Bioenergy model

This model has a focus on the inherent energies of the body. Several types of techniques use this model in whole or in part. A variety of energies are addressed, such as improvement of cranial and sacral motions through osteopathy in the cranial field. Fluid fluctuations may be addressed. Thermal diagnosis is a part of visceral manipulation.

E. Psychobehavioral model

The goals of this model are to influence perceptions of pain, illness, and disability. Some mental/emotional conditions, particularly anxiety and stress, respond well to hands-on treatment. Often there is a release of emotions, such as laughing or crying, during an osteopathic treatment. Any patient who has had pain for a period of time will eventually be affected emotionally and this can interact with the soma to create a cycle of pain–anxiety–pain, with anger or fear frequently being involved.

Models of manipulation are exactly that, models. In the treatment of any given individual, a mixture of models may be appropriate. Always, it is imperative to "listen" to the feedback from the patient's tissues to determine when and where a particular type of technique will be used. The choice of technique is dependent on what works best for the patient receiving the treatment and the condition, as well as the skills of the treating physician.

**REFERENCES**

DiGiovanna EL. *An Encyclopedia of Osteopathy.* Indianapolis, IN: American Academy of Osteopathy, 2002.

DiGiovanna EL, Schiowtiz S. *An Osteopathic Approach to Diagnosis and Treatment, 2nd ed.* Philadelphia: Lippincott-Raven, 1997.

Greenman PE. *Principles of Manual Medicine, 2nd ed.* Baltimore: Williams & Wilkins, 1996.

# Myofascial (Soft Tissue) Techniques

*Toni Spinaris and Eileen L. DiGiovanna*

**M**yofascial techniques are a group of specific maneuvers that are directed toward the soft tissues of the body, particularly the muscles and fasciae. For this reason, they are also referred to as *soft tissue techniques*. These can be used as the primary modality of treatment or in combination with or preparation for other methods.

The term *myofascial* comes from the root words *myo*, meaning "muscle," and *fascia*, which is self-explanatory. Muscle and fascia are most commonly thought of as the tissues treated by these techniques, but all of the fibroelastic connective tissues, as well as skin, tendons, ligaments, cartilage, blood, and lymph, may be affected.

There are several goals that may be achieved through the use of myofascial techniques. Among others, these include:

1. Relaxation of contracted muscles, which decreases the oxygen demand of the muscle, decreases pain, and allows normalized range of motion across a joint.
2. Increased circulation to an area of ischemia, therefore supplying blood carrying oxygen and nutrients to the tissues and removing harmful metabolic waste products.
3. Increased venous and lymphatic drainage, thereby decreasing local swelling and edema.
4. A stimulatory effect on the stretch reflex in hypotonic muscles.

The schematic diagram in Figure 12-1 explains the tissue changes that lead to impaired mobility and function, pain, and soft tissue changes seen and felt in the human body at various stages. The initiating insult or trauma may be subtle or quite dramatic. Cailliet defines *trauma* as "a wound or injury with implication of a force applied externally or internally causing a tissue reaction. Pain is the resultant which has varying degrees of intensity and effective interpretation with numerous avenues of transmission."

The initiating trauma may be anything that causes soft tissue irritation. The irritation is most frequently interpreted as pain. The body's usual reaction to pain is an increase in muscle tension. A vicious cycle ensues: a positive feedback mechanism informed by pain leads to increased muscle tension, which leads to increased pain, and so on. The increase in muscle tension plays an important role in tissue ischemia. The cycle continues, with tissue ischemia hindering provision of nutrients to the tissue and permitting buildup of waste products in the tissues. These waste products act as noxious stimuli, causing further irritation of the tissues, pain, and inflammation.

To this point, the process can be thought of as acute. If the process continues, it may become chronic. The next step is fibrous tissue reaction. If this occurs, it is believed to be permanent, which makes the soft tissue damage less reversible. An effect of the fibrous reaction is limited muscle elongation or stretch, which allows muscle shortening to develop, which in turn may

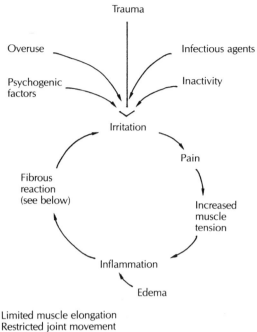

Trauma

Overuse

Infectious agents

Psychogenic factors

Inactivity

Irritation

Pain

Fibrous reaction (see below)

Increased muscle tension

Inflammation

Edema

Limited muscle elongation
Restricted joint movement
Limited tendon function
Fascial shortening

■ **FIG. 12-1** Cycle of soft tissue changes/pain/soft tissue changes after traumatic insult.

limit movement across a joint. Other effects are limitation in tendon function and fascial shortening. All lead to a decrease in the functional ability of the body part and person.

Myofascial techniques are useful in breaking the pain–muscle tension–pain cycle. Increasing the circulation to and drainage from the tissues may aid in diminishing the inflammatory response.

Some of the physiologic principles applied in myofascial techniques include the following:

1. **Extensibility of the connective tissues.** Connective tissue placed under prolonged mild tension shows plastic elongation.
2. **Stretch reflex.** The stretch of a muscle excites the muscle spindle mechanism, resulting in reflex contraction of that muscle. This is to be avoided when applying passive myofascial techniques to contracted or contractured muscles. It can be avoided by applying slow, even force and releasing that force slowly and evenly. However, the stretch reflex is to be used during active myofascial

techniques for the purpose of stimulating muscle tone in hypotonic muscles.
3. **Heat.** Heat applied to a muscle usually results in an increase in elastic response of the muscle to stretch.
4. **Muscle spindle reflex.** This is used in active resistive myofascial techniques. If the extrafusal fibers contract less than the intrafusal fibers, the muscle spindle will maintain a stretch reflex, further exciting the extrafusal fibers.
5. **Golgi tendon organ reflex.** This is used in active myofascial techniques. When the tension on the tendon becomes extreme, the inhibitory effect from the Golgi tendon organ can cause sudden relaxation of the entire muscle.
6. **Reciprocal inhibition.** This is used in active myofascial techniques with or without resistance. When a stretch reflex stimulates one muscle, it simultaneously inhibits the antagonist muscle; e.g., if the stretch reflex excites the biceps, reciprocal inhibition inhibits the triceps.
7. **Crossed extensor reflex.** This is used in active myofascial techniques with resistance. When a stretch reflex excites one muscle, it simultaneously relaxes the contralateral agonist muscle. Motion is created that crosses from one side of the spine to the other in an X pattern; e.g., the stretch reflex excites the right biceps, and the crossed extensor reflex relaxes the left biceps.

## Passive and Active Techniques

The physician uses passive myofascial techniques with the patient relaxed. Passive techniques entail application of a manual traction force in one of four directions:

1. Linear pull at either end of the muscle
2. Linear pull at both ends of the muscle at the same time
3. Pushing the muscle in a direction perpendicular to the long axis of the muscle fibers, thus creating stretch
4. Pulling the muscle in a direction perpendicular to the long axis of the muscle fibers, thus creating stretch

In **active** techniques, the patient assists the physician by actively contracting certain muscles under the guidance of the physician. There are two forms of active myofascial techniques. **Active direct** techniques are those in which the patient is asked to contract the involved muscle. These techniques use the Golgi tendon organ reflex to result in relaxation of the involved muscle(s). In these techniques, the physician applies isometric resistance to the contraction. (*Isometric resistance:* The physician applies resistance to the patient's contraction such that little shortening of the muscle is permitted but a great increase in muscle tension results.)

**Active indirect** techniques are those in which the patient is asked to contract the ipsilateral antagonist muscles or the same muscles on the contralateral side. This method uses either the reciprocal inhibition or the crossed extensor reflexes to relax the muscles being treated. In these techniques, the physician typically applies isokinetic resistance to the patient's contraction. (*Isokinetic resistance:* The physician applies a resistive force such that the muscle contraction increases very little with the gradual decrease in muscle length; i.e., the joint is allowed to move and the resistance is gradually increased.)

## General Considerations

There are a few general rules to follow when applying myofascial techniques.

1. The patient should be in a position of comfort and be relaxed.
2. The physician should be in a position of comfort and be at ease.
3. The physician should minimize energy expenditure and use body weight whenever possible instead of upper arm strength.
4. The force must be of low intensity, slowly applied and maintained for 3 to 4 seconds, and is slowly released.
5. The force applied must not create pain or other discomfort.
6. Always push or pull muscle away from bone, because it is uncomfortable when soft tissue is pressed against bone.
7. Avoid rubbing or irritating the patient's skin by the friction of your fingers or hands.
8. Use leverage whenever possible.
9. When treating muscles with myofascial techniques, the physician's fingerpads and the thenar and hypothenar eminences are used to apply pressure.
10. When a transverse force (push or pull) is applied across a muscle body, a counterforce may also be used to maintain the patient's position.
11. The stretch may be applied along the length of the muscle or perpendicular to the muscle.
12. Compression may be used in areas of multiple muscle layers to reach the deeper tissues.

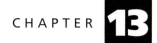

# Muscle Energy

*Dennis J. Dowling*

As a physician, Fred Mitchell, Sr, DO, FAAO, first formulated muscle energy technique. Later, in cooperation with Neil Pruzzo, DO, and Peter Moran, DO, he developed a tutorial program. A collection of descriptive techniques was published in *An Evaluation and Treatment Manual of Osteopathic Muscle Energy Procedures* in 1979. Dr. Mitchell's work appears to have been based on that of another osteopathic physician, T. J. Ruddy, DO, who used pulse-timed procedures in and around the head and neck as treatment.

Many osteopathic practitioners had used similar techniques over the decades, but the work by Mitchell, Moran, and Pruzzo was the first coordinated, unifying work. Since then, another work, *Outline of Muscle Energy Techniques* by Kenneth Graham, DO, has become available. Dr. Mitchell's son, Fred Mitchell, Jr., DO, FAAO, has recently developed a series of books detailing the theory and practice of muscle energy in a comprehensive fashion.

A basic tenet of the muscle energy modality is that muscles cause and/or maintain somatic dysfunctions. For type II somatic dysfunctions, the small spurt-and-shunt muscles such as the rotator brevis or the intertransversii may become or remain in a state of hypertonicity. This allows some regional motion but restricts single intervertebral motion.

A type II somatic dysfunction may also be theorized to occur because of locking of the involved facets. In this case, the position of the vertebrae may cause stress on the small muscles that respond by contracting. After treatment with techniques such as high-velocity, low-am-plitude thrusting techniques, the joint may be more mobile, but the tonicity of these small muscles may not be reduced. The continued, inappropriate contraction may return the vertebral or other joint to its dysfunctional position. This pattern may account for the need to treat patients several times per week if articulatory techniques are the sole ones employed. Thus, by using muscle energy techniques, one can improve or resolve the reflex maintaining dysfunction. These techniques can also be utilized prior to or in combination with other techniques such as high-velocity, low-amplitude thrust.

It is postulated that muscle energy, when used directly on involved restrictions, utilizes the Golgi tendon reflex. The physician localizes the muscles surrounding and acting across a joint by placing the joint into its barrier or restriction in all involved planes. The patient is instructed to move that portion of his or her body toward the diagnosed relative freedoms of the joint. The physician resists by using an isometric counterforce. This is held for 3 to 5 seconds. After complete relaxation, the joint is further moved into the new barriers and the whole procedure is repeated as often as is necessary until the physiologic limits are restored. This generally requires three to five repetitions. A passive repositioning must occur after the last sequence to adequately restore more normal motion.

After the technique is completed, the region is re-evaluated. The Golgi tendon reflex is activated by the resisted contraction and the muscles relax by neurophysiological reflex. Another theory is that a temporary muscle fatigue takes place and that simple contraction–relaxation allows for further stretching without reflex contraction of the inappropriately contracted muscles.

Diagnosis requires that testing be localized to the target joint. Restriction of motion is the primary criterion, but asymmetry, soft tissue tension changes, and tenderness may be used to further localize and corroborate the diagnosis. There are specific muscle energy techniques for each region of the body. However, a few basic principles apply to all areas. Once one knows the joint, the origins, insertions, and actions of the muscles, the findings of the relative freedoms, and the restrictions of motion, a treatment can be formulated.

Dr. Graham summarized some of the principles in his book. The following is a paraphrase of his eight essential steps.

1. Accurate structural *diagnosis* must be made. Each location can be defined by its somatic dysfunction diagnosis. An example would be $C4ES_RR_R$ or $C4ES_RR_R$, which informs us that flexion, side-bending, and rotation left are the barriers to be engaged.
2. Engage the *restrictive barrier* in all three planes. Spinal motion would involve restriction in flexion–extension, side-bending, and rotation. Appendicular restrictions frequently involve flexion–extension, supination–pronation (external–internal rotation), and abduction–adduction. The barrier engagement should not cause distress to the patient. Even though the final effect is greater motion at a joint, the physician must be aware of the soft tissue muscular barrier. Some physicians describe this as "feather edge" barrier placement.
3. Unyielding *counterforce* (operator force = patient force) in the form of isometric resistance is necessary to activate the Golgi tendon reflex. Inaccuracy could lead to counterproductive force.
4. Appropriate patient *muscle effort:*
   a. Correct amount of force, which is light to moderate in effort (ounces to pounds)
   b. Correct direction of effort (away from the restrictive barrier)
   c. Correct duration of effort (3–5 seconds)

5. *Complete relaxation* after the muscle effort (both operator and patient relax their forces simultaneously). Generally, a few seconds are necessary for sufficient muscular relaxation in order that there is no activation of stretch receptors.
6. *Repositioning* to the new restrictive barrier in all three planes; the physician monitors motion with palpation. In most cases, this will involve maintaining monitoring with one hand throughout the whole treatment. Reengagement in most cases will involve small motions in each direction.
7. Steps 3 through 6 are *repeated* three to five times or until normal range is attained.
8. The region is *retested* (structural diagnosis is repeated).

Dr. Graham also notes some of the most common errors made by physicians when they are first learning and practicing muscle energy techniques:

1. The physician does not accurately monitor with palpation of the involved joint.
2. The patient uses a muscle contraction that is too forceful. This may prevent the treatment from being localized because other muscles and joints are recruited. The larger muscles may override the smaller muscles" effort and reduce the effectiveness. Conversely, too little effort may not activate the target muscles enough.
3. The muscle contraction is too short in duration. In this case the Golgi tendon organ would not be activated. If one supposes a simple contract–relax mechanism, there may not be enough fatigue to allow stretch.
4. The patient is not allowed to totally relax before repositioning into new restrictive barriers. This may lead to inefficient localization, or the new barriers may not be engaged at all.
5. The examiner forgets to re-evaluate the dysfunction. Any improvement may not be noted. Further treatment may or may not be necessary.

The muscle energy techniques are very effective and well tolerated in many conditions and by a wide age range of patients. Spasm, either primary or secondary, that is reduced will almost always be accompanied by some reduction of pain.

Muscle energy techniques may also be used over wider regions, especially for type I group curve spinal dysfunctions. In this case, the barriers of side-bending and rotation are applied and the region does not move from neutral in the sagittal plane (there is no flexion or extension component). The same principles as stated previously are employed. Whether used segmentally or regionally, these forms of muscle energy are direct, in that barriers are engaged, and active, in that the patient performs some activity.

Other forms of muscle energy can likewise be employed. Active indirect techniques of muscle energy employ a crossed extensor reflex. Contraction of antagonist muscles results in reflex relaxation of the target agonist muscles. Typically, the target muscles are large regional muscles. Initially, the region is placed into its relative freedoms and the target muscles are shortened. The patient is directed to push toward the barriers. The physician provides an isokinetic counterforce that allows movement toward the barrier. In other words, the patient pushes against resistance but slowly moves in the prescribed directions. After pushing as far as possible without discomfort, the patient is instructed to relax. The physician then gently pushes a few degrees more into the barriers. The region is again repositioned into the relative freedoms and the procedure is repeated at least twice, with each successive time involving more effort on the part of the patient and coordinated resistance on the part of the physician. Crossed extensor or reciprocal inhibition results in reflex activation of inhibitory interneurons, which limit or prevent motor neurons from activating muscle.

Isolytic procedures involve lengthening involved muscles while the patient actively contracts them. In theory, adhesions and fibrotic changes could be broken and the muscle permitted to perform in a more physiologic manner.

Isotonic contractions can be of an eccentric or concentric fashion and generally involve large regional muscle groups. This type of muscle energy is directed toward the development of muscle strength, stamina, enlargement, and/or definition. Many of the well-known exercise apparatuses use this principle. Concentric activity occurs when the patient overcomes a force by the continued constant tone of the muscle accompanied by muscle shortening. In the case of eccentric isotonic contraction, the muscle is stretched while maintaining relatively the same tone. During forward bending from the waist, the muscles of the back activate to help maintain fluidity of motion and balance while gravity and the flexor muscle promote the motion. Machinery-assisted exercise is more efficiently used when the patient exerts a smooth range of motion while maintaining tension in both agonist and antagonist groups.

## REFERENCES

Graham K. *Outline of Muscle Energy Techniques.* Tulsa, OK: Oklahoma College of Osteopathic Medicine, 1985.

Greenman PE. Models and mechanisms of osteopathic manipulative medicine. *Osteopath Med News* 1987;IV: 11–14,20.

Guyton AC. *Textbook of Medical Physiology.* Philadelphia: W.B. Saunders, 1986.

Hutton RS, Nelson DL. Stretch sensitivity of Golgi tendon organs in fatigued gastrocnemius muscle. *Med Sci Sports Med* 1986;18(1):69–74.

Mitchell FL Jr, Moran PS, Pruzzo NA. *An Evaluation and Treatment Manual of Osteopathic Muscle Energy Procedures.* Valley Park, MO: Mitchell, Moran, and Pruzzo Association, 1979.

Stauffer EK, et al. Responses of Golgi tendon organs to concurrently active motor units. *Brain Res* 1986;375: 157–162.

Thistle HG, Hislop HJ, Moffroid M. Isokinetic contraction: A new concept of resistive exercise. *Arch Phys Med Rehabil* 1967;48:279–282.

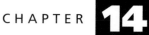

# Counterstrain

*Eileen L. DiGiovanna*

Lawrence Jones, an osteopathic family practitioner in Oregon, developed the counterstrain technique. In 1955, he chanced on its discovery during the treatment of a patient with severe psoas spasm who had not responded to previous chiropractic or conventional osteopathic manipulation. After positioning the patient into a position of comfort, he left him on the table for a time and, when the man arose, he was pain-free. Dr. Jones spent many years perfecting the technique before introducing it to the profession.

In his text, *Strain and Counterstrain,* Jones offers two definitions of the technique:

1. "Relieving spinal or other joint pain by passively putting the joint into its position of greatest comfort."
2. "Relieving pain by reduction and arrest of the continuing inappropriate proprioceptor activity. This is accomplished by markedly shortening the muscle that contains the malfunctioning muscle spindle by applying mild strain to its antagonists."

The physiologic basis of counterstrain is based on the presumption that somatic dysfunction has a neuromuscular basis (Fig. 14-1) (see Chapter 6). With trauma or muscle effort against a sudden change in resistance, or with muscle strain incurred by resisting the effects of gravity (e.g., bending over) for a period of time, one muscle is strained and its antagonist is hypershortened. When the shortened muscle is suddenly stretched, the annulospiral receptors of the muscle spindles in that muscle are stimulated, causing a reflex contraction of the already shortened mus-

cle. The proprioceptors in the short muscle now fire impulses as if the shortened muscle were being stretched. Because this inappropriate proprioceptive response can be maintained indefinitely, a somatic dysfunction has been created. The joint is restricted, within its physiologic range of motion, from achieving full range of motion by this shortened muscle. It is therefore an active process rather than a static injury, such as is usually associated with strain (Fig.14-2).

In counterstrain, the diagnosis is made by finding reflex "tender points." Each involved ligament, joint, or muscle has its own specific tender points, anterior or posterior, depending on the joint somatic dysfunction. The point may lie in the shortened muscle or in a more distant area to which it has been referred reflexively. It is a palpable tissue texture change and comprises a tense, fibrotic area approximately the size of a dime. It is tender to an amount of pressure that would not normally cause pain. The tender points may very well be related to trigger points (Travell points) and acupuncture points; there are marked similarities in distribution.

The treatment technique is positional and Dr. Jones originally called his technique "spontaneous release by positioning." According to Jones, positioning the joint in the position that shortens the involved muscle will relieve the pain and dysfunction. Therefore, the joint is positioned in such a manner that pressure on the tender point no longer elicits tenderness. This most often results in a palpable softening of the tissues. Students first learning palpatory skills may rely on feedback from the patient regarding

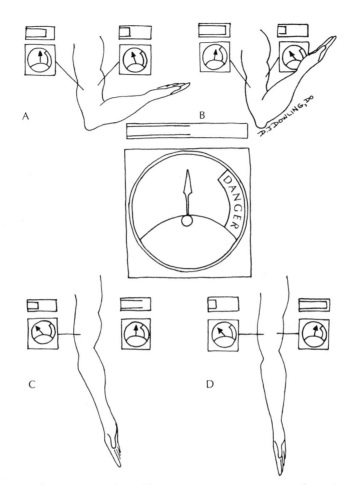

■ **Fig. 14-1** Muscular activity. Bar gauge represents extent of muscle fiber stretch and circular gauge indicates impulses from muscle stretch receptors. **(A)** Arm flexed. **(B)** Arm hyperflexed. **(C)** Arm extended. **(D)** Arm hyperextended.

a decrease in tenderness when proper positioning is attained. As palpatory skills increase, it is possible to rely solely on the tissue changes that occur.

The technique is passive in that the patient is requested to allow the muscle being treated to relax completely. It is indirect because the joint is positioned into its ease of motion (away from the barrier).

To position the joint, the physician makes a gross adjustment toward the position of comfort and then fine-tunes. For example, the joint may require flexion to reduce the degree of pain, and then a little rotation or side-bending to remove the remaining tenderness. Jones refers to the final position as the "mobile point." The position is held for 90 seconds, the amount of time usually required for the proprioceptive firing to decrease in frequency and amplitude and for the mechanoreceptors to reduce stimulation of muscle contraction.

The next step is important. The joint is returned slowly to its neutral position. The slow motion prevents re-initiation of the inappropriate proprioceptive firing. The point should be monitored at all times because it is possible to palpate the changes occurring in the muscle, and therefore perhaps less than 90 seconds may be needed for treatment. The degree of tenderness remaining in the tissues should be re-assessed.

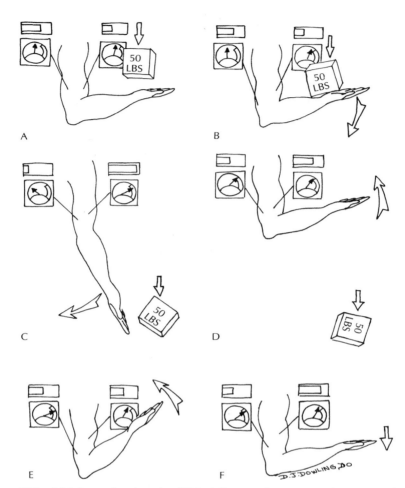

■ **Fig. 14-2** Cause of tender point. **(A)** Both flexors and extensors are in easy normal position. **(B)** Force is suddenly exerted counter to the flexors, forcing the arm into extension. **(C)** Fibers and stretch receptors indicate that a danger point has been reached. Extensor fibers are hypershortened. **(D)** Arm is relatively flexed, exciting the muscle stretch receptors. **(E)** Rapid rate of flexion overstimulates extensor stretch receptors. **(F)** Arm is in same position as in **A**, but stretch receptors continue to respond as if muscle were being rapidly stretched.

The patient is cautioned that some muscle soreness may result, but because this is not a somatic dysfunction, the muscle will return to normal quickly. A contraindication to use of this technique may include an inflammatory process at the location of the tender point indicating the presence of other possible problems.

Counterstrain treatment is an extremely effective and nontraumatic treatment. It is especially good for elderly or hospitalized patients, and any others for whom gentleness is desirable. Patients who have experienced an acute strain respond well. Certain positions may be uncomfortable or undesirable for some patients, so the physician must use judgment when selecting the treatments.

### REFERENCES

Jones LH. *Strain and Counterstrain.* Indianapolis, IN: American Academy of Osteopathy, 1981.

Jones LH, Kusunose R, Goering E. *Jones Strain-Counterstrain.* Boise, ID: Jones Strain-CounterStrain, Inc, 1995.

Yates HA, Glover JC. *Counterstrain Handbook of Osteopathic Technique.* Tulsa, OK: Y Knot Publishers, 1995.

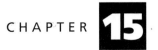

# Facilitated Positional Release

*Stanley Schiowitz*

Facilitated positional release was developed by the author of this chapter. He first presented it to the profession in an article in the *Journal of the American Osteopathic Association*, "Facilitated Positional Release," in 1990.

This technique uses a modification of indirect myofascial release techniques, enhanced by placing the region in the neutral position and adding a facilitating force of compression or torsion. The advantage of this technique is its ease of application and speed of response. In addition, if the desired results do not occur immediately, it may be repeated or other methods of treatment can be added.

This treatment is directed toward the normalization of hypertonic muscles, both superficial and deep. It is probable that most of the vertebral joint motion restrictions diagnosed as somatic dysfunctions are caused and/or maintained by hypertonicity of the small, deep, intervertebral muscles. These hypertonic muscles respond well to facilitated positional release, thus immediately restoring normal joint function.

When treating dysfunctions in the posterior spinal region, the modification of the sagittal posture is to create a flattening of the anterior–posterior spinal curve in the region or segment to be treated. Thus a mild, localized, reduction of normal cervical and lumbar lordosis or thoracic kyphosis is established. An attempt is made to approach the spinal neutral position as defined by Fryette, that is, the position of any area of the spine in which the facets are idling, in the position between the beginning of flexion and the beginning of extension.

A facilitating force is then added that consists of compression, torsion, or a combination of the two. Occasionally, it may be necessary to use a traction force rather than compression.

The muscles to be treated are placed into their specific freedoms of motion, i.e., shortening. Two types of muscles are involved: larger superficial, easily palpable muscles and smaller, deep muscles. Place the posterior, superficial muscles into extension and ipsilateral lateral flexion. If muscle hypertonicity is found anteriorly, then forward bending is usually required. Some muscles have a contralateral side-bending function or a rotary component; these muscles must be placed in their individual shortened positions. Careful localization of the component motions of facilitation, forward and backward bending, side-bending, and rotation to the area of the hypertonicity will produce more accurate results. The deep muscles should be placed in the directions of the named intersegmental somatic dysfunction being treated.

A plausible explanation for the effectiveness of this treatment relates to the action of the muscle spindle gamma loop when the gain is suddenly decreased. According to Carew, with a sudden decrease in load, the spindles in the muscle become unloaded and the Ia fiber discharges from these spindles cease and no longer excite motor neurons controlling the extrafusal muscle fiber. The muscle then begins to relax until it lengthens. This physiologic change may well account for the immediate effect felt when facilitating force is used in these techniques.

There are three basic steps involved:

1. The physician modifies the patient's sagittal posture in the region to be treated.
2. A facilitating force is applied.
3. The large muscle is shortened or the somatic dysfunction is placed into its freedoms of motion.

## Technique for Superficial Muscle Hypertonicity in the Spine

1. The patient assumes a relaxed position.
2. The physician flattens the anteroposterior spinal curve of the area to be treated.
3. The physician places the muscle into its ease of motion (i.e., shortened).
4. The physician applies a facilitating force (compression, torsion, or a combination of these forces).
5. Steps three and four may be applied in reverse order depending on the specific technique.
6. The position is held for 3 to 4 seconds.
7. Release the position and reevaluate.

## Technique for Hypertonicity of Deep Intervertebral Muscles

The steps are the same as for treating superficial muscle hypertonicity, except for step three. The physician places the vertebra into its planes of freedom of motion. For example, a somatic dysfunction diagnosed as $C5FS_RR_R$ is treated by placing the fifth cervical vertebra into a position of flexion, right side-bending, and right rotation with respect to the sixth cervical vertebra.

Springing, which exaggerates the freedoms of motion, may be added to completely release articular dysfunctions.

## Technique for Hypertonic Muscles in the Extremities

The patient will be in either the supine or the prone position.

The physician places the involved articulation into its position of "easy normal," i.e., freely moveable, with ligaments relaxed.

1. The physician applies compression toward the articulation. This should shorten the involved muscle.
2. Abduction/adduction are added as needed in the direction of the action of the muscle being treated.
3. If abduction is added, place the articulation into external rotation up to the hypertonic muscle region. If adduction is added, place the articulation into internal rotation up to the hypertonic muscle region.
4. The position is held for 3 to 4 seconds
5. Release the position and reevaluate.

**REFERENCES**

Carew TJ. The control of reflex action. In: Kandel ER, Schwartz JH, eds. *Principles of Neural Science,* 2nd ed. New York:, Elsevier, 1985.
DiGiovanna EL, Schiowitz S. *An Osteopathic Approach to Diagnosis and Treatment, 2nd ed.* Philadelphia: Lippincott-Raven, 1997.
Schiowitz S. Facilitated positional release. *J Am Osteopath Assoc* 1990;901:145–155.

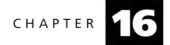

# Still Technique

*Dennis J. Dowling, DO, FAAO.*

There is a common statement in osteopathic lore that Dr. Andrew Taylor Still never wrote a technique book. It is true that he attempted, instead, by way of his writings, to guide his students to an understanding of structure and function and then to the application of the treatment that was most appropriate. He resisted the idea that they should do exactly as he had done. He desired thinking osteopathic physicians rather than mimics.

Part of the original resistance to the establishment of the first school was the impression that the treatment provided by the "Old Doctor" was peculiar to him. His continued success became the magnet that drew patients and students to him. It is no wonder that the latter attempted to emulate him. Once the school was established, he had felt disappointment with some of his early students. He called them "engine wipers" because they could clean the surface problems without truly understanding the inner workings of the human machine. It was important to Dr. Still that those who practiced osteopathic medicine develop treatments for the individual. However, it is not truly accurate to say that he never showed a technique or wrote down a description. He buried his descriptions in what he considered the more important components, the philosophy and principles of his new science. Some maneuvers are embedded in *Osteopathy: Research and Practice* and *The Philosophy and Mechanical Principles of Osteopathy*. He also, obviously, could not keep his followers from observing some of the methods that he did use, especially when they would see him repeat them.

There is even a very brief movie clip of a few seconds with Dr. Still demonstrating a treatment for either a shoulder or a rib on the porch of a house in Kirksville. He frequently referred to the "pops and cracks" that the joints sometimes made in response to the manipulations. Whether these were caused by articulatory or positioning maneuvers, he felt that the goal was to restore function. He also admonished his followers to diagnose and find the health of the human patient.

Despite his own hesitations in being descriptive of adjustments, some of Dr. Still's students wrote down their own observations in books and articles. One of these was Charles Hazzard, DO, a graduate from the American School of Osteopathy in the late nineteenth century. Dr. Hazzard produced his own work and credited all to Dr. Still. His observations were a continuation of Dr. Still's own descriptions. There is a consistency of approach that sets it apart as a unique modality. Some of the applications have survived down through the decades outside of the Hazzard book after having been passed along from parent to child, osteopathic physician or mentor to apprentice. However, they existed as localized specific treatments, not an organized systematic approach.

It was not until Richard Van Buskirk, DO, PhD, published an article in 1996 that a true recognition was offered of a technique that was uniquely developed and applied by Dr. Still. Dr. Van Buskirk first became intrigued by the possibility while a faculty member and then as a student at the West Virginia School of Osteopathic

Medicine. This led him to investigate further the writings of Dr. Still and his students. Sometimes he was able to correlate these with demonstrations by other practitioners. A more thorough compilation appeared in the publication, *The Still Technique Manual,* in 1999.

In terms of procedure, the Still technique most resembles facilitated positional release (FPR) developed by Stanley Schiowitz, DO, FAAO. Those educated in this method generally have little or no difficulty in learning the eponymous "Still" technique. Dr. Van Buskirk has stated that FPR is most like the indirect portion of the Still technique, but does not include the final articulatory portion of the Still technique. This is true if one were to only learn FPR from the writings of Dr. Schiowitz and others. However, the actual practice of FPR frequently includes a challenge toward the barrier at its completion. This is most notable in the FPR treatment for first rib dysfunction, a technique that differs from the Still technique version only in the location of the physician, not the procedure. The Still technique also relies on accurate segmental diagnosis of somatic dysfunction. Using this information, the application of the Still technique is relatively simple and elegant at the same time. The steps are:

1. The patient is passive throughout all procedures.
2. The diagnosis of the joint and the position at which the surrounding tissue is least taut are determined.
3. The joint and tissue are moved into the directions of ease in all planes.
4. The position is slightly exaggerated so as to increase the relaxation of the affected myofascial elements.
5. A force that is vectored parallel to the part of the body that is being used as a lever (i.e., head & neck, arm, leg, trunk) is applied to the point of further relaxing the involved tissues. Traction or compression are the most common forces applied for a few seconds.
6. While maintaining the vector force, the region and dysfunction are brought towards the barrier directions and then back through the restrictions.
7. The force and motion will commonly mobilize the joint and release the tissue to the point that there may be a sudden release as reflected by a "pop," "click," or other such noise.
8. The forces are released and the region is brought back to neutral for reassessment of the dysfunction.

The Still technique is a passive technique. The fact that it is a passive method as opposed to an active one is only one aspect of separation. The beginning, consisting of positioning into the freedoms, is an indirect factor. Then, the movement into the directions of the restrictions converts it to a direct technique. It addresses the arthrodial and soft tissue components of the somatic dysfunction.

Finally, whether being applied to an interphalangeal joint or a shoulder, the applied principles remain. There are some standard descriptions of treatment to certain areas that are meant to be a guide. However, the true application is in the ability to examine, adapt, and individually apply the method.

**REFERENCES**

Hazzard C. *The Practice and Applied Therapeutics of Osteopathy, 3rd revised ed.* Kirksville, MO: Journal Printing, Co., 1905.

Schiowitz S. Facilitated positional release. *J Am Osteopath Assoc* 1990;90:145–155.

Still AT. *Osteopathy: Research and Practice.* Kirksville, MO: Journal Printing Co., 1910 (Reprint: Seattle, WA: Eastland Press, 1992).

Still AT. *The Philosophy and Mechanical Principles of Osteopathy.* Kansas City, MO: Hudson Kimberly Publishing Co., 1902 (Reprint: Kirksville, MO: Osteopathic Enterprise).

Van Buskirk RL. A manipulative technique of Andrew Taylor Still. *J Am Osteopath Assoc* 1996;96:597–602.

Van Buskirk RL. *The Still Technique Manual.* Indianapolis, IN: American Academy of Osteopathy, 1999.

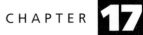

# Articulatory and Thrusting Techniques

*Eileen L. DiGiovanna*

Articulatory techniques are direct, passive techniques in which no thrusting force is used. They can be considered low-velocity and low-amplitude. They are generally performed within the physiologic range of motion of any given joint and tend to be repetitive to free all planes of motion within the joint.

Most *thrusting techniques* are direct techniques in that the dysfunctional unit is placed into at least one of its restrictive barriers to motion and the physician thrusts through that barrier. The techniques are considered passive because the physician provides the treating force and the patient remains passive.

## High-Velocity, Low-Amplitude Techniques

The best known of all manipulative techniques are the high-velocity, low-amplitude thrusting techniques. In these techniques, the physician positions the patient in such a way that the restricted joint is placed into its restrictive barrier(s) to motion. The physician then quickly applies a small to moderate amount of force to the joint in such a way as to move it through the barriers. Improved joint motion should result very quickly.

To achieve the best results with as little discomfort as possible, the surrounding soft tissues should be relaxed before the thrusting force is applied. Myofascial (soft tissue) techniques or other nonthrusting techniques are used for this purpose. When the muscles and soft tissues are relaxed, less force is needed to move the joint and the treatment will be less uncomfortable.

High-velocity, low-amplitude techniques may have been the first type of manual medicine ever devised. They are the therapeutic maneuvers most commonly used by chiropractors and osteopathic physicians, as well as other practitioners of manual medicine.

## Low-Velocity, High-Amplitude Techniques

In some thrusting techniques, a greater force is applied slowly with the goal of moving the joint through the barrier. Care must be taken to avoid joint or soft tissue damage. These techniques, when applied skillfully, are quite useful, but the force must be carefully controlled. Again, relaxation of the soft tissues before force is applied makes the procedure safer and less uncomfortable.

## Springing Techniques

Springing techniques are similar to high-velocity, low-amplitude techniques except that a full force is not applied. The joint is positioned as before, then gently sprung several times against its barriers. This maneuver gently nudges the joint to move through its restrictive barrier. The springing force is much less than that applied in high-velocity, low-amplitude techniques.

With repeated springing thrusts against the barrier, the joint may be moved as effectively as with high-velocity, low-amplitude thrusting but with less possibility of adverse effect. Springing techniques are useful in more painful joints, older persons, and children, and whenever a stronger force is contraindicated.

## General Principles of Thrusting Techniques

1. Prepare the joint to be treated by relaxing the soft tissues so that the joint may be moved more easily with less resistance from the soft tissues.
2. Place the joint into its restrictive motion barriers. If only one barrier is to be engaged, it is essential that all other joint motions be "locked" out.
3. Once a joint has been placed into its motion barriers, this position must be held firmly by the physician and the "locking" thus created not lost as the force is applied.
4. The physician must control the force.. Excessive force should never be applied in the hope that the joint will move. Only force sufficient to create the motion desired should be used. Force should never replace skill.
5. Treatment must be localized and applied to the specific restricted joint. A "shotgun" approach to an entire area of the spine is inappropriate and harmful.

## Pops and Cracks

Particularly with high-velocity, low-amplitude techniques, a popping or cracking sound may be heard, similar to the sound made by cracking the knuckles. Some observers believe the sound is caused by the breaking of a vacuum in the joint, others believe that it is caused by release of a nitrogen bubble. Whatever its cause, eliciting this noise is not essential to the correction of a dysfunction. Feeling the joint move is more important than hearing it pop.

Many patients feel that the treatment is successful only if they hear this sound; others are frightened by it, fearing bones may be breaking. The patient must be assured that the sound is harmless, as well as unnecessary.

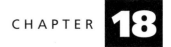

# Myofascial Release Concepts

*Dennis J. Dowling and Paula Scariati*

Fascia is a connective tissue substance sheet or band of fibrous tissue that lies deep to the skin and invests all structures of the body. Every nerve, bone, muscle, and organ is covered with some form of fascia. The term, which is Latin for band or bandage, is descriptive of the pervading presence of the material. If all of the other structures, visceral and somatic, were somehow dissolved, a ghostly fascial image would persist and retain recognizable form.

## Function

Some authors (Kuchera and Kuchera) have described the functions of fascia as the four Ps: packaging, protection, posture, and passageways. There is a rich nervous supply to the fascia, and all nerves perforate or are encompassed by fascia. Muscles—smooth, cardiac, and skeletal—are enveloped by it. Contraction and motion of the muscles are guided by fascia, and the balance of structures is maintained by stresses distributed throughout. As an encasement and as a tether, fascia protects underlying structures. Usually this means that forces are absorbed or redistributed. Because of its reactivity to forces, its configuration may change and precede changes in other structures, such as the muscles. The processes of circulation, both vascular and lymphatic, are maintained and regulated through fascial influence. When change does occur in the structure of fascia, with reorganization, directionality, and thickening, all of the functions may be altered and/or reduced. Sudden stretching of fascia may be accompanied by a sensation of burning pain and irritation of membranous components and may result in sharp or stabbing sensations. Regional muscles may contract in reflex to these stimuli.

## Organization

Much of the regional and localized named fasciae are artificially divided. Fascia forms a continuity and is a form of connective tissue. The cellular components include fibroblasts, osteoblasts, chondroblasts, osteocytes, chondrocytes, reticular cells, mast cells, and formed elements of blood.

There are two types of general connective tissue: loose and dense. Dense tissue may be regular or irregular. *Dense regular connective tissue* has either long or overlapping layers. Tendons and ligaments are formed of dense connective tissue. The dermis, organ capsules, periosteum, and perichondrium are forms of *dense irregular connective tissue*. The fibers are mesh-like, lack a distinct pattern, and are oriented in many different directions.

*Loose connective tissue* is found in subcutaneous fascia, in the lamina propria beneath epithelium, and in the mesenteries. There is a rich assortment of nonfibrous material such as fibroblasts, mast cells, and macrophages contained throughout. Any formed blood element, with the exception of erythrocytes and platelets, may exist in this tissue.

## Components

*Fibroblasts* prepare and secrete collagen, elastin, and other proteoglycans. When there is increased need for repair, they can proliferate to accommodate the increased demand. In conjunction with macrophages, known as histiocytes, they comprise the reconstructive component of reconstruction. The macrophages phagocytose debris and are developed from monocyte precursors.

*Collagens* are composed of many smaller fibers and are the most abundant and widely distributed proteins in the body. Although they are typically soft and flexible, they contribute high tensile strength to many structures. Four classes exist as determined by location and type: I is found in dermis, tendon, and bone; II forms cartilage; III is located in the cardiovascular tract, gastrointestinal tract, and integument; and IV is in the basement membranes of epithelium.

The protein *elastin* is the major component of elastic fibers. They have a distinct ability to be stretched and then return to their original disposition without being permanently deformed. Abundant in regions subjected to cyclical expansion and relaxation, they appear in cardiac, pulmonary, and skin structures. Stressors such as cigarette smoke and sunlight break down the elastic fibers of elastin.

All connective tissues have a spatial fill-in material of varying amounts known as *amorphous ground substance*, which is a mixture of macromolecules known as proteoglycans and glycoproteins. Both contain carbohydrates and proteinaceous material. Glycosaminoglycans are of several types, with some regional specificity. Along with proteoglycans, they give a large net negative charge to the amalgam and can bind to large amounts of water. This allows for free diffusion of smaller molecules throughout; it also gives the amorphous ground substance a gel-like consistency.

Both nutrients and waste products diffuse through the liquid material. Approximately 70% of connective tissue is composed of water, of which the ground substance is primarily responsible. Hyaluronic acid, a component of ground substance, is very hydrophilic. This aspect gives the fascia a colloid-like capacity. Intermittent or low-force impulses can create wave-like fluid mechanics that are distributed and then dissipate. *Drag* is the amount of resistance to motion as determined by internal molecular resistance.

Sudden focal force evokes a more rigid reaction. Injury or constant tension may reduce the water component, leaving the remaining components drier and relatively stiffer. Adhesions, which are abnormal cross-linkages between collagen fibers, are then more likely to occur. The relatively late adaptations to significant or sustained forces are the fibrotic changes and the development of directionality of the substance. Both of these result in a tougher, more resistant change of the substance.

As a connective tissue, *adipose* is subcutaneous and found around some internal organs. An energy storage site, it also serves as an insulator against temperature extremes and as support for some structures. A rich blood supply and reticular mesh are found, and the relative size of each of the cells varies, depending on the activity and nutritional status of the individual.

## Types

Fascia is also described as superficial, deep, and subserous. A continuous layer of *superficial fascia* lies beneath and is continuous with the skin's dermis layer. Two layers exist, with a potential space between capable of accommodating fluid accumulation. Superficial fascia invests the outer components of skeletal muscle and helps to give form to the skin. In concept, it is a sac that helps to insulate and separate the body from the external environment. Small fibrils act as anchors from the skin to the deeper fascia. Forces directed through palpation perpendicular to these tethers but parallel to the deep fasciae allow the examiner to appreciate a sense of resistance ("*drag*" or "bind") or freedom ("*ease*") to movement.

The *deep fascia* serves more of a compartmentalization role. Woven in a tighter, more compact fashion, it encapsulates and separates muscles and visceral organs. Variously named regions of fascia are the locations of thicker, deep fascia. The fibrous pericardium, parietal pleura, perineurium, and perimysium are some forms. The septa of the muscles are also examples. These coverings give some form and guidance to the structures they envelop. A condition such as "shin splints" or other compartment syndromes may result from ischemia because of muscular enlargement within a confining space.

*Subserous fascia* is a loose, fibroelastic connective tissue. The visceral pleura, pericardium, peritoneum, and other capsular coverings of the visceral organs are representative examples. The tissue is also subject to inflammatory and infectious processes such as pleuritis or peritonitis. Pericarditis can severely tamponade the function of the heart.

## Interconnection

Rather than exist in a segregated fashion, the various fasciae show continuous communication. Suspensory ligaments of the heart and other organs represent continuities. The recently discovered connection between the dura and the rectus capitis posterior minor is an example of the continuity and interrelatedness of bodily structures. The inguinal ligament is a reflection of the in-rolled lower edge of the external oblique muscle aponeurosis.

As connective tissue, other elements such as the blood and osseous structures of the body act to maintain communication among the various areas of the body. Blood is a connective tissue in its ability to remove, replace, nourish, and deliver to all regions of the body. The musculoskeletal system allows interaction of various parts of the body and helps in the process of fluid flow. The replacement and maintenance of elemental substances such as calcium are dependent on the storage sites in the bone, and the process of hematopoiesis occurs in the marrow.

Bones must be thought of as more like plastic than like stone. They have a good deal of flexibility and can accommodate and distribute stresses within a certain capacity of tolerance. The amount, interval, and impulse of the force, as well as the vector, direction, and individual structure, age, and nutritional status of the bone help to determine the result. Sudden forces may create bending, as in a green-stick fracture in children, or rupture of the components and related structures. Sometimes the force is transmitted to surrounding or underlying structures of other types. It is difficult to conceive of any instance when a fracture of bone does not involve also soft tissue injury of the regional structures.

Head trauma may avoid frank skull fracture but result in disruption of blood vessels, damage to the underlying meninges, or contusion of the brain. Constant or intermittent forces of relatively less intensity may result in deformation and/or reformation of bone.

According to Wolff's law, alteration of function results in a change in the structure of bone. The mastoid processes are barely existent in a newborn infant but become larger, knob-like projections from the temporal bone by adulthood. Hypertrophy of the inion most likely indicates chronic tension introduced by the trapezius and splenii muscles. Asymmetric or even symmetric stressors on bone or other bodily components bring about long-term changes in structure.

The principle of Wolff's law also applies to the fascial tissue. When subjected to stress, previously ambiguous tissue develops directionality. The ability to return to a more elastic state is hampered or eliminated. The longer the force and the responsive reaction continue, the less likely the tissue is to reformulate itself. Fiber adhesions develop from both the approximation of tissue and inflammatory processes. As an acute process, the compression that the material undergoes is protective. Contraction and reformation restrict and resist further destruction. With removal of the irritating event, the body's self-healing mechanisms help restore the tissue's capacity. However, inappropriate persistence of the reaction or further injury results in more chronic changes and perhaps even scarring. Fasciae retain a memory of the forces that have been inflicted through the reorganization of tissue. These histochemical changes may occur parallel to the vector force when there is shearing of the fascia or perpendicular when there is focal impact. Conditions such as fibromyalgia may represent chronic inflammatory changes at multiple sites. In other words, the connective tissues easily exhibit a structure–function interrelationship. The corollary of abnormal function promoting development of abnormal structure is apparent.

## Reconstruction

The repair and proliferation of the type and amount of tissue have multiple determinants.

Tobacco, sun exposure, and age reduce the facility to produce elastin. Piezoelectric currents develop because of ionic charges after irritation or injury. Fibroblasts align along the electric fields and determine the direction of repair and proliferation. Certain specialized fasciae such as the thoracolumbar fascia, tentorium cerebri, and the falx cerebri show lines of force based on chronic normal stresses.

## Patterns of Fascial Strain

As a compensatory organ, the fascia absorbs and distributes forces. When examining patients for somatic dysfunction, one often sees patterns to the findings. Most frequently, areas of restriction are found at transitional zones, with an apparent preference for alteration from side to side from one region to the next successive one. J. Gordon Zink called these *compensatory patterns*. He found that 80% of the people he examined who described themselves as "well" exhibited this pattern. The remaining group of "well" people also showed an alternating sequence but in the exact opposite directions. He termed these *common* and *uncommon compensatory patterns*, respectively. The patterns are outlined in Table 18-1.

Some subjects may not show a preference to one side or other and have tissue that is equally responsive bilaterally. These are fairly healthy and adaptive tissues.

The reason for the compensatory patterns may be handedness, eye dominance, or foot preference. Postural imbalance such as leg length discrepancies and eye-level imbalance may also play a role. The tendency to move in one direction results in attempts to maintain a center of gravity and a balance of all forces to attain equilibrium. Some authors have even suggested a ge-

netic basis in the natural formation of helical patterns, even as small as DNA.

Individuals who did not fit either of these compensatory patterns were noted to have *uncompensated patterns*, in which there may be no alternation or the alteration is incomplete. Dr. Zink reasoned that the compensated patterns were more adaptive and that these individuals responded more favorably to any stress or illness. Injuries tend to exaggerate already existent patterns. People with uncompensated patterns were more likely to have experienced trauma, were slower to recover from illness, and required more chronic treatment.

## Therapeutic Considerations

All manipulative medicine interventions rely on the physical interaction of the physician with the somatic elements of the patient. The process is guided by various considerations. All of the soft tissues have a tolerance for stretch based on their condition, within certain limits. Some of the structures, such as muscle, have the ability to contract. They may do so under voluntary control or reflexively. Injury, chronicity, nutritional status, and position all affect responsiveness. The origins and insertions of the tendons and ligaments determine available motion. The fascia shows decreased elasticity with age and relatively undiminished contractility. The nature of the surrounded structures, regional force and tension requirements, and nutritional status further modify the stretch or contract reactivity. The bones act as levers, both in their function and when used by the physician therapeutically.

Connective tissue release modalities have been called *myofascial release* techniques historically. In truth, they are "myo-fascial-tendon-ligament-osseous-viscera" techniques. Most of the

## TABLE 18-1 COMMON AND UNCOMMON COMPENSATORY PATTERNS

|  |  | OCCIPITOATLANTOID | CERVICOTHORACIC | THORACOLUMBAR | LUMBOSACRAL |
|---|---|---|---|---|---|
| Common | (CCP) | L | R | L | R |
| Uncommon | (UCCP) | R | L | R | L |

practitioners of these techniques have used the responsiveness of the tissue as a guide for further introduction of therapeutic assistance.

Practically all of the modalities are passive in that the patient is to make no conscious effort at moving a region. When active involvement is requested, it is usually to facilitate relaxation, either through a contract/relax response or reflexively through reciprocal inhibition. In both of these situations, the patient's involvement is in short pulses.

The modalities can be described as either direct or indirect. *Direct* techniques bring the region in question into one or more of the relative barriers to motion, with the intent that the tissue relaxes and stretches toward the physiologic limits. A response called *creep* has been used to describe the relaxation of myofascial tissue to a gentle force load and the decreased resistance to subsequent applications. Varieties of *indirect* techniques all position the region into the various freedoms. Some are static in that the position is held. Others are dynamic and use either continuous motion in response to feedback experienced by the physician or the application of facilitating forces or motions. After treatment, reassessment or mobilization into the barriers is engaged. Some of these modalities and specific techniques are also described in other sections of this book.

## Myofascial Release Techniques

*Counterstrain* is a myofascial release technique originally described as "spontaneous release by positioning." A tender point is noted on palpation and the region or entire body is positioned into freedoms for the purpose of shortening muscles. The positions are typically held for 90 to 120 seconds or until a mobile point reaction is noted. Subsequent tissue softening and/or reduced tenderness are noted.

*Facilitated positional release* involves positioning a region or joint into neutral, unloading the joint, adding a facilitating force (compression and/or torsion), adding motion in all three planes of freedom, and monitoring for release. The time interval is a few seconds.

*Functional techniques* appear to have started with Dr. Still. Palpation of specific joint and tis-

sue compliance determines positioning in three cardinal planes, translation in two planes (transverse and anterior or posterior), and compression or traction. An additional element is reaction to a respiratory component (inhalation or exhalation).

*Torque unwinding* is an unpublished modality, which has been taught at seminars. It has a theoretical construct of bodily cubes with regions of restriction being reflected on opposing surfaces caused by vectors of force resulting from injury. Treatment involves bringing the two ends into alignment, mimicking the position of the original injury, and waiting for release and/or adding slight oscillatory torsional forces into both locations at the same time. These techniques are attempts to balance the stress load by adding limited forces in the direction opposite to the original vector of injury.

*Balanced ligamentous release (ligamentous articular release)* uses the palpating hands as both monitors and fulcrums. The regions of the joints and ligaments are balanced to create relaxation and gapping. Release occurs as the tissue further relaxes and more normal motion is established.

*Unwinding* is a dynamic technique. The patient gives constant feedback to the examiner while moving a portion of the body in response to sensations of movement. The technique can be localized using impulses of drag and ease over wider regions. The neck or extremities can be treated regionally or used as levers to manipulate the trunk. The physician facilitates the process by resisting influences such as gravity while following small muscular motions or fascial ease.

*Direct fascial release* requires that a torsion, compression, and/or traction force be maintained into the barrier while one waits for a release (fascial creep). After this occurs, the region can be moved in all planes more easily.

*Cranial osteopathy* is a form of fascial release that attempts to balance forces of the five components, as proposed by William Garner Sutherland.

*Visceral manipulations* use manual techniques (the physician's contact with the somatic system) to balance forces that create stresses on the visceral organs.

The *Still technique* is a recently "rediscovered" application of manipulative techniques believed to have been used by Dr. Still. It combines indirect technique with a subsequent quick articulatory procedure. It shares a great similarity to facilitated positional release. Sometimes the only differences between the two are the positions of the patient and physician.

*Progressive inhibition of neuromuscular structures* and other forms of *inhibition* are techniques that may address fascial restrictions by use of inhibitory forces.

*Trigger band* technique, as described by Stephen Typaldos, DO, is a direct form involving very deep pressures. The practitioner exerts significant force by using an instrument or fingers along involved tissue in a basically linear fashion from an area of relative dysfunction toward the more involved region.

*Biodynamic* method, described by James Jealous, DO, is a system of osteopathic diagnosis and treatment using monitoring and facilitation of the innate health–restorative forces, which occur in polyrhythmic motion cycles. *Bioelectric Fascial Release*, described by Judith O'Connell, DO, FAAO, is also a form of fascial release using and directing inherent forces.

*Integrated neuromusculoskeletal release* (INR) can be considered a fusion technique in that it uses fascial release, functional technique, and isometric–isotonic muscular efforts. This technique was developed by Robert Ward, DO, FAAO, with the focus on bringing about stretch and reflexive relaxations in areas of dysfunction.

Even though these modalities are mentioned as distinct units, their use may be overlapping. The physician may switch from one to another to adapt to tissue response.

## ■ EXAMPLES OF MYOFASCIAL TECHNIQUES

### Cervical Spine Functional Technique

1. **Patient position:** supine.
2. **Physician position:** seated at the head of the table.
3. **Technique:**
   a. The physician places the index finger of either hand on the transverse process of the vertebra to be released.
   b. Range of motion of the vertebral unit is

assessed in all three planes: flexion–extension, side-bending, and rotation.
   c. Response to translation laterally in the coronal plane and anteriorly/posteriorly along the sagittal plane is assessed.
   d. Tissue responsiveness at the monitoring site is assessed for compression or traction.
   e. The vertebra is positioned in all three cardinal planes of freedom.
   f. The two directions of translation are added.
   g. Respiration is used to determine tissue relaxation. If the tissue feels more relaxed during inhalation, then the patient is instructed to take a deep breath and hold it. If exhalation is the freer modifier, then the patient takes a breath and exhales fully and maintains full exhalation for several seconds.
   h. The physician follows the vertebra into the direction of ease at each release.
   i. The region is reassessed.

### Thoracic Spine/Upper Extremity Unwinding

1. **Patient position:** supine.
2. **Physician position:** standing or seated at the side of the table along the side to be treated.
3. **Technique:**
   a. The physician grasps the patient's forearm with both hands.
   b. The patient's arm is brought to approximately 90 degrees of shoulder flexion.
   c. Slight tension is introduced by traction and the whole arm is subjected to a mild amount of torsion by internally and then externally rotating the arm.
   d. The tension is reduced and effort is directed toward supporting the arm against gravity.
   e. Tissue responsiveness at the monitoring site is assessed.
   f. The physician allows the arm to drift in any or all directions. If the extremity hits a barrier, there will be a tendency for the muscles to tighten. The physician should attempt to use the least amount of interaction necessary.

g. As the movement becomes more active, the physician can give less and less support.

h. If a pattern of movement is repeated three times or more, the physician should hold the arm at one or another extreme of the movement and hold it in place. Any tugging motion that leads to the same repetitive motion should be resisted by maintaining the extremity in place.

i. Elimination of the resistance should occur when the extremity begins to move in a direction that does not fit the previous pattern.

j. The endpoint occurs when the arm comes to rest alongside or across the patient's abdomen. Palpated impulses to movement should be absent.

k. The region is reassessed.

l. Large movements of the shoulder involve the thoracic spine, whereas smaller conical types of movement may support only regional extremity movement.

## Scapula Release

1. **Patient position:** lying on side, with the side to be treated facing upward.
2. **Physician position:** standing, facing the patient.
3. **Technique:**
   a. The physician abducts the patient's arm and places his caudad arm (relative to the patient) between the patient's arm and his chest wall.
   b. The physician grasps the patient's scapula at the medial edge and inferior angle with his caudad hand and the medial edge and superior medial angle with his cephalad hand (Fig. 18-1).
   c. With a slight amount of traction, the scapula is tested in the following directions:
      (1) Cephalad (elevation) and caudad (depression)
      (2) Lateral (distraction) and medial (retraction)
      (3) Rotation clockwise and counterclockwise
   d. The scapula is placed into all three direc-

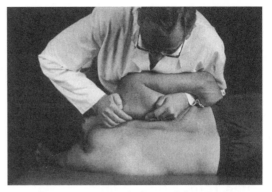

■ **FIG. 18-1** Fascial release of the scapula.

tions of freedom successively and held in place.

   e. The physician waits for a further loosening into one or more directions of freedom, indicating a release.
   f. The region is reassessed.

## Sacral Balancing

1. **Patient position:** supine.
2. **Physician position:** seated to one side of the patient facing toward the patient's head.
3. **Technique:**
   a. Depending on the patient's comfort, one of the following two positions can be used:
      (1) Both knees bent, feet flat on the table, separated and adducted.
      (2) Legs extended.
   b. The physician places the hand of the arm that is closer to the patient beneath the patient's sacrum. The physician's fingertips extend to the patient's sacral base and the apex of the sacrum rests between the physician's thenar and hypothenar eminences. The hand contours to the sacrum. The physician rests his forearm on the table.
   c. The physician places the forearm of his other arm across the ASISs of the patient's pelvis. The physician's arm, which is now close to the patient's head, rests on the ipsilateral ASIS while the hand holds the outer edge of the opposite iliac crest.
   d. A medial force is engaged across these two contact points with this arm.

e. The physician monitors the motion of the sacrum during inhalation and exhalation. The sacral base moves posteriorly in inhalation and anteriorly in exhalation.

f. The physician evaluates the motion for symmetry and quality.

g. The physician attempts to balance the sacrum in all directions of ease.

h. When symmetry is established, the physician assesses the efficacy of the treatment.

## Knee Torque Unwinding

1. **Patient position:** supine.
2. **Physician position:** seated or standing to one side of the patient facing toward the patient's head.
3. **Technique:**

   a. The physician finds a point of tenderness, motion restriction, or tissue tension at any given location about the knee.

   b. The physician should imagine that the knee is encased in a cube.

   c. Drawing an imaginary line diagonally across from the location of the original point, the physician must realize that this point is a reflection of the original point. Palpating the original point, tapping it, and feeling for a resonance of the impulse may also find the second point. If the point is two fingerbreadths below the upper edge of the cube, the resonance point will be two fingerbreadths above the lower edge of the opposite face of the cube. The same relationship is maintained for the point relative to the lateral edges of the cube.

   d. One or two fingers of each hand cover each point.

   e. A rotary motion is introduced at both locations at the same time. The preferred manner is to rotate one side clockwise while the other moves counter-clockwise, and

then reverse directions. The angle of the rotary motion is narrow, and the oscillation of motion is a few cycles per second for up to a minute.

f. Alternating points found on opposite faces of imaginary cubes can be located throughout the lower extremity.

g. The region is reassessed.

## REFERENCES

Barral JP, Mercier P. *Visceral Manipulation.* Seattle: Eastland Press, 1988.

Bowles CH. Functional technique: a modern perspective. In: Beal MC, ed. *The Principles of Palpatory Diagnosis and Manipulative Technique.* Newark, OH: American Academy of Osteopathy, 1992:174–178.

DiGiovanna E. *Encyclopedia of Osteopathy.* Indianapolis, IN: American Academy of Osteopathy, 2001.

Dowling DJ. Progressive inhibition of neuromuscular structures (PINS) technique. In: *Chaitow L, ed. Modern Neuromuscular Techniques.* New York: Churchill Livingstone, 2003:225–250.

Dowling DJ. Progressive inhibition of neuromuscular structures (PINS) technique. In: *Ward RC, ed. Foundations for Osteopathic Medicine, 2nd ed.* Philadelphia: Williams & Wilkins, 2003.

Greenman PE. *Principles of Manual Medicine.* Baltimore: Williams & Wilkins, 1989.

Jones LH. Spontaneous release by positioning. In: Beal MC, ed. *The Principles of Palpatory Diagnosis and Manipulative Technique.* Newark, OH: American Academy of Osteopathy, 1992:179–185.

Kuchera WA, Kuchera ML. *Osteopathic Principles in Practice, 2nd ed.* Columbus, OH: Greyden Press, 1994.

O'Connell J. *Bioelectric Fascial Release.* Indianapolis, IN: American Academy of Osteopathy, 2000.

Typaldos S. Introducing the fascial distortion model. *American Academy of Osteopathy Journal* 1994:4(2).

Van Buskirk RL. A manipulative technique of Andrew Taylor Still. *J Am Osteopath Assoc* 1996;96:597–602.

Van Buskirk RL. *The Still Technique Manual.* Indianapolis, IN: American Academy of Osteopathy, 1999.

Wallace EM. *Torque Unwinding.* Presented at the Convocation of the American Academy of Osteopathy, Nashville, 1995.

Ward RC. Integrated Neuromusculoskeletal Release. In: Ward RC, ed. *Foundations for Osteopathic Medicine, 2nd ed.* Philadelphia: Williams & Wilkins, 2003.

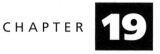

# Ligamentous Articular Strain Technique and Balanced Ligamentous Tension Technique

*Wm. Thomas Crow*

Ligamentous articular strain (LAS) technique and balanced ligamentous tension (BLT) techniques are two techniques derived from what were once called "general osteopathic techniques." They both are primarily indirect techniques that affect connective tissues of the body: fascia, ligaments, tendons, and, indirectly, lymphatic and blood flow. Both terms come from the phrase from William Garner Sutherland that "ligamentous articular strains are treated by using balanced ligamentous tension." The reason that both names have persisted is the various osteopathic physicians who taught them called their methods of treatment by either term.

Balanced ligamentous tension techniques have usually been associated with a very light touch, and the use of respiratory cooperation, although ligamentous articular strain techniques usually have more force applied and the use of respiratory cooperation is not always used. In general terms, the amount of force used in BLT is approximately 1 to 3 lbs, whereas LAS techniques may be as high as 40 lbs. However, both of them have three components in common:

1. DISENGAGEMENT
2. EXAGGERATION
3. BALANCE

## ■ DISENGAGEMENT

To "disengage," the osteopathic physician must use either compression or decompression. Push-ing a joint or tissue together or pulling it apart generally accomplishes this. The more common approach is the use of compression. Once disengaged, the joint or tissue will move. The osteopathic physician uses palpation to bring the tissue to a neutral point.

## ■ EXAGGERATION

After disengagement, the joint or tissue is taken into the direction of the injury. This exaggerates the position of the diagnosis of relative freedom. Because the joint or tissue was taken beyond its physiologic barrier and remained dysfunctional by the injury, it fails to return to its physiologic position. Close to the point of injury is the most likely location to find the dysfunction. By approaching the dysfunction with exaggeration of its relative freedom, a balance point is determined.

## ■ BALANCE POINT

Establishing the balance point leads to the resolution of the somatic dysfunction. The first points are determined by palpation and diagnosis. This is where the treatment begins. A balance point is established, much in the same manner as one balances a plate, a pencil, or anything on the end of one's finger. All of the parameters of pull are brought to a state of balance. Balance consists of not taking the tissues beyond the elastic limits, and yet it is not light touch. A vital resilience should still be present in the tissue after enough pressure is applied to accomplish a release. The key to successful treatment is this delicate balance of all the ligaments, all the strains, and all the other tissues, fascia, etc.

LAS and BLT techniques were originally published in the 1949 *Year Book of the Academy of Applied Osteopathy* as "The Osteopathic Technique of Wm. G. Sutherland" written by H.A. Lippincott, DO. Dr. Sutherland credited the origin of these techniques to Dr. Still.

Carl Phillip McConnell, DO, MD, who had been treated by Still and was on the faculty of the American School of Osteopathy, wrote in his book *The Practice of Osteopathy*:

> Disengage the articular points that have become locked. Reduce the dislocation by retracing the path along which the parts were dislocated. One can readily see that a dislocated ball and socket joint could be reduced only by the dislocated bone retracing the path through which it left its socket as the capsular ligament would at once prevent its returning to the socket by any path other than that taken when dislocated. This applies to all dislocations to a greater or lesser extent.

This was the first written documentation to discuss Dr. Still's technique found in sources from other than Dr. Still himself. A description for the treatment from Dr. Still states,

> One asks how much do you pull a bone to replace it? I reply, pull it to its proper place and leave it there.

The phenomenon of "popping" is also addressed:

> One man advises to pull out a bone to attempt to set until they pop. That popping is no criterion to go by. Bones do not always pop when they go back into their proper place, nor does it mean they are properly adjusted when they do pop. If you pull your finger you will hear a sudden noise. The sudden and forcible (sic) separation of the ends of the bones that form the joint causes a vacuum and the air entering from about the joint to fill the vacuum causes the explosive noise.

Dr. Still continues,

> It matters not from which one it is or how far it has been forced from its socket, you must first loosen it at its attachments at its articulating end, always bearing in mind that when a bone has left its proper articulation the surrounding muscles and ligaments are irritated and keep up a continual contracture.

He further states,

> Without going into further detail I will say that all dislocations, partial or complete, can be adjusted by this rule: First loosen the dislocated end from other tissues, then gently bring it back to its original place.

In 1915, Dr. Edythe Ashmore, a student of Dr. Still, wrote "Osteopathic Mechanics," in which she describes osteopathic techniques. "General Rules—The articulating surfaces must retrace the path they took in their displacement." In addition, she states, "There are two methods commonly employed by osteopathists in the correction of lesions the older of which is the traction method, the later the direct method or thrust." She goes further in a footnote, stating, "The term 'direct' is preferred for the reason that the imitators of osteopathy have given to the word 'thrust' an objectionable meaning of harshness."

Then, she writes about "*the old method*"—ligamentous articular strain. The new method that came to represent thrust was high-velocity–low-amplitude (HVLA). "Those who employ the traction method secure the relaxation of the tissues about the articulation by what has been termed exaggeration of the lesion, a motion in the direction of the forcible (sic) movement which produced the lesion, as if its purpose were to increase the deformity."

C. P. McConnell, DO, stated, "this disengages the tissues that are holding the parts in the abnormal position." The movement bringing this about is a reaction. "The exaggeration is held, traction made upon the joint, replacement initiated and then completed by reversal of the forces."

Dr. Ashmore goes on to describe the method used by Dr. Still.

> Technic: In all spinal technic it is my custom to have the patient exercise his own natural forces rather than the application of mine. There are no thrusts, no jerks nor the application of another or distal end of the anatomy as a lever. The principle is that used and taught by Dr. Still, namely, exaggeration of the lesion to the degree of release and then allowing the ligaments to draw the articulations back into normal relationship. This same method is applied in sacroiliac technic.

One may easily note the similarity of descriptions between Drs. Ashmore's and Lippincott's detailing of Sutherland's technique.

> Since it is the ligaments that are primarily involved in the maintenance of the lesion it is they, not mus-

cular leverage, that are used as the main agency for reduction. The articulation is carried in the direction of the lesion position as far as is necessary to cause tension of the weakened elements of the ligamentous structure to be equal to or slight in excess of the tension of those that are not strained. This is the point of balanced tension. Forcing the articulation back and away from the direction of lesion strains the ligaments that are normal and unopposed, and if it is done with thrust or jerks there is definite possibility of separating fibers of ligaments from their bony attachments. When the tension is properly balanced, the respiratory or muscular cooperation of the patient is employed to overcome the resistance of the defense mechanism of the body to the release of the lesion.

## ■ LIGAMENTOUS ARTICULAR STRAIN TECHNIQUE FOR THE TERES MINOR

1. **Patient position**: Lateral recumbent with affected shoulder up
2. **Physician position**: Standing behind the patient
3. **Technique**:
   a. The physician uses the thumb of his caudad hand and places his thumb at the posterior axillary fold.
   b. The physician's other hand is placed over the ilium with the thumb in the region of the quadratus lumborum.
   c. The physician then places pressure on the teres minor while stabilizing the ilium (Fig. 19-1).
   d. The thumb of the upper hand should be over the area of maximum spasm.

e. Steady pressure is maintained by the upper hand. The amount of force is usually approximatley 20 to 30 lbs of force.
   f. The hold can be released when the spasm has relaxed.
   g. The area is reassessed

## ■ BALANCED LIGAMENTOUS TENSION TECHNIQUE FOR THORACIC VERTEBRAE—SIDE-BENDING ROTATION (Example T4 F $S_L$ $R_L$)

1. **Patient position**: Seated on the table
2. **Physician position**: Standing behind the patient
3. **Technique**:
   a. The physician places the thumb on the side of the somatic dysfunction rotation over the transverse process of the next lower vertebra on that side (left thumb on T5 left transverse process in this example).
   b. The physician's other thumb is placed on the transverse process of the somatic dysfunction on the side opposite to the rotation (right thumb on T4 right transverse process). This is also placed a little more forward to bring the vertebra into a relative flexion with the one below.
   c. The patient is directed to raise the shoulder on the side opposite to the dysfunction side-bending (patient raises the right shoulder in this example). This creates side-bending into the somatic dysfunction relative freedom (Fig. 19-2).

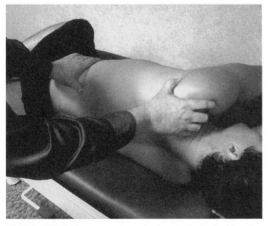

■ **FIG. 19-1** Ligamentous articular strain technique for the teres minor.

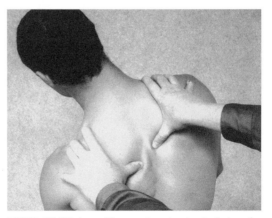

■ **FIG. 19-2** Balanced ligamentous tension technique for the thoracic spine.

d. The point of balanced tension is located, monitored, and "the respiratory cooperation may be in either inhalation or exhalation—inhalation if the ligamentous imbalance is mainly on the side of convexity and exhalation if on the concavity." (Lippincott)

e. The patient is brought back to a neutral position and the somatic dysfunction is reassessed

**REFERENCES**

Ashmore EF. *Osteopathic Mechanics: A Textbook.* Kirksville, MO: Journal Printing Co, 1915:72.

Lippincott HA. *The Osteopathic Technique of Wm. G. Sutherland, D.O. Yearbook of the Academy of Applied Osteopathy, reprint.* Indianapolis, IN: American Academy of Osteopathy, 1949.

McConnell CP. *Practice of Osteopathy,* 1899. Kirksville, MO: Journal Printing Co, 1906:58.

Still AT. *Osteopathy: Research and Practice.* Kirksville, MO: The Journal Printing Co, 1910:52.

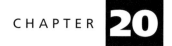

# CHAPTER 20

# Functional Techniques

*Stanley Schiowitz*

Functional techniques can be described as low-force, nonthrusting techniques for the treatment of vertebral motion restrictions that utilize indirect positioning to create a gradual release of restrictive tensions at the dysfunctional segment.

Historically, the use of functional techniques can be dated back to A. T. Still. It is noted that Harold Hoover, DO, one of the early pioneers in the use of functional methodologies, was using the techniques learned from the teachings of Still. Over time, these functional techniques lost popularity in favor of thrusting techniques. The schools found the thrusting techniques easier to teach, and most practitioners found that patients more readily accepted these methods and looked forward to hearing the "popping" sound that was created.

In the early 1950s, Harrison Fryette's findings on spinal motions, as well as Irvin M. Korr's research reports on the neural relationship of the somatic dysfunction, created an atmosphere for the resurgence of the acceptance of these techniques. It was believed that a scientific explanation had been found that would explain the rationale of why and how the results could be obtained. In 1951, Hoover was invited to New England to present a program on his approach to the diagnosis and treatment of somatic dysfunctions. He called the methods taught a functional approach to the treatment of segmental restrictions. The next year, a New England branch of the Academy of Applied Osteopathy was formed. This group of physicians spent the next 5 years studying and formalizing both functional palpatory diagnosis and the application of functional methods of treatment.

To properly use these techniques, a diagnosis has to be made, and the positioning of the segment involved must be into its freedoms of motions creating an indirect technique. William Johnston, DO defines an indirect technique as "the method of moving one bone or segment slightly in the direction away from the direction of correction until the resistance of holding tissues and fluids is partially overcome and the tensions are bilaterally balanced; then allowing the released ligaments and muscles themselves to aid in pulling the part towards normal. Other body forces including that of respiration may be employed."

Functional techniques apply palpatory information derived as the segment is passively placed into its three planes of motion. The general methodology is to place one hand on the segment involved; this is the palpatory or "listening" hand. The other hand is used to passively move the patient in a manner that creates motion of the segment in the three planes. This is called the "motive" hand. The palpatory hand assesses the motion being created, diagnosing any restrictions of motion present. The "motive" hand positions the patient, increasing the segmental motion in the direction of its ease of motions. The patient may be asked to slowly inhale and exhale. As the palpatory hand feels release of the restrictions, the patient's position is modified to allow for an increase in the segmental motion into its freedoms. This is repeated until full freedom of motion is restored.

It is readily understandable that the application of functional techniques requires that the physician be well versed in palpatory procedures. He/she must be able to separate the feelings of segmental motion from those created by the tissues surrounding the segment as it is placed into position. However, the results obtained and the patient's appreciation of the gentleness and ease of its application will reward mastery of these methods

## REFERENCES

Bowles CH. *Functional Techniques: A modern perspective.* Colorado Springs: Academy of Applied Osteopathy, 1964.

DiGiovanna EL. *An Encyclopedia of Osteopathy.* Indianapolis: American Academy of Osteopathy, 2001.

Fryette HH. *Principles of Osteopathic Techniques.* Colorado Springs: Academy of Applied Osteopathy, 1954.

Hoover HV. *Collected Papers.* Colorado Springs: Academy of Applied Osteopathy, 1969.

Johnston WL. Functional Technique. In: Ward RC, ed. *Foundations for Osteopathic Medicine. 2nd ed.* Philadelphia: Lippincott Williams & Wilkins, 2003.

Korr IM. The neural basis of the osteopathic lesion. *J Am Osteopath Assoc* 1947. Reprinted in The Collected Papers of Irvin M. Korr. Colorado Springs: American Academy of Osteopathy, 1979: 120–127.

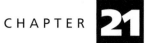

# Osteopathy in the Cranial Field

*Hugh Ettlinger and Bonnie Gintis*

The cranial concept was originally conceived and developed by William Garner Sutherland from 1899 until his death in 1954. Sutherland's teachings are a direct extension of the principles of osteopathy as taught by Andrew Taylor Still at the American School of Osteopathy.

Dr. Sutherland's study began after careful examination of a disarticulated skull. He first identified a design for motion in the structure of the sutures. After lengthy study, he concluded that motion must be the response to an involuntary mechanism. He named this mechanism the *primary respiratory mechanism* (PRM).

This chapter introduces the basic principles of the cranial concept and the primary respiratory mechanism, according to the teaching models presented in *Osteopathy in the Cranial Field and Teachings in the Science of Osteopathy*. It should be used as a stepping-stone to a more in-depth study of the field. In addition to didactic study, individual perceptual training is a mandatory adjunct to the study of this aspect of osteopathy.

## The Primary Respiratory Mechanism

The primary respiratory mechanism is perceptible in the cranium and throughout the body. Its action is part of the normal physiology of the living human body. It has two alternating phases referred to as *inhalation* and *exhalation* phases. The primary respiratory mechanism is not a wave that travels from head to foot.

The following five phenomena function together as the primary respiratory mechanism.

1. The fluctuation of the cerebrospinal fluid (CSF) and the potency of the tide.
2. The mobility of the intracranial and intraspinal membranes and the function of the reciprocal tension membrane
3. The inherent motility of the central nervous system
4. The articular mobility of the cranial bones
5. The involuntary mobility of the sacrum between the ilia

Together, these five phenomena reflect a structure–function relationship that exists not only between the central nervous system and its container but also throughout the entire living human body.

## Phases of the Primary Respiratory Mechanism

The *inhalation* and *exhalation* phases of the primary respiratory mechanism can be sensed simultaneously throughout the five phenomena and the entire body. During the inhalation phase, midline bones flex and paired bones externally rotate, moving the basicranium superiorly. The resultant increased transverse diameter of the cranium is accompanied by a simultaneous decrease in anteroposterior diameter and a decrease in vertical dimension (Fig. 21-1). The foramen magnum moves relatively superiorly drawing the sacral base posteriorly by means of its dural attachment at the second sacral segment. The shape of the space that contains the CSF and the fluid itself are affected by the alternating phases of the primary respiratory mechanism. The dural membranes change shape

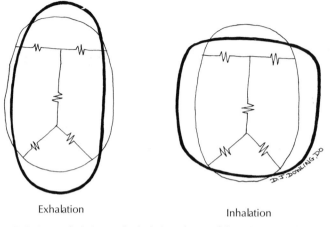

Exhalation

Inhalation

■ **FIG. 21-1** Inhalation and exhalation phases of the primary respiratory mechanism.

around a suspended, automatically shifting fulcrum, maintaining balance and constant tension during the phases of the primary respiratory mechanism. There is a rhythmic coiling and uncoiling of the brain and spinal cord during the phases of the primary respiratory mechanism. In the exhalation phase, these motions are reversed. The study of the primary respiratory mechanism begins with examination of each of its five phenomena.

## The Fluctuation of the Cerebrospinal Fluid and the Potency of the Tide

The fluctuation of the CSF is considered the first principle in the primary respiratory mechanism. Within the fluid is a potency or force that manifests as a fluctuant movement. Dr. Sutherland referred to this force as the "breath of life."

> Within the cerebrospinal fluid there is an invisible element that I refer to as the Breath of Life as a fluid within this fluid, something that does not mix, something that has potency as the thing that makes it move. Is it really necessary to know what makes the fluid move?
> (*Teachings in the Science of Osteopathy*, W. G. Sutherland, p.14)

Although Dr. Sutherland did not theorize on the origin of the breath of life and the fluctuation that it produces, he did clearly distinguish it from the actions created by arterial pulse and respiration (Fig. 21-2).

## The Mobility of the Intracranial and Intraspinal Membranes and the Function of the Reciprocal Tension Membrane

The reciprocal tension membrane (RTM) refers to the function of the mobility of intracranial and intraspinal membranes, the pia, arachnoid, and dura. Understanding the development and the anatomy of the membranes helps illustrate their function (see Section X, Chapter 102). The intracranial membranes are intimately related to the fascia throughout the rest of the body.

The internal layer of the dura surrounds the brain and comes together in two layers to form the falx cerebri, the tentorium cerebelli, and the falx cerebri.

The RTM is a single unit of structure and function. All membranes change shape during the phases of the primary respiratory mechanism. Membranes balance and maintain a constant level of tension during the phases of the PRM.

## The Inherent Motility of the Central Nervous System

There is a rhythmic expansion and contraction of the brain and spinal cord during the phases of the primary respiratory mechanism. This change of shape occurs simultaneously with movement of membrane, bone, and fluid during

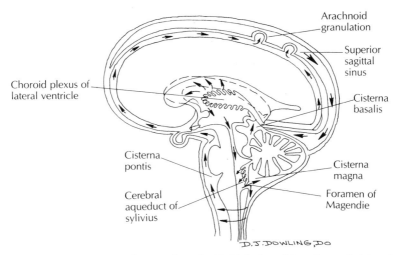

■ **FIG. 21-2** Circulation of the cerebrospinal fluid. (Adapted from Netter F. *Atlas of Human Anatomy*. Summitt, NJ: Ciba Geigy, 1989:plate 103.)

the phases of the PMR. This coiling and uncoiling of the nervous system occurs about a fulcrum located at the lamina terminalis, the most anterior point of the primitive neural tube.

Because every cell in the body is affected by the phases of the PRM, there is a parallel effect within the peripheral nervous system, because the peripheral nerves and their associated structures respond to the phases of inhalation and exhalation.

## The Articular Mobility of the Cranial Bones

The study of cadaveric bone specimens has enabled anatomists to obtain extensive information regarding the form of bone but has led to inaccurate information regarding its function. According to *Gray's Anatomy*, "Bones from preserved cadavers yield misleading values, especially in regards to plastic deformation, but also in elasticity, hardness, and compressive and tensile properties."

Living bone is approximately 60% water. Its properties are closer to other connective tissues than cadaveric study would lead one to believe. The limited mobility allowed by sutures makes the plasticity of bone a relatively important source of motion for the cranium. The thin, flat bones of the cranium are well suited to plastic deformity.

Structure of the cranial sutures allows various types of motion between contiguous bones. The nature of the sutures is discussed further in Section X, Chapter 102, as is the motion characteristics of the various cranial bones.

## Involuntary Mobility of the Sacrum Between the Ilia

The axis of motion of the sacrum can be considered using a variety of different reference points. It will vary depending on whether one considers its voluntary postural motions, its motion response to breathing, or its involuntary motion in response to the PRM.

The sacrum rocks on a transverse axis through the articular pillar of the second sacral segment posterior to the sacral canal. This motion must be differentiated from respiratory sacral motion, which is caused by spinal motion and contraction of the pelvic diaphragm. The axis of involuntary sacral motion lies anterior to the sacral canal and passes through the body of S2 at the junction of the short and long arms of the L-shaped sacral articulation.

## Methodology

Osteopathy in the cranial field is performed with the hands placed in defined locations on the cranium. After diagnosis of dysfunctions, the hands gently guide the cranial bones into more normal patterns of motion or release restrictions to motion.

Because of the close functioning of the sacrum with the cranial motions, the sacrum may also be used as an entry point for diagnosis and treatment of dysfunctions amenable to osteopathy in the cranial field.

## Indications for Use of Osteopathy in the Cranial Field

Because the primary respiratory mechanism is perceived throughout the living human body, it is possible to reach dysfunctions and pathologies in a vast array of locations. Multiple systems and organs of the body can be affected by use of osteopathy in the cranial field. See Section X, Chapter 106 for some of the practical applications.

**REFERENCES**

*Gray's Anatomy.* London: Churchill Livingstone, 1995.

Magoun HI. *Osteopathy in the Cranial Field, 3rd ed.* Kirksville, MO: Journal Printing Co, 1976.

Sutherland WG. *Teachings in the Science of Osteopathy.* Cambridge, MA; Rudra Press, 1990.

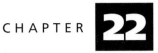

# Chapman's Reflex Points

*John D. Capobianco*

## ■ INTRODUCTION

Chapman's points are viscerosomatic reflexes discovered by their namesake, Frank Chapman, in the early part of the twentieth century. These reflexes, or "gangliform" contractions, or excessive tissue congestion, reflect visceral dysfunction and are mediated by the sympathetic arm of the autonomic nervous system. Excessive sympathetic tone from an irritated, diseased, or stressed organ leads to lymphatic stasis manifesting as myofascial nodules, which may feel boggy, ropy, shotty, and/or thickened. These points almost always exhibit tenderness on palpation. Chapman's reflexes are excellent diagnostic tools to the osteopathic physician and they may also be used to break positive feedback cycles through somatovisceral pathways to restore health.

## ■ HISTORY

A student of Andrew Taylor Still, Frank Chapman graduated the American School of Osteopathy in 1897. Chapman's thoughts and methods did not appear in a vacuum. As a student of the "Old Doctor," he learned the role of the fascia and the importance of the lymphatics in health and disease. Still admonished, "The fascia is the place to look for the cause of disease . . ." and "All nerves go to and terminate in that great system the fascia." Still also stated that, "Finer nerves dwell with the lymphatics than even with the eye" and goes on to say that, "the lymphatic system is the universal system of irrigation."

Chapman never lived to see his work completed. His wife, Ada Chapman, and brother-in-law, Charles Owens, along with W. F. Link published his work in the 1930s. Drs. Fred Mitchell Sr. and Jr. shed additional clarity on Chapman's work during subsequent publications of Owens' treatise *An Endocrine Interpretation of Chapman's Reflexes*. Chapman's work influenced many osteopathic masters, including Drs. William Garner Sutherland, Beryl Arbuckle, Harold Magoun Sr., Fred Mitchell Sr. and Jr., Robert Fulford, and William and Michael Kuchera.

## ■ DIAGNOSIS

There are approximately 50 distinct Chapman's reflexes, ranging from points for the eye to the prostate. These points are bilateral and are located on the anterior and posterior regions of the body. This would account for nearly two hundred separate neurolymphatic reflexes. The "neuro" indicates that the autonomic nervous system mediates these reflexes. "Lymphatic" is used because all vasculature, including the lymphatic vessels, are under sympathetic control.

The student should acquaint himself with *groupings* of reflexes rather than memorizing each specific point. Anteriorly, these gangliform contractions, or excessive tissue congestion, which manifest as edematous or ropy, are usually located in the intercostal space "between the anterior and posterior layers of the anterior intercostal fascia." These rib segments are associated with the corresponding sympathetic innervation of the involved viscera. For example, the sympathetic fibers to the sinuses originate in the cell

**113**

bodies of the first through fourth thoracic spinal segments. Sinusitis, or any ear, nose, or throat pathology, therefore, would manifest as altered tissue texture along the clavicle and first two ribs.

The principles of Chapman's reflexes are based on anatomy and physiology. These gangliform contractions may feel hard, boggy, and tender and are usually the size of a "BB" pellet or a pea that has been split in half. These tissue texture changes may be felt on the periosteum of the rib or clavicle. An acute reflex point is more likely to feel boggy or edematous. A more chronic gangliform contraction will likely feel ropy or stringy. Chapman's reflexes do not radiate pain like trigger points and are not necessarily associated with remote somatic dysfunction, as are Jones's counterstrain points. Although these neurological reflexes exhibit pain on palpation, *tenderness is not the sole criterion for a Chapman's point; rather, it is lymphatic congestion and altered myofascial texture.*

Posteriorly, Chapman's reflexes are located in the soft tissues between the spinous process of a vertebra above and the transverse process of a vertebra below. For example, the posterior Chapman's point for the heart is located between the spinous and transverse process of the second and third thoracic vertebrae. The posterior points have the feel of a classic viscerosomatic reflex; the operator will palpate what feels like a rubbery nodule. If the physician attempts to articulate a vertebral somatic dysfunction and the spine "bounces" away from the force, the possibility of a viscerosomatic reflex should be considered.

Chapman's reflexes are also located along the extremities. This is because of the fact that the upper and lower extremities are innervated by T2-8 and T11-L2, respectively. The arm and leg share sympathetic fibers with the viscera. For example, the colon and thigh are innervated by the sympathetic cell bodies of T11-L2. If the patient has colitis, the resulting Chapman's reflex will manifest as quarter-sized or half-dollar-sized "shotty plaque(s)" along the outer thigh. Likewise, disorders of the eye may exhibit tissue texture changes along the anterior superior aspect of the humerus.

A common misconception is that the anterior Chapman's points (Fig. 22-1) are used for diagnosis and the posterior points (Fig. 22-2) are used for treatment. Any of the points may be used for diagnosis or treatment as desired.

In his analysis of Chapman's work, Dr. Fred Mitchell states, "A light touch is essential, as these centers may be exquisitely tender and palpatory sense is better maintained with the light touch."

One anterior point of interest in surgical diagnosis is the reflex for appendicitis. This is located along the tip of the right twelfth rib. This reflex may help the osteopathic physician in the emergency department to distinguish appendicitis from a different surgical problem such as a ruptured ovarian cyst, mesenteric adenitis, or ureterolithiasis. However, because one spinal cord segment innervates more than one organ, Chapman's reflexes are considered to be *more sensitive than specific* indicators of disease.

## ■ TREATMENT

In the text, *An Endocrine Interpretation of Chapman's Reflexes*, Owens stressed the importance of first treating the pelvis. Later, Dr. Beryl Arbuckle explained that the pelvis houses not only the ganglion impar, the most distal aspect of the sympathetic nervous system, but also the ovaries and testes. Owens emphasized the role of hormones on total body homeostasis. According to the original text, the diagnosis of an innominate dysfunction was made by assessing the inguinal (Poupart's) ligament for any thickening. This "foundation" of the spine was treated in a manner similar to what is later described by Mitchell, Moran, and Pruzzo as a direct engagement of the barrier that involves a de-rotation of the involved innominate.

When the operator is ready to approach specific Chapman's points, a gentle rotary motion is induced over each point, using the finger pad, for a period of approximately 15 seconds. Treatment, however, may take a few seconds or last 2 minutes. The pressure should be firm, although not enough to elicit a sustained grimace from the patient. The end point of a reflex treatment by the physician's "thinking, knowing, feeling, sensing" fingers is the dissolution of

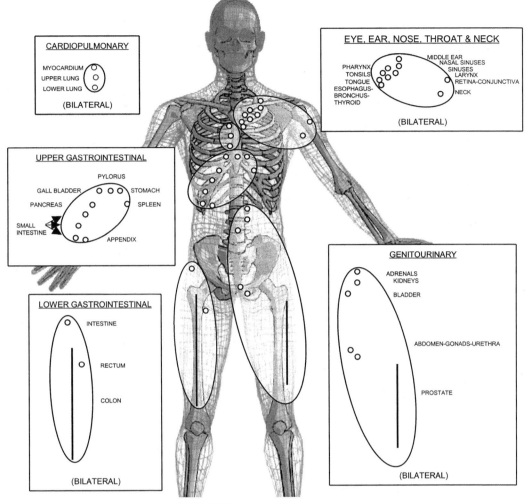

**■ FIG. 22-1** Anterior Chapman's points.

edema and lessening of tension in the myofascial tissues. A decrease in pain is more the result, rather than the aim, of treatment.

## ■ NEUROENDOCRINE—IMMUNE CONNECTION

Chapman was one of the first to describe the interrelatedness of the "neuroendocrine–immune" systems with the introduction of the concept of the "pelvic–thyroid" syndrome. Years later, Arbuckle included the term "adrenal," coining the term "pelvic-thyroid-adrenal syndrome" (PTAS). To Chapman and Owens, the thyroid was the master gland of immunity. As

previously mentioned, treating the pelvis was vital because of the proximity of the ganglion impar to the coccyx. Moreover, the ovaries and testes produce sex steroid hormones, specifically estrogen, progesterone, and testosterone. These hormones interact not only with immunocytes but also with the adrenal and thyroid glands. The sex hormones have receptors in the thyroid gland, influence thyroid stimulating hormone (TSH), and may increase thymocyte proliferation. The thyroid in turn enhances reproductive function. Thyroid hormone not only permeates every cell in the body but also is important in myelin production for the nerves. Proper thyroid function is necessary for immunocyte prolifera-

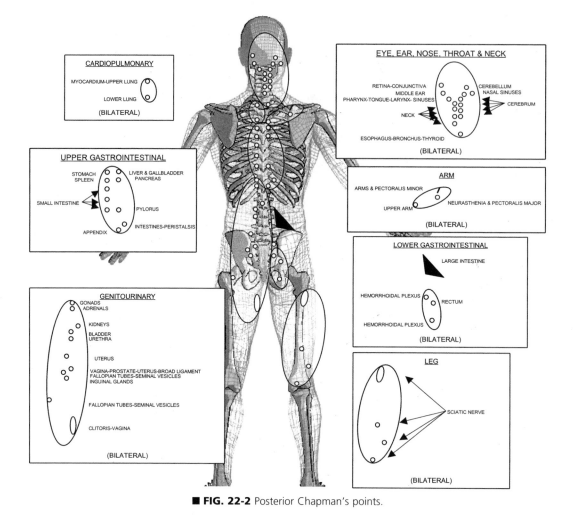

**■ FIG. 22-2** Posterior Chapman's points.

tion. Moreover, thyroid hormone has a sympatheticomimetic effect.

Excess adrenergic tone may lead to organic vasoconstriction. It is good to remember Still's admonition, "The rule of the artery is absolute, universal, and it must be unobstructed, or disease will result." Cortisol, secreted by the adrenal gland, may affect the thyroid by inhibiting TSH secretion. On an immune cellular level, lymphocytes are miniature producers of endocrine substances evidenced by the fact that they can secrete TSH in addition to progesterone, corticotrophin-releasing hormone (CRH), and adrenocorticotrophic hormone (ACTH). Each aspect of the neuroendocrine triad functions on a metabolic stillpoint, which promotes homeo-

static balance; for example, excess cortisol production is an immunosuppressant.

Chapman's reflexes for gonads can be located anteriorly along the upper border of the pubic bone, just lateral to the symphysis. Posteriorly, reflexes for the gonads are found between the spinous and transverse processes of T8 and T10, and T10 and T11, respectively. The anterior reflex for the adrenal gland is found 1 inch lateral and 2.5 inches superiorly from the umbilicus. The thyroid reflex resides in the second intercostal space, along the sternal border. The posterior point for the adrenal is located between the spinous process of T11 and the transverse process of T12. The posterior Chapman's reflex for the thyroid can be found along the transverse process of T2.

Chapman's reflex treatment is easy to administer; it is delivered rapidly and safely. Most importantly, Chapman's reflexes are effective in many of the systemic disorders encountered in the general practice of osteopathic medicine.

## REFERENCES

Arbuckle BE. *Reflexes, The Selected Writings of Beryl E. Arbuckle,* D.O., F.A.C.O.P. Indianapolis, IN: American Academy of Osteopathy, 1994 (revised edition).

Beal MC. Viscerosomatic reflexes: A review. *J Am Osteo Assoc* 1985.

Brown EA. Clinical Aspects of the Chapman's Reflexes. In: Northup TL, ed. *Academy of Applied Osteopathy Yearbook,* Ann Arbor, MI: Edwards Brothers, Inc, 1949.

DiGiovanna EL and Schiowitz S. *An Osteopathic Approach to Diagnosis and Treatment, 2nd ed.* Philadelphia: Lippincott-Raven, 1997.

Kuchera, ML, Kuchera WA. *Osteopathic Considerations in Systemic Dysfunction,* revised 2nd ed. Columbus, OH: Greyden Press, 1994.

Magoun HI. *Practical Osteopathic Procedures.* Kirksville, MO: The Journal Printing Company, 1978.

Mitchell Jr. FL. The Influence of Chapman's Reflexes and the Immune Reactions. In: Stark EH, ed. *Clinical Review Series in Osteopathic Medicine.* Acton, MA: Publishing Sciences Group, Inc, 1975.

Mitchell Jr. FL, Moran PS, Pruzzo NA. *An Evaluation and Treatment Manual of Osteopathic Muscle Energy Procedures.* Valley Park, MO: Mitchell, Moran, and Pruzzo, 1979.

Owens C. *An Endocrine Interpretation of Chapman's Reflexes* (1937). Carmel, CA: Academy of Applied Osteopathy, 1969 (reprint).

Patriquin DA. Chapman's Reflexes. In: Ward RC, ed. *Foundations for Osteopathic Medicine.* Baltimore: Williams and Wilkins, 1997.

Pottenger FM. *Symptoms of Visceral Disease,* seventh ed, St. Louis, MO: CV Mosby Co, 1953.

Sherwood L. *Human Physiology.* Belmont, CA: Wadsworth Publishing Company, 1997.

Soden CH. Lecture Notes on Chapman's Reflexes. In: Northup TL, ed. *Academy of Applied Osteopathy Yearbook.* Ann Arbor, MI: Edwards Brothers Inc, 1949

Still AT. *Autobiography of Andrew T. Still (1908).* Kirksville, MO: American Academy of Osteopathy, 2000 (reprint).

Thorpe RG. *Osteopathic Manipulative Therapy for Infections.* Osteopathic Annals. InsightPublishing Co, Inc, 1980.

Thorpe RG. *Psychodynamics of Stress and Relationships with the Musculoskeletal System, Osteopathic Annals.* Insight Publishing Co, Inc, 1973.

Truhlar RE. Doctor A.T. *Still in the Living.* Cleveland, OH: privately printed, 1950:54–55, 80–83.

Willard FH, Mokler DJ, Morgane PJ. Neuroendocrine-Immune System and Homeostasis. In: Ward RC, ed. *Foundations for Osteopathic Medicine.* Baltimore: Williams and Wilkins, 1997.

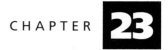

# Inhibition and Progressive Inhibition of Neuromusculoskeletal Structures (PINS) Techniques

*Dennis J. Dowling*

## ■ INHIBITION

Inhibition, as defined by the *Glossary of Osteopathic Terminology*, is "a term that describes steady pressure to soft tissues to effect relaxation and normalize reflex activity." This use of "steady pressure to soft tissues" is perhaps one of the earliest techniques of manual treatment. There may be other names used but the method is practically the same. Inhibition is most commonly performed by pressing the fingers or other body part against a region of the patient's body with a constant mild-to-moderate amount of force on regions of spasm or hypertonic muscle. Some have even used instruments of wood, plastic, rubber, stone, metal, or other substance as a means of either self-application or protecting the hand.

Initially, the patient may report pain, spasm, or decreased function, but one goal of the treatment is to decrease the tonicity of the muscles. Patient symptoms appear to be directly related to the amount of increased muscular tone. The larger, more superficial muscles are easily identified, especially when hypertonicity exists. Even though a patient can be in any position, having them lie supine or prone will facilitate the process. A muscle, such as the trapezius, can be easily palpated in the cervical, shoulder, and upper thoracic regions. The trapezius between the shoulder and neck can be grasped, or other

portions can be pressed or pinched. When in spasm, it is generally found to be firmer than normal muscle tissue. The patient may report an increase in sensitivity or tenderness. If the force is maintained at a constant pressure for a period of seconds to minutes, the sensitivity gradually decreases and the structures relax.

Inhibition is also theorized to affect other bodily structures and functions. There is a relationship between musculoskeletal structures and the viscera, via their common innervation from the spinal cord.

The skin and subcutaneous tissue in the region may have a "doughy" consistency and the pain sharp and throbbing when the change is acute. Over a period of time, the alterations reflect the chronicity such as fibrotic muscles and thinner, paler, and cooler skin. The spectrum of pain may range from insensitivity ("anesthetic") to altered sensitivity ("paresthesia") to hypersensitivity. Inhibitory pressure provided by the physician may initially result in a transitory increase in spasm or sensitivity followed by subsequent reduction of some or all of these components. If there is persistent visceral abnormality, then the results of inhibition at the somatic level may be short lived. When a musculoskeletal injury is the origin, a somatovisceral reflex may occur. Inhibitory treatment of the musculoskeletal structures may bring about longer lasting results.

Inhibition applied to the suboccipital and

sacral regions is directed at resetting parasympathetic activity. The parasympathetic system is the other half of the autonomic nervous system. Upgraded parasympathetic activity results in increased gastrointestinal motility, decreased sphincter closure, reduction of heart rate, constriction of pupils, and sleepiness among other reactions. Persistent conditions such as nausea, vomiting, diarrhea, dysmenorrhea, and dyspepsia are parasympathetic in nature. Dysfunction of the upper cervical, occipital, and sacral regions may reflect or result in inappropriate parasympathetic activity. Inhibitory treatment results in reduction of the more superficial musculoskeletal tone and congestion and by extension theoretically downregulates the more internal mechanisms.

Andrew Taylor Still, MD, had chronic headaches as a young man. Still treated himself with a rope swing. He lowered the rope to a few inches above the ground, slung a blanket across it, and then positioned himself with his neck, at the base of the skull, directly on the blanket. He subsequently fell asleep and when he awakened he felt refreshed and pain-free. This method may represent inhibition as well as a positional intervention. Dr. Still included some descriptions of both inhibition and stimulation methods in some of his early writings.

## ■ PROGRESSIVE INHIBITION OF NEUROMUSCULAR STRUCTURES

Progressive inhibition of neuromuscular structures (PINS) is a variant of "inhibition." The physician must, by monitoring throughout the procedure, note changes in the soft tissues caused by the dysfunction. There are instances when an osteopathic physician treats noticeable dysfunctions with many techniques but the problem persists. One part may be more noticeable to both the patient and the doctor because it is the more symptomatic, whereas the other, lesser component may be the initiator or maintainer of the dysfunction. These are factors that act to resist resetting or the treatment. A nexus exists to hold the pattern. This has been known within the profession colloquially and archaically as the *"key lesion."* In theory, treatment of this allowed the pattern of dysfunction to unravel. PINS is a

systematic approach using inhibition to discover and treat the anchor of dysfunction. As a more focused approach it is used to determine patterns of dysfunction. Theoretically, these dysfunctions are not just local but are a series or stream of components that persist.

The PINS system allows for versatility that is based on the physician's ability to use anatomical and clinical knowledge to determine treatment. A point is located in the region of the dysfunction. The primary point will exhibit sensitivity other than would be expected by the amount of pressure exerted. Then a related point within an underlying structure is also determined. The application of functional anatomy determines the course in selecting the next sensitive point. The physician's knowledge of the typical and variant courses of nerves, fascial bands, muscles, and other structures must be augmented by clinical decision-making skills for efficacy and accuracy. The physician exerts a mild amount of pressure progressively from one point to the other.

Patients participate in the PINS treatment by describing their response to sensitivity.

## Procedure

The development of an appropriate and specific diagnostic and treatment protocol using PINS requires the following:

1. Examination precedes treatment in all instances.
2. The components comprising a somatic dysfunction must be determined. The mnemonic "S-T-A-R" can be used to track the different aspects:

   [S]Sensitivity changes
   [T]Tissue texture changes
   [A]Asymmetry
   [R]Restriction of motion

3. A "primary sensitive" point is located by examination of the patient's symptom. If a significant one is not found, then the physician widens the search to contiguous areas.
4. Another point, designated as the "endpoint" is located distal or proximal to the primary point. If the primary point is at the origin of a muscle, the endpoint may be at the

insertion. The reverse can also be true. Sometimes the primary point is located in the belly of the muscle. In that case, both ends of the attachments to bone may reveal the location of an endpoint. Ligaments have points that are also fairly close to one another. The path between one point and another in fascia may seem to cross other structures. The more specialized the fascia, the more palpable and tendinous it is.

5. Some pathways follow superficial and deep pathways of nerves. The primary point can be found at the beginning of one nerve and the endpoint at the beginning of the other if more than one nerve innervates a region. Usually, the chosen primary point will most likely be nearer to the patient's symptoms. The endpoint may also elicit symptoms but to a lesser extent. At the two ends of the same problem, both and all intervening points must be addressed.

For the purpose of proceeding in a logical fashion, the point that is more sensitive is designated as the initial "primary." The other point, which is found on the other extreme, is considered as the "endpoint."

6. The physician establishes a muscular, fascial, and/or neurological pathway between the primary sensitive point and the endpoint. The primary-to-endpoint line may be curved, straight, or zigzag. The direction of treatment may be from distal to proximal, or proximal to distal.

7. A connection between the two points using knowledge of anatomy is drawn, especially:
   a. Nerve innervation
   b. Muscle origins and insertions
   c. Fascia
   d. Ligamentous attachments
   e. Bones (although the bones are the deepest of the musculoskeletal structures, they and their components should be considered as connective tissue as well)
   f. Vascular and lymphatic

8. Both the primary point and the endpoint are pressed simultaneously using a few ounces of pressure by a finger pad on each hand. The physician can identify the primary point as the "first point" for the patient. The pressure is enough to elicit the patient's symptoms and should be of equal amount. The patient may experience a mild to moderate increase in sensitivity initially, but this diminishes fairly rapidly. The physician should also determine the soft tissue response to pressure:
   a. Acute dysfunctions may be more sensitive than chronic ones. A hypertonic muscle will usually be more sensitive to pressure than the contralateral muscle.
   b. The longer that a muscle has been hypertonic, the larger that muscle will be compared to the contralateral side.
   c. Larger muscles do not necessarily indicate dysfunction but size does indicate use.
   d. Hypertonic muscles that have been so for some time may not be quite so sensitive to pressure. A more sensitive but less hypertonic muscle indicates a problem. This does not necessarily indicate the laterality of the problem. Both sides can be dysfunctional. The physician should initially treat the more dysfunctional tissue, re-examine, and treat the less involved side as well.
   e. The patient should be in a comfortable position.

9. The pressure exerted on both the primary and endpoints should be equal. Patients should be reassured that the reason for the asymmetry is the apparent dysfunction or hyperactivity of the involved tissue.

10. The physician maintains constant pressure on the endpoint throughout the treatment.
   a. Another finger is used to locate a "secondary point." If the index finger is on the primary point, then the middle finger can be used to palpate the secondary point.
   b. A secondary point is generally found approximately 2 to 3 centimeters away from the primary point into the direction of the endpoint. The physician can identify the secondary point as "the second point" for the patient. This will typically follow the predicted course of an anatomical structure (innervating nerve, along the direction of the muscle fibers, or following fascial planes).

11. Equal pressure is exerted onto both the primary and secondary points while maintaining pressure on the endpoint.
12. The patient cooperates by informing the physician as to which of the two points (primary versus secondary or "first versus second") is more sensitive. The physician can state, "I am pressing on two points that are close together. Please tell me which of the two, the "first" (physician may move the finger slightly) or the "second," is more sensitive.
13. If the second point is more or equally sensitive as compared to the first:
    a. Pressure is relieved and removed from the first point (primary);
    b. Constant pressure is maintained on the second (secondary), sensitive point for 20 to 30 seconds.
    c. The sensitivity at any point does not have to be completely gone before moving to the next point. It is important that the next point is more sensitive.
    d. The initial pressure on a new "secondary" point will usually cause a response of increased tension and sensitivity. This usually returns to baseline after a few seconds, as noted. The amount of time depends on the soft tissue response.
       There are a few considerations if the primary point persists as the more sensitive of the two contiguous points:
    e. Maintain pressure at the location of the primary point.
    f. The physician moves the finger pressing on the secondary point more laterally or medially. A point may be found that has more or the same sensitivity as the primary point by searching slightly out of line with the targeted endpoint (the anatomical structure, which is being inhibited, may have slight variations in the specific course in this individual).
    g. Once a secondary point that is equally or more sensitive is located, pressure is released from the primary point and maintained on the new secondary point as described.

    h. The secondary point then becomes the new "first" point in the continuing sequence of treatment toward the endpoint.
14. Before searching or inhibiting any subsequent points, the physician should wait approximately 20 to 30 seconds.
15. If no secondary point can be located despite searching in a 2-centimeter radius from the primary point, then the clinician maintains pressure on the primary point (or the new "primary" point) for an additional 30 seconds. Sometimes, certain points require further inhibition before progress can be made. After doing so, a new secondary point may be located where previously there was less sensitivity.
16. The endpoint receives inhibition throughout and up to the end of the treatment. Often the patient will forget that this point is being inhibited and it may lose all sensitivity.
17. The process is continued successively until the ultimate "second" point is 2 centimeters from the endpoint.
18. Once there are the two final points being inhibited, the physician determines the amount of dysfunction that persists at the end and secondary point locations. It may have reduced or disappeared totally.
19. If the dysfunction, including the endpoint persists, the physician can choose to treat the dysfunction with another modality. *PINS* technique can be the sole approach to the somatic dysfunctions that were found or can be used in conjunction with any other modality of osteopathic manipulative treatment. Determining this is:
    a. The persistence of the dysfunction or related components after treatment.
    b. The ability of the physician to perform other modalities of treatment.
    c. The need or capability of the patient to accept additional treatment.
20. Some soreness or other symptom may persist despite sufficient treatment. The physician should determine termination of treatment based on the findings for the individual. It should not be based on the

patient's subjective symptoms. Overtreatment can cause as many problems as undertreatment.

21. The somatic dysfunction is always reassessed.
22. The patient should be advised that despite the relative comfort of the treatment, there may be a post-treatment reaction. These reactions are relatively minor, transient, and self-limited, and generally consist of soreness, aching, and/or fatigue. In patients prone to bruising, or when there are certain other predisposing factors (i.e., medication), ecchymoses can occur. This can also occur if excessive pressure has been used. Generally, all of these side effects will resolve in 24 to 48 hours.

The patterns presented within this book are only examples. The optimum approach is for the osteopathic physician to use the principles presented herein and apply them to the patient rather than memorize specific patterns. However, some patterns are consistently found. This may be caused by typical habits of activity that result in the same or similar findings and results across groups of patients.

## REFERENCES

Dowling DJ, Scariati PD. Neurophysiology relevant to osteopathic principles and practice. In: DiGiovanna, Schiowitz, eds. *An Osteopathic Approach to Diagnosis and Treatment,* 2nd ed. Philadelphia: Lippincott-Raven, 1997:33.

Dowling DJ, S.T.A.R.: a more viable alternative descriptor system of somatic dysfunction, *The AAO Journal* 1998; 8(2):34–37.

Dowling DJ. Progressive inhibition of neuromuscular structures (PINS) technique. *J Am Osteopath Assoc* 2000;100: 285–286, 289–298.

Dowling DJ. Progressive inhibition of neuromuscular structures (PINS) technique. In: Chaitow L. *Modern Neuromuscular Techniques.* Edinburgh: Churchill Livingstone, 2003:225–250.

Dowling DJ. Progressive inhibition of neuromuscular structures (PINS) technique. In Ward RC, ed. *Foundations for Osteopathic Medicine,* 2nd ed. Philadelphia: Lippincott Williams & Wilkins, 2003.

Educational Council on Osteopathis Principles. *Glossary of Osteopathic Terminology.* Chicago: AOA Yearbook and Directory of Osteopathic Physicians, 1998.

Ehrenfeuchter WC. Soft tissue techniques. In: Ward RC, ed. *Foundations for Osteopathic Medicine.* Baltimore: Williams & Wilkins, 1997:781–794.

Still AT. *The Philosophy and Mechanical Principles of Osteopathy.* Kansas City, MO: Hudson-Kimberly Pub. Co, 1902: 101.

Still AT. *Autobiography of A. T. Still, revised ed.* Kirksville, MO: Published by the author, 1908:32.

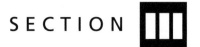

# Cervical Spine

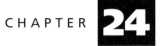

# CHAPTER 24

# Cervical Anatomic Considerations

*Stanley Schiowitz and Jonathon Fenton*

The cervical spine articulates at its cephalic end with the skull at the occipitoatlantal articulation and at its caudal end with the first thoracic vertebra. As a total unit, it has extreme mobility, with the mid-cervical articulations able to approach subluxation. The cervical spine is made up of seven cervical vertebrae. Functionally, it is divided into two areas: the articulations between the occiput, atlas, and axis, and the articulations between the third through seventh cervical vertebrae.

## ■ OCCIPITOATLANTAL JOINT

The occipitoatlantal articulation consists of the superior articular facets of the atlas and the two occipital condyles. The superior facets of the atlas face backward, upward, and medially, and are concave in both anteroposterior and transverse diameters. The surfaces of the occipital condyles match the facets of the atlas, and the joint is best thought of as a sphere (the occiput) gliding on the articular surfaces of the atlas (Fig. 24-1). The freely movable occiput is limited by its muscular and ligamentous attachments, which make flexion–extension the primary motion, producing a small-amplitude nodding of the head. Flexion of the occiput on the atlas is accompanied by a posterior translatory slide of the occiput; extension is accompanied by an anterior translatory slide.

Side-bending and rotation of the occipitoatlantal joint always occur in opposite directions, in part because of the position of the lateral atlanto-occipital ligament. When the occiput rotates left on the atlas, the lateral atlanto-occipital ligament causes the occiput to slide (translate) to the left and therefore side-bend to the right (Fig. 24-2). Somatic dysfunctions of the occipitoatlantal joint most often involve the minor motions of side-bending with contralateral rotation.

## ■ ATLANTOAXIAL JOINT

The atlantoaxial articulation is specially adapted for (nearly) pure rotation. In addition to the inferior articular facets of the atlas and the superior articular facets of the axis, movement other than rotation is limited by the anteriorly located odontoid process (dens) of the axis. The odontoid process is held close to the anterior arch of the atlas by the transverse ligament of the atlas, which allows only a slight amount of flexion of the atlas on the axis.

There is no true lateral flexion at the atlantoaxial joint, only a wobble created by the articulation of the superior axial and inferior atlantal articular facets. Unlike most facets, these four facets are all convex in shape (Fig. 24-3). During rotation of the atlas on the axis to the right, the left articular facet of the atlas in effect slides uphill on the left articular facet of the axis, while on the right the atlas slides downhill on the axis. This wobble motion is not true lateral flexion.

Somatic dysfunction at the atlantoaxial joint occurs in rotation.

The complex of the occipitoatlantal plus the atlantoaxial joints is known as the *suboccipital*

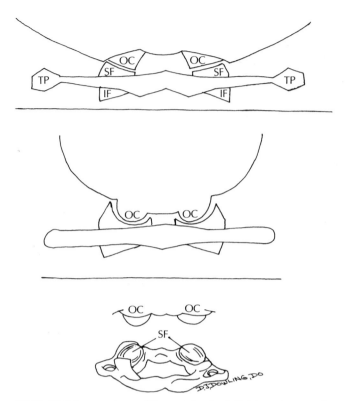

■ **FIG. 24-1** Bony anatomy of the occipitoatlantal joint, posterosuperior view. OC, occipital condyl; SF, superior facet; IF, inferior facet; TP, transverse process.

*articulation.* Its range of motion makes it function as a universal (swivel) joint. Many consider the suboccipital articulation the final compensator of the spine, by which the body adjusts to any dysfunctions occurring below. Compensatory adjustment is needed to keep the eyes level in two planes and to promote binocular vision.

The articulation between the second (C2) and third (C3) cervical vertebrae sustains tremendous stress because of its position between the final compensator above and the rest of the spine below. Therefore, it is a common location for chronic somatic dysfunction. These are usually compensatory to structural imbalance that has occurred below it. These imbal-

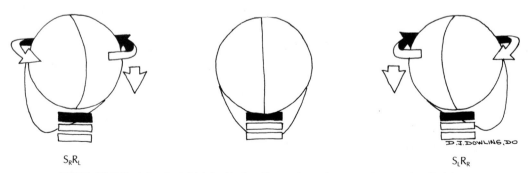

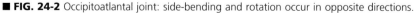

■ **FIG. 24-2** Occipitoatlantal joint: side-bending and rotation occur in opposite directions.

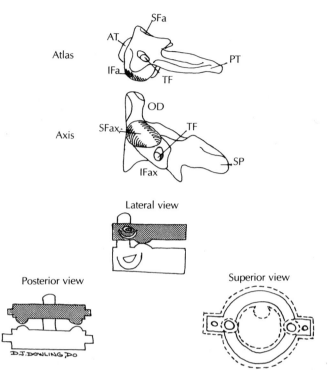

■ **FIG. 24-3** Atlantoaxial articulation. AT, anterior tubercle; PT, posterior tubercle; TF, transverse foramen; SP, spinous process; Ifa, inferior facet of axis; Sfa, superior facet of atlas; Sfax, superior facet of axis.

ances must be corrected to resolve the C2–C3 somatic dysfunction.

## Third to Seventh Cervical Vertebrae (C3–C7)

This portion of the cervical spine allows for a great deal of motion, with special adaptation to meet the demands of mobility and stability placed upon it. The cervical intervertebral disks are the relatively thickest of the spinal disks; the ratio of disk height to vertebral body height in this section of the spinal column is 2:5. The disks are wedge-shaped and thicker anteriorly than posteriorly (Fig. 24-4). In conjunction with the anteroposterior convexity of the vertebral endplates, the wedge shape maintains the flexible cervical lordosis.

The facet joints in this area are located posterolaterally. Two articulating facets, one superior and one inferior, form the palpable articu-

lar pillars. The superior articular facets face backward and upward. The plane of the facet joints lies midway between the horizontal and frontal planes in normal lordosis (Fig. 24-5). This orientation causes rotation and side-bending to be coupled motions, normally occurring in the same direction. When the cervical spine is placed in a more backward bending position, the facets are more oriented in the frontal plane, where side-bending is the primary mo-

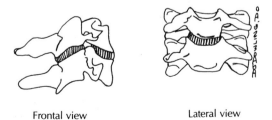

Frontal view        Lateral view

■ **FIG. 24-4** Cervical intervertebral disk between C3 and C4.

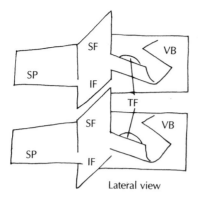

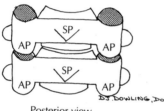

**■ FIG. 24-5** Orientation of articular facets of C3 and C4 vertebrae. SP, spinous process; SF, superior facet; IF, inferior facet; VB, vertebral body; AP, articular pillar; TF, transverse foramina.

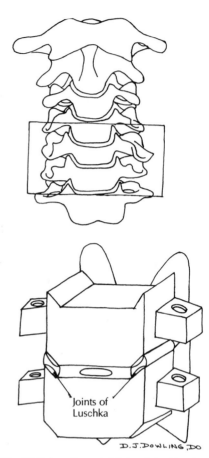

**■ FIG. 24-6** Location of joints of Lushka (unciform joints), anterior view.

tion. When the neck is brought into a forward bending position, the plane of the facets becomes more horizontal, and rotation is the major motion.

The cervical vertebrae C3 to C7 move least in flexion-extension. In flexion the inferior articular facets of the upper vertebrae must slide up the superior articular facets of the lower vertebrae, up a 45-degree incline. The normal lordotic curve in this area places the cervical spine in partial extension; the cervical spine has no neutral position.

To assist in maintaining some measure of stability in the face of the large amounts of motion possible in the mid-cervical spine, a specialized set of synovial joints has developed as an adaptation for upright posture in humans. These joints, known as the *unciform* joints or the *joints of Luschka,* are located on the lateral edges of the cervical vertebral bodies (Fig. 24-6). The lateral lips of two adjacent vertebrae articulate and are contained within a small

synovial capsule. These joints develop at age 8 to 10 years.

The unciform joints (joints of Luschka) act as guide rails for the motions of flexion–extension. They also limit the lateral translatory motion (side slip) that occurs simultaneously with the coupled motions of side-bending and rotation. When one vertebra side-bends and rotates on another, that vertebra will translate laterally in the opposite direction. In the cervical spine, this lateral translatory motion would be excessive to the point of subluxation were it not for the unciform joints.

Somatic dysfunctions in the C3 to C7 joints occur in the coupled rotary motions of side-bending and rotation, and in lateral translation. Dysfunctions of translatory motion that accompany rotary dysfunctions create a complicated dysfunction, *side slip.*

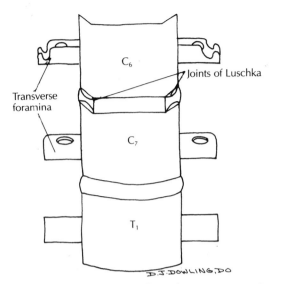

■ **FIG. 24-7** Seventh cervical vertebra. Note anatomic similarity superiorly to sixth cervical vertebra and inferiorly to first thoracic vertebra.

## Seventh Cervical–First Thoracic Joint (C7–T1)

The anatomy of the seventh cervical vertebra is transitional, resembling cervical vertebral anatomy superiorly and thoracic vertebral anatomy inferiorly (Fig. 24-7). At the cervicothoracic (C7–T1) junction, cervical lordosis normally ends and thoracic kyphosis begins. As a result, the forces placed on this area are quite complex and of a different nature from forces sustained higher or lower in the spine. Somatic dysfunction of the cervicothoracic junction is quite common and difficult to treat. Dysfunctions in these articulations will often involve the first ribs.

### REFERENCES

Fryette H. *Principles of Osteopathic Techniques.* Carmel, CA: Academy of Applied Osteopathy, 1954.

Kapandjii IA. *The Physiology of the Joints, Vol 3. The Trunk and Vertebral Column.* Edinburgh: Churchill Livingston, 1973.

Schiowitz S, DiGiovanna E. *An Osteopathic Approach to Diagnosis and Treatment.* Philadelphia: Lippencott-Raven, 1997.

Warwick RW. *Grays Anatomy. 35th British Ed.* Philadelphia: W.B. Saunders, 1973.

White A, Panjabi MM. *Biomechanics of the Spine.* Philadelphia: J.B. Lipincott, 1978.

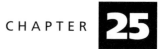

# Evaluation of the Cervical Spine

*Eileen L. DiGiovanna*

Evaluation of the cervical spine begins with a history of the patient's symptom and a thorough examination of the patient. A history of trauma to the neck is especially important. Pain and decreased range of motion are the most common complaints relative to the cervical spine.

## ■ OBSERVATION

The physician should observe the position in which the patient's head is carried—forward or back of the shoulders, tilted to one side, or rotated with the chin away from the midline. The lordotic curve should be inspected for an increased lordosis or a flattening of the curve.

Any evidence of trauma, such as bruising, abrasions, or lacerations, should be noted, as should scars that may indicate an old injury or surgery of the neck.

The physician should be aware of the manner in which the patient moves in general, with special attention given to the cervical spine when the symptom is relative to that region.

## ■ GROSS MOTION TESTING

Gross motion of the cervical spine is tested with the patient in a seated position and the physician standing behind him or to his side. Each direction of motion is tested while monitoring at the cervicothoracic junction (between C7 and T1) or at the distal shoulder.

### Forward Bending (Flexion)

1. The physician places one hand on the patient's head and the other monitors the cervicothoracic junction (Fig. 25-1).

2. The head is gently pushed forward until motion is felt at the monitoring finger or the patient's chin touches the manubrium.
3. Purely cervical motion ends when there is upward motion felt at the cervicothoracic junction.
4. The angle of displacement from the upright position is noted. This should normally be 80 to 90 degrees.

### Backward Bending (Extension)

1. The physician places one hand on the patient's forehead and the other monitors at the cervicothoracic junction (Fig. 25-2).
2. The head is gently pushed backward until motion is felt at the monitoring finger.
3. Purely cervical motion ends when there is downward motion felt at the cervicothoracic junction.
4. The angle of displacement from the upright position is noted. This is usually 45 degrees.

### Side-Bending

1. The physician places one hand on the side of the patient's head and the other monitors at the cervicothoracic junction or at the lateral shoulder (Fig. 25-3).
2. The head is gently pulled to one side and the angle of displacement from the upright position is noted. Purely cervical motion ends when there is upward motion felt at the contralateral shoulder. The hands are reversed and the head is moved to the opposite side and that angle of displacement is noted. This

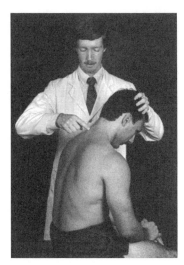

■ **FIG. 25-1** Gross motion testing of the cervical spine, forward bending.

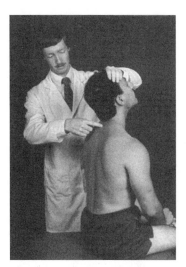

■ **FIG. 25-2** Gross motion testing of the cervical spine, backward bending.

is normally 40 to 45 degrees. The two angles should be compared for a restriction in one direction or in both directions.

## Rotation

1. The physician places one hand on the left frontal area and the other monitors at the cervicothoracic junction (Fig. 25-4).
2. The head is rotated to the right and the degree of rotation is noted.

3. Purely cervical motion ends when there is forward motion felt at the contralateral shoulder.
4. The hands are reversed with one hand on the right frontal area and other monitoring at the cervicothoracic junction.
5. The head is then rotated to the left and the degree of rotation is noted, normally 45 to 60 degrees.
6. The two sides are compared for a restriction in one or both directions.

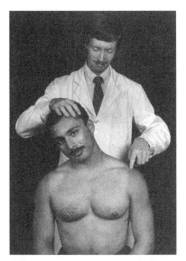

■ **FIG. 25-3** Gross motion testing of the cervical spine, side-bending.

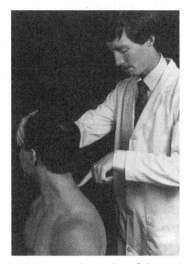

■ **FIG. 25-4** Gross motion testing of the cervical spine, rotation.

## ■ PALPATION

Although palpation may be performed with the patient seated, it is best to have the patient supine. This allows relaxation of the postural muscles of the neck, making it easier to palpate more deeply. The physician is then seated at the head of the table.

The physician palpates superficially at first and then more deeply into the tissues. The texture of the tissues is evaluated including bogginess, ropiness, or a change in tone of the muscles. Although the tissues posteriorly are being evaluated for an indication of the presence of somatic dysfunction, the anterior neck tissues should be evaluated as well. The scalene muscles and the sternocleidomastoid muscles can give important clues regarding cervical pain or motion restriction.

The physician will also note any asymmetry of position of the articular pillars of the spine. In the cervical spine, the transverse processes are small and deep to the articular pillars, making them less valuable as diagnostic landmarks. Thus the articular pillars are palpated for this purpose.

Occasionally, severe arthritic changes around the facet joints may be palpable. The physician will also note any masses, such as cysts or lipomas, that may be palpated.

## ■ INTERSEGMENTAL RANGE OF MOTION TESTING

In the evaluation of the cervical spine for somatic dysfunction, the intersegmental motion between vertebrae is extremely important. There are several ways the cervical spine may be tested for individual vertebral motion. For all these methods, the patient will be supine with the physician seated at the head of the table.

### Intersegmental Motion Testing

I. Occipitoatlantal Joint (O-A)
  1. The physician cups the occiput in his hands and slides his fingers into the occipital sulcus lateral to the midline (Fig. 25-5).
  2. The physician will evaluate the depth of the sulci bilaterally. A sulcus that is shal-

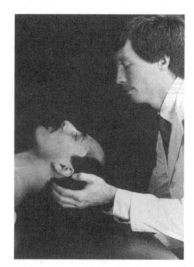

■ **FIG. 25-5** Intersegmental motion testing of the occipitoatlantal joint.

low when compared with the opposite one indicates side-bending of the occiput to that side.
  3. The head is then bent forward and the depth of the sulci is noted.
  4. The head is then bent backward and the depth of the sulci is noted.
  5. The change in the depth of the sulci is compared in flexion and extension of the occiput. The position in which the sulci are most symmetrical is the freedom of motion and the position in which the sulci are most asymmetrical is the restriction.

Example: If the right sulcus is deeper than the left and its depth increases with flexion and the two sulci are most symmetrical in extension of the occiput, the diagnosis is O-A E $S_L R_R$. Conversely, if the right sulcus is deeper than the left and its depth increases with extension and the two sulci are most symmetrical in flexion, the diagnosis is O-A F $S_L R_R$.

II. Atlanto-axial Joint (A-A)
  1. The physician cups the patient's head in the palm of his hand and slides his fingers along the occipital sulcus laterally until he palpates the tips of the mastoid processes. Tissue texture changes are noted. Then he moves his fingers just inferior and lateral to them and onto the

tips of the transverse processes of the atlas, which lie between the tips of the mastoid processes and the angles of the jaw (Fig. 25-6).

2. The patient is instructed to nod his head forward, thus locking the O-A joint.
3. The physician then rotates the head to the right and to the left to test the freedom of rotation of the A-A joint. The range of rotational motion is compared bilaterally for symmetry. Any decrease on one side compared to the other indicates a restriction in rotation of the A-A joint.

Example: If the head rotates more freely to the right than to the left, the diagnosis is A-A $R_R$. If the head rotates more freely to the left, the diagnosis is A-A $R_L$.

**III.** C2 Through C7

1. The physician cups the patient's head in the palms of his hands and places a monitoring finger of each hand on the articular pillar of the vertebra being evaluated. These are best palpated in the groove between the paravertebral muscle masses.
2. C2–C3 is approximately 1 cm below the occipital sulcus.
3. The patient is asked to side-bend the head in each direction and the palpating

fingers will be able to identify the sliding motion. If there is an asymmetry such that one articular pillar is more posterior than the other, it will indication a rotation to that side.

4. Motion-testing side-bending (Fig. 25-7) Maintaining contact with the articular pillars, introduce side-bending until motion is felt at the fingertips.
   a. Note the displacement of the head from the midline.
   b. Greater motion to one side than the other indicates a side-bending restriction on the side of the decreased motion. Note the fluidity and amount of motion.
5. Flexion/Extension (Fig. 25-8)
   a. Maintaining firm contact with the articular pillars, flex the neck until motion is felt at the segment being tested.
   b. Return the neck to a neutral position and then extend the neck until motion is palpated with the monitoring finger at the involved segment.
   c. Note any asymmetry of motion at the segment. If the motion is restricted in flexion, it is an extension dysfunction. If motion is restricted in extension, it is a flexion dysfunction.

## Rotoscoliosis Motion Testing

When a cervical vertebra side-bends, it also rotates in the same direction. A somatic dysfunction will exhibit restrictions in side-bending and

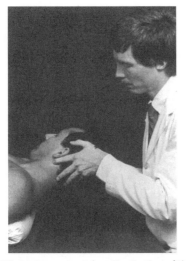

■ **FIG. 25-6** Intersegmental motion testing of the atlantoaxial joint.

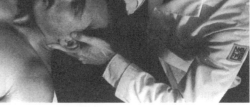

■ **FIG. 25-7** Intersegmental motion testing of C2 through C7, side-bending.

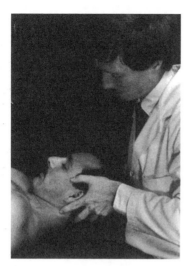

■ **FIG. 25-8** Intersegmental motion testing of C2 through C7, flexion-extension.

rotation in the same directions except in unusual circumstances, which are usually traumatic in nature, as well as in flexion or extension. Rotoscoliosis is a method of motion testing that used this principle for diagnostic purposes. For this method, the patient is supine and the physician is seated comfortably at the head of the table.

1. C2 through C7
   a. The physician cups the patient's head in the palms of his hands and places one finger of each hand on the involved articular pillars.
   b. The physician flexes the patient's head and neck until motion is felt at the palpating finger.
   c. If the posteriorly rotated articular pillar becomes more posterior, the vertebra has restricted motion in flexion. This also confirms freedom of rotation.
   d. The head and neck are then extended until motion is felt at the palpating finger. If the pillars become more symmetrical, this confirms that the restriction is in flexion and the freedom of motion is in extension.
   e. Example: If the posteriorly rotated articular pillar of C4 was palpated on the right and the rotation became worse in flexion and more symmetrical in extension, the diagnosis would be C4 $ES_RR_R$.

2. Atlantoaxial Motion Testing
   The atlantoaxial joint never leaves the neutral position, because extension is limited by bony apposition and the odontoid ligament limits flexion. Therefore, the major motion of this joint is rotation.
   a. The physician cups the patient's occiput in the palms of his hands.
   b. The patient's neck is fully flexed, locking all the cervical vertebrae to prevent motion of the vertebral column below the atlantoaxial joint.
   c. While maintaining full flexion, the head is rotated to the right and to the left and a comparison of fluidity and amount of motion is noted. (Fig. 25-9).
   d. Example: If rotation is greater to the right than to the left, the diagnosis would be AA $R_R$.

## Translatory Motion Testing

Rotoscoliosis motion testing evaluates the rotation of the vertebrae. Translatory motion testing evaluates side-bending motion. Lateral translation of the vertebra is coupled with side-bending in the opposite direction. Translatory motion of C4 toward the right is coupled with side-bending of C4 to the left. For most cervical vertebrae, side-bending and rotation are coupled and occur

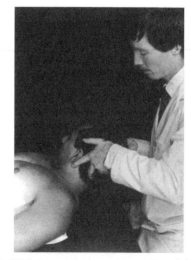

■ **FIG. 25-9** Rotoscoliosis motion testing of the atlantoaxial joint.

in the same direction. These principles can be used to evaluate the ability of the cervical vertebrae to move. A common mistake is to observe increased tissue tension at the finger introducing translation and interpret that as a barrier. Often, there is increased tissue response over a posterior articular pillar, because that is the side-bending and rotation side. The direct pressure from the translating finger may cause an increase in tissue tension, which the inexperienced examiner may erroneously take as meeting the barrier. The focus must be on the deeper articular response and the amount or asymmetry of motion is the determination when performing Translatory testing in the cervical region. Translatory motion testing is performed with the patient supine and the physician seated comfortably at the head of the table.

1. C2 through C7
   a. The physician cups the patient's occiput in the palms of his hands and places a monitoring finger of each hand bilaterally on the articular pillars of the segment to be tested.
   b. The physician uses the monitoring finger of his right hand to push the vertebra in a lateral translation to the left. He then pushes the vertebra in a lateral translation to the right. This translatory motion creates side-bending of the vertebra to the opposite side (Fig. 25-10).
   c. Example: If C4 is translated towards the right, it will side-bend to the left and rotate to the left.

d. The physician notes the ease and amount of translation. The two sides are compared.
e. The physician then flexes the patient's neck until motion is felt at the monitoring fingers and repeats the translatory push to each side, comparing the two.
f. The physician then extends the patient's neck until motion is felt at the monitoring fingers and repeats the translatory push to each side, comparing the two.
g. Example: If the translation of C4 is equal bilaterally with the neck flexed but a restriction is felt when pushing to the right when the neck is extended, the diagnosis would be C4 $FS_LR_L$. Remember that the motions will be symmetrical in the directions of the somatic dysfunction and restrictions will be felt in the opposite directions.

2. Occipitoatlantal Joint
   a. The physician cups the patient's occiput in the palms of his hands while placing a monitoring finger of each hand bilaterally in the occipital sulci.
   b. The neck is flexed slightly until motion is felt at the monitoring fingers.
   c. The head is moved laterally to the left and to the right. Translation to the right is coupled with side-bending to the left (Fig. 25-11).

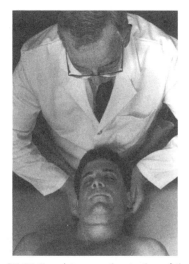

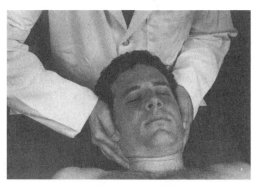

■ **FIG. 25-10** Translatory motion testing of C2 through C7.

■ **FIG. 25-11** Translatory motion testing of the occipitoatlantal joint.

d. Side-bending to the left is coupled with rotation of the occiput to the right.

e. Interpretation: Because rotation is opposite to side-bending at the occipitoatlantal joint, there are four possible designations for the somatic dysfunction found: OA $FS_RR_L$, OA $FS_LR_R$, OA $ES_RR_L$, and OA $ES_LR_R$.

f. Example: If there is normal translation to the left in flexion and decreased translation to the left in extension, the somatic dysfunction is designated OA $FS_LR_R$ (occiput restricted in right side-bending and left rotation while in the extended position).

## Neurologic Testing

Impingement of cervical nerve roots is often the cause of numbness or paresthesias of the upper extremities. When nerve root involvement is suspected, a neurologic evaluation is essential. Because only C5 through C8 innervate the arm, they will be the nerve roots evaluated in a neurologic examination. Motor weakness of the intrinsic muscles of the neck will assist in identifying impingement of motor nerves to the cervical spine. Muscle strength testing of the muscles of the upper extremity is also useful in the neurologic evaluation. Sensory testing can be performed over the following areas of the upper extremity:

1. C5—lateral arm
2. C6—lateral forearm, thumb, index finger, and the lateral half of the middle finger
3. C7—middle finger
4. C8—medial forearm, fourth and fifth fingers

The deep tendon reflexes of the upper extremities indicate the integrity of some of the cervical nerve roots.

1. C5—Biceps reflex, tested on the biceps tendon at the elbow (also has a small component of C6)
2. C6—Brachioradialis reflex, tested on the tendon of the brachioradialis in the forearm just proximal to the wrist.
3. C7—Triceps reflex, tested on the triceps tendon over the posterior olecranon process

**REFERENCES**

DiGiovanna EL. Schiowitz S. *An Osteopathic Approach to Diagnosis and Treatment.* Philadelphia: Lippincott-Raven, 1997.

Fryette H. *Principles of Osteopathic Technique.* Colorado, CO: American Academy of Osteopathy, 1954.

Hoppenfeld S. *Physical Examination of the Spine and Extremities.* Norwalk, CT: Appleton-Lange, 1976.

Kapandji IA. *The Physiology of the Joints , Vol 3. The Trunk and the Vertebral Column,* Edinburgh: Churchill-Livingstone, 1974.

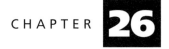

# Myofascial Techniques

*Toni Spinaris and Eileen L. DiGiovanna*

This chapter describes *passive, direct active, and indirect active myofascial techniques* used to treat cervical somatic dysfunction as well as muscle or fascial tension in the cervical region. These techniques may entail a passive linear or perpendicular stretch of the neck muscles or an active use of neuromuscular methods to create relaxation of the suboccipital and paravertebral muscles.

## ■ PASSIVE TECHNIQUES

*Passive techniques* are performed by the physician on a relaxed patient. The purpose of the passive techniques described is to place a stretch on the posterior extensor muscles of the cervical region. The stretch must be slowly applied and slowly released to prevent activation of the Golgi organ tendon reflex. When performed in this manner, the stretched muscles tend to relax and the tone of the muscle is returned to a more normal state.

### Linear Traction Applied to Suboccipital Muscles

1. **Patient position:** supine.
2. **Physician position:** standing or seated at the head of the table.
3. **Technique:**
   a. The physician cups her palms to support the patient's occiput.
   b. The physician's fingers are placed in the occipital sulcus bilaterally.
   c. For best results, the patient's neck should be straight or bent slightly forward.
   d. The physician's elbows should be in near or full extension, so that they can be used as long levers. This position allows the physician to use her weight as the force of traction, by rocking backward on her feet or, if seated, on her buttocks, rather than relying on upper body strength (Fig. 26-1).
   e. The traction is slowly and uniformly applied, maintained for a few seconds, and slowly released.
   f. The technique may be repeated without repositioning of the physician's fingers.
4. Hints for performing technique:
   a. The physician's feet should be placed far enough from the table so that she may rock back and thus apply traction without changing her stance. If seated, move the stool back from the table to allow body motion.
   b. The physician should avoid creating friction by sliding her fingers over the patient's skin. This is uncomfortable for the patient.
   c. See that the patient is comfortable and relaxed.
   d. This technique may be performed from a seated position as well (Fig. 26-2).

### Suboccipital Technique

A similar technique can be used in the suboccipital region. In this technique, the physician's fingers stretch the tissues of the occipital sulcus laterally as linear traction is applied.

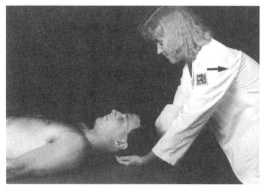

■ **FIG. 26-1** Linear stretch with the physician standing.

1. **Patient position:** supine.
2. **Physician position:** seated at the head of the table.
3. **Technique:**
   a. The physician places her index and middle fingers in the occipital sulcus bilaterally but medially so that the middle fingers meet at the midline.
   b. The occiput is cupped in the physician's palms.
   c. The patient's neck is maintained in a straight or slightly forward bent position.
   d. The physician applies linear traction slowly by rocking back on her buttocks.
   e. Maintaining linear traction, the physician rolls her finger laterally away from the

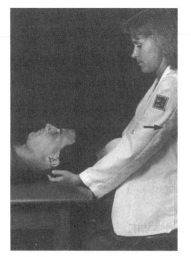

■ **FIG. 26-2** Linear stretch with the physician seated.

midline. With the longitudinal axis of the forearm as the rotational axis, the fingers remain in the occipital sulcus but gradually roll out laterally.
   f. The physician's wrist, forearm, hand, and fingers are maintained in straight alignment and work as a single unit.
   g. The technique may be repeated as needed.

## Linear Traction Applied to Lower Cervical Muscles

1. **Patient position:** supine.
2. **Physician position:** standing or sitting at the head of the table.
3. **Technique:**
   a. The physician places her fingers on the patient's posterior neck muscles bilaterally at any cervical level and maintains a firm contact.
   b. The physician applies a linear traction force to the musculature, slowly and uniformly, by rocking back on her feet or buttocks.
   c. The patient's neck is held straight or slightly forward bent as the traction is applied.
   d. Slowly release by rocking forward.
   e. Some perpendicular stretch may be added by pushing the fingers ventrally while maintaining the traction.

## Linear Stretch to Posterior Cervical Muscles

1. **Patient position:** supine.
2. **Physician position:** standing or sitting at the head of the table.
3. **Technique:**
   a. The physician cradles the occiput in one hand and cups the patient's chin with the other hand (Fig. 26-3).
   b. The physician applies a linear traction force along the longitudinal axis of the cervical spine with the hand holding the occiput. The hand cupping the chin is primarily used to stabilize the neck and hold it slightly bent forward. The main force of traction is applied to the occiput.
   c. This may be repeated as necessary until the muscles soften.

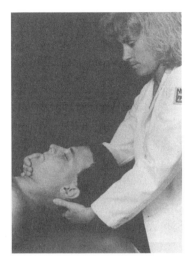

■ **FIG. 26-3** Linear stretch of posterior extensor neck muscles, cupping the chin.

## Perpendicular Stretch of Muscles

1. **Patient position:** supine.
2. **Physician position:** standing at the patient's side opposite the side to be treated.
3. **Technique:**
   a. The physician places one hand on the patient's forehead to act as a stabilizing counterforce to the treating hand.
   b. The physician places her other hand across the patient's body and grasps the posterior cervical muscles of the opposite side (Fig. 26-4).

c. A gentle stretch is applied to the muscle body by pulling it away from the spinous processes laterally and ventrally.
d. The stretch is maintained for a few seconds, and then slowly released. The maneuver may be repeated as needed. The hand stretching the muscles may move up and down the cervical spine.
e. Additional stretch may be achieved by rotating the patient's head away while pulling on the muscle.

## Bilateral Linear Stretch Applied to Both Ends of Muscle

1. **Patient position:** supine.
2. **Physician position:** standing at the head of the table.
3. **Technique:**
   a. The physician crosses her forearms under the patient's occiput and neck so that the patient's head is fully supported on the physician's forearms and the physician's hands are pressing down on the patient's contralateral shoulders (Fig. 26-5).
   b. The physician gently and slowly lifts her arms, creating a lever-fulcrum effect that puts linear traction on both ends of the muscles. The patient's neck should be bent forward to a comfortable position of

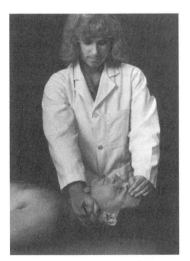

■ **FIG. 26-4** Unilateral perpendicular stretch.

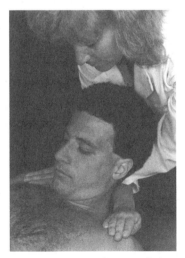

■ **FIG. 26-5** Crossed arms technique.

maximum stretch. Careful control of the force must be used.

c. This position is held for a few seconds and slowly brought back to neutral.

d. When repeating the technique, the physician should bend the neck forward a bit more than the previous time. Each repetition of the technique should increase the range of motion.

4. **Modification—active direct technique:**

a. While the physician is fully supporting the head at the maximal stretch, she may ask the patient to push back against her arms.

b. The physician resists this motion with an isometric counterforce.

c. The patient is allowed to push for 3 seconds, and then told to relax.

d. The physician allows the patient 3 to 6 seconds of relaxation, and then bends the neck forward to the new point of maximal stretch.

## Unilateral Linear Stretch Applied to Both Ends of Muscles

1. **Patient position:** supine.
2. **Physician position:** standing at the head of the table.
3. **Technique:**

a. The physician places one forearm on the side of the neck to be treated, under the patient's head, with the hand on the patient's contralateral shoulder. The patient's head should be fully supported.

b. The physician places her other hand on the patient's head, on the side to be treated.

c. The physician slowly and gently lifts the head up, forward-bending the neck (Fig. 26-6). The head is rotated away to give a stretch on the muscles opposite the rotation.

## Suboccipital Muscle Treatment

1. **Patient position:** supine.
2. **Physician position:** standing or seated at the side of the table facing the patient.
3. **Technique:**

a. The physician places one forearm under the patient's neck in the suboccipital sul-

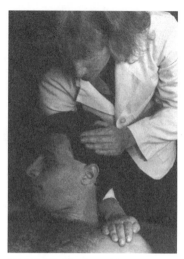

■ **FIG. 26-6** Unilateral linear stretch.

cus so that the patient's neck rests on the radical edge of the forearm.

b. The other hand is placed on the patient's forehead and gentle pressure is applied downward toward the table. The forearm can be rolled towards the patient's head for further suboccipital muscle stretch. (Fig. 26-7).

## ■ ACTIVE DIRECT TECHNIQUES

*Active direct techniques* use the *Golgi tendon reflex* to cause relaxation in the treated muscle. These techniques are described for the suboccipital

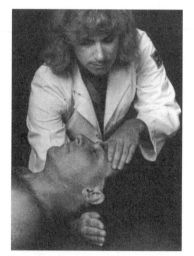

■ **FIG. 26-7** Linear stretch of suboccipital muscles.

muscle region and for unilateral occipital and paravertebral muscles.

## Suboccipital Muscle Region

1. **Patient position:** supine.
2. **Physician position:** seated at the head of the table with her forearms resting on the table, palms facing up.
3. **Technique:**
   a. The physician places her fingertips in the patient's occipital sulcus, allowing the occiput to rest in her palms.
   b. The patient gently pushes his head into the physician's palms, with the physician's fingertips being used as a fulcrum, avoiding neck extension.
   c. As the patient pushes into her palms, the physician resists this motion with an isometric counterforce (Fig. 26-8).

The muscles involved in this technique include the bilateral suboccipital muscles: the rectus capitis posterior major, rectus capitis posterior minor, obliquus capitis inferior, and obliquus capitis superior.

4. **Modification**
   a. The same technique can be applied to the lower extensor muscles of the cervical region. The physician places her fingers more caudally.

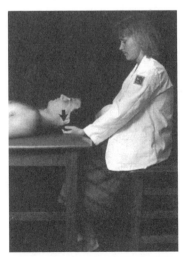

■ **FIG. 26-8** Active direct myofascial technique to suboccipital region with isometric resistance.

b. The patient may push his head into the physician's palms with slightly greater force the lower down the neck one is treating, because the muscles enlarge.

## Unilateral Occipital Muscle Active Technique

1. **Patient position:** supine.
2. **Physician position:** seated at the head of the table with forearms resting on the table, palms up.
3. **Technique:**
   a. The physician places her fingertips in the occipital sulcus on the side to be treated.
   b. The physician's other hand guides the patient's head into side-bending over the fulcrum of her fingers.
   c. The patient tries to side-bend his head farther into the freedom of motion (toward the dysfunctional side).
   d. The physician resists this motion by applying an isometric counterforce with her palm.
   e. The physician should be able to feel the involved muscle contracting.
4. **Modification:** The physician may instruct the patient to push his head gently backward toward the table. This motion is similarly resisted with an isometric counter force.

## Unilateral Single Paravertebral Muscle Treatment—Side-bending and Rotation

1. **Patient position:** supine.
2. **Physician position:** seated at head of table.
3. **Technique:**
   a. The physician places her index or middle finger on the involved muscle. This is the monitoring finger.
   b. With her other hand, the physician grasps the patient's head under the occiput and bends it backward, side-bends, and rotates it ipsilaterally until motion of the involved muscle is felt by the monitoring finger.
   c. The patient attempts to push his head into further backward bending and ipsilateral side-bending and rotation.

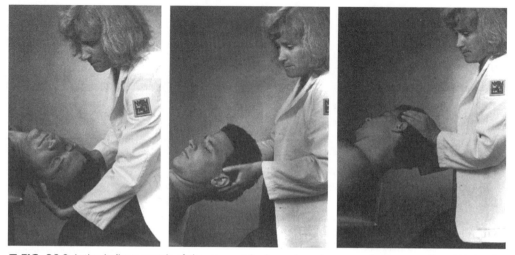

■ **FIG. 26-9** Active indirect stretch of the paravertebral muscles using crossed extensor reflex. **(A)** Starting position. **(B)** Midway through the maneuver, with the patient attempting to bring his chin to his right shoulder as the physician applies isokinetic resistance. **(C)** A passive stretch ends the technique.

d. The physician resists this motion with an isometric counterforce for no more than 2 seconds. Relax and repeat the process.

## ■ ACTIVE INDIRECT TECHNIQUES

*Active indirect techniques* use *reciprocal inhibition* or the *crossed extensor reflex.* They are described for the paravertebral muscles.

1. **Patient position:** supine with his head off the end of the table.
2. **Physician position:** seated at the head of the table, fully supporting the patient's head.
3. **Technique:**
   a. The physician places the palm of one hand on the patient's ipsilateral parieto-occipital area so that the patient's head is fully supported.
   b. The palm of the other hand is placed on the other side of the head. No pressure is placed on the patient's ear.

c. The physician places the patient's head in a position of backward bending, side-bending, and rotation toward the side of the hand on the occiput (Fig. 26-9A). (Discontinue if patient experiences any dizziness.)

d. The patient is instructed to bring his neck into flexion at the same time as pushing his chin to the opposite shoulder (Fig. 26-9B).

e. The physician applies isokinetic resistance to this motion with her hand on the temporoparietal region.

f. The physician stops the patient's effort at the limit or if there is pain.

g. The physician then gently applies a passive stretch of the patient's neck, manually increasing the desired muscle stretch (Fig. 26-9C).

h. The patient relaxes. The physician returns to the starting position and repeats the maneuver.

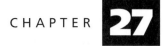

# Muscle Energy Techniques

*Nancy Brous*

This section describes muscle energy techniques used to treat dysfunctions of the occipitoatlantal joint, rotational dysfunctions of the atlantoaxial joint, and single dysfunctions of a typical cervical vertebral joint. The procedure should be repeated as many times as is necessary to restore motion to the physiological barrier. However, the techniques are usually repeated a minimum of three times, with the motion barrier engaged at each repetition.

## ■ OCCIPITOATLANTAL DYSFUNCTION

### Dysfunction in Flexion

*Example: OA $FS_RR_L$*

1. **Patient position:** supine.
2. **Physician position:** seated at the head of the table.
3. **Hand position:** The physician's monitoring hand cradles the patient's occiput. Two fingers of the monitoring hand are in the patient's occipital sulci (medial and inferior to mastoid). The physician's other hand is placed on the inferior aspect of the patient's chin.
4. **Technique:**
   a. The physician extends the patient's head back over his monitoring hand until motion is felt at the occipitoatlantal joint (Fig. 27-1).
   b. With the monitoring hand, the physician side-bends the occiput left and rotates it right until motion is felt at the occipitoatlantal joint.

c. The patient is instructed to push his chin towards his chest against the isometric resistance of the physician (into the freedom of motion) for approximately 3 to 5 seconds. *Ounces* of force are used to achieve the desired results.
   d. The patient relaxes for 3 to 5 seconds.
   e. The physician re-engages the motion barrier each time and repeats steps a through d at least twice more.
   f. The patient's head is returned to neutral and the dysfunction is reassessed for change.

### Dysfunction in Extension

*Example: OA $ES_RR_L$*

1. **Patient position:** supine.
2. **Physician position:** seated at the head of the table.
3. **Hand position:** The physician's monitoring hand cradles the patient's occiput. Two fingers of the monitoring hand are in the patient's occipital sulci. The physician's other hand is placed on the anterior aspect of the patient's chin.
4. **Technique:**
   a. The physician flexes the patient's head forward until he feels motion at the monitoring hand (Fig. 27-2).
   b. With his monitoring hand, the physician side-bends the patient's neck left and rotates it right until motion is felt at the occipitoatlantal joint.
   c. The patient is instructed to push his chin forward against the isometric resistance of

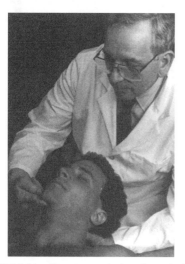

■ **FIG. 27-1** Muscle energy technique for a dysfunction in flexion of the occipitoatlantal joint.

the physician for approximately 3 to 5 seconds. *Ounces* of force are used to achieve the desired result.

d. The patient relaxes for 3 to 5 seconds.

e. The physician re-engages the motion barrier each time and repeats steps a through d at least twice more.

f. The patient's head is returned to neutral and the dysfunction is reassessed for change.

■ **ATLANTOAXIAL DYSFUNCTION**

*Example: AA $R_R$*

1. **Patient position:** supine.
2. **Physician position:** seated at head of table.
3. **Technique:**

   a. Because the motion at the atlantoaxial joint involves primarily rotation, the physician need only address the motion barrier of rotation.

   b. The physician supports the back of the patient's head with his palms. The fingertips of the second digit of each hand placed at the level of the atlas laterally can monitor AA motion. The pads of the fingers are gently placed between the descending ramus of the mandible and the mastoid process.

   c. The physician fully flexes the patient's neck and head forward until locking occurs below the A-A joint.

   d. Keeping the patient's neck bent forward, the physician rotates the head toward the side of the restricted rotation and engages the motion barrier (left).

   e. The physician then places the palm of his hand on the side of the patient's cheek and temple opposite to the restriction. (Fig. 27-3).

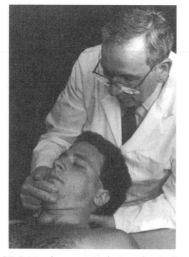

■ **FIG. 27-2** Muscle energy technique for dysfunction in extension of the occipitoatlantal joint.

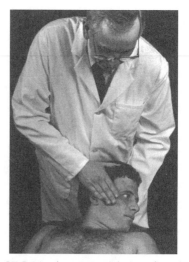

■ **FIG. 27-3** Muscle energy technique for atlantoaxial rotation restriction.

f. The patient is instructed to turn his head with a pure rotary force against the isometric resistance provided by the physician's hand on the patient's cheek.

g. After 3 to 5 seconds, the patient is instructed to relax and the physician simultaneously stops applying the counterforce.

h. Once the patient has completely relaxed for at least 3 to 5 seconds, the physician increases the rotation of the head and neck into the restriction direction, engaging a new motion barrier.

i. Steps f through h are repeated at least three times. Symmetry of motion at the atlantoaxial joint is rechecked.

j. The patient's head is returned to neutral position and the dysfunction is reassessed for change.

## ■ TYPICAL CERVICAL VERTEBRAL DYSFUNCTIONS (C2–C7)

*Example: C4 $ES_RR_R$*

1. **Patient position:** supine.
2. **Physician position:** seated at the head of table.
3. **Technique:**
   a. The physician places the fingertip of the index finger of the monitoring hand against the posterior lateral pillar at the level of the involved segment (left side) (Fig. 27-4A).

   b. The physician introduces flexion of the neck to treat an extension dysfunction, or extension to treat a flexion dysfunction. The motion is monitored and localized to the particular level being treated by monitoring until the motion barrier is engaged.

   c. Side-bending is introduced by placing a medial translatory force on the side of the restricted segment, resulting in side-bending into the barrier (left).

   d. Rotation is introduced by rotating the patient's head and neck into the restriction (left) until motion is felt at the monitored segment. All three barriers are engaged (Fig. 27-4B).

   e. The patient is directed to move into a freedom of motion by having the patient bring his ear to his shoulder, causing a side-bending away from the barrier. (The physician could also ask the patient to rotate his head toward the freedom.) These actions are performed against isometric resistance provided by the physician's hand against the patient's cheek for 3 to 5 seconds.

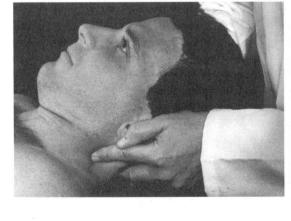
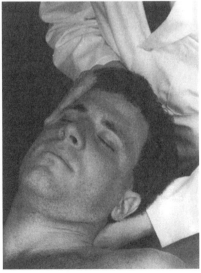

■ **FIG. 27-4** Muscle energy technique for dysfunction in extension of a typical cervical vertebra. **(A)** Note position of monitoring finger. **(B)** Rotation is introduced into barrier to motion of a typical cervical vertebra.

f. The patient relaxes and the physician simultaneously stops applying the counterforce for 3 to 5 seconds.

g. The physician engages the new motion barriers in all three planes by increasing the side-bending, rotation, and flexion (or extension) further into the restrictive barrier.

h. The procedure, steps e through g, should be repeated as many times as is necessary to restore motion to the physiological barrier. This is generally a minimum three times.

i. The patient's head is returned to neutral and the dysfunction is reassessed for change.

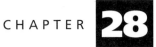

# CHAPTER 28

# Counterstrain Techniques

*Eileen L. DiGiovanna and Lillian Somner*

The treatment of tender points by the Jones counterstrain method requires that the patient be completely relaxed. The goal is to shorten the involved muscle, hold it in this shortened position for 90 seconds, and then return the patient to a neutral position.

Each patient is a unique individual. Remember that the positioning given is useful for the majority of patients. If the described position does not provide relief from tenderness, it may require modification for that patient.

## ■ ANTERIOR TENDER POINTS

The anterior tender points are diagrammed in Figure 28-1. The typical cervical tender points are located on the anterolateral tip of the articular pillars of the cervical vertebrae or in the lateral muscle mass. C1 has an atypical tender point located high on the posterior edge of the ascending ramus of the mandible. This is close to the tip of the transverse process of C1. The tender point for C7 is located on the superior surface approximately 1 inch lateral to the medial end of the clavicle and is likely related to the attachment of the sternocleidomastoid muscle. The C7 tender point is quite common. The point for C8 is located on the medial tip of the clavicle in the sternal notch. Obviously there is not an eighth cervical vertebra; however, there is innervation from an eighth cervical nerve. This latter point is uncommon.

Two mnemonics assist the student in remembering the positioning of the vertebral joint being treated:

STAR = side-bending toward and rotation away from the tender point.
SARA = side-bending and rotation away from the tender point.

1. **Patient position:** supine.
2. **Physician position:** seated at the head of the table.
3. **Technique:**
   a. C1: Rotate the head away from the tender point (Fig. 28-2). There is no flexion, extension, or side-bending.
   b. C2 and C3: Slight flexion, rotation, and side-bending away from the tender point (SARA).
   c. C4: Create flexion to the vertebra, then side-bend and rotate away from the tender point (Fig. 28-3) (SARA). This tender point is unusual in that it frequently requires extension rather than flexion.
   d. C5 and C6: Create flexion with side-bending and rotation away from the tender point (Fig. 28-4) (SARA).
   e. C7: Create moderate to strong flexion of the neck to the C7 level (force is not applied to the head), slightly rotate away, and slightly side-bend toward the tender point (Fig. 28-5) (STAR).
   f. C8: Create flexion of the neck, side-bending, and rotation away from the tender point (SARA).

It is important to remember that although SARA (side-bend away, rotate away) is used to treat most anterior cervical tender points, adjustment may need to be made for individual pa-

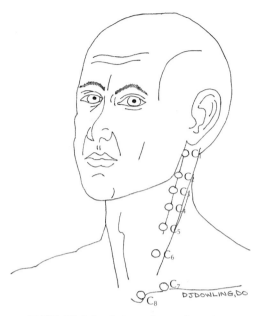

■ **FIG. 28-1** Cervical anterior tender points.

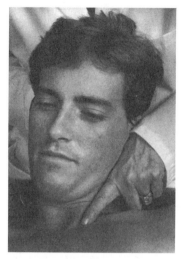

■ **FIG. 28-4** Treatment of left anterior tender point of C7. Note flexion with slight rotation away and side-bending toward the tender point.

tients who require some variation, particularly of the side-bending component.

# ■ POSTERIOR TENDER POINTS

The posterior cervical tender points are shown in Figure 28-6. They are generally located on the interspinous ligaments between the spinous processes or slightly medial or lateral to them,

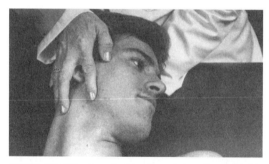

■ **FIG. 28-2** Treatment of tender point on the right side of C1. The head is rotated away from the tender point.

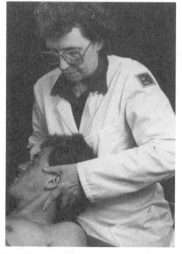

■ **FIG. 28-5** Treatment of anterior tender point for C8. Note marked flexion with side-bending and rotation away.

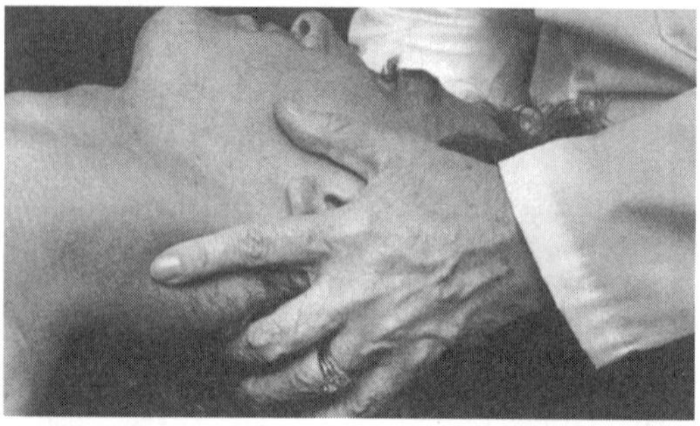

■ **FIG. 28-3** Treatment of tender point on the left side of C4. Side-bending and rotation are away from the tender point. Shown with extension.

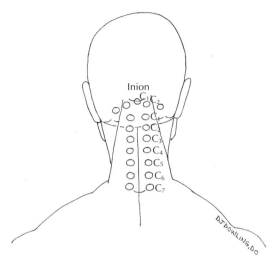

■ **FIG. 28-6** Posterior cervical tender point locations.

or on the articular pillars more laterally. C1 has tender points just below the inion and in the muscle masses laterally on the nuchal line.

1. **Patient position:** supine.
2. **Physician position:** seated at the head of the table.
3. **Technique:** While carefully monitoring with one finger on the tender point, the physician positions the neck, as noted, until the point is no longer tender. This position is held for 90 seconds, slowly returned to a neutral position, and re-evaluated.

a. C1: Treated in marked flexion for midline (inion) tender point with greatest flexion occurring just below the occiput by putting a forward pressure on the forehead rather than only to the back of the head. For the lateral tender points, some extension with rotation and side-bending away from the tender point is provided.

b. C2 tender points: Create extension of the neck to the segment to be treated with slight side-bending and rotation away from the tender point (SARA).

c. **Articular pillar points:**
   (1) C4 to C7: Create extension with rotation and side-bending away from the tender point (SARA).
   (2) C3: Create flexion with rotation away and side-bending toward the tender point (STAR). Occasionally C3 will require extension. This tender point may be present with either a flexed or an extended somatic dysfunction. Flexion is used most commonly.
   (3) C8: Create marked flexion with side-bending and rotation away from the tender point.

Some adjustment of the side-bending, rotation, or flexion–extension component may be required in some patients. It is more imperative to achieve a position of comfort than to follow a written prescription.

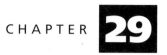

# Facilitated Positional Release

*Stanley Schiowitz*

$A$ll facilitated positional release techniques for treating cervical region dysfunctions are begun with a slight flattening of the cervical lordosis.

## ■ SUPERFICIAL MUSCLE HYPERTONICITY, POSTERIOR RIGHT SIDE, IN REGION OF C4 VERTEBRA

1. **Patient position:** supine.
2. **Physician position:** seated at the head of the table.
3. **Technique:**
   a. The patient moves up the table until his head and neck are off the table and supported by the physician. (The head may be supported by a pillow on the physician's lap.)
   b. With the thumb, palm, and middle finger of the left hand, the physician cradles the patient's neck. His middle finger is on the tissue to be treated. The rest of the hand helps support the patient's neck.
   c. The patient's head is firmly supported in the palm of the physician's right hand, which will be used in the ensuing maneuvers.
   d. The physician gently bends the head and neck forward to flatten the cervical lordosis.
   e. From this starting position, the physician gently applies axial compression on the patient's occiput, with the vector of force directed through the patient's head toward his feet (Fig. 29-1). Less than 1 pound of

force is sufficient—just enough to be felt at the physician's left index finger.
   f. Maintaining axial compression, the physician bends the patient's neck backward, then side-bends it up to the physician's left index finger (Fig. 29-2). This maneuver causes shortening and relaxation of the muscle being treated.
   g. This position is held for 3 seconds and then released and the area of interspinous dysfunction reevaluated.

### Somatic Dysfunction—C4 ES$_R$R$_R$

1. **Patient position:** supine, as described in aforementioned technique.

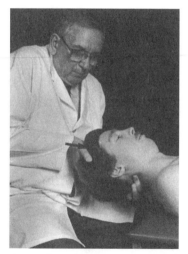

■ **FIG. 29-1** Facilitated positional release treatment of superficial muscle hypertonicity of cervical region; application of axial compression.

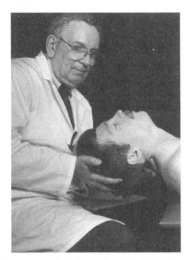

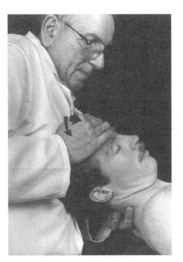

■ **FIG. 29-2** Facilitated positional release treatment of muscle hypertonicity in the cervical region with extension and right side-bending added.

■ **FIG. 29-3** Facilitated positional release treatment for C4 flexion dysfunction with right side-bending and rotation.

2. **Physician position:** seated at the head of the table, with hands placed as described in aforementioned technique.
3. **Technique:**
   a. The physician places his finger at the articular facet of C4 on C5.
   b. After flattening the curve and adding a compressive force, the physician moves the patient's neck into extension and rotation to the right.
   c. The physician then adds right lateral flexion of C4 on C5.
   d. Immediate release of the articulation should be felt.
   e. The position is held for 3 seconds, returned to the original position, and reassessed.

## Somatic Dysfunction—C4 FS$_R$R$_R$

1. **Patient position:** supine as described in first technique.

2. **Physician position:** seated at the head of the table, with hands placed as in aforementioned techniques.
3. **Technique:**
   a. The physician gently bends the patient's neck forward to flatten the sagittal curve.
   b. From this starting position, the physician applies compression.
   c. Maintaining compression, the physician gently increases the forward bending until flexion of C4 on C5 is felt by the monitoring finger. (With compression maintained, the degree of forward bending of the neck needed to achieve the necessary vertebral flexion is greatly reduced.)
   d. The physician adds right rotation and lateral flexion, up to the monitoring finger (Fig. 29-3).
   e. After feeling an articular release, the physician holds the position for 3 seconds, then releases it and reevaluates the dysfunction.

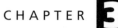

# Still Techniques

*Dennis J. Dowling*

This chapter describes the techniques of the Still technique for treating somatic dysfunctions of the cervical spine—atypical (OA & AA) and typical (C2–C7). The patient may be treated either in the seated position or in the supine position. Compression is used for both positions but traction may be used when the patient is supine. Occasionally, the portion of the treatment involving movement towards the barriers may result in an articulatory "pop."

## ■ OA SOMATIC DYSFUNCTION (OA $S_R$ $R_L$)—SEATED

1. **Patient position:** seated.
2. **Physician position:** standing facing the patient.
3. **Technique:**
   a. The physician places the pad of the index or middle finger of his monitoring hand on the side of the side-bending component in the basiocciput at the level of the shallow occipital sulcus (the left finger contacts the patient's right shallow occipital sulcus in this example). The palm of that hand contours to and supports the side of the patient's head.
   b. The physician places the palm of his other hand on top of the patient's head with the fingers contouring to the patient's head.
   c. The physician side-bends the patient's head towards the monitoring finger at the basiocciput. Because the motion is coupled at the OA joint, slight rotation away from the shallow sulcus will occur. The physician can further exaggerate this if

necessary. Slight flexion or extension is added, depending on the diagnosis of the dysfunction, finishing the position into the relative freedoms of the somatic dysfunction (Fig. 30-1).

   d. The physician puts approximately 5 pounds of downward pressure toward the monitoring finger with the hand on the top of the patient's head.
   e. While maintaining the compression, the head is gently carried through sagittal plane neutral and towards the flexion or extension barrier, then through neutral position and into the barrier directions (side-bending left and rotating right in this case).
   f. The patient's head and neck are brought back to the neutral position and the OA joint is reassessed.

## ■ OA SOMATIC DYSFUNCTION (OA $S_R$ $R_L$)—SUPINE/COMPRESSION

1. **Patient position:** supine.
2. **Physician position:** seated at the head of the table.
3. **Technique:**
   a. The physician places the pad of his index or middle finger of his monitoring hand on the side of the side-bending component in the basiocciput at the level of the shallow occipital sulcus (the right finger contacts the patient's right shallow occipital sulcus in this example). The palm of that hand contours to and supports the side of the patient's head and the remain-

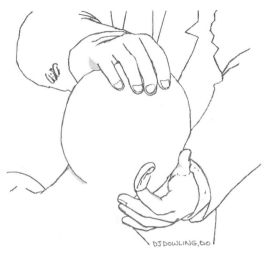

■ **FIG. 30-1** Still technique OA somatic dysfunction (OA S$_R$ R$_L$), seated.

ing fingers support the patient's head beneath the occiput.

b. The physician places the palm of his other hand on top of the patient's head with the fingers contouring to the patient's head.

c. The physician side-bends the patient's head toward the monitoring finger at the basiocciput. Because the motion is coupled at the OA joint, slight rotation away from the shallow sulcus will occur. The physician can further exaggerate this if necessary.

d. Slight flexion or extension is added, depending on the diagnosis of the dysfunction, finishing the position into the relative freedoms of the somatic dysfunction (Fig. 30-2).

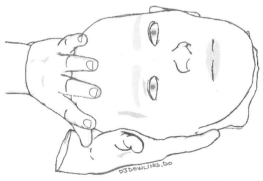

■ **FIG. 30-2** Still technique OA somatic dysfunction (OA S$_R$ R$_L$), supine/compression.

e. The physician puts approximately 5 pounds of downward pressure toward the patient's feet with the hand on the top of the patient's head toward the monitoring finger.

f. While maintaining the compression, the head is gently carried through the sagittal plane neutral and toward the flexion or extension barrier, then through neutral position and into the barrier directions (side-bending left and rotating right in this case).

g. The patient's head and neck are brought back to the neutral position and the OA joint is reassessed.

## ■ OA SOMATIC DYSFUNCTION (OA S$_R$ R$_L$)—SUPINE/TRACTION

1. **Patient position:** supine.
2. **Physician position:** seated at the head of the table.
3. **Technique:**
   a. The physician places the pad of his index or middle finger of his monitoring hand on the side of the side-bending component in the basiocciput at the level of the shallow occipital sulcus (the right finger contacts the patient's right shallow occipital sulcus in this example). The palm of that hand contours to and supports the side of the patient's head.
   b. The physician places the palm of his other hand against the opposite side of the patient's head and one or two fingers are placed beneath the patient's chin.
   c. The physician side-bends the patient's head towards the monitoring finger at the basiocciput. Because the motion is coupled at the OA joint, slight rotation away from the shallow sulcus will occur. The physician can further exaggerate this if necessary.
   d. Slight flexion or extension is added, depending on the diagnosis of the dysfunction, finishing the position into the relative freedoms of the somatic dysfunction (Fig. 30-3).
   e. The physician puts approximately 5 pounds of traction with the contacts of the

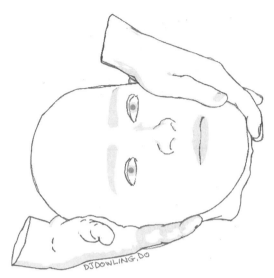

■ **FIG. 30-3** Still technique OA somatic dysfunction (OA $S_R$ $R_L$), supine/traction.

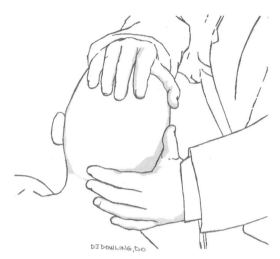

■ **FIG. 30-4** Still technique AA somatic dysfunction (AA $R_R$), seated.

palms of his hands that are against the patient's head and pulls parallel to the table and toward the physician.

f. While maintaining the traction, the head is gently carried through sagittal plane neutral and toward the flexion or extension barrier, then through neutral position and into the barrier directions (side-bending left and rotating right in this case).

g. The patient's head and neck are brought back to the neutral position and the OA joint is reassessed.

## ■ AA SOMATIC DYSFUNCTION (AA $R_R$)—SEATED

1. **Patient position:** seated.
2. **Physician position:** standing facing the patient.
3. **Technique:**
   a. The physician places the pad of his index or middle finger of his monitoring hand at the transverse process of the atlas located between the mastoid process and the mandibular ramus (the left finger contacts the patient's right atlas transverse process in this example). The palm of that hand contours to and supports the side of the patient's head and the remaining fingers wrap around the rest of the patient's neck.

b. The physician places the palm of his other hand on top of the patient's head with the fingers contouring to the patient's head.

c. The physician rotates the patient's head towards the monitoring finger until tissue relaxation is noted.

d. The physician puts approximately 5 pounds of downward pressure toward the monitoring finger with the hand on the top of the patient's head (Fig. 30-4).

e. While maintaining the compression, the head is gently carried through neutral position and into the barrier directions (rotating left in this case).

f. The patient's head and neck are brought back to the neutral position and the AA joint is reassessed.

## ■ AA SOMATIC DYSFUNCTION (AA $R_R$)—SUPINE

1. **Patient position:** supine.
2. **Physician position:** seated at the head of the table.
3. **Technique:**
   a. The physician places the pad of his index or middle finger of his monitoring hand at the transverse process of the atlas located between the mastoid process and the mandibular ramus (the right finger contacts the patient's right atlas transverse process

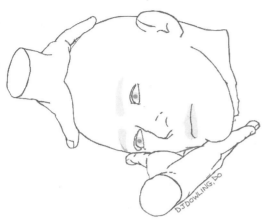

■ **FIG. 30-5** Still technique AA somatic dysfunction (AA $R_R$), supine.

in this example). The palm of that hand contours to and supports the side of the patient's head and the remaining fingers support the patient's head beneath the occiput.

b. The physician places the palm of his other hand on top of the patient's head with the fingers contouring to the patient's head.

c. The physician rotates the patient's head toward the monitoring finger until relaxation is noted.

d. The physician puts approximately 5 pounds of downward pressure toward the monitoring finger with the hand on the top of the patient's head.

e. While maintaining the compression, the head is gently carried through neutral position and into the barrier directions (rotation left in this case) (Fig. 30-5).

f. The patient's head and neck are brought back to the neutral position and the AA joint is reassessed.

## ■ TYPICAL CERVICAL SOMATIC DYSFUNCTION (C5 $S_R$ $R_R$)—SEATED

1. **Patient position:** seated.
2. **Physician position:** standing facing the patient.
3. **Technique:**
   a. The physician places the pad of his index or middle finger of his monitoring hand on posterior articular pillar at the level of the somatic dysfunction (the left finger contacts the patient's posterior C5 articular pillar in this example). The palm of that hand contours to and supports the side of the patient's head and the remaining fingers wrap around the patient's neck

   b. The physician places the palm of his other hand on top of the patient's head with the fingers contouring to the patient's head.

   c. The physician side-bends and rotates the patient's head towards and to the level of the monitoring finger.

   d. Flexion or extension is added, depending on the diagnosis of the dysfunction, finishing the position into the relative freedoms of the somatic dysfunction.

   e. The physician puts approximately 5 pounds of downward pressure toward the monitoring finger with the hand on the top of the patient's head (Fig. 30-6).

   f. While maintaining the compression, the head is gently carried through sagittal plane neutral and toward the flexion or extension barrier, then through neutral position and into the barrier directions (side-bending left and rotating left in this case).

   g. The patient's head and neck are brought back to the neutral position and the cervical somatic dysfunction level is reassessed.

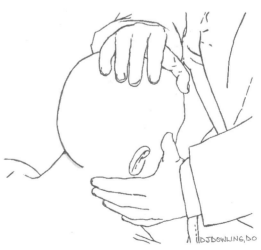

■ **FIG. 30-6** Still technique typical cervical somatic dysfunction (C5 $S_R$ $R_R$), seated.

## ■ TYPICAL CERVICAL SOMATIC DYSFUNCTION (C5 $S_R$ $R_R$)—SUPINE/COMPRESSION

1. **Patient position:** supine.
2. **Physician position:** seated at the head of the table.
3. **Technique:**
   a. The physician places the pad of his index or middle finger of his monitoring hand on posterior articular pillar at the level of the somatic dysfunction (the right finger contacts the patient's posterior C5 articular pillar in this example). The palm of that hand contours to and supports the side of the patient's head and the remaining fingers support the patient's head and neck.
   b. The physician places the palm of his other hand on top of the patient's head with the fingers contouring to the patient's head.
   c. The physician side-bends and rotates the patient's head toward and to the level of the monitoring finger.
   d. Flexion or extension is added, depending on the diagnosis of the dysfunction, finishing the position into the relative freedoms of the somatic dysfunction.
   e. The physician puts approximately 5 pounds of downward pressure toward the monitoring finger with the hand on the top of the patient's head (Fig. 30-7).
   f. While maintaining the compression, the head is gently carried through the sagittal plane neutral and toward the flexion or extension barrier, then through neutral position and into the barrier directions (side-bending left and rotating left in this case).
   g. The patient's head and neck are brought back to the neutral position and the cervical somatic dysfunction level is reassessed.

## ■ TYPICAL CERVICAL DYSFUNCTION (C5 $S_R$ $R_R$)—SUPINE/TRACTION

1. **Patient position:** supine.
2. **Physician position:** seated at the head of the table.
3. **Technique:**
   a. The physician places the pad of his index or middle finger of his monitoring hand on posterior articular pillar at the level of the somatic dysfunction (the right finger contacts the patient's right CS articuler pillar in this example). The palm of that hand contours to and supports the side of the patient's head.
   b. The physician places the pad of his index or middle finger of his other hand on the opposite articular pillar at the same level as the somatic dysfunction (the left finger contacts the patient's left articular pillar of C5 in this case). The palm of that hand contours to and supports the side of the patient's head.

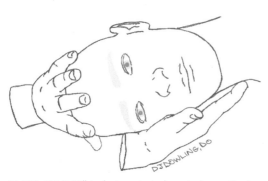

**■ FIG. 30-7** Still technique typical cervical somatic dysfunction (C5 $S_R$ $R_R$), supine/compression.

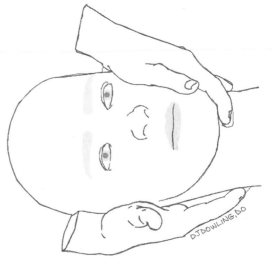

**■ FIG. 30-8** Still technique typical cervical somatic dysfunction (C5 $S_R$ $R_R$), supine/traction.

c. The physician side-bends and rotates the patient's head toward the monitoring finger at the posterior articular pillar.

d. Flexion or extension is added, depending on the diagnosis of the dysfunction, finishing the position into the relative freedoms of the somatic dysfunction.

e. The physician puts approximately 5 pounds of traction with the contacts of the palms of his hands that are against the patient's head and pulls parallel to the table and towards the physician (Fig. 30-8).

f. While maintaining the traction, the head is gently carried through sagittal plane neutral and towards the flexion or exten-sion barrier, then through neutral position and into the barrier directions (side-bending left and rotating left in this case).

g. The patient's head and neck are brought back to the neutral position and the OA joint is reassessed.

**REFERENCES**

Van Buskirk RL. A manipulative technique of Andrew Taylor Still. *J Am Osteopath Assoc* 1996;96:597–602.

Van Buskirk RL. *The Still Technique Manual.* Indianapolis, IN: American Academy of Osteopathy, Indianapolis, 1999.

Van Buskirk RL. Treatment of somatic dysfunction with an osteopathic manipulative method of Dr. Andrew Taylor Still. In Ward RC, ed. *Foundations for Osteopathic Medicine.* Philadelphia: Lippincott Williams & Wilkins, 2003: 1094–1114.

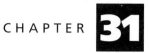

# PINS Techniques for the Cervical Spine

*Dennis J. Dowling*

This chapter describes PINS techniques for treating somatic dysfunctions of the cervical region. The examples provided are not the only ones that are possible (Figures 31-1 and 31-2). They are fairly common. Occasionally, patterns in the cervical region may continue into or from adjacent regions. The patient is most commonly treated in the supine position but could be treated seated or prone. The physician should be positioned comfortably facing the region to be treated or at the head of the table. The principles and methods of PINS can be applied:

1. Locate a sensitive point in the region of the symptoms.
2. Analyze the structures that are deep to that point
3. Locate another sensitive point at the other end of a connecting structure (i.e., muscle, ligament, nerve, etc.). The more sensitive point is the primary point and the less sensitive point is the endpoint.
4. Apply inhibitory pressure to both points for 30 seconds or more. The soft tissue at the more sensitive point will typically lessen in tension.
5. Beginning at the more sensitive of the two points, locate another sensitive point approximately 2 to 3 centimeters toward the less sensitive point.
6. Repeat the procedure progressively toward the endpoint.
7. Reassess the status of the dysfunction. Deter-

mine whether additional treatment or the application of other modalities is necessary

## ■ FRONTALIS-OCCIPITALIS/ TRIGEMINAL (OPHTHALMIC DIVISION)—GREATER OCCIPITAL NERVE

1. Technique:
   a. The physician places the pad of his index or middle finger on superior orbital ridge near the trochlear notch. A finger of the physician's other hand locates a sensitive point in the suboccipital triangle. The point can be on the same or opposite side of the head.
   b. The pattern of intervening points can be straight or curved (muscle pattern) or zigzag (nerve pattern).
2. Clinical Correlation:
   a. Eye pain
   b. Headache
      (1) Tension headache
      (2) Migraine headache
   a. Visual symptoms (eye pain, blurring, increased lacrimation)
   b. Unilateral cephalgic pain
   c. Sinusitis

## ■ SPHENOID—TEMPORAL

1. Technique:
   a. The physician places the pad of his index or middle finger lateral to the eyebrow at

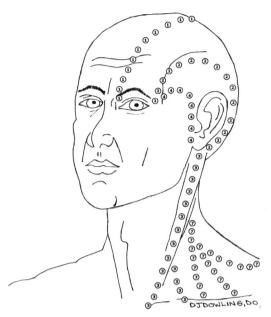

■ **FIG. 31-1** PINS cervical point patterns, anterior, *1, frontalis–occipitalis/trigeminal (ophthalmic division), greater occipital nerve; 2, sphenoid–temporal; 3, sterno-cleidomastoid; 4, sphenoid–temperomandibular joint; 7, scalenes.*

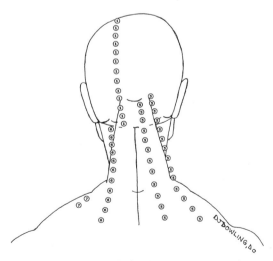

■ **FIG. 31-2** PINS cervical point patterns, posterior. *2, sphenoid–temporal; 5, trapezius; 6, levator scapular; 7, scalenes (posterior scalene approximate position of points anterior to trapezius).*

the location of the greater wing of the sphenoid. A finger of the physician's other hand locates a sensitive point in the occipitomastoid suture or on the mastoid process of the temporal bone. The point may be at the level of the lateral arch of the atlas.

b. The pattern of intervening points is generally curved (muscle pattern) or zigzag (nerve pattern). When it is lower, the pattern may follow the squamous suture of the temporal and parietal bones. A higher pattern may follow the temporalis muscle edge.

c. Occasionally, some of the intervening points may be located in the belly of the temporalis muscle and then be directed towards the coronoid process of the mandible and not at the occipitomastoid suture.

2. Clinical Correlation:
   a. Eye pain
   b. Headache
      (1) Tension headache
      (2) Migraine headache
   a. Visual symptoms (eye pain, blurring, increased lacrimation)
   b. Unilateral cephalgic pain
   c. Otitis externa or media
   d. Jaw pain—TMJ Dysfunction

## ■ STERNOCLEIDOMASTOID (SCM)

1. Technique:
   a. The physician places the pad of his index or middle finger on the mastoid process. A finger of the physician's other hand locates a sensitive point at the jugular notch on the manubrium. The point may be at the medial third of the clavicle where the deeper portion of the SCM attaches.
   b. The pattern of intervening points is generally straight (muscle pattern) following the sternocleidomastoid muscle.

2. Clinical Correlation:
   a. Jaw pain—TMJ Dysfunction
   b. Tension headache
   c. Otitis externa or media
   d. Pain on swallowing

## ■ SPHENOID— TEMPEROMANDIBULAR JOINT

1. Technique:
   a. The physician places the pad of his index or middle finger lateral to the eyebrow at the location of the greater wing of the sphenoid. A finger of the physician's other hand locates a sensitive point over the temporomandibular joint.
   b. The pattern of intervening points generally follows the sphenoid, zygomatic, and temporal bone sutures.
2. Clinical Correlation:
   a. Jaw pain—TMJ Dysfunction
   b. Bruxism
   c. Otitis externa or media
   d. Toothache

## ■ TRAPEZIUS

1. Technique:
   a. The physician places the pad of his index or middle finger on or lateral to the inion. A finger of the physician's other hand locates a sensitive point in the thoracic region, the scapula, or toward the lateral posterior clavicular region.
   b. The pattern of intervening points generally follows a straight or curved path (muscle) or zigzag (spinal accessory nerve).
2. Clinical Correlation:
   a. Headache
   b. Cervicalgia (neck pain)
   c. Upper back pain

## ■ LEVATOR SCAPULA

1. Technique:
   a. The physician places the pad of his index or middle finger on the lateral and posterior upper cervical spine. A finger of the physician's other hand locates a sensitive point on the upper medial border of the scapula.
   b. The pattern of intervening points generally follows a fairly straight path following the course of the muscle.
2. Clinical Correlation:
   a. Headache
   b. Cervicalgia (neck pain) especially on rotation of neck with radiation to occiput
   c. Upper back pain
   d. Shoulder pain

## ■ SCALENES

1. Technique:
   a. The physician places the pad of his index or middle finger on the lateral and middle cervical spine. A finger of the physician's other hand locates a sensitive point in the lower and lateral cervical region. The anterior scalene point is posterior to the medial clavicle. The middle scalene is lateral, at approximately the middle of the clavicle. The posterior scalene is further lateral and posterior but anterior to the trapezius.
   b. The pattern of intervening points generally follows a fairly straight path following the course of each of the muscles.
2. Clinical Correlation:
   a. Headache
   b. Cervicalgia (neck pain)
   c. Shoulder pain
   d. Upper extremity radicular symptoms (from compression of the brachial plexus by the anterior and middle scalenes)
   e. Respiratory relationship (inhalation dysfunctions of the upper two ribs)

### REFERENCES

Dowling DJ. Progressive inhibition of neuromuscular structures (PINS) technique. *J Am Osteopath Assoc* 2000;100: 285–286, 289–298.

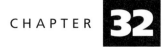

# Thrusting Techniques

*Eileen L. DiGiovanna and Barry Erner*

This section describes the application of high-velocity, low-amplitude thrusting techniques to correct somatic dysfunctions of the cervical spine. The vertebra may be placed into one or all of its barriers to motion. Frequently with this technique, however, only one plane of motion is addressed. When this motion restriction is corrected, the other planes of restriction respond as well. After placing the vertebra into its restrictive barrier, the physician applies a rapid, gentle force through a very short distance to pass through the barrier.

Especially in the cervical spine, it is imperative to localize precisely to the joint being treated and use a controlled force, sufficient only to move the involved joint the necessary amount. Force should never be substituted for skill.

Cervical high-velocity, low-amplitude technique is most effectively performed on joints in which the end-feel at the restrictive barrier is firm. A rubbery end-feel does not respond as well to the minimal forces that should be used in the cervical spine.

At all times, the head and neck should be kept in the midline and never hyperextended. Any extension that is used should be only at the joint to be treated.

## ■ OCCIPITOATLANTAL JOINT DYSFUNCTION

1. **Patient position:** supine.
2. **Physician position:** standing at the head of the table toward the side of the freedom of rotation.
3. **Technique:**

a. The patient's head may rest on the physician's non-thrusting hand or forearm. The neck is flexed slightly by the hand or forearm.
b. The metacarpophalangeal joint of the thrusting hand is placed on the occiput just above the sulcus.
c. The occiput is allowed to extend just over that finger in a backward nod. The extension should occur *only* at the involved joint, not the entire neck.
d. The occiput is rotated and side-bent into its barriers, taking up the slack in the soft tissues. These motions should be simultaneous so that rotation will be minimal.
e. A thrust is given as a coupled side-bending and rotational force directed toward the eye (Fig. 32-1).

*The neck should always be maintained in the midline, never allowing the head to be moved laterally. This technique should not be performed if rotation of the head and neck causes dizziness, lightheadedness, or pain.*

## ■ ATLANTOAXIAL JOINT DYSFUNCTION

1. **Patient position:** supine.
2. **Physician position:** standing at the head of the table toward the involved side.
3. **Technique:**

a. The physician cups the lateral aspect of the patient's chin in his non-thrusting hand for support only.
b. The physician's thrusting finger is posi-

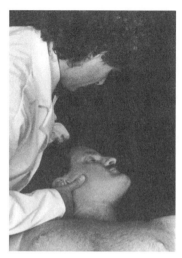

■ **FIG. 32-1** High-velocity, low-amplitude thrusting technique for somatic dysfunction of the occipitoatlantal joint.

tioned behind the posteriorly rotated articular pillar.

c. The physician rotates the head into the motion barrier, keeping the head in the midline. No extension should be permitted.

d. The physician exerts a rapid rotary thrust through the rotational restrictive barrier (Fig. 32-2). The force should move only the involved joint, not the entire neck.

*This procedure should not be performed if rota-*

*tion of the head and neck cause dizziness, lightheadedness, or pain.*

## ■ C3 TO C7 SOMATIC DYSFUNCTION

1. **Patient position:** supine.
2. **Physician position:** standing at the head of the table.
3. **Technique:**
   a. The physician flexes the neck to the level of the vertebra being treated.
   b. The physician places his second metacarpophalangeal joint behind the posteriorly rotated articular pillar.
   c. The vertebra being treated is allowed to extend over the thrusting finger. The head and neck should be well supported so that the entire neck does not extend.
   d. The neck is simultaneously rotated toward the barrier and side-bent, at the involved joint, up away from the table. All the slack is taken out of the soft tissues. The side-bending will prevent over-rotation of the joint.
   e. The physician exerts a rapid, short rotary thrust (Fig. 32-3).

*It is important to keep the head in the midline at all times when performing this technique. The technique may be modified to engage all three barriers to motion before performing the thrust. This technique should not be performed if rotation of the*

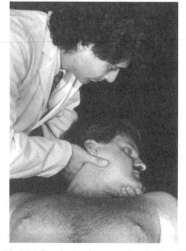

■ **FIG. 32-2** High-velocity, low-amplitude thrusting technique for somatic dysfunction of the atlantoaxial joint.

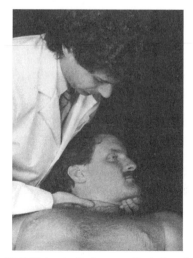

■ **FIG. 32-3** High-velocity, low-amplitude thrusting technique for somatic dysfunction of cervical spine, C3–C7.

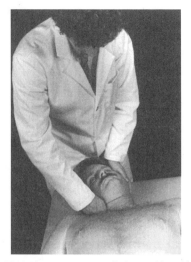

■ **FIG. 32-4** Alternate HVLA technique with a side-bending thrust.

*head and neck cause dizziness, lightheadedness, or pain. Force should never be substituted for skill.*

The direction of thrust varies with the level of vertebra being treated. For the upper cervical region, the thrust is toward the eye, the middle cervicals are thrust straight across the neck, and the thrust through the lower cervicals is directed down toward the chest.

## ■ CERVICAL SOMATIC DYSFUNCTION, ALTERNATIVE TECHNIQUE

1. **Patient position:** supine.
2. **Physician position:** standing at the head of the table.
3. **Technique:**
   a. The physician places the lateral aspect of the second metacarpophalangeal joint of the thrusting hand on the articular pillar contralateral to the posteriorly rotated one.
   b. The other hand is placed along the opposite side of the patient's head. (The chin may be cupped to maintain rotation, but the thrust must never be made through the chin.)
   c. Engage the barriers of extension-flexion, rotation, and side-bending.
   d. The physician exerts a rapid side-bending thrust through the involved vertebra (Fig. 32-4).

# Exercise Therapy

*Stanley Schiowitz and Albert R. DeRubertis*

The exercises described can be used to increase regional cervical motion (muscle stretch, extensibility), to increase regional strength (muscle contractility), or to restore structural symmetry. Many cervical muscle functions and structural changes involve the thoracic region. It is suggested that the physician review the section in Chapter 9, Exercise Therapy, and Chapter 44, Exercise Therapy for the Thoracic Spine, when writing an exercise prescription for the cervical area.

## ■ REGIONAL STRETCH

### Forward Bending

1. **Patient position:** seated or standing, with the back erect.
2. **Instructions:**
   a. Drop your head forward; let its weight (gravity) pull it down.
   b. Add anterior (flexor) muscle contraction to bring your chin to your chest.
   c. Place both hands behind your head and passively pull your head down, chin to chest (Fig. 33-1). Do not create pain.
   d. Hold this position for 5 to 15 seconds. Relax, rest, and repeat.

### Backward Bending

1. **Patient position:** seated or standing, with the back erect.
2. **Instructions:**
   a. Drop your head backward; let its weight pull it back.

b. Add posterior (extensor) muscle contraction to increase the backward bending.
   c. Place both hands on your forehead and passively push your head back (Fig. 33-2). Do not create pain.
   d. Hold this position for 5 to 15 seconds. Relax, rest, and repeat.

### Side-Bending

1. **Patient position:** seated or standing, with the back erect.
2. **Instructions:**
   a. Without moving your shoulders, drop your head to the right; let its weight pull your right ear toward the right shoulder.
   b. Add right-sided muscle contraction to increase the side-bending.
   c. Place your right hand over your head, palm on the left side of your head, and passively pull your head down to the right (Fig. 33-3). Try not to introduce rotation motion. Do not create pain.
   d. Hold this position for 5 to 15 seconds. Relax, rest and repeat. For left side-bending, reverse the instructions.

### Rotation

1. **Patient position:** seated or standing, with the back erect.
2. **Instructions:**
   a. Without moving your shoulders, turn your head to the right as far as you can, using right rotation muscle contraction.
   b. Place your right hand in front of your fore-

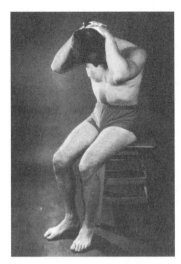

■ **FIG. 33-1** Exercise therapy for the cervical spine: forward bending.

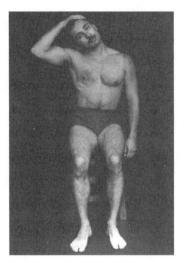

■ **FIG. 33-3** Exercise therapy for the cervical spine: side-bending.

head with the palm on the left side of your head. Passively pull your head to the right as far as possible (Fig. 33-4). Do not create pain.

*Note:* In steps a and b, keep the chin in one horizontal plane. Avoid adding lateral bending motion.

  c. Hold this position for 5 to 15 seconds. Relax, rest, and repeat. For left rotation, reverse directions.

## ■ REGIONAL STRENGTH

The exercises for promoting cervical strength use static contraction. Exercises are described for flexor muscles, extensor muscles, side-bending muscles, and rotator muscles.

### Flexor Muscles

1. **Patient position:** seated or standing, with the back erect.

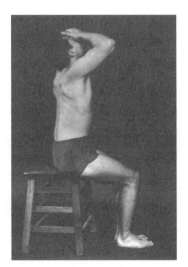

■ **FIG. 33-2** Exercise therapy for the cervical spine: backward bending.

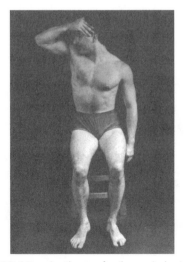

■ **FIG. 33-4** Exercise therapy for the cervical spine: rotation.

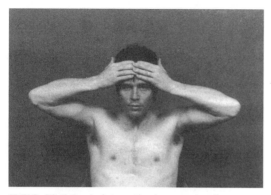

■ **FIG. 33-5** Cervical strengthening exercise: flexor muscles.

2. **Instructions:**
   a. Place both your palms on your forehead.
   b. Push your head forward against your palms. Resist the forward push to prevent all head motion (Fig. 33-5).
   c. Hold for 4 seconds, then relax.
   d. Repeat the exercise, gradually increasing the strength of the contracting force and hand resistance. Do not create pain. Do not hold a static contraction beyond 5 seconds.

## Extensor Muscles

1. **Patient position:** seated or standing, with the back erect.
2. **Instructions:**
   a. Place both hands behind your head.
   b. Push your head backward against your resisting hands (Fig. 33-6). Prevent all head motion.

c. Hold for 4 seconds, then relax.
d. Repeat the exercise, gradually increasing the strength of the contracting force and hand resistance. Do not create pain. Do not hold a static contraction for more than 5 seconds.

## Side-Bending Muscles

1. **Patient position:** seated or standing, with the back erect.
2. **Instructions:**
   a. Place your right hand on the right side of your head, above the ear.
   b. Push your head to the right against your resisting right hand (Fig. 33-7). Prevent all head motion.
   c. Hold for 4 seconds, then relax.
   d. Repeat the exercise, gradually increasing the strength of the contracting force and hand resistance. For left side-bending, reverse directions. Do not create pain. Do not hold a static contraction for more than 5 seconds.

## Rotator Muscles

1. **Patient position:** seated or standing, with the back erect.
2. **Instructions:**
   a. Place your right hand on the right side of your forehead.
   b. Turn your head to the right against your resisting right hand (Fig. 33-8). Prevent all head motion.

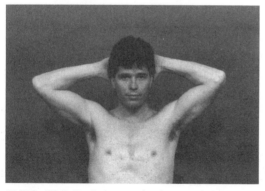

■ **FIG. 33-6** Cervical strengthening exercise: extensor muscles.

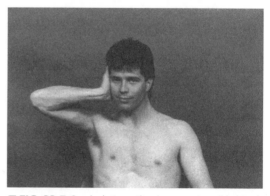

■ **FIG. 33-7** Cervical strengthening exercise: side-bending muscles.

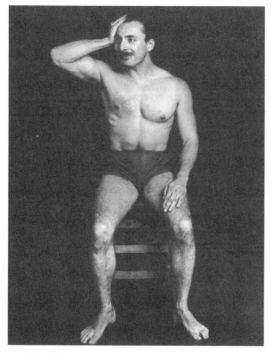

■ **FIG. 33-8** Cervical strengthening exercise: rotator muscles.

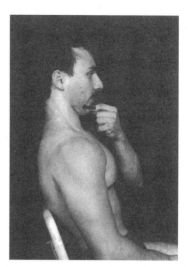

■ **FIG. 33-10** Second exercise for cervicothoracic asymmetry.

c. Hold for 4 seconds, then relax.
d. Repeat the exercise, gradually increasing the strength of the contracting force and hand resistance. For left rotation, reverse directions. Do not create pain. Do not hold a static contraction for more than 5 seconds.

## ■ CERVICOTHORACIC ASYMMETRY

Exercises for cervicothoracic asymmetry are designed to reduce excessive cervical lordosis and

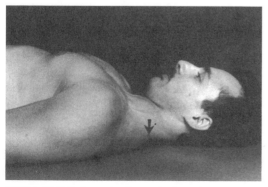

■ **FIG. 33-9** First exercise for cervicothoracic asymmetry.

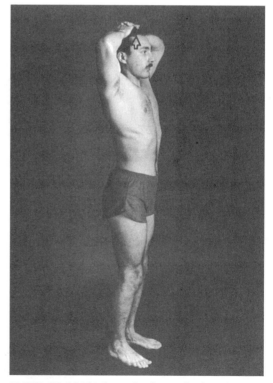

■ **FIG. 33-11** Third exercise for cervicothoracic asymmetry.

upper thoracic kyphosis (dowager's hump). Three exercises are described.

### Exercise 1

1. **Patient position:** supine on solid flat surface.
2. **Instructions:**
   a. Tuck in your chin.
   b. Try to push your neck down, flattening your neck against the surface (Fig. 33-9).
   c. Hold for 4 seconds, relax, and repeat.

### Exercise 2

1. **Patient position:** seated in a chair with back pressed firmly against the back of the chair. A pillow may be used to maintain a low back lordotic curve if necessary.
2. **Instructions:**
   a. Tuck in your chin.
   b. With one hand, push your chin toward the back of your neck, trying to flatten the neck. Your chin must be kept in one horizontal plane (Fig. 33-10).
   c. Hold for 4 seconds, relax, and repeat.

### Exercise 3

1. **Patient position:** standing.
2. **Instructions:**
   a. Stand straight with your back and neck stretched as tall as possible.
   b. Tuck in your chin.
   c. Place both hands on top of your head.
   d. Push your head up toward your hands, lengthening your neck. Keep your chin in one horizontal plane (Fig. 33-11).
   e. Hold for 4 seconds, relax, and repeat.

*Note:* Do not increase your lumbar lordosis. Once this procedure has been mastered, keep your hands down and practice standing and walking with your chin and neck in this position, as often as possible.

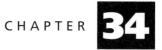

# Practical Applications and Case Histories

*Eileen L. DiGiovanna*

## ■ TRAUMA

The cervical spine is frequently involved in trauma caused by the flexibility of the neck with a heavy head sitting atop the small vertebrae. With the rapid motion of modern vehicles, acceleration/deceleration injuries of the neck are quite common. As the neck is snapped forward and backward, the long muscles tend to have their fibers torn, with associated bleeding into the muscles. However, it is important to remember that "whiplash injury" is not a problem of the cervical spine alone, because the entire body has abnormal forces applied to it. Osteopathic manipulation is a major part of the treatment of the patient with whiplash injuries.

## ■ POSTURE

Posture is significant to any problem of the cervical spine. If the head is carried too far forward or too far back, abnormal stresses are placed on the supporting cervical muscles. A slouching of the upper back and shoulders carried forward lead to an increase in the cervical lordosis with muscular strains. In women with long, thin necks and weak supporting muscles, there is a greater risk of injury and the development of somatic dysfunctions. Working, especially in stressful conditions, with the head and neck bent forward, commonly leads to abnormal tensions in the muscles with the development of pain and somatic dysfunction.

## ■ STRESS

The cervical region musculature is commonly involved in stress-related reactions. During times of stress, individuals tend to tense the neck and upper back muscles, elevate the shoulders, and as a result have pain and stiffness of the neck and upper back. Some patients tend to "carry the weight of the world" on their shoulders, and the trapezius tenses. Often, tender points and trigger points develop in this muscle. Trigger points in the trapezius usually refer pain to the head. Teaching the patient techniques to cope with stress is important in the treatment of stress-related somatic dysfunctions.

## ■ HEADACHE

Tension headaches begin in the neck and scalp muscles. These muscles tense during stress or with poor posture. Spasm and somatic dysfunctions follow. The spasm leads to ischemia of the involved muscles and there is a build-up of metabolic wastes. Pain, described as a headache, then occurs.

Other types of headaches, including migraines, often have elements of muscle tension and somatic dysfunction. Somatic dysfunction of the upper cervical spine causes pain behind the eyes. Migraine headaches are frequently associated with abnormal motions or restrictions of the temporal bones. Any patient with headache should be evaluated for somatic dysfunctions of the cranium and cervical spine with treatment of any found.

## ■ TEMPOROMANDIBULAR JOINT DYSFUNCTION

Temporomandibular joint (TMJ) dysfunction may be caused by or may cause dysfunctions of the cervical spine. The neck must always be evaluated in cases of TMJ pain and restriction of motion. The sternocleidomastoid muscle is often involved in these dysfunctions along with the muscles of mastication.

## ■ SINUSITIS

Sinusitis is almost always in conjunction with somatic dysfunction of the upper cervical spine Sympathetic innervation to the sinus areas arises from the upper cervical region. An occipitoatlantal somatic dysfunction is the most common. Treating the cervical somatic dysfunctions and performing sinus drainage techniques help to relieve pain as well as assist in drainage of the sinuses.

## ■ LEVATOR SCAPULAE DYSFUNCTION

The levator scapula muscle is frequently involved in neck and posterior shoulder pain. Spasm of this muscle often occurs due to overuse in persons using computers or typewriters. These individuals need to be evaluated for correct posture and ergonomic working conditions. Taking time to stretch and relax the cervical muscles helps prevent this common problem. Untreated, trigger points tend to form in this muscle leading to increased pain and disability.

## ■ TORTICOLLIS (WRYNECK)

Torticollis or wryneck is a shortening of a muscle on one side of the neck, usually the sternocleidomastoid. The head is pulled toward the affected side and rotated in the opposite direction. This often has a congenital component and is seen in infants and young children. Neuromuscular problems may cause torticollis. Many times no specific cause can be found, especially in adults.

Torticollis may require the injection of botulinum toxin, which paralyzes the contractured muscle and allows the head to return to a normal position. Osteopathic manipulation may relieve many of these cases.

## ■ CASE 1: WHIPLASH INJURY TO THE CERVICAL SPINE

Mary K. is a 30-year-old woman in whom neck pain and stiffness developed after an automobile accident. She had stopped for a red light when a car larger than her own struck her from behind. She was wearing a seat belt and sustained no injuries that she noted at the time of the accident. Several hours later, she began to feel an ache in her neck and it became difficult for her to bend her head forward or to either side.

At the time of her first visit, she reported a slight headache and a feeling of nausea, as well as the neck pain and stiffness. She had been well until the time of the accident and was using no regular medications. She seldom experienced headaches and had no past history of musculoskeletal problems or injuries.

Her physical examination was unremarkable for any problems other than findings related to the neck injury. The posterior neck musculature was tense and tender to palpation. Motion was grossly restricted in flexion, side-bending, and rotation bilaterally. There was some muscle tension and tenderness in the upper back to about the level of T4. A neurologic examination was normal. The cranial rhythm was sluggish and there was a tendency toward a right side-bending dysfunction of the basi-occiput.

An x-ray of the cervical spine was normal except for a flattening of the cervical lordosis.

Mary was treated initially with cranial manipulation for a decreased rhythm of the cranial rhythmic impulse, given a soft collar, and told to use ice and rest for 48 hours. She was to take a nonsteroidal anti-inflammatory medication as needed for pain. She was then to return for a follow-up evaluation in 48 hours.

At the second visit she still reported a slight headache, but the muscles were less tense and tender. Somatic dysfunctions were diagnosed: $C3ES_RR_R$ and $C7S_LR_L$. She was treated with counterstrain and muscle energy techniques. She was told to stop using the collar and to begin gentle isometric strengthening exercises. At the third visit, she was feeling much better. The C3 dysfunction had returned but the muscles were more relaxed. This dysfunction was treated with facilitated positional release and some gentle muscle energy used on the remaining tensions in the muscles. She was discharged, pain-free, after the third visit.

## Discussion

"Whiplash" is commonly used to describe a soft tissue injury caused by acute hyperextension–hyperflexion of the cervical spine. These injuries are identified as *whiplash, acceleration injuries*, and *cervical strain/sprain*. Motor vehicle accidents account for the majority of this type of injury. When a vehicle is struck from the rear, the unsupported head and neck are thrown into hyperextension, followed quickly by a hyperflexion. The soft tissues bear the brunt of the forces. There is a sudden elongation of relaxed, unprepared muscles. The intrafusal muscle fibers, which normally monitor muscle length, are stretched and produce—by a reflex reaction—a strong contraction of the involved muscle. This contributes to the recoil of the neck. If the stretch is great enough, there will be a tearing of the fibers. There may be some bleeding into the muscle tissue. Edema and microhemorrhage lead to an irritability of the muscles leading to spasm. While hyperflexion results in damage to the posterior muscles, hyperextension will injure the anterior ones. Trigger points may develop in involved muscles. Some compression of the vertebrae may occur and anterior or posterior translation frequently will occur.

Other symptoms such as headache, nausea, dizziness, or paresthesias may be present. Because the entire body is involved with the forces that cause the hyperflexion and hyperextension, it is important to evaluate the entire spine. The sacrum is frequently involved in somatic dysfunction. If the sacral dysfunction is not treated, it tends to maintain disability in cases that fail to respond to treatment. Dysfunctions of the cranium are commonly present after an acceleration/deceleration injury. The occiput and sacrum tend to exhibit the same restrictions to motion. The temporal bones are especially vulnerable to the forces transmitted through the sternocleidomastoid muscles.

Radiological studies may be necessary to rule out occult fractures or dislocations despite the fact that the majority of films show only an alteration in the cervical lordosis, either a flattening or an actual reversal of the curve. A significant reversal of the curve undoubtedly indicates some degree of structural damage.

The initial phase of whiplash injury is characterized by muscle contraction and limitation of head and neck motion. Soft tissues feel warm and boggy. These tissues require ice for the first 18 hours after the injury, to stop the microhemorrhages, and rest for 24 to 48 hours to allow healing to begin. Moist heat may be used at home after that time. A soft collar may be used to prevent unwanted motion of the neck for the first 24 to 48 hours. It should be removed after that time so that the cervical muscles do not lose strength. Areas adjacent to those most severely injured should be treated with osteopathic manipulation, particularly the cranium and the sacrum. Nonsteroidal anti-inflammatory medication may be given, if appropriate, to ease the discomfort.

Once the acute inflammation has subsided, some tissue tension will still remain. Range of motion will improve but may still be limited. The patient may now be treated with appropriate osteopathic manipulative techniques to the injured area or wherever somatic dysfunction is found. Muscle energy, counterstrain, lymphatic drainage techniques, cranial, and facilitated positional release techniques may be used judiciously. Thrusting techniques should not be used until the soft tissues are no longer boggy and warm. If necessary, they may be used to correct stubborn somatic dysfunctions with firm barriers to motion.

Adjunctive therapy may be used as necessary, including the treatment of trigger points. The patient should be encouraged to exercise the cervical spine and any other involved areas to promote muscle relaxation and strengthening. Physical therapy may be necessary to assist patients with their exercise program.

## ■ CASE 2: TORTICOLLIS

Alyssa R. was a 4-year-old girl who was brought to the clinic by her mother and father. Alyssa had a stiffness of her neck and held her head tilted to the right. Her parents reported no history of injury. The child had not reported pain, but the mother noticed that when she was playing she sat with her head tilted. The mother observed her over time and she always maintained this position except when asleep. If her mother tried to bend her head to the left, the child said that it hurt and would begin to cry. She had been evaluated by a pediatric neurologist who had told the parents that she might have some form of muscular dystrophy, although the tests were negative to that point. He recommended a reevaluation in 6 months.

The mother reported a normal, vaginal birth history with normal development and activity. Alyssa was an only child but had many friends in preschool, some of whom came to her home to play.

Alyssa was a bright, cooperative child. When asked to bend her head to the left, she tried but said it hurt and was unable to do so. Forward and backward bending and side-bending to the right were normal. Left side-bending and rotation to the right and left were all restricted. The cervical muscles, especially on the right, were tense and ropy. The neurologic examination was normal, as was the rest of her physical examination. The cranial examination was normal. The rest of the musculoskeletal examination was normal, with no evidence of scoliosis.

The mother brought in cervical spine x-rays that had been taken previously and they were normal.

Alyssa was treated with gentle soft tissue techniques and muscle energy techniques at the first visit. Counterstrain was used on a tender point found at C3 on the left. The mother was shown how to gently stretch the neck into side bending to the left and was instructed to do this several times during the day. On each return visit, Alyssa showed gradual improvement. There was no evidence of contracture of any muscles, which could have led to permanent disability.

On one return visit, during questioning, the mother did admit to the fact that she and her husband had had some loud arguments. She did not think Alyssa had heard but could not be sure. This may have been a stressful situation for Alyssa if she had overheard her parents.

## Discussion

Torticollis is often caused by a neurologic condition and this must be ruled out before manipulative treatment. In this case, no neurologic condition could be diagnosed. In infants, it can be the result of positioning in the womb; but in this case, Alyssa was too old for that to be considered. Osteopathic treatment is helpful even in the case of a neurologic problem and may be used.

Children may need to be distracted during treatment. Holding a favorite toy or having the parent hold one in front of them may help. The muscles should be gently stretched. Use of muscle energy techniques is especially useful if the child is old enough to follow instructions. Thrusting techniques should not be used on children with torticollis.

As in this case, stress can be the major contributing factor. Having the mother perform regular stretching exercises at home has a physical benefit and an emotional one. Emotions are very much reciprocal with musculoskeletal problems, each affecting the other.

**REFERENCES**

Bailey RW, Sherk HH, Dunn EJ. *The Cervical Spine*. Philadelphia: JB Lippincott, 1983.

DiGiovanna E, Schiowitz S. *An Osteopathic Approach to Diagnosis and Treatment*. Philadelphia: Lippincott-Raven, 1997.

Esses SI. *Textbook of Spinal Disorders*. Philadelphia: JB Lippincott, 1995.

Foreman SM, Croft AC. *Whiplash Injuries, The Cervical Acceleration/Deceleration Syndrome*, 2nd ed. Baltimore: Williams & Wilkins, 1995.

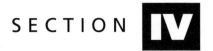

# Thoracic Spine

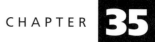

# Thoracic Spine Anatomic Considerations

*Jonathan F. Fenton and Donald E. Phykitt*

The thoracic spine is a relatively immobile area, compared with the cervical or lumbar spine. The immobility has two anatomic causes. First, considerable stability is provided by the intimate connection of the thoracic spine to the thoracic cage, the ribs and sternum, via the costovertebral articulations. Second, the ratio of intervertebral disk height to vertebral body height is small (1:5), which greatly reduces intersegmental motion. By contrast, the disk height-to-vertebral body height ratios in the cervical and lumbar regions are 2:5 (permitting greatest motion) and 1:3, respectively.

Although the thoracic spine normally displays a gentle kyphosis, a C-shaped curve, convex posteriorly. This is mainly caused by the wedge shape of the vertebral bodies, which are slightly higher at the posterior edge than at the anterior edge. The degree of kyphosis can vary with age and postural habits as well as with pathologic conditions, such as osteoporosis.

Although the thoracic spine has characteristic features that distinguish it from the cervical and lumbar spinal regions, it is mainly a transitional zone between the cervical and lumbar regions, as evidenced by the steady increase in height of the vertebral bodies from T1 to T12. Moreover, the inferior articular facets of T12 correspond to those in the lumbar area to allow proper articulation with L1. The different forms of articulation play a considerable role in the amplitude of various physiologic motions in the thoracic spine.

## ■ OSTEOLOGY

### Vertebral Body

The transverse diameter of the thoracic vertebral body is approximately equal to its anteroposterior diameter. The vertebral body is slightly higher at the posterior edge than at the anterior edge, contributing to normal kyphosis in the area. The anterior and lateral edges of the body are hollow.

The posterolateral corners of the superior and inferior vertebral plateaus bear the costal articular facets. These facets are oval, set into the body at an oblique angle, and lined by cartilage. They articulate with the heads of the ribs. Of the thoracic vertebrae, only T12 has costal articular facets only at the superior plateau.

### Articular Facets

The superior articular facets face backward, upward, and laterally. They are rotated approximately 60 degrees from the horizontal plane and 20 degrees from the frontal plane. In the transverse dimension, they are convex.

The inferior articular facets face forward, downward, and medially. In the transverse dimension, they are concave. The inferior articular facets of T12 resemble those of a lumbar vertebra in that they face laterally and anteriorly and are convex transversely.

### Transverse Processes

The transverse processes of the thoracic vertebrae face laterally and slightly posteriorly; they are easily palpated. They bear costal articular facets at the anterior aspects of their bulbous tips, the point of articulation with the costal tubercles of the corresponding ribs.

## The Spinous Process

The spinous processes face posteriorly and inferiorly, the degree of inferior angulation varying with the area of the thoracic spine. The *"rule of 3s"* is used to locate a vertebra's spinous process in relation to its transverse process.

## Rule of 3s

1. The upper three thoracic vertebrae (T1, T2, T3) have spinous processes that project directly posteriorly; therefore, the tip of the spinous process is in the same plane as the transverse processes of that vertebra.
2. The next three vertebrae (T4, T5, T6) have spinous processes that project slightly downward; therefore, the tip of the spinous process lies in a plane halfway between that vertebra's transverse processes and the transverse processes of the vertebra below it.
3. The next three vertebrae (T7, T8, T9) have spinous processes that project moderately downward; therefore, the tip of the spinous process is in a plane with the transverse processes of the vertebra below it.
4. The last three thoracic vertebrae (T10, T11, T12) have spinous processes that project from a position similar to T9 and rapidly regress until the orientation of the spinous process of T12 is like that of T1. That is, the spinous process of T10 is near the plane of the transverse processes of the vertebra below it, the spinous process of T11 is halfway between its own transverse processes and the transverse processes of the vertebra below it, and the spinous process of T12 projects directly posteriorly in the plane of its own transverse processes.

## ■ RIB ARTICULATIONS

## Costovertebral Articulations

The articular facets on the vertebral bodies are really demifacets (i.e., partial facets). The entire facet consists in the demifacet on the superior aspect of one vertebra and the demifacet on the inferior aspect of the vertebra above it.

The heads of the second through twelfth ribs articulate with the bodies of the corresponding vertebrae and the one above, as well as with the corresponding intervertebral disk. However, the first rib articulates only with the superior aspect of T1. The costovertebral articulation is a synovial joint, with a joint capsule that is strengthened by the radiate ligament (see Costovertebral Ligaments).

## Costotransverse Articulations

The costotransverse articulation is a joint representing the articulation of the tubercle of a rib with the transverse process of the corresponding vertebra. The joint is surrounded by a weak capsule that is greatly strengthened by the costotransverse ligaments.

## Anterior Articulations

The anterior ends of the ribs are joined to its costal cartilage by the costochondral joint. The costal cartilage articulates anteriorly in a number of stenochondral joints with different formations.

1. The first rib is joined to the manubrium by a cartilaginous joint.
2. The cartilage of the second rib articulates with joints on both the manubrium and the body of the sternum by way of synovial joints.
3. The cartilages of the third through seventh ribs create small synovial joints with the body of the sternum.
4. The eighth through tenth costal cartilages do not directly join the sternum but connect with the seventh rib costal cartilage immediately above.
5. The eleventh and twelfth costal cartilages are free. These ribs are known as the floating ribs.

## ■ LIGAMENTOUS ATTACHMENTS

Seven ligaments connect adjacent vertebrae in the thoracic spine.

1. The anterior longitudinal ligament is attached to the anterior surface of all vertebral bodies.

2. The posterior longitudinal ligament runs down the posterior surface of all vertebral bodies.
3. Intertransverse ligaments pass between the transverse processes in the thoracic spine.
4. Capsular ligaments are attached just beyond the margins of the adjacent articular processes.
5. Ligamenta flava (arcuate, flaval, or yellow ligaments) extend from the anteroinferior border of the laminae above to the posterosuperior borders of the laminae below.
6. Interspinous ligaments connect adjacent spinous processes; they extend from the root to the apex of each spinous process.
7. The supraspinous ligament originates in the ligamentum nuchae and continues along the tips of the spinous processes.

## Costovertebral Ligaments

There are two kinds of costovertebral ligaments, interosseous ligaments and radiate ligaments, with the latter consisting of three bands. Interosseous ligaments are attached to the head of the rib between the two articular demifacets and to the corresponding intervertebral disk. In the radiate ligaments, the superior band of tissue runs from the head of the rib to the vertebral body above. The inferior band runs from the head of the rib to the corresponding vertebral body, and the intermediate band runs from the head of the rib to the corresponding intervertebral disk.

## Costotransverse Ligaments

There are three kinds of costotransverse ligaments, determined by anatomic location with respect to the ribs and vertebrae—interosseous, posterior, and superior. The interosseous costotransverse ligament runs from the transverse process to the posterior surface of the neck of the corresponding rib. The posterior costotransverse ligament runs from the tip of the transverse process to the lateral border of the corresponding costal tubercle. The superior costotransverse ligament runs from the inferior border of the transverse process to the superior border of the neck of the underlying rib.

## ■ THORACIC SPINAL MOTION

### Intervertebral Motion, Excluding Ribs

#### Extension (Least Motion)

In extension, the vertebrae approximate posteriorly. The inferior articular process of the superior vertebra glides posteriorly and inferiorly on the inferior vertebra. Motion is limited by approximation of the articular processes and spinous processes. These structures are sharply inclined posteriorly and inferiorly, and in normal anatomic relation are almost touching. The anterior longitudinal ligament is stretched, and the posterior longitudinal ligament, the ligamenta flava, and the interspinous ligaments are relaxed.

#### Flexion (Second Least Motion)

During flexion, the interspace between vertebrae increases posteriorly. The inferior articular process of the superior vertebra glides anteriorly and superiorly. Motion in the flexed spine is limited by the tension developed in the interspinous ligaments, the ligamenta flava, and the posterior longitudinal ligament.

#### Lateral Flexion (Second Greatest Motion)

In lateral flexion, the articular surfaces on each side of a vertebra glide in opposite directions: on the contralateral side they glide upward, as in flexion; on the ipsilateral side they glide downward, as in extension. Lateral flexion to one side is accompanied by axial rotation to the opposite side, for three reasons: (1) one articular surface glides anteriorly while the other glides posteriorly; (2) compression developed in the intervertebral disk, the anterior aspect of the unit, causes the vertebral body to move in the direction opposite to that of side-bending; and (3) lateral flexion tends to stretch the contralateral ligaments, located at the posterior aspect of the unit, which causes these ligaments to move toward the midline posteriorly to minimize their lengths.

Motion in the laterally flexed thoracic spine is limited by the impact of the articular processes on the ipsilateral side and by the tension developed in the contralateral ligamenta flava and intertransverse ligaments.

### Rotation (Greatest Motion)

In rotation, the orientation of the thoracic articular facets allows them to glide relative to each other with an axis of rotation near the center of the vertebral body. Thus, one vertebra can rotate around an axis, producing a simple twisting of the thoracic intervertebral disk. In contrast, the facets of the lumbar vertebrae are aligned such that the axis of rotation is at the spinous process. For rotation to occur, one vertebral body must glide laterally with respect to its adjacent vertebrae. This results in shearing forces at the intervertebral disk. The articulation at T12–L1 is identical to the articulations found in the lumbar spine, so that the degree of rotation is greatly reduced. For the thoracic spine, motion in rotation is limited by multiple ligamentous tensions.

### ■ STABILITY AFFORDED BY THE COSTAL CAGE

There are two mechanisms by which the ribs tend to increase the stability (and decrease the motion) of the thoracic spine. The first mechanism involves the articulation of the head of the ribs with the body and transverse processes of the vertebrae. The second mechanism increases the spine's moment of inertia via an increase in the transverse and anteroposterior dimensions of the spine structure. This results in increased resistance to motion in all directions.

Although no studies have compared the motion of the thoracic spine with and without intact costovertebral joints, White and Panjabi et al. have determined that the costovertebral joint plays a critical role in stabilizing the thoracic spine during flexion and extension.

The rib cage as a whole greatly enhances the stiffness of the spine, despite the flexibility of the individual components of the rib cage—the ribs, sternum, and their joints. Using a mathematical model of the thoracic and lumbar spine and the rib cage, Andriacchi et al. performed computer simulations to determine the effect of the rib cage

on the stiffness of the normal spine during flexion, extension, side-bending, and axial rotation. They also studied the effect of removing one or two ribs or the entire sternum from an intact thorax. The stiffness properties of the spine were found to be greatly enhanced by the presence of an intact rib cage for all four motions, especially extension. The percentage increase in the stiffness of the spine with an intact rib cage, as compared with the spine and ligaments alone, was 27% for flexion, 132% for extension, 45% for lateral bending, and 31% for axial rotation. Removal of the sternum virtually nullified the stiffening effect of the costal cage. Removal of one or two ribs had minimal effect.

Thus, the intact thoracic cage, rather than individual elements or articulations, is a major factor contributing to the increased stability of the thoracic spine.

### ■ OVERALL MOTION OF THE THORACIC SPINE

The thoracic spine is a transitional region between the relatively more mobile cervical and lumbar regions. It is designed for rigidity and support of vital structures. The extent of each of the four physiologic motions varies throughout the region because of variable effects of the costal cage and changes in vertebral osteology from a cervical-like osteology to a lumbar-like osteology.

*Flexion and extension.* Flexion and extension are the least of the motions of the thoracic spine and occur to the smallest extent in the upper thoracic spine, gradually increasing in amplitude in the lower thoracic spine. This transition is largely caused by the stiffening effect of the costal cage in the upper thoracic spine, which is most evident during extension. The first seven ribs are attached directly to the sternum, promoting greatest stability. The next three ribs are only indirectly attached via costal cartilage. The last two ribs are not attached at all anteriorly and therefore resemble the cylinder with a strip cut out, providing considerably less stability than the ribs higher in the costal cage.

The motions of flexion and extension in the thoracic spine are further limited by costovertebral articulations. This stabilization is lost at T11–T12 and T12–L1, because the eleventh and twelfth rib articulates only with the same numbered body, thus losing the support found when a rib articulates with two adjacent vertebrae.

## Lateral Bending

Lateral bending is the second greatest motion in the thoracic spine. The amplitude of motion remains fairly constant throughout the region but is restricted by articular impingement, by ligamentous attachments (including costovertebral and costotransverse ligaments), and by the resistance afforded by the intact costal cage.

## Rotation

Rotation is the greatest motion in the larger part of the thoracic spine (T1–T10). The amplitude of rotation is markedly decreased in the lower part of the region. The articular orientation of the thoracic vertebrae allows them to rotate about a point in the center of the vertebral body. The articular orientation of the lower thoracic vertebrae, however, is similar to that of the lumbar vertebrae and permits rotation only about a point near the spinous process. This rotation is greatly resisted by shearing forces in the intervertebral disk. The extent of rotation is further diminished by the resistance afforded by the intact costal cage.

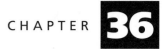

# Evaluation of the Thoracic Spine

*Eileen L. DiGiovanna and Donald E. Phykitt*

## ■ OBSERVATION

Observation of the thoracic spine should be performed from the back and from each side. One should observe for any abnormal curvature of the spinal column. *Kyphosis*, an increase in the normal anteroposterior curvature of the spine, or *scoliosis*, an abnormal lateral curve should be looked for. Kyphosis is sometimes manifested in the upper thoracic spine as the *dowager's hump* so frequently seen in osteoporosis, especially in older women. Flattening of the thoracic spine may be seen in the presence of muscle spasm or somatic dysfunction. See Chapters 48, 58, and 78 for a further discussion of these postural changes and their significance.

The skin should be inspected for any signs of trauma or surgical scars. Skin lesions should be noted. The erythema test and skin drag test can be performed as possible indicators of somatic dysfunction.

## ■ PALPATION

The soft tissues of the thoracic area should be palpated for texture changes: skin, fascia, subcutaneous tissues, and muscle. Large muscle hypertonicity or small localized areas of muscle tension should be noted. Areas of tenderness or specific Jones tender points or trigger points should be noted.

Bony landmarks may be palpated, especially looking for asymmetries of position of the spinous processes and transverse processes. It is important to recall the *rule of 3s* when attempting to identify specific locations of asymmetries; the transverse processes are not always at the same level as the vertebral body and spinous process. Bony landmarks of the scapula are useful in evaluating muscle attachments and vertebral levels. The inferior angle of the scapula lies at the level of T7 and the spine of the scapula at the level of T3. The twelfth rib may be used to identify T12 and the *vertebra prominens* (C7) may be used to locate T1 just below it, also a prominent spinous process.

## Tissue Texture Changes and Symmetry

1. **Patient position:** seated comfortably, with the hands on the thighs and the cervical spine in neutral position.
2. **Physician position:** standing behind the patient.
3. **Technique:**
   a. The physician slides one finger along the spinous processes from T1 to T12. *Note:*
      (1) Deviation from midline.
      (2) Any change in the size of the space between spinous processes.
      (3) Displacement of the spinous processes in the sagittal plane.
      (4) Point tenderness along the spinous processes.
   b. Place the pads of the second and third fingers on each side of the spinous process of T1, over the transverse processes. Slide them down from T1 to T12. *Note:*
      (1) Tissue texture changes (firmness, bogginess).
      (2) Posterior prominence of transverse processes.

(3) Change in size of space between transverse processes.

(4) Deviation of spinous process from the midline.

## ■ GROSS MOTION TESTING

The thoracic spine should be evaluated for regional restrictions to motion. Because of the length of this region—12 vertebrae—it is helpful to divide the region into three segments: upper thoracic spine (T1–T4), mid-thoracic spine (T5–T8), and lower thoracic spine (T9–T12).

### Side-Bending, T1–T12

1. **Patient position:** seated.
2. **Physician position:** standing behind patient.
3. **Technique:**
   a. The physician places his hands on the patient's shoulders with the web of the thumb and first finger over the acromion. The thumb rests posteriorly, pointing to T12, and the fingers rest anteriorly.
   b. To evaluate *right* side-bending:
      (1) The physician exerts *downward* pressure accompanied by *left* translatory force on the *right* shoulder (Fig. 36-1A). The resulting force is transmitted downward through the body of T12.
      (2) Note the ease and degree of side-bending (normal = approximately 20 degrees) and the smoothness of the right lateral curve created in the thoracic spine.
   c. To evaluate *left* side-bending:
      (1) The physician exerts *downward* pressure accompanied by a *right* translatory force on the *left* shoulder. The resulting force will be directed downward through the body of T12.
      (2) Note the ease and degree of side-bending (normal = approximately 20 degrees) and the smoothness of the left lateral curve created in the thoracic spine.
   d. Compare the degree of side-bending in each direction.
   e. Note the presence and location of any pain experienced by the patient during these maneuvers.

### Side-Bending, T1–T8

1. **Patient position:** seated.
2. **Physician position:** standing behind the patient.

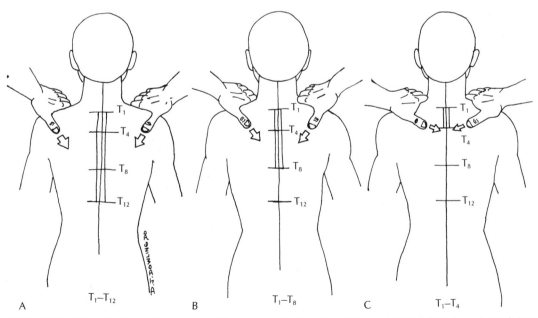

■ **FIG. 36-1 (A)** Localization of force induced for thoracic side-bending. T1 through T12. **(B)** T1 through T8. **(C)** T1 through T4.

3. **Technique:**
   a. The technique is similar to that described for side-bending of T1–T12, with the following modifications. The physician's hands are placed with the web of the thumb and first finger halfway between the base of the patient's neck and the acromion process. The thumbs point toward T8. Greater force is required to induce side-bending in the T1–T8 region. The resulting force exerted by the physician is directed downward and through the body of T8 (Fig. 36-1*B*).
   b. Compare the degree of side-bending (left versus right) and note any difference (normal = approximately 10 degrees).
   c. Observe the smoothness of the lateral curve created.

## Side-Bending, T1–T4

1. **Patient position:** sitting.
2. **Physician position:** standing behind patient.
3. **Technique:**
   a. The technique is similar to that described for testing side-bending of T1–T12 and T1–T4, with the following modifications. The physician's hands are placed with the web of the thumb and first finger as close as possible to the patient's shoulders at the base of the neck. The thumbs point toward T4. Greater force is required to induce side-bending than in the previous two tests. The force induced by the physician is directed downward and through the body of T4 (Fig. 36-1*C*).
   b. Compare the degree of side-bending (right versus left) and note any differences (normal = approximately 5 degrees).
   c. Note: Asymmetry in side-bending (right versus left) can be caused by single dysfunctions, group curves, or myofascial tension in the area being examined.

Discrepancies in findings between areas of the thoracic spine (T1–T12, T1–T8, or T1–T4) may indicate an area of dysfunction and should prompt the physician to examine this area more closely with the techniques of rotoscoliosis testing and intersegmental motion testing, described later.

## Rotation of the Thoracic Spine

1. **Patient position:** seated, straddling the table, with his back near the end of the table.
2. **Physician position:** standing behind patient.
3. **Technique:**
   a. The physician places a hand on each of the patient's acromion processes.
   b. Rotation is induced by the physician drawing one shoulder toward himself while simultaneously pushing away the opposite shoulder (Fig. 36-2).
      (1) *Right rotation:* The physician draws the right shoulder toward himself while pushing away the left shoulder.
      (2) Left rotation: The physician draws the left shoulder toward himself while pushing away the right shoulder.
   c. Note:
      (1) The degree of rotation in each direction. This is best measured by noting the deviation of the shoulder line from the frontal plane. Normal rotation is approximately 40 degrees in each direction.
      (2) The symmetry of right rotation versus left rotation.
      (3) The presence and location of pain during this maneuver.

## Forward Bending/Backward Bending

It is quite difficult to separate the motions of forward and backward bending in the thoracic

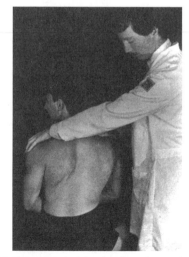

■ **FIG. 36-2** Position for thoracic rotation.

spine from the same motions in the lumbar spine. Therefore, these motions are considered for the combined thoracolumbar region, and the technique is described in Section V, Chapter 47.

## ■ SEGMENTAL TESTING

*Rotoscoliosis testing* and *intersegmental motion testing* are two diagnostic modalities for evaluating somatic dysfunction at a vertebral level. They can be used alone or in conjunction with each other, according to physician preference.

Rotoscoliosis testing evaluates the rotational position of the vertebrae with respect to the position of the transverse processes. This position is evaluated with the spine in neutral position, in flexion, and in extension.

Vertebrae involved in a group curve will exhibit the greatest positional rotation in neutral position. From Fryette's first principle, side-bending and rotation should occur in opposite directions. Single somatic dysfunctions exhibit the greatest positional rotation in either flexion or extension. From Fryette's second principle, side-bending and rotation should occur in the same direction. Furthermore, in single somatic dysfunctions, the freedom of motion (the direction for which the dysfunction is named) in flexion or extension will be opposite to the position in which the rotation is exaggerated.

The positions described in the following sections are the positions in which the patient is examined. Examples of examination findings and the corresponding diagnoses are given at the end of the chapter.

## ■ THE DOMINANT EYE

The dominant eye is the eye through which most information about the outside world is conveyed. A dominant eye develops in every person soon after birth and does not change for the duration of life. It has no relationship to handedness. It is helpful for the physician to identify his or her dominant eye so that that eye may be brought to the level being inspected for the most accurate information.

### Technique for Determining Dominant Eye

1. Make a circle by opposing your thumb and index finger.
2. Fully extend the arm in front of you.

3. With both eyes open, locate an object at least 10 feet away so that it is enclosed in the circle formed by your two fingers.
4. Maintaining this position, close each eye alternately, until the object remains in the circle.
5. The dominant eye is the one that "sees" the object as within the circle. The nondominant eye "sees" the object as outside the circle.

## ■ ROTOSCOLIOSIS TESTING

### Type II Somatic Dysfunction, T1–T3

1. **Patient position:** seated.
2. **Physician position:** standing behind the patient.
3. **Technique:**
   a. The physician uses **the second and third fingers of one hand** to palpate the tips of the transverse processes, located one-half inch lateral to and at the same level of the corresponding spinous process (Fig. 36-3).
   b. Evaluate for the presence of pain, increased myofascial tension, and one transverse process (right or left) more posterior than the other. The latter can be detected either by palpating a more posterior transverse process or by sensing a decreased tissue depth on the side of the posterior transverse process.

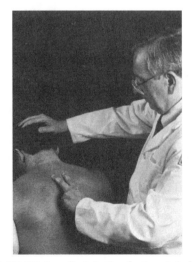

■ **FIG. 36-3** Rotoscoliosis testing for type II dysfunction in the upper thoracic.

c.  At each level, have the patient begin with the neck fully flexed. Instruct the patient to slowly bring his head back into neutral position and then into full extension.

d.  Observe the changes under your palpating fingers. *Note* the position (flexion, extension) in which the maximum positional rotation occurs, and the direction of positional rotation (side of the posterior transverse process).

e.  Repeat these steps for T2 and T3.

## Type II Somatic Dysfunction, T4–T12

Rotoscoliosis testing in the region of T4–T12 is identical to testing in the upper thoracic region, with the exception of differences in patient position for the different physiologic motions.

### Extension

1.  **Patient position:** prone, resting on his elbows. The upper thoracic musculature should be relaxed to allow full extension and to facilitate palpation (Fig. 36-4).

2.  **Physician position:** standing at the side of the patient, facing the patient's head. The physician's dominant eye is closer to the patient.

3.  **Technique:** described under Flexion, which follows.

### Flexion

1.  **Patient position:** seated, with the feet supported on the floor or a stool. The hands are locked behind the neck and the patient is instructed to bend forward as far as possible (Fig. 36-5).

2.  **Physician position:** standing in front of or behind patient.

3.  **Technique:** (for all lower thoracic rotoscoliosis diagnoses):

a.  The physician uses the thumbs or index fingers to palpate the tips of the transverse processes, located one-half inch to one inch lateral to the spinous processes.

b.  Evaluate the posterior transverse processes. Increased musculature in this region makes direct palpation of transverse processes difficult. Posterior rotation will most likely be detected from a decreased tissue depth.

c.  The physician positions himself so that he can visualize the midline of the patient's back parallel to the spine. *Note* the relative heights of the palpating fingers. Are they even? Is one finger more posterior?

d.  Begin by examining the entire lower thoracic region in neutral position and noting findings. Then instruct the patient to move up into extension, and note findings in this position. Finally, instruct the pa-

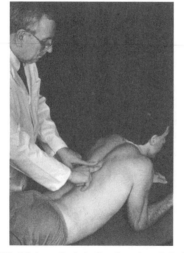

■ **FIG. 36-4** Rotoscoliosis testing for a type II dysfunction in mid-thoracic region, patient prone and extended.

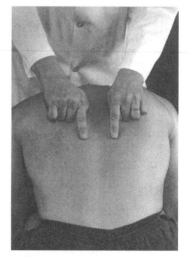

■ **FIG. 36-5** Rotoscoliosis testing for a type II dysfunction in the mid-thoracic region, patient seated and flexed.

tient to move into flexion, and note findings in this position.

e. After evaluating the lower thoracic region in all three positions, note in which position rotation was greatest at each vertebral level. It may be necessary to reevaluate one or more levels to determine the position in which the transverse process was most posterior.

## Type I Somatic Dysfunction

Evaluation of the thoracic spine for the detection of type I dysfunctions entails three different kinds of examinations:

1. Static symmetry. Observation from behind the patient may reveal side-bending of a group of vertebrae, asymmetry in the *height* of paired landmarks (e.g., shoulders), or asymmetry in the *prominence* of paired landmarks (e.g., scapulae).
2. Regional motion testing. The physician observes for asymmetric side-bending. Restricted motion to the side of the convexity is common.
3. Rotoscoliosis testing. The diagnosis of type I dysfunctions is based on detecting three or more adjacent vertebrae whose positional rotation is greatest in neutral. Testing is performed separately for the upper and lower thoracic regions.

### Upper thoracic region (T1–T3)

1. **Patient position:** seated.
2. **Physician position:** standing behind patient.
3. **Technique:**
   a. The patient is instructed to sit up straight, thus placing the vertebrae in neutral position.
   b. Using the thumbs, the physician palpates the transverse processes of T1 bilaterally.
   c. The physician determines which transverse process is more posterior.
   d. Repeat these steps at T2 and T3.

### Lower Thoracic Region (T4–T12)

1. **Patient position:** prone, head resting on chin and facing forward, arms either at the side or hanging down from table (Fig. 36-6).
2. **Physician position:** standing at the side of the patient, facing the patient's head. The

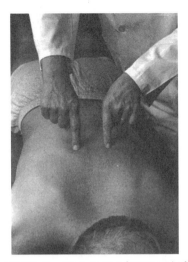

■ **FIG. 36-6** Rotoscoliosis testing for type I dysfunction, lower thorax, neutral position.

physician's dominant eye is closer to the patient.
3. **Technique:** Repeat test as described for rotoscoliosis testing for type II dysfunctions, T4–T12.

### Alternative Methods of Rotoscoliosis Testing, T4–T12

The methods described here are alternatives to conventional rotoscoliosis testing. Their advantages include ease and speed of diagnosis. The patient remains in a single position in all three methods. Furthermore, the physician can more readily compare findings in neutral, flexion, and extension. These techniques require greater palpatory skill and should be used only after much experience and correlation with other findings.

### Alternate Technique 1

1. **Patient position:** seated on a stool with the feet resting firmly on the ground, shoulder width apart.
2. **Physician position:** standing behind the patient.
3. **Technique:**
   a. The physician's thumbs are used to palpate the tips of the transverse processes bilaterally (Fig. 36-7).
   b. At each vertebral level, evaluation begins with the patient in neutral position (sitting

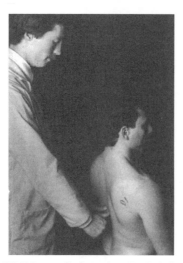

■ **FIG. 36-7** Rotoscoliosis testing, T4–T12, hand position.

straight up). *Note* pain, tissue changes, and vertebral rotation, as in conventional rotoscoliosis testing of T4–T12.

c. With the physician's thumbs at the same vertebral level, the patient is asked to bend over as far as possible. *Note* changes in vertebral positional rotation.

d. With the physician's thumbs at the same level, the patient is asked to sit up and position himself in extension.
   (1) To evaluate T4–T8, ask the patient to thrust his chest out as far as possible.
   (2) To evaluate T9–T12, ask the patient to thrust his abdomen out as far as possible.
   (3) Note changes in vertebral positional rotation.

e. Note in which position (neutral, flexion, or extension) vertebral positional rotation is greatest.

f. Repeat these steps for all levels, T4 through T12.

## Alternate Technique 2

1. **Patient position:** prone, head resting on chin, arms at sides.
2. **Physician position:** standing at the patient's side, with the dominant eye closer to the patient.

3. **Technique:**
   a. The physician's thumbs or index fingers are used to palpate the tips of the transverse processes bilaterally.
   b. At each level, the physician begins by palpating the vertebra in the neutral position by pressing straight down on the transverse processes.
      (1) Note tissue tension and vertebral positional rotation, as described for the conventional method.
      (2) Visualize the relative heights of thumbs, as described for the conventional method.
   c. With the thumbs at the same level, the physician evaluates the vertebrae in flexion.
      (1) Roll the thumbs superiorly and press down on the superior aspect of the transverse processes, thus placing the vertebrae into flexion (Fig. 36-8).
      (2) Evaluate as described.
   d. With the thumbs at the same level, the physician evaluates the vertebrae in extension.
      (1) Roll the thumbs inferiorly and press down on the inferior aspect of the transverse processes, thus placing the vertebrae into extension (Fig. 36-9).
      (2) Evaluate as described.
   e. Determine in which position (neutral, flexion, extension) the greatest positional rotation is found.
   f. Repeat these steps at all levels, T4 through T12.

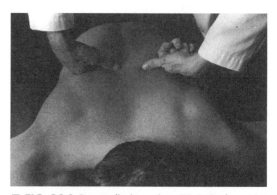

■ **FIG. 36-8** Rotoscoliosis testing, T4–T12 alternative technique 2, flexion testing.

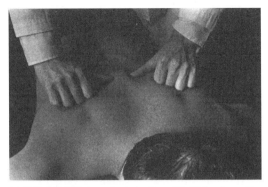

**■ FIG. 36-9** Rotoscoliosis testing, T4–T12, alternative technique 2, extension testing.

### Alternate Technique 3

1. **Patient position:** prone, head resting on chin, arms at sides.
2. **Physician position:** standing at the patient's side.
3. **Technique:**
   a. The physician places his hand on the patient's back with his fingers perpendicular to the patient's spine. One finger is placed in the interspinous space above and one finger in the interspinous space below the vertebra being evaluated.
   b. **Note:**
      (1) Symmetry of interspinous spaces above and below vertebra in question.
      (2) Lateral deviation of spinous process of vertebra in question.
      (3) Anteroposterior deviation of spinous process of vertebra in question.
   c. **Interpretation:**
      (1) Flexion (freedom of motion) dysfunction:
         a. Superior interspinous space narrower.
         b. Inferior interspinous space wider.
         c. Spinous process more prominent.
      (2) Extension dysfunction:
         a. Superior interspinous space wider.
         b. Inferior interspinous space narrower.
         c. Spinous process less prominent.
      (3) Neutral dysfunction (group curve):
         a. Superior and inferior interspinous spaces equal.

(4) Rotation:
   a. Spinous process deviated to the side opposite that of vertebral rotation.

**Example:** The spinous process of T6 is more prominent and rotated to the left; the space between the spinous processes of T5 and T6 is narrower than the space between the spinous processes of T6 and T7. The diagnosis is T6 flexion, rotation, and side-bending to the right.

   d. Repeat these steps at each level, T4 through T12.

### ■ EXAMPLES OF ROTOSCOLIOSIS FINDINGS AND CORRESPONDING DIAGNOSES

#### Example 1

Transverse process of T8 is posterior on the right and most prominent in flexion. Diagnosis: T8 E $S_R R_R$.

#### Example 2

Transverse processes of T4–T10 are posterior on the right and most prominent in neutral position. Diagnosis: T4–10 N $S_L R_R$.

#### Example 3

The same finding as in example two, except that the transverse process of T7 is posterior on the left and most prominent in extension. Diagnosis: group curve (T4–T10 N $S_L R_R$) with a single somatic dysfunction (T7 F $S_L R_L$) at the apex. *Note:* Single somatic dysfunctions can occur within a group curve. They are most common at the apex (center) and the ends of a curve.

### ■ INTERSEGMENTAL MOTION TESTING

Intersegmental motion testing is another method of determining the motion between two vertebrae as one is moved on the other. This assists in determining motion restrictions involved in somatic dysfunction.

### Intersegmental Motion Testing, T1–T4

1. **Patient position:** seated comfortably, with the hands on the thighs and the cervical spine in neutral position.

2. **Physician position:** behind and to one side of the patient. The hand farther from the patient (the motion-inducing hand) is placed on top of the patient's head. The position of the other hand (the palpating hand) varies with the motion being tested and is described for the individual cases.

3. **Technique:**

   a. In evaluating **flexion–extension,** the physician's palpating hand is placed so that the fingers are oriented horizontally and pointing away from the physician. The pad of the third finger lies in the interspinous space of the level being tested (i.e., for testing T1, it lies in the interspinous space between T1 and T2). The pads of the second and fourth digits lie in the interspinous spaces one level above and one level below, respectively. The patient's head is passively bent forward and backward until motion is palpated at the level in question, but not at the level below (Fig. 36-10). *Note* symmetry of flexion versus extension at the vertebral level.

   **Interpretation:** The dysfunction is named for the direction (flexion or extension) where greater motion is detected.

   b. To evaluate **rotation,** the physician places one or two fingers on either side of the spinous process, over the transverse processes of the vertebrae being tested. The patient's head is bent forward or backward (the direction in which least motion was detected on flexion–extension testing) down to the level in question. The patient's head is then rotated to the left until full motion is palpated at the transverse process in question (Fig. 36-11). This process is repeated to the right. *Note* symmetry of rotation right versus rotation left.

   **Interpretation:** The dysfunction is named for the direction of greater rotation.

   c. To evaluate side-bending, the physician places one finger on both sides of the spinous process, between the transverse processes of the level being tested and the level below. The patient's head is bent forward or backward (in the direction of least motion) down to the level being tested, then is bent laterally to both sides (Fig. 36-12). Side-bending is detected as separation or approximation of the transverse processes under the palpating fingers. *Note* symmetry of right side-bending versus left side-bending.

   **Interpretation:** The dysfunction is named for the direction of greater side-bending.

   Note that side-bending on intersegmental motion testing is greatly restricted by the ribs

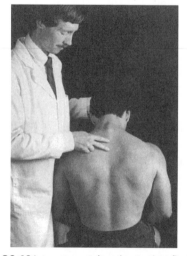

■ **FIG. 36-10** Intersegmental motion testing, flexion–extension T1–T4.

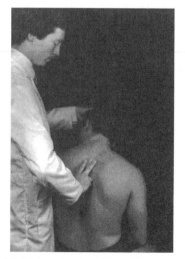

■ **FIG. 36-11** Intersegmental motion testing, rotation, T1–T4.

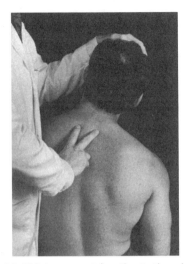

■ **FIG. 36-12** Intersegmental motion testing, side-bending, T1–T4.

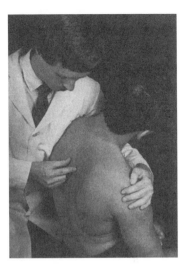

■ **FIG. 36-13** Intersegmental motion testing, rotation, T5–T12.

and may be difficult to evaluate. In normal spines or in group curves, side-bending is in the direction opposite the direction of rotation. In type II single-segment somatic dysfunctions, side-bending occurs in the same direction as rotation. The diagnosis of a side-bending limitation relies primarily on the finding of asymmetric motion in flexion–extension and in rotation.

## Intersegmental Motion Testing, T5–T12

The methods of diagnosing intersegmental dysfunction in the lower thoracic spine are quite similar to the techniques used in the upper thoracic spine. The patient position is the same except that the patient must sit up straight. The positions of the palpating hand are the same. However, the physician is positioned differently with respect to the patient, and different techniques are used to induce motion in the lower thoracic spine. Only these differences are described.

1. **Patient position:** as for intersegmental motion testing of the upper thoracic spine.
2. **Physician position:** behind and to one side of patient. The hand closer to the patient serves as the palpating hand. The other arm is positioned so that the axilla rests on the patient's near shoulder. The arm reaches across the patient's sternum and the hand grasps the patient's far shoulder.
3. **Technique:**
   a. **Flexion** is induced by applying a downward and slightly anterior force to both of the patient's shoulders.
   b. **Extension** is induced by applying a caudal and slightly posterior force to both of the patient's shoulders.
   c. **Rotation** is induced by rotating the shoulders in the desired direction (Fig. 36-13).
   d. **Side-bending** is induced by exerting a caudal force to one shoulder (the side ipsilateral to the desired side-bending), accompanied by a translatory force to the opposite side.

Palpation and interpretation are identical to those described for intersegmental motion testing of the upper thoracic spine.

### REFERENCES

DiGiovanna EL. Schiowitz S. *An Osteopathic Approach to Diagnosis and Treatment*, 2nd ed. Philadelphia: Lippincott-Raven, 1997.

Fryette H. *Principles of Osteopathic Technique*. Colorado Springs: Academy of Applied Osteopathy, 1954.

Kapandji IA. *The Physiology of the Joints, vol 3. The Trunk and the Vertebral Column*. Edinburgh: Churchill Livingstone, 1974.

Warwick R, Williams P. *Gray's Anatomy*, 35th British ed. Philadelphia: W.B. Saunders, 1973.

White A, Panjabi MM. *Biomechanics of the Spine*. Philadelphia: J.B. Lippincott, 1978.

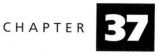

# Thoracic Myofascial Techniques

*Eileen L. DiGiovanna and Toni Spinaris*

The soft tissue techniques described in this chapter are good general techniques for relaxing and stretching the muscles of the thoracic and shoulder girdle. They may be used as the only treatment for a soft tissue hypertonicity and tension or to prepare the tissues for other types of osteopathic manipulative techniques.

## ■ PASSIVE TECHNIQUES

### Perpendicular Stretch

Perpendicular stretch techniques can be used to treat any muscles of the thoracolumbar region that run parallel to the spinous processes, including the erector spinae and their subdivisions.

1. **Patient position:** prone, with the head turned to the side of greater comfort.
2. **Physician position:** standing at the side of the table and opposite the side being treated.
3. **Technique:**
    a. The physician places the thumb and thenar eminence of one hand at the medial edge of the muscle to be treated and lateral to the spinous processes. The thumb is parallel to the spinous processes (Fig. 37-1).
    b. He then places the thenar eminence of the other hand over the thumb of the first hand (Fig. 37-2).
    c. The physician applies a slow, gentle pressure downward (toward the table) and laterally. The pressure is held for 3 seconds and gently released.

*Note:* The direction of the force is lateral and parallel to the table. Do not press down into the muscle belly when using this technique.

    d. The physician may shift his hands up or down the spine to treat different areas of the thoracolumbar region.
    e. The technique may be repeated several times.

### Treatment of Muscles Running Along Suprascapular Area from Cervical Region to Shoulder (e.g., Trapezius)

1. **Patient position:** prone, with the head turned toward the physician.
2. **Physician position:** standing at the side of the table and patient, and opposite to the side being treated, near shoulder level.
3. **Technique:**
    a. The physician places the thumb and thenar eminence of one hand perpendicular and slightly caudad to the fibers being treated.
    b. The other hand may reinforce the first or may be placed beside it to extend the area of treatment.
    c. The physician applies a slow gentle force downward and perpendicular to the muscle fibers (Fig. 37-3). This force is maintained for 3 seconds and gently released.

*Note:* Always push the muscle perpendicular to the fibers. Do not allow the hands to slip and cause friction on the skin.

    d. The technique may be repeated several times.

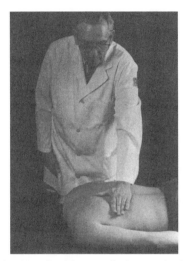

■ **FIG. 37-1** Myofascial perpendicular stretch, thumb position. For illustration, fingers point direction of push but are usually relaxed.

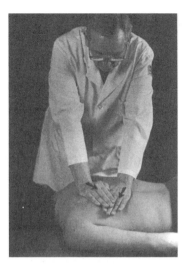

■ **FIG. 37-2** Myofascial perpendicular stretch, both hands in place.

## Treatment of Superior Border of Trapezius

1. **Patient position:** prone, with the head turned to the side of most comfort.
2. **Physician position:** standing at the side of the table and opposite the side being treated, near shoulder level.
3. **Technique:**
   a. The physician places his hand, which is closer to the patient's feet, over the patient's shoulder on the side to be treated.
   b. The fingers of the other hand are wrapped around the superior border of the trapezius, grasping the muscle border.
   c. The physician applies gentle traction on the trapezius while applying a downward counterpressure on the shoulder. The direction of traction should be upward from the table and perpendicular to the muscle fibers (Fig. 37-4).
   d. The traction is held for 3 seconds and gently released.

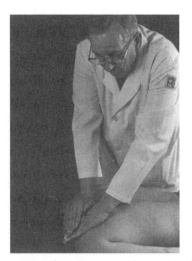

■ **FIG. 37-3** Myofascial perpendicular stretch of trapezius.

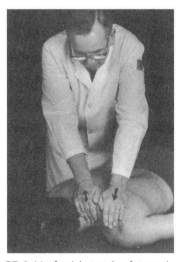

■ **FIG. 37-4** Myofascial stretch of trapezius, patient prone.

e. The physician may slide his treating hand closer to the patient's neck or shoulder in order to treat other parts of the muscle.

f. The technique may be repeated several times.

**Modification:** The same technique can be performed with the patient supine (Fig. 37-5).

## Treatment of Subscapular Muscles (e.g., Serratus Anterior)

1. **Patient position:** prone, with the head turned away from physician.
2. **Physician position:** standing at the side to be treated, slightly cephalad to the scapula.
3. **Technique:**
   a. The patient places his hand (on the side to be treated) behind his back until the scapula abducts away from the rib cage.
   b. The physician wraps his fingers around the medial border of the scapula (Fig. 37-6).
   c. A gentle upward and lateral traction is applied, pulling the scapula away from the rib cage. This force is maintained for 3 seconds and gently released.
   d. The technique may be repeated several times.

## Parallel Stretch

1. **Patient position:** prone, with the head turned to the side of greatest comfort.

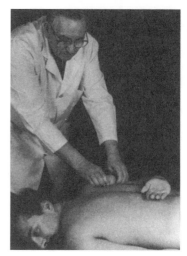

■ **FIG. 37-6** Subscapular muscle, myofascial stretch.

2. **Physician position:** standing at the side of the table opposite the side of being treated.
3. **Technique:**
   a. The physician's forearms are crossed and heels of his hands are placed on the body of the muscle with the fingers of each hand parallel to each other. One hand is directed cephalad, the other is directed caudad (Fig. 37-7).
   b. A gentle downward pressure is applied as the hands are separated.

*Note:* To avoid excessive stretching of the skin, the hands are placed approximately 1 inch apart, then moved together to create slack in the skin. This will bring the hands to the position shown in Figure 37-7.

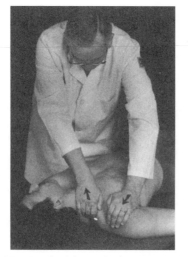

■ **FIG. 37-5** Myofascial stretch of trapezius, patient supine.

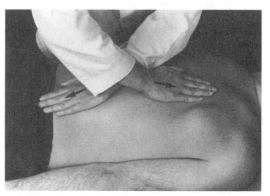

■ **FIG. 37-7** Parallel stretch of long muscle.

## Perpendicular Traction for Thoracic Region

1. **Patient position:** lying on his side, the side to be treated facing up. The hips and knees are flexed 90 degrees.
2. **Physician position:** standing at the side of the table and facing the patient.
3. **Technique:**
   a. The physician places her hands around the patient's scapula, allowing the patient's arm to hang over hers.
   b. Using her fingerpads, the physician gently grasps the muscle to be treated (erector spinae, trapezius), separating it from the spine.
   c. The physician rocks her body backward while simultaneously applying a lateral and anterior (with respect to the patient) traction on the muscle (Fig. 37-8). The traction is held for 3 seconds and released.

*Note:* The physician's hands should not slide over the patient's skin, because this will cause friction and irritation. To avoid fatigue, the physician should use leverage and rock her body rather than apply the traction force with her arms.

   d. The physician can move her hands (and body) caudad and cephalad to treat other muscle groups.

## Perpendicular Traction for the Thoracolumbar Area

1. **Patient position:** lying on his side, the side to be treated facing up. The knees and hips are flexed 90 degrees.

2. **Physician position:** standing at the side of the table, facing the patient. Her thighs rest against patient's knees.
3. **Technique:**
   a. The physician grasps the paravertebral muscles to be treated.
      (1) The fingers are directed perpendicular to the muscle fibers being treated.
      (2) The tips of the fingers are between the spinous processes and the muscle being treated.
   b. The physician rocks her body backward while simultaneously applying a gentle lateral and anterior traction to the muscle (Fig. 37-9).
      The physician exerts a counterforce with her thighs against the patient's knees.
   c. The traction is held for 3 seconds and gently released.
   d. The physician can move her hands up or down the back to treat other parts of the paravertebral musculature.

## Modification of Thoracolumbar Technique

1. **Patient position:** same as described.
2. **Physician position:** same as described, except the physician need not place her thighs against the patient's knees.
3. **Technique:**
   a. The physician grasps the muscle to be treated, as described.
   b. The physician braces her cephalad (with respect to the patient) elbow against the patient's axilla and the other elbow against

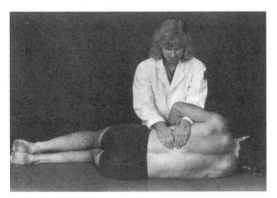

■ **FIG. 37-8** Perpendicular stretch, lateral recumbent.

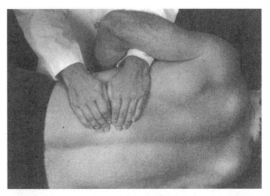

■ **FIG. 37-9** Perpendicular stretch of paravertebral muscles, patient lateral recumbent.

the patient's hip. The elbows should not dig into the patient's body.

c. The physician applies a gentle traction to the muscle while simultaneously pressing downward and cephalad on the axilla and downward and caudad on the hip (Fig. 37-10). This induces both a parallel stretch and perpendicular traction on the muscle.

## Medial Scapular Area (Levator Scapulae, Rhomboids, Superior Trapezius)

1. **Patient position:** lying on his side, with the side to be treated facing up.
2. **Physician position:** standing at the side of the table, facing the patient.
3. **Technique:**
   a. The physician grasps the medial scapular muscles with her cephalad (with respect to the patient) hand and places the patient's arm over hers, toward the patient's head.
   b. The physician's other hand is placed over the inferior portion of the scapula and is used to stabilize the patient.
   c. Gentle traction is applied in a direction perpendicular to the muscle fibers (Fig. 37-11).
   d. The traction is held for 3 seconds and gently released.

## Subscapular Area

1. **Patient position:** lying on his side, the side to be treated facing up.
2. **Physician position:** standing at the side of the table, facing the patient.

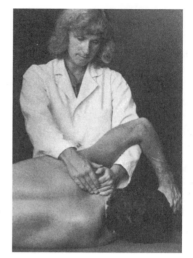

■ **FIG. 37-11** Medial scapular stretch, lateral recumbent.

3. **Technique:**
   a. The physician places her cephalad (with respect to the patient) hand over the patient's suprascapular area and grasps the upper medial border of the scapula with her fingers.
   b. With her other hand, the physician reaches under the patient's arm and grasps the inferior angle and border of the scapula (Fig. 37-12).
   c. The physician applies gentle traction laterally and caudally (relative to the patient), lifting the scapula into abduction and away from the rib cage.
      (1) The physician may also try to insert her fingers under the scapula and pull the scapula away from the rib cage (as

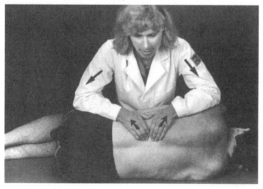

■ **FIG. 37-10** Thoracolumbar bi-directional stretch.

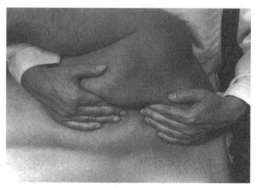

■ **FIG. 37-12** Subscapular stretch.

previously described and illustrated in Fig. 37-6).

    (2) This technique must be performed gently so as to not cause the patient discomfort.

  d. The traction is held for 3 seconds and gently released.

## ■ ACTIVE DIRECT TECHNIQUES

In the active direct techniques described, the patient pushes his hand toward the floor. The first two techniques can be used to treat the paravertebral muscles, the rhomboids, the levator scapulae, and the trapezius muscle.

## Technique I

1. **Patient position:** lying on his side, the side to be treated facing up.
2. **Physician position:** standing at the side of the table, facing the patient.
3. **Technique:**
  a. With her caudad hand, the physician palpates (monitors) the muscles to be treated.
  b. The other hand grasps the patient's upper arm at the elbow such that the arm is fully supported. The patient's arm is flexed at the elbow and the fingers point toward the floor.
  c. Once the area to be treated has been localized (see later), the physician instructs the patient to push his fingers toward the floor (Fig. 37-13).
  d. The physician provides an isometric resistive counterforce to the patient's arm with her cephalad hand.
  e. To localize the muscle fibers to be treated, she monitors the muscles with her caudad hand during the isometric contraction. The localization is controlled by the position (caudad or cephalad) of the patient's arm during isometric contraction.
    (1) The further cephalad the physician positions the patient's elbow during contraction, the further cephalad are the fibers that will contract (i.e., be treated).
    (2) The further caudad the physician positions the elbow, the further caudad are the fibers being treated

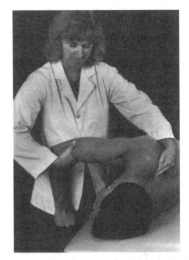

■ **FIG. 37-13** Active direct myofascial technique for thoracolumbar muscles. Patient pushes arm toward floor while physician gives isometric resistance.

    (3) The caudal hand monitors for muscle contraction localized to the fibers being treated.
  f. The isometric contraction is held for 3 seconds, then the patient is instructed to relax.
  g. This technique can be repeated at the same location, or the elbow can be repositioned to treat a different area.

## Technique II

In the technique described, the patient pushes his elbow toward the ceiling while the physician applies an isometric counterforce.

1. **Patient position:** lying on his side, the side to be treated facing up.
2. **Physician position:** standing at the side of the table, facing the patient.
3. **Technique:**
  a. The physician's caudad hand monitors the muscle being treated, as in the previous technique.
  b. The patient's arm is positioned as in the previous technique (elbow flexed, fingers pointing toward the floor). The physician grasps the dorsal aspect of the patient's elbow, the part closest to the ceiling (Figs. 37-14 and 37-15).
  c. The physician instructs the patient to push his elbow to the ceiling while she provides

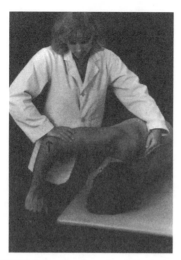

■ **FIG. 37-14** Active direct myofascial technique for thoracolumbar muscles. Patient pushes arm toward ceiling while physician gives isometric resistance.

an isometric resistive force with her cephalad (with respect to the patient) hand.
  d. With this technique the area being treated is in a direct line with the long axis of the patient's upper arm (Fig. 37-16).
    (1) If the patient's elbow is placed more cephalad, the fibers being treated are located more caudad.
    (2) If the elbow is placed more caudad, the fibers being treated are located more cephalad.

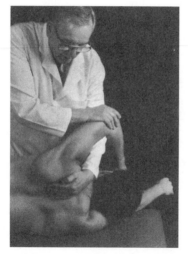

■ **FIG. 37-15** Active direct technique with arm supported.

  e. The isometric force is maintained for 3 seconds; then the patient is instructed to relax.
  f. The technique can be repeated at the same location, or the elbow can be repositioned to treat another area.

### Active Direct Technique III: Scapula

This technique is good as an initial treatment to facilitate general relaxation of the entire scapular area.

1. **Patient position:** lying on his side, the side to be treated facing up.
2. **Physician position:** standing at side of table, facing the patient.
3. **Technique:**
  a. The physician grasps the superior border of the scapula with her cephalad (with respect to the patient) hand and the inferior angle with her other hand. The patient's arm rests on her caudad arm.
  b. The physician gently presses her sternum against the patient's shoulder.
  c. Using the weight of her upper torso against the patient's shoulder, the physician gently pushes the scapula medially and either superiorly or inferiorly (whichever motion is more free). The scapula is held in this position.
  d. The patient pushes his shoulder straight up against physician's chest while she applies downward isometric resistive force.
  e. The contraction is maintained for 3 seconds; then the patient relaxes.
  f. The physician moves the scapula further medially and either superiorly or inferiorly.
  g. The technique is repeated three times.

### ■ ACTIVE INDIRECT TECHNIQUE

The active indirect technique described is a generalized technique for all the muscles in the upper and middle thoracic region.

1. **Patient position:** supine.
2. **Physician position:** standing at the side of the table near the patient's head, on the side opposite that being treated.
3. **Technique:**
  a. The patient grasps the wrist on the side being treated with his other hand. He is

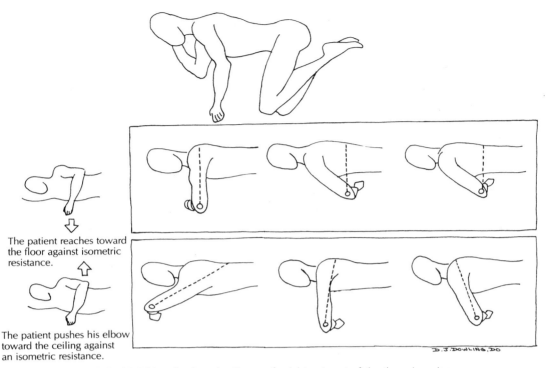

The patient reaches toward the floor against isometric resistance.

The patient pushes his elbow toward the ceiling against an isometric resistance.

■ **FIG. 37-16** Localization of active myofascial treatment of the thoracic region.

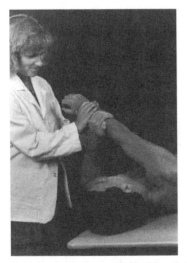

■ **FIG. 37-17** Active indirect myofascial technique for the thoracic region. The physician provides an isokinetic resistance to the patient's left arm pull. Passive stretch added at end.

then instructed to rotate his upper torso away from the physician while keeping his lower body flat on the table.

b. The physician reaches across the table and holds the patient's opposite wrist.

c. The patient pulls the arm he is holding (the one opposite the physician) across his body toward the physician, thus rotating his torso toward the physician.

d. The physician provides an isokinetic counterforce to this motion (Fig. 37-17).

e. The patient's active motion will end when his upper torso is fully rotated to the side of the physician.

f. The patient is instructed to relax.

g. The physician applies a passive stretch to increase the rotation while stabilizing the lower body at the opposite anterosuperior iliac spine.

h. The technique is repeated three times, with the physician providing increasingly greater counterforce each time.

# Muscle Energy of the Thoracic Spine

*Eileen L. DiGiovanna and Dennis J. Dowling*

This section describes the application of techniques to group curves and single-segment somatic dysfunctions in the thoracic spine. All of the techniques begin with the patient sitting erect and his feet adequately supported on the floor.

## ■ TYPE I GROUP CURVE (EXAMPLE T1–T10 N $S_R$ $R_L$)

1. **Patient position:** seated, feet on the floor
2. **Physician position:** standing behind the patient and to the side of the convexity of the group curve.
3. **Technique:**
   a. The physician monitors at the apex of the curve being treated with the hand that is closer to the convexity (i.e., physician's right hand monitors at T5 on left side).
   b. The physician places the forearm of his other arm on the patient's shoulder on the side of the convexity (i.e., physician's left arm on patient's left shoulder). He may use his axilla instead of the forearm.
   c. With the arm that is on the patient's shoulder, the physician induces side-bending toward the convexity and rotation away from the convexity (i.e., side-bends the patient to the left and rotates to the right) down to the monitored apex (Fig. 38-1).
   d. A translatory force should be applied toward the concavity if the aforementioned movement unbalances the patient. *Note*

that the spine is kept in neutral position (i.e., no flexion or extension).
   e. The patient is then directed to side-bend toward the concavity (the freedom of motion) for 3 to 5 seconds by attempting to raise the shoulder on the side of the curve convexity).
   f. The physician provides isometric resistance, producing a static contraction.
   g. The patient is directed to relax. This is typically maintained for 3 to 5 seconds but may be slightly longer if necessary.
   h. The physician further side-bends and rotates the patient until motion is felt at the new barriers.
   i. The procedure is repeated at least three times.
   j. A passive stretch is added after the last repetition.

## ■ TYPE II SINGLE-SEGMENT SOMATIC DYSFUNCTION

### Upper Thoracic Region (T1–T4) (Examples T3 $ES_RR_R$ or T3 $FS_RR_R$)

1. **Patient position:** seated, with feet on the floor.
2. **Physician position:** standing behind the patient and to the side of the motion barriers (i.e., physician stands to the left).
3. **Technique:**
   a. The physician's hand closest to the patient's spine monitors the somatic dys-

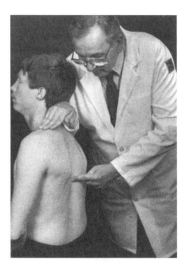

■ **FIG. 38-1** Muscle energy treatment for a type I group curve, convex right.

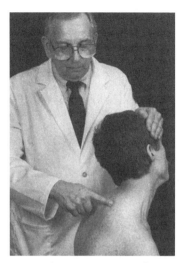

■ **FIG. 38-2** Muscle energy treatment for an upper thoracic type II somatic dysfunction.

function at the involved vertebra on the transverse process (i.e., physician's right hand monitors at T3 left transverse process).

b. The physician's other hand holds the patient's head, or the arm is wrapped around it turban-style to control its motion and to provide a resistance to the patient's motion.

c. The patient's neck is either flexed or extended to its motion barrier, while the physician monitors at the vertebra being treated.

d. The patient's head is then side-bent and rotated into the barriers to motion (side-bent and rotated left) until localized to the monitored somatic dysfunction (Fig. 38-2).

e. The patient is instructed to side-bend or rotate his head toward the freedom of motion (Fig. 38-3) for 3 to 5 seconds.

f. The physician provides isometric resistance, producing a static contraction.

g. The patient is directed to relax. This is maintained for 3 to 5 seconds typically but may be slightly longer if necessary.

h. The physician further side-bends and rotates the patient's neck into the barrier directions until motion is felt at the new barrier.

i. The procedure is repeated at least three times.

j. A passive stretch is added after the last repetition.

## Middle and Lower Thoracic Region (Example T7 F $S_L$ $R_L$ or T7 E $S_L$ $R_L$)

1. **Patient position:** seated, with the feet on the floor.

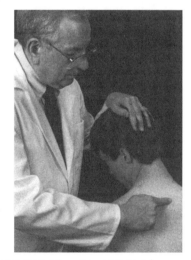

■ **FIG. 38-3** Muscle energy treatment for an upper thoracic type II somatic dysfunction. The barriers to flexion have been engaged, with left rotation and side-bending of the patient's head.

2. Physician position: standing behind the patient and to the side of the motion barriers (i.e., physician stands to the right).
3. **Technique:**
   a. The physician's finger is placed on the involved vertebra at the transverse process to monitor the somatic dysfunction (i.e., physician's left hand monitors at T7 right transverse process).
   b. The physician places the forearm of his other arm on the patient's shoulder on the barrier side (i.e., physician's right arm on patient's right shoulder) He may use his axilla instead of the forearm.
   c. The patient is flexed or extended to the motion barrier. Extension may be achieved by asking the patient to sit up straight or to stick his abdomen out (Fig. 38-4). Flexion is achieved by having the patient slump forward (Fig. 38-5). Motion should be localized to the involved segment.
   d. With the axilla or arm that is on the pa-

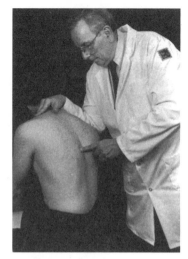

■ **FIG. 38-5** Muscle energy treatment for an extension type II somatic dysfunction of the middle and lower thoracic region. The barriers to flexion have been engaged, with right rotation and side-bending of the patient.

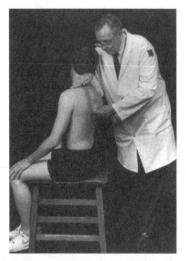

■ **FIG. 38-4** Muscle energy treatment for a flexion type II somatic dysfunction of the middle and lower thoracic region. The barriers to extension have been engaged, with right rotation and side-bending of the patient.

tient's shoulder, the physician side-bends and rotates the patient into the motion barriers at the involved segment (i.e., side-bends and rotates the patient to the right).
   e. If the dysfunction is low enough that side-bending unbalances the patient, a translatory force in the opposite direction may be used to keep the patient stable on the table.
   f. The patient is instructed to side-bend or rotate his shoulder toward a freedom of motion for 3 to 5 seconds.
   g. The patient is directed to relax. This is maintained for 3 to 5 seconds typically but may be slightly longer if necessary.
   h. The physician further side-bends and rotates the patient's torso into the barrier directions until motion is felt at the new barrier.
   i. The procedure is repeated at least three times.
   j. A passive stretch is added after the last repetition.

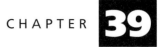

# Thoracic Counterstrain Techniques

*Eileen L. DiGiovanna*

$S$ome of the counterstrain tenderpoints correspond to vertebral segment dysfunctions. As in other areas of the body, when counterstrain treatment is used in the thoracic spine, the positions are held for 90 seconds. The patient is returned to a neutral position slowly, without any muscle contraction on his part, and the tender point is reassessed.

## ■ ANTERIOR TENDER POINTS

Figure 39-1 shows the locations of the anterior tender points for the thoracic spine. All anterior tender points are treated with flexion as the major movement in positioning. Fine-tuning of the position will be by side-bending and/or rotation.

## ■ UPPER THORACIC SPINE (T1–T4)

1. **Patient position:** supine. The head and upper torso rest on the physician's knee so that the upper thoracic spine is flexed to the desired level.
2. **Physician position:** standing at the head of the table and resting his knee on the table. One hand monitors the tender point.
3. **Technique:** Pure flexion is usually all that is necessary. However, some slight side-bending and rotation modification may help localize and reduce the point tenderness (Fig.39-2).

## ■ MID-THORACIC SPINE (T5–T8)

Mid-thoracic dysfunctions may require such marked flexion that flexion of the upper body alone may not be sufficient. Flexion may be increased if the patient's hips are bent and the spine is allowed to flex from the lumbar area into the lower thoracic area.

1. **Patient position:** supine, upper body supported by pillows, hips bent to 90 degrees, with lower legs resting on the physician's knee.
2. **Physician position:** at the side of table, one foot on the table with the knee bent, supporting the patient's lower legs on her thigh.
3. **Technique:** Patient is flexed up by bringing the knees toward the abdomen while monitoring the tender point. When tenderness is relieved, the position is held for 90 seconds.

   **Modifications:**

1. The technique may be performed with the patient in a lateral recumbent position with hips and knees flexed; the physician flexes the patient's torso until the tender point is relieved.
2. Another alternative is similar to that used for the upper thoracics, with the upper back supported by the physician's knee (Fig. 39-3).

## ■ LOWER THORACIC SPINE (T9–L1)

1. **Patient position:** supine, with knees and hips flexed and supported by the physician's knee. A pillow may be placed under the hips and upper back to aid flexion if necessary.
2. **Physician position:** standing at the side of the table next to the side of the tender point, one foot on the table and supporting the patient's legs.

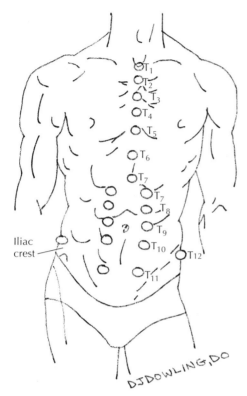

**FIG. 39-1** Locations of anterior thoracic tender points.

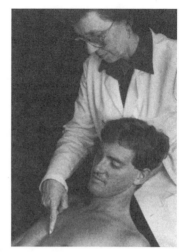

**FIG. 39-3** Counterstrain technique for anterior tender points: mid-thoracic spine.

3. **Technique:** The patient's knees and hips are flexed and the physician supports the patient's thighs on her thigh. Pressure is applied cephalad as the knees are rotated toward the side of dysfunction (Fig. 39-4).

## Posterior Tender Points

Figure 39-5 shows the locations of the posterior tender points. All posterior tender points are treated in extension with the patient prone. The

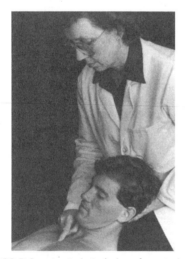

**FIG. 39-2** Counterstrain technique for anterior tender points: upper thoracic spine.

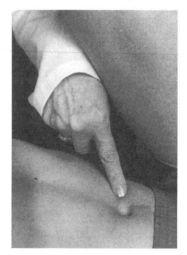

**FIG. 39-4** Counterstrain technique for anterior T10 tender point: knees rotated to side of tender point.

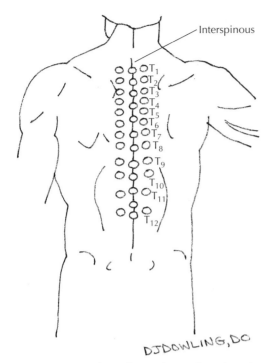

Interspinous

DJDOWLING,DO

■ **FIG. 39-5** Locations of posterior tender points: thoracic spine.

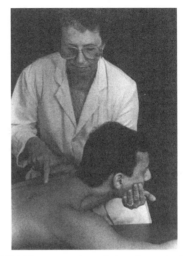

■ **FIG. 39-7** Counterstrain technique for posterior tender point: mid-thoracic spine. Tender point is to the right; slight rotation is induced to the left.

patient's position varies only so that motion may be localized to a given point.

## ■ UPPER THORACIC SPINE (T1–T2)

1. **Patient position:** prone, with arms at his side.
2. **Physician position:** standing on the side of the patient opposite the tender point.
3. **Technique:** One hand supports the patient's chin; the other hand monitors the tender

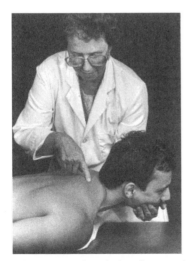

■ **FIG. 39-6** Counterstrain technique for posterior tender points: upper thoracic spine.

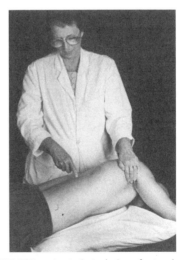

■ **FIG. 39-8** Counterstrain technique for tender point of lower thoracic spine.

point on the opposite side of the spinous process. The head and neck are extended to the involved segment (Fig. 39-6). Rotation and side-bending will be away from the point.

## ■ MID-THORACIC SPINE (T3–T5)

1. **Patient position:** same as described, except the arms are extended over the head.
2. **Physician position:** standing at side of patient opposite the side of the tender point.
3. **Technique:** same as described (Fig. 39-7), with slight rotation.

## ■ LOWER THORACIC SPINE (T6–L2)

1. **Patient position:** prone, arms extended above head.

2. **Physician position:** standing at side of patient opposite the side of the tender point. The cephalad (with respect to the patient) hand supports the patient's axilla on the side of the tender point.
3. **Technique:** Rotation and side-bending are induced through pull on the axilla to the opposite side and cephalad, with care not to irritate the skin and other tissue. Extension may be facilitated by placing pillows under the patient's chest (Fig. 39-8).

**Modification:**

The physician may use the pelvis to increase the rotation of a spinous process that is already rotated to one side. This relieves a tender point directly on the spinous process.

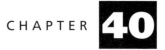

# Facilitated Positional Release

*Stanley Schiowitz*

Facilitated Positional Release in the thoracic region may be performed with the patient in either a seated position or in a prone position. If the patient is treated in a prone position, use of a pillow will be necessary. The pillow is placed under the patient's abdomen or head and neck to assist in flattening the thoracic kyphosis.

## ■ SUPERFICIAL MUSCLE HYPERTONICITY (LEFT POSTERIOR REGION OF T7 VERTEBRA)

1. **Patient position:** seated.
2. **Physician position:** standing behind and to the side of the involved muscle (the left of the patient).
3. **Technique:**
   a. The physician places his right index finger on the site of the dysfunction.
   b. The physician's left arm is placed on the patient's left shoulder with the elbow at the lateral aspect to allow direction and control of the patient's motion. The physician's forearm rests behind the patient's neck.
   c. The patient is instructed to sit up straight until the thoracic kyphosis flattens slightly.
   d. If necessary, the patient is told to push his chest out until backward bending is created up to the monitoring finger, for further flattening of the thoracic spine.
   e. The physician applies compression with his forearm near the patient's neck. The vector of force is aimed straight down parallel to the spine (Fig. 40-1).
   f. Maintaining the backward bending and

compression, the physician creates side-bending down to the monitoring finger by pressing down with his left arm (Fig. 40-2).
   g. The position is held for 3 seconds and then released.
   h. The dysfunction is reevaluated.

## ■ SOMATIC DYSFUNCTION—T7 $ES_LR_L$

1. **Patient position:** seated.
2. **Physician position:** standing behind and to the side of the dysfunction (the left of the patient).
3. **Technique:**
   a. The physician's monitoring finger is at the posterior transverse process.
   b. The physician's left arm is placed on the patient's left shoulder with the elbow at the lateral aspect to allow direction and control of the patient's motion. The physician's forearm rests behind the patient's neck.
   c. The patient is instructed to sit up straight until the thoracic kyphosis flattens slightly.
   d. If necessary, the patient is told to push his chest out until backward bending is created up to the monitoring finger, for further flattening of the thoracic spine.
   e. The physician applies compression with his forearm near the patient's neck. The vector of force is aimed straight down parallel to the spine.
   f. Maintaining the backward bending and

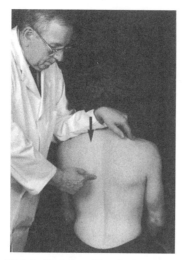

■ **FIG. 40-1** Facilitated positional release treatment for thoracic superficial muscle hypertonicity; application of compression at the left cervico-thoracic junction.

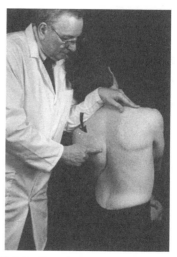

■ **FIG. 40-2** Facilitated positional release treatment for thoracic superficial muscle hypertonicity; left side-bending added.

compression, the physician creates side-bending down to the monitoring finger by pressing down with his left arm, to increase extension and add rotation to the left side-bending component.

  g. The position is held for 3 seconds and then released. The dysfunction is reevaluated.

To treat a flexion dysfunction (T7 F SR$_L$), flexion of spine is added after the compressive

forced is applied. Side-bending and rotation are introduced to the left down to the dysfunction. Otherwise the technique is the same as for an extension dysfunction.

### ■ PRONE TECHNIQUE—T3 ESR$_R$

1. **Patient position:** prone.
2. **Physician position:** standing beside the table, opposite the side of the dysfunction.

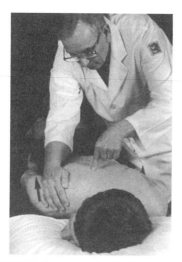

■ **FIG. 40-3** Facilitated positional release treatment for T3 extension somatic dysfunction, patient prone. The physician applies a caudad and parallel pull, creating compression and side-bending.

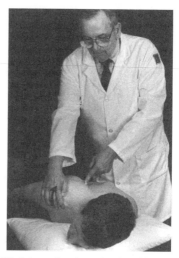

■ **FIG. 40-4** A torsional motion is added, turning the shoulder upward and creating compression, side-bending, and rotation.

3. **Technique:**
   a. The physician places the index finger of his cephalad hand at the posterior transverse process of T3. With the patient prone, mild flattening of the thoracic kyphosis is usually created. If not, a pillow is placed under the patient's head and neck.
   b. With his caudad hand, the physician grasps the patient's shoulder over the acromion process. With his hand on the superior aspect of the shoulder girdle, he pulls the shoulder, parallel to the table and toward the patient's feet, until force is felt at the monitoring finger (Fig. 40-3). This creates right side-bending.
   c. Maintaining this force, the physician straightens up, thereby pulling the patient's shoulder backward off the table, creating right rotation.
   d. These combined motions create compression, extension, side-bending, and rotation up to the monitoring finger (Fig. 40-4).
   e. The position is held for 3 seconds, then released; the dysfunction is reevaluated.

This technique, with the patient in the prone position, can be used to treat hypertonic muscles of the thoracic region and upper lumbar region. The physician places the index finger at the site of hypertonicity and creates the same forces down to the monitoring finger. For lower vertebrae, the flattening of the region may be created by placing a pillow under the abdomen.

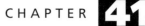

# Still Techniques

*Dennis J. Dowling*

This chapter describes Still techniques for treating somatic dysfunctions of the thoracic spine. Type I (regional) and type II (segmental, single) somatic dysfunctions occur within the thoracic region and are treated by positioning into the directions of ease of the diagnostic components.

T1 and possibly T2 may be treated in much the same manner as the typical cervical vertebral somatic dysfunctions, with the exception that the rotation and side-bending are into the same direction. Although the primary position of application is with the patient seated, the patient may also be treated in the side-lying position. Compression is used for both. Occasionally, the portion of the treatment involving movement towards the barriers may result in an articulatory "pop." The descriptions are for the specific side-bending and rotation components with flexion and extension as modifications into the appropriate directions.

## ■ TYPE II T1 SOMATIC DYSFUNCTION (T1 $S_L$ $R_L$)—PATIENT SEATED

1. **Patient position:** seated.
2. **Physician position:** standing facing the patient; closer to the side of the dysfunction (right side in this example).
3. **Technique:**
   a. The physician places the pad of the index or middle finger of his monitoring (right) hand on the side of the posterior transverse process of the somatic dysfunction (the right finger contacts the patient's left T1 transverse process in this example). The palm of that hand contours to the patient's (left) shoulder.

   b. The physician places the palm of his other hand on top of the patient's head with the fingers contouring to the patient's head.
   c. The physician side-bends the patient's head towards the monitoring finger at the posterior transverse process. Simultaneously, slight rotation towards the posterior transverse process is introduced. Slight flexion or extension is added, depending on the diagnosis of the dysfunction, finishing the position into the relative freedoms of the somatic dysfunction (Fig. 41-1).
   d. The physician puts approximately 5 pounds of downward pressure toward the floor with the hand on the top of the patient's head towards the monitoring finger. There should be relaxation of the palpated soft tissue noted.
   e. While maintaining the compression, the head is gently carried through sagittal plane neutral and towards the flexion or extension barrier, then through neutral position and into the barrier directions (side-bending right and rotating right in this case).
   f. The patient's head and neck are brought back to the neutral position and the T1 joint is reassessed.

## ■ UPPER THORACIC TYPE II SOMATIC DYSFUNCTION (T3 $S_R$ $R_R$)—PATIENT SEATED

1. **Patient position:** seated.
2. **Physician position:** standing in front of and facing the patient.

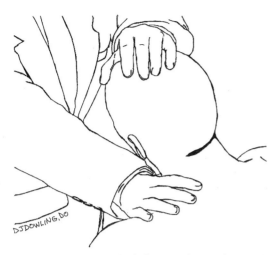

■ **FIG. 41-1** T1 Somatic dysfunction (T1 $S_L$ $R_L$), seated.

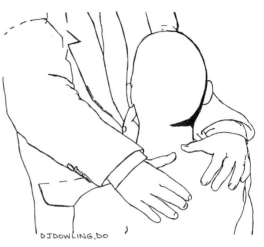

■ **FIG. 41-2** Upper thoracic type II somatic dysfunction (T3 $S_R$ $R_R$), patient seated (physician anterior to patient).

3. **Technique:**
   a. Both of the physician's forearms are placed on the patient's shoulders as close to the patient's neck as is possible.
   b. The physician places the pad of his index or middle finger of his monitoring hand on the transverse process on the side of the side-bending/rotation component of the somatic dysfunction (the left finger contacts the patient's T3 right transverse process in this example).
   c. The physician introduces a downward pressure through the patient's shoulders with slightly more pressure exerted on the side of the dysfunction. The proximal part of the physician's forearm on the involved side, which is anterior to the patient's shoulder, pushes the shoulder on that side posterior. These motions introduce side-bending and rotation into the direction of the relative freedoms.
   d. Slight flexion or extension is added, depending on the diagnosis of the dysfunction, finishing the position into the relative freedoms of the somatic dysfunction (Fig. 41-2).
   e. The physician puts approximately 5 pounds of downward pressure with both forearms on the patient's shoulders towards the monitoring finger.
   f. While maintaining the compression, the patient's upper body is gently carried through the sagittal plane neutral and towards the flexion or extension barrier, then through neutral position and into the other barrier directions (side-bending left and rotating left in this case).
   g. The patient's body is brought back to the neutral position and the thoracic somatic dysfunction is reassessed.

## ■ THORACIC TYPE II SOMATIC DYSFUNCTION (T6 $S_R$ $R_R$)—PATIENT SEATED (PHYSICIAN POSTERIOR TO PATIENT)

1. **Patient position:** seated.
2. **Physician position:** standing behind the patient.
3. **Technique:**
   a. The physician places the pad of his index or middle finger of his monitoring hand on the transverse process on the side of the side-bending/rotation component of the somatic dysfunction (the right finger contacts the patient's T6 right transverse process in this example). The palm of that hand contours to and supports the patient's back.
   b. The patient is instructed to take his or her hand on the side of the somatic dysfunction and reach anteriorly and across to hold the contralateral shoulder.

c. The physician places his axilla on the contralateral shoulder and reaches the non-monitoring hand anterior and across to hold the shoulder on the side of the dysfunction (the physician's left axilla is on the patient's left shoulder and the physician's left hand is upon the patient's right shoulder).

d. The physician side-bends and rotates the patient down to and toward the posterior transverse process. The physician can further exaggerate this if necessary until softening of the underlying tissue is noted.

e. Slight flexion or extension is added, depending on the diagnosis of the dysfunction, finishing the position into the relative freedoms of the somatic dysfunction (Fig. 41-3).

f. The physician puts downward compression with the contacts of the palm of his (left) hand and (left) axilla that are on the patient's shoulders until further soft tissue is noted at the monitoring finger.

g. While maintaining the compression, the patient's body is gently carried through sagittal plane neutral and towards the flexion or extension barrier, then through neutral position and into the barrier directions (side-bending left and rotating left in this case).

h. The patient's body is brought back to the neutral position and the thoracic somatic dysfunction is reassessed.

# ■ LOWER THORACIC TYPE II SOMATIC DYSFUNCTION (T9 $S_R$ $R_R$)—PATIENT SEATED (PHYSICIAN ANTERIOR TO PATIENT)

1. **Patient position:** seated.
2. **Physician position:** standing facing the patient.
3. **Technique:**

a. The physician places the pad of the index or middle finger of his monitoring hand at the posterior transverse process of the somatic dysfunction by passing the monitoring hand beneath the patient's axilla and then posteriorly to the patient's back (the left finger contacts the patient's right T9 transverse process in this example). The palm of that hand contours to and supports the patient's back in this region.

b. The physician places the forearm of his opposite arm on the patient's contralateral shoulder as close to the patient's neck as possible (the physician's right forearm is on the patient's left shoulder in this example).

c. The physician rotates and side-bends the patient's body towards the monitoring finger until tissue relaxation is noted. Slight flexion or extension is added, depending on the diagnosis of the dysfunction, finishing the position into the relative freedoms of the somatic dysfunction.

d. The physician puts approximately 5 pounds of downward pressure with the arm on top of the patient's shoulder towards the monitoring finger creating compression (Fig. 41-4).

e. While maintaining the compression, the body is gently carried through neutral position and into the barrier directions (side-bending left and rotating left in this case).

f. The patient's body is brought back to the neutral position and the thoracic somatic dysfunction is reassessed.

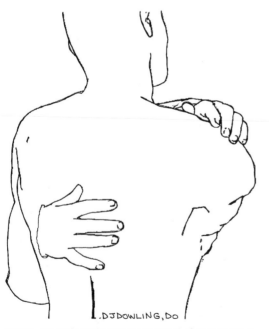

■ **FIG. 41-3** Thoracic type II somatic dysfunction (T6 $S_R$ $R_R$), patient seated (physician posterior to patient).

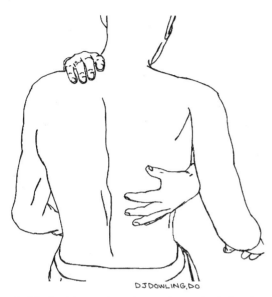

■ **FIG. 41-4** Lower thoracic type II somatic dysfunction (T9 S$_R$ R$_R$), patient seated (physician anterior to patient).

# ■ LOWER THORACIC TYPE II SOMATIC DYSFUNCTION (T9 S$_R$ R$_R$)—PATIENT SEATED (PHYSICIAN ANTERIOR TO PATIENT) ALTERNATIVE

1. **Patient position:** seated.
2. **Physician position:** standing anterior to patient.
3. **Technique:**
   a. The patient places the palms of both hands on his lap and leans slightly forward.
   b. The physician reaches his hands beneath both of the patient's axillae laterally, then passes them behind the patient and then places the pads of his index or middle fingers of both hands at the transverse processes either at or one segment below the level of the somatic dysfunction (the fingers contact the same level if it is a flexion and one level below if it is an extension somatic dysfunction). The palms of the hands and the remaining fingers contour to and support the patient's back.
   c. The patient's head and shoulders rest on the physician's chest. The physician's upper arm/shoulder on the side of the so-matic dysfunction make contact with the patient's shoulder on that side.
   d. The patient's body is rotated backwards on the side of the posterior transverse process by drawing the transverse process on the opposite side forward. Side-bending is created by the physician's arm on the opposite side lifting the opposite axilla upwards.
   e. The physician draws the fingers and hand toward himself creating flexion or extension. (The fingers on the same level as the somatic dysfunction will create relative flexion. When the fingers are below the level of the somatic dysfunction, this will create relative extension at the dysfunction level.)
   f. The physician puts approximately 5 pounds of downward pressure with the upper arm/shoulder that is in contact with the patient's shoulder on the somatic dysfunction side.
   g. While maintaining the compression, the body is gently carried through neutral position, anterior pressure on the transverse processes is released and the region is brought into the barrier directions (rotation and side-bending left in this case) (Fig. 41-5).
   h. The patient's body is brought back to the neutral position and the thoracic somatic dysfunction is reassessed.

# ■ LOWER THORACIC TYPE II SOMATIC DYSFUNCTION (T8 S$_R$ R$_R$)—PATIENT LATERAL RECUMBENT

1. **Patient position:** lying on side with somatic dysfunction side up.
2. **Physician position:** standing beside the table facing the patient.
3. **Technique:**
   a. The patient's arm on the side of the somatic dysfunction is flexed and abducted and the hand is placed on his or her own neck.
   b. The physician places his cephalad arm (the one closer to the patient's head) through the opening created by the pa-

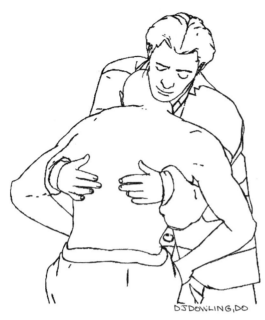

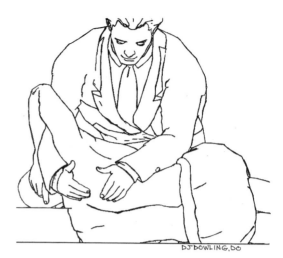

■ **FIG. 41-6** Lower thoracic type II somatic dysfunction (T8 $S_R$ $R_R$), patient side-lying (physician anterior to patient).

■ **FIG. 41-5** Lower thoracic type II somatic dysfunction (T9 $S_R$ $R_R$), patient seated (physician anterior to patient) alternative.

tient's bent arm and places the palm and fingers of that hand over the scapula on that side.

c. The physician places the pad of his index or middle finger of the other (caudad) monitoring hand on the posterior transverse process at the level of the somatic dysfunction (the left finger contacts the patient's right posterior T8 transverse process in this example). The palm and fingers of this hand contour to the patient's body and maintain position of the trunk throughout much of the treatment. The physician may rest his elbow or forearm on the patient's iliac crest on that side as well (left elbow on right hip).

d. Flexion or extension is added, depending on the diagnosis of the dysfunction. If the somatic dysfunction is a flexion dysfunction, the physician uses the hand on the patient's shoulder and scapula to first introduce flexion of the spine to that level. If the direction of the somatic dysfunction is extension, then the physician initially pushes the patient's shoulder posteriorly.

e. By pushing the patient's shoulder posteriorly, the physician rotates the patient's

upper body towards the direction of the freedom of motion of the somatic dysfunction. Compression (approximately 5 pounds of pressure) and side-bending are introduced by the physician using his cephalad arm to push the patient's shoulder (right in this example) toward the posterior transverse process by finishing the positioning into the relative freedoms of the somatic dysfunction. (Fig. 41-6)

f. While maintaining the compression, the physician uses his caudad arm on the patient's hip and rolls the pelvis posterior. The cephalad hand and arm pull the patient's shoulder anteriorly and the scapula up toward the patient's head and reverses the flexion or extension (side-bending left and rotating left in this case into the barrier directions)

g. The patient's body is brought back to the neutral position and the thoracic somatic dysfunction level is reassessed.

## ■ THORACIC TYPE I GROUP CURVE SOMATIC DYSFUNCTION (T1-9 N $S_R$ $R_L$)—PATIENT SEATED

1. **Patient position:** seated.
2. **Physician position:** standing facing the patient.

3. **Technique:**
   a. Both of the physician's forearms are placed on the patient's shoulders as close to the patient's neck as is possible.
   b. The physician places the pad of his index or middle finger of his monitoring hand on the transverse process on the side of the apex of the group curve on the convex side (the right finger contacts the patient's T5 left transverse process in this example).
   c. The physician introduces a downward pressure through the patient's shoulders with slightly more pressure exerted on the side of the group curve side-bending (physician's left arm pushes the patient's right shoulder downwards in this example). Simultaneously, the physician's other arm pushes the patient's other shoulder posteriorly creating rotation opposite to side-bending (physician's right arm pushes the patient's left shoulder posteriorly in this example).
   d. The patient is kept in neutral while the physician puts bilateral compression through the patient's shoulders towards the group curve apex (Fig. 41-7).
   e. While maintaining the compression, the patient's upper body is gently carried into the side-bending and rotation barrier directions (side-bending left and rotating right in this case).
   f. The patient's body is brought back to the neutral position and the group curve is reassessed.

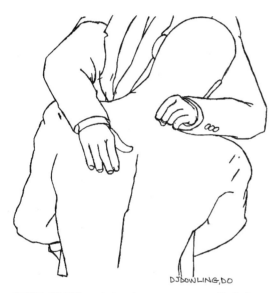

**■ FIG. 41-7** Thoracic type I group curve somatic dysfunction (T1–9 N $S_R$ $R_L$), patient seated (physician anterior to patient).

### REFERENCES

Van Buskirk RL. A manipulative technique of Andrew Taylor Still. *J Am Osteopath Assoc* 1996;96:597–602

Van Buskirk RL. *The Still Technique Manual.* Indianapolis, IN: American Academy of Osteopathy 1999.

Van Buskirk RL. Treatment of somatic dysfunction with an osteopathic manipulative method of Dr. Andrew Taylor Still. In Ward RC, ed. *Foundations for Osteopathic Medicine.* Philadelphia: Lippincott Williams & Wilkins, 2003: 1094–1114

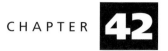

# PINS Techniques For The Thoracic Spine

*Dennis J. Dowling*

This chapter describes PINS techniques for treating somatic dysfunctions of the thoracic region. The examples provided are not the only ones that are possible (Fig. 42-1). However, they are fairly common. Occasionally, patterns in the thoracic region may continue into or from adjacent regions. The patient is most commonly treated in the prone position but could be treated seated. The physician should be positioned comfortably facing the region to be treated or alongside the table. The principles and methods of PINS can be applied:

1. Locate a sensitive point in the region of the symptoms.
2. Analyze the structures that are deep to that point
3. Locate another sensitive point at the other end of a connecting structure (i.e., muscle, ligament, nerve, etc.). The more sensitive point is the primary point and the less sensitive point is the endpoint.
4. Apply inhibitory pressure to both points for 30 seconds or more. The soft tissue at the more sensitive point will typically lessen in tension.
5. Beginning at the more sensitive of the two points, locate another sensitive point approximately 2 to 3 centimeters toward the less sensitive point.
6. Repeat the procedure progressively toward the endpoint.
7. Reassess the status of the dysfunction. Determine if additional treatment or the application of other modalities is necessary

## ■ RHOMBOIDS/SERRATUS POSTERIOR SUPERIOR

1. **Technique:**
   a. The physician places the pad of his index or middle finger on the medial border of the scapula. A finger of the physician's other hand locates a sensitive point superior and medial to that point near the spinous processes.
   b. The pattern of intervening points is usually straight but the depth of pressure may indicate the muscles involved (deeper is the serratus and the rhomboids are more shallow).
2. **Clinical Correlation:**
   a. Neck pain
   b. Back pain

## ■ PARAVERTEBRAL MUSCLES

1. **Technique:**
   a. The physician places the pad of his index or middle finger lateral to the spinous processes. A finger of the physician's other hand locates a sensitive point either cephalad or caudad. The point may be at the level medial to the twelfth rib.
   b. The pattern of intervening points is generally slightly curved or straight (muscle pattern).
2. **Clinical Correlation:**
   a. Back pain
   b. Flank pain

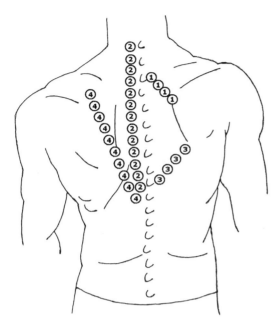

■ **FIG. 42-1** PINS thoracic point patterns; *1, rhomboids/ serratus posterior superior; 2, paravertebral muscles; 3, serratus posterior inferior; 4, trapezius.*

    (1) Nephrolithiasis (can mimic or be re-
        lated to renal calculi)
    (2) Cholelithiasis/cholecystitis (on the right)

## ■ SERRATUS POSTERIOR INFERIOR

1. **Technique:**
   a. The physician places the pad of his index
      or middle finger on a point in the lower

thoracic region lateral to the transverse processes. A lateral sensitive point may be found at a higher and more lateral position in the rib cage.
   b. The pattern of intervening points is gener-
      ally straight (muscle pattern) but may be
      slightly zigzag in following the course of
      the knife-like serratus muscles.
2. **Clinical Correlation:**
   a. Back pain
   b. Rib pain
   c. Flank pain

## ■ TRAPEZIUS

1. **Technique:**
   a. The physician places the pad of his index
      or middle finger laterally near the under-
      side of the spine of the scapula. A finger
      of the physician's other hand locates a sen-
      sitive point medially near the spinous pro-
      cess of T12.
   b. The pattern of intervening points gener-
      ally follows the lateral border of the trape-
      zius.
2. **Clinical Correlation:**
   a. Back pain
   b. Shoulder pain

### REFERENCES

Dowling DJ. Progressive inhibition of neuromuscular struc-
    tures (PINS) technique. *J Am Osteopath Assoc* 2000;100:
    285–286, 289–298.

# Thoracic Spine Thrusting Techniques

*Eileen L. DiGiovanna, Dennis J. Dowling, Barry S. Erner, and Paula D. Scariati*

This chapter describes high-velocity, low-amplitude thrusting techniques for treating somatic dysfunctions of the thoracic spine by region—upper, middle, and lower spine. For most of the techniques, the patient is supine; a variation is illustrated in which the patient is seated.

The technique described for the mid-thoracic spine may be used for any area of the thoracic spine that is amenable to using it. The reason to use the other types of techniques is because of the fact that sometimes the upper or lower thoracic spine is arched away from the table surface and firm contact of the physician's hand and the spine with the table surface is difficult. Flexing the upper or lower areas brings them in closer contact with the table. The physician should use his or her judgment as to which technique to use.

## ■ UPPER THORACIC SOMATIC DYSFUNCTION (T1–T3)

1. **Patient position:** supine.
2. **Physician position:** standing at the side of the table opposite the side of the posteriorly rotated transverse process.
3. **Technique:**
   a. The patient places his clasped hands behind his neck and approximates his elbows. The physician places his thrusting hand on the elbows and his chest over the dorsum of the hand.
   b. The physician palpates the restricted seg-

ment with his fulcrum hand and rests its posterior transverse process on the thenar eminence of the fulcrum hand.
   c. With his other hand, the physician grasps the patient's elbows and rolls the patient slightly toward his feet so the transverse process more firmly rests upon the physician's thenar eminence.
   d. The patient is asked to inhale deeply and then exhale completely.
   e. At the end of exhalation, the physician exerts a rapid anteroposterior thrust through the patient's arms onto the transverse process resting on his thenar eminence (Fig. 43-1).
   f. The somatic dysfunction is reassessed.

## ■ MID-THORACIC SOMATIC DYSFUNCTION

1. **Patient position:** supine.
2. **Physician position:** standing at the side of the table opposite the side of the dysfunction.
3. **Technique:**
   a. The patient crosses his arms over his chest. The arm on the side of the posterior transverse process is the arm that is placed uppermost. The arms should not intertwine, but the uppermost should rest on the lower
   b. The physician side-bends the patient's upper torso down to the region of the dysfunction and away from the posterior transverse process.

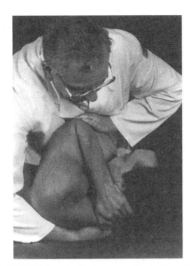

■ **FIG. 43-1** High-velocity low-amplitude thrusting technique for upper thoracic somatic dysfunction.

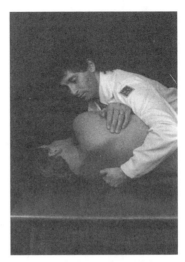

■ **FIG. 43-2** Hand placement for mid-thoracic high-velocity low-amplitude thrusting technique.

c. The physician palpates the restricted segment and rests its posterior transverse process on the thenar eminence of his fulcrum hand (Fig. 43-2).

e. With his other hand, the physician grasps the patient's elbows and rolls the patient's body forward and creates a greater contact onto his thenar eminence. The physician places his chest over his own thrusting hand, which rests on the patient's elbows.

f. The physician may exert a slight amount of downward pressure to spring slightly onto the somatic dysfunction to judge the

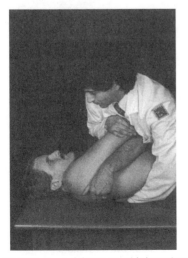

■ **FIG. 43-3** Downward thrust on mid-thoracic segment.

accuracy of localization in preparation for the thrust.

g. The patient is instructed to inhale deeply and exhale completely.

h. At the end of full exhalation, the physician exerts a rapid downward thrust through the patient's arms into the transverse process resting on his thenar eminence (Fig. 43-3). Controlled body weight is used as the thrusting force onto the physician's hand and forearm and through these to the patient's body.

i. The somatic dysfunction is reassessed.

*Note: This technique has the colloquial title of "Kirksville Krunch" in honor of the first school of osteopathy.*

■ **LOWER THORACIC SOMATIC DYSFUNCTION**

1. **Patient position:** supine.
2. **Physician position:** standing at the side of the table opposite to the side of the posteriorly rotated transverse process.
3. **Technique:**
   a. The patient crosses his arms over his chest. The upper arm is the arm on the side of the posterior transverse process.
   b. The physician palpates the restricted segment and rests its posterior transverse process on the thenar eminence of his fulcrum hand.

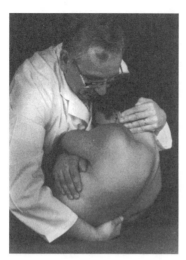

■ **FIG. 43-4** High-velocity low-amplitude thrusting technique for lower thoracic somatic dysfunction.

c. With his other hand, the physician grasps the patient behind the shoulders and cradles him, creating and localizing flexion down to the restricted segment.

d. The physician places his chest on top of the patient's crossed arms. A thin pillow may be placed between the patient's arms and the physician's chest.

e. The physician may exert a slight amount of downward pressure to spring slightly onto the somatic dysfunction to judge the accuracy of localization in preparation for the thrust.

f. The patient is asked to inhale fully, and then exhale completely.

g. At the end of exhalation, the physician rolls the patient over his thenar eminence and exerts a rapid thrust, creating a vector force through to the posterior transverse process (Fig. 43-4).

h. The somatic dysfunction is reassessed.

## ■ ALTERNATIVE TECHNIQUES FOR THORACIC SOMATIC DYSFUNCTION

### Alternative 1

1. **Patient position:** on the table reclined with back supported by the physician's knee and thigh.

2. **Physician position:** standing at the head of the table, with one knee on the table.

3. **Technique:**

   a. The physician places his knee under the posterior transverse process of the restricted segment.

   b. The patient is instructed to reach back and grasp his hands together around the physician's waist.

   c. The physician grasps the patient beneath the scapulae bilaterally.

   d. The patient is asked to inhale fully, then exhale completely.

   e. At the end of exhalation, the physician exerts an upward cephalad traction force with his hands while simultaneously rolling the patient over his knee (Fig. 43-5).

   f. The somatic dysfunction is reassessed.

### Alternative 2

1. **Patient position:** seated on a stool or table with his feet flat on the floor.

2. **Physician position:** standing behind the patient.

3. **Technique:**

   a. The physician places his foot on the side of the patient's posterior transverse process onto the table or stool.

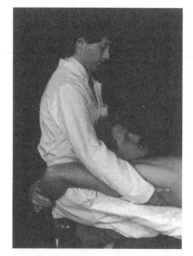

■ **FIG. 43-5** Alternative thrusting technique for thoracic spine somatic dysfunction, patient supine.

b. A pillow is placed between the posterior transverse process of the somatic dysfunction and the physician's bent knee for comfort.

d. The patient is instructed to interlock his fingers of both hands behind his neck.

e. The physician localizes the posterior transverse process and places his knee on it (with the right knee for a right-sided lesion).

f. The physician grasps the patient's forearms by sliding his arms underneath the patient's axillae and holding on the dorsal surface of the patient's wrists.

g. The physician's arms rest firmly against the patient's chest at the level of the axillae.

h. The patient is asked to inhale fully, then exhale completely.

i. At the end of exhalation, the physician exerts an upward cephalad force through the patient's axillae while simultaneously rolling the patient's spine over his knee (Fig. 43-6). Some forward thrust move-

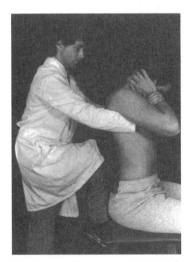

■ **FIG. 43-6** Alternative thrusting technique for thoracic spine somatic dysfunction, patient seated.

ment of the physician's knee may also be used.

j. The somatic dysfunction is reassessed.

## Alternative 3

1. **Patient position:** prone
2. **Physician position:** standing beside the table facing the patient.
3. **Technique:**

a. The physician places either the thenar or the hypothenar eminence of one hand on the posterior transverse process of the somatic dysfunction. The fingers of the thrusting hand are to be parallel to the spine and directed cephalad.

b. The physician places either the thenar or hypothenar eminence of the other hand on the transverse process of the same thoracic level but on the side opposite to the posterior transverse process. The fingers of this thrusting hand are to be parallel to the spine and directed caudad.

c. The hands can be brought together slightly to reduce the stretch of the patient's skin.

d. The patient is instructed to inhale deeply and exhale completely.

e. At the end of full exhalation, the physician introduces the thrust.

f. The physician's hand on the side of the posterior transverse process exerts an anterior-downward-cephalad force .

g. The hand on the other side maintains a slight counterbalance pressure or downward–caudad force.

h. The somatic dysfunction is reassessed.

*Note: This technique has the colloquial title of "Texas Twist" because of the twisting motion or is known as the "crossed pisiform" technique because of the contact point of the technique in some applications.*

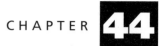

# Exercise Therapy

*Stanley Schiowitz and Albert R. DeRubertis*

The thoracic region is much more complex than the cervical region. It consists of the thoracic spine, rib cage, shoulder girdle, and the intricate musculature that accompanies the functioning of each of these. Prescribing exercise treatment for dysfunctions of any of these areas should include recognition of their interdependence. Pain and limited motion in one segment can be secondary to dysfunction of another.

Regional motions and functions can be divided as follows:

1. Thoracic spine: forward bending, backward bending, rotation, side-bending.
2. Scapula: elevation, protraction, retraction, and rotation.
3. Ribs: individual ribs have rotary elevating or depressing motions. The entire thorax, however, expands in the anteroposterior plane (pump handle motion) and in the frontal plane (bucket handle motion).

## ■ REGIONAL STRETCH

### Forward Bending

1. **Patient position:** seated, with back upright.
2. **Instructions:**
   a. Drop your head forward, allowing its weight to create forward bending.
   b. Allow the forward bending to continue gradually into the thoracic region, from the first thoracic vertebra down. Do not create pain.
   c. To increase stretch, maintain your body in its position of forward bending, drop

both hands between your legs, and reach for the floor (Fig. 44-1). Do not change or increase your forward-bending position.
   d. Hold for 5 to 15 seconds, then slowly return to upright position.
   e. Relax, rest, and repeat.

### Backward Bending

1. **Patient position:** seated, with back upright and hands at sides.
2. **Instructions:**
   a. Drop your head backward, allowing its weight to create backward bending.
   b. Allow the backward bending to continue into the thoracic region.
   c. To increase stretch, push out your chest and abdomen and point your hands downward and backward toward the floor (Fig. 44-2). Do not change or increase your backward bending position.
   d. Hold for 5 to 15 seconds. Slowly return to the upright position.
   e. Relax, rest, and repeat.

### Side-Bending

1. **Patient position:** standing, back upright, hands at sides.
2. **Instructions:**
   a. Tilt your head, neck, and thoracic region to the right as you walk your right hand down your right leg toward the floor (Fig. 44-3).

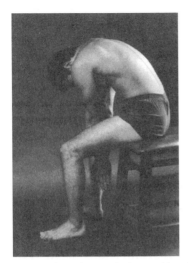

■ **FIG. 44-1** Thoracic stretch: forward bending.

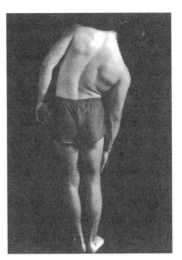

■ **FIG. 44-3** Thoracic stretch: side-bending.

b. To increase stretch, raise your left arm over your head and try to touch the top of your right shoulder.

c. Hold for 5 to 15 seconds. Slowly return to the upright position.

d. Relax, rest, and repeat.

e. To stretch the left side laterally, reverse the instructions.

## Rotation

1. **Patient position:** seated, facing backward, on an armless chair, with legs straddling the seat.

2. Instructions:

a. Fold your arms in front of your chest, each hand holding the opposite elbow.

b. Slowly turn your head, then your neck, and then your back to the right, as far as possible without pain. Do not change your seated position.

c. To increase stretch, with your right hand pull your left elbow toward the right, increasing the rotary motion (Fig. 44-4).

d. Hold for 5 to 15 seconds. Slowly return to the starting position.

e. Relax, rest, and repeat.

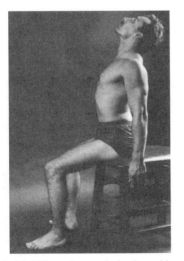

■ **FIG. 44-2** Thoracic stretch: backward bending.

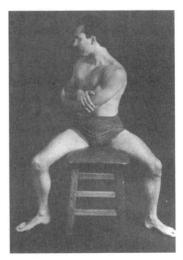

■ **FIG. 44-4** Thoracic stretch: rotation.

f. To stretch in left rotation, reverse the instructions.

## ■ UPPER BACK STRETCH

### Passive Stretch

1. **Patient position:** seated.
2. **Instructions:**
   a. Raise your left elbow to shoulder level and place that hand over your right shoulder.
   b. Place your right hand on your left elbow and gently push it toward your back (Fig. 44-5). This will create a passive left upper back stretch.
   c. Maintain at maximum painless stretch for 5 to 15 seconds. Return to starting position.
   d. Relax, rest, and repeat.
   e. To stretch the right side, reverse the instructions.

### Active Stretch

#### Exercise 1

1. **Patient position:** prone, forehead touching the table.
2. **Instructions:**
   a. Abduct shoulders to 90 degrees and bend elbows to 90 degrees. Hands, elbows, and arms rest on the table (or floor).

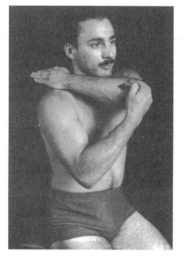

■ **FIG. 44.5** Passive upper back stretch: patient seated.

b. Simultaneously raise both upper extremities off the table, including the hands, elbows, and arms (Fig. 44-6).
c. Hold for 5 to 15 seconds.
d. Return arms to table, relax, rest, and repeat.

*Note:* Modifying the degree of shoulder abduction will change the area of the back that is stretched.

#### Exercise 2

1. **Patient position:** prone, forehead touching the table.
2. **Instructions:**
   a. Place both arms, elbows straight and palms down, raised over your head.
   b. Simultaneously raise both upper extremities off the floor, including the hands, elbows, and arms (Fig. 44-7).
   c. Hold for 5 to 15 seconds.
   d. Return arms to table, relax, rest, and repeat.

#### Exercise 3

1. **Patient position:** sitting, with back upright.
2. **Instructions:**
   a. Stretch both arms over your head, with fingers interlocked.
   b. Press both arms backward.
   c. Tilt your upper body to one side (Fig. 44-8). Hold for 5 seconds, then tilt upper body to other side.
   d. Return to starting position. Relax, rest, and repeat.

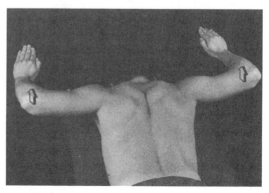

■ **FIG. 44-6** Active upper back stretch: patient prone.

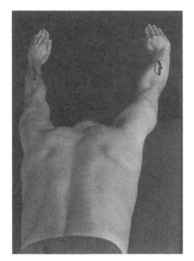

**FIG. 44-7** Active upper back stretch: patient prone.

## ■ KYPHOSIS

*Exercise 1*

1. **Patient position:** supine, knees flexed, with a small pillow under the mid-thoracic region
2. **Instructions:**
   a. Clasp your hands behind your neck.
   b. Try to touch the shoulder blades together at the midline (Fig. 44-9).
   c. Hold for 5 to 15 seconds.
   d. Relax, rest, and repeat.

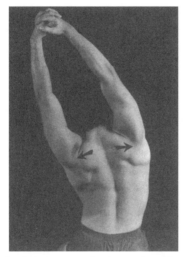

**FIG. 44-8** Active upper back stretch: patient seated.

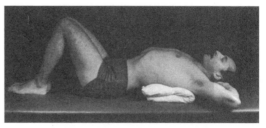

**FIG. 44-9** Stretch for kyphosis.

*Exercise 2*

1. **Patient position:** same as in previous exercise.
2. **Instructions:**
   a. Bring both arms fully extended over your head.
   b. Press your forearms and elbows down toward the table (Fig. 44-10).
   c. Hold for 5 to 15 seconds.
   d. Relax, rest, and repeat.

*Exercise 3*

1. **Patient position:** seated, back upright.
2. **Instructions:**
   a. Hold broomstick or pole at each end, your hands facing forward.
   b. Raise the pole over your head.
   c. Tuck in your chin and, holding your neck in a fixed position, bring the pole down between your shoulder blades (Fig. 44-11).
   d. Hold for 5 to 15 seconds. Return to starting position.
   e. Relax, rest, and repeat.

## ■ SCAPULAR MOTIONS
### Elevation Stretch (Shrug)

1. **Patient position:** standing, back upright, arms extended down at sides.

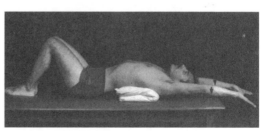

**FIG. 44-10** Stretch for kyphosis.

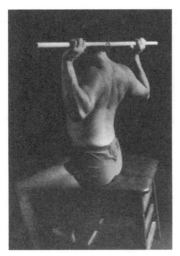

■ **FIG. 44.11** Stretch for kyphosis using pole.

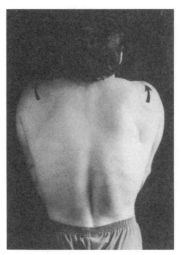

■ **FIG. 44-13** Scapular protraction.

2. **Instructions:**
   a. Raise your shoulders straight up, trying to touch them to your ears (Fig. 44-12).
   b. Hold for 5 to 15 seconds.
   c. Slowly return to starting position.
   d. Slowly relax, rest, and repeat.

## Protraction Stretch

1. **Patient position:** standing, back upright, arms extended at sides.

2. **Instructions:**
   a. Raise your shoulders straight up, trying to touch your ears.
   b. Roll your shoulders forward, separating the shoulder blades (Fig. 44-13).
   c. Hold for 5 to 15 seconds.
   d. Slowly relax, rest, and repeat.

## Retraction Stretch

1. **Patient position:** standing, back upright, arms extended at sides.

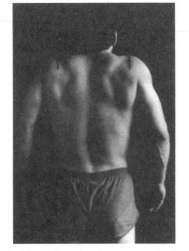

■ **FIG. 44-12** Scapular elevation stretch (shrug).

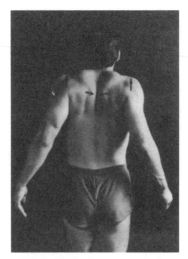

■ **FIG. 44-14** Scapular retraction.

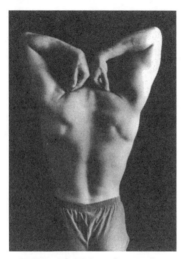

**■ FIG. 44-15** Scapular rotation.

2. **Instructions:**
   a. Raise your shoulders straight up, and try to touch your ears.

b. Roll your shoulders backward, trying to bring the shoulder blades together (Fig. 44-14).
   c. Hold for 5 to 15 seconds.
   d. Slowly relax, rest, and repeat.

The previous two exercises can be modified to create increased strength and stretch. Perform the shrug maneuver; then, with your shoulders elevated, proceed into the anterior and posterior shoulder roll.

## Rotation

1. **Patient position:** standing, back upright.
2. **Instructions:**
   a. Place both hands on your shoulders and raise your arms away from the body (abduct) to 135 degrees (Fig. 44-15).
   b. Maintain this raised position.
   c. Hold for 5 to 15 seconds.
   d. Relax, rest, and repeat.

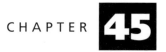

# Thoracic Spine Practical Applications and Case Histories

*Eileen L. DiGiovanna*

The thoracic spine is subject to many conditions that affect the cervical and lumbar spine including somatic dysfunction, herniation of an intervertebral disk, arthritis, and other bony and soft tissue injuries and degenerative processes. Osteoporosis commonly manifests in the thoracic spine, with vertebral compression fractures and formation of the *dowager's hump,* caused by microfractures of the anterior bodies of the vertebrae leading to a forward bending of the upper thoracic spine. This chapter discusses some of the conditions most commonly affecting the thoracic spine.

Somatic dysfunction of the thoracic spine is especially significant because of the close association of the sympathetic nervous system with the costovertebral area of this spinal region. Through this association, somatic dysfunctions may have an affect on the major internal organs of the body and disease processes of many internal organs may manifest as viscero-somatic reflex somatic dysfunctions in the thoracic region. The thoracic spine, therefore, plays a significant role in diagnosis and treatment of other than purely musculoskeletal disorders.

## ■ TRAUMA

Trauma is not common in the thoracic spine unless there has been severe impact to the spine, as in vehicular accidents or some sports. Vertebral fracture in the thoracic region is most commonly associated with osteoporosis. Herniation of the thoracic intervertebral disks is not common and is often associated with scoliosis of this region.

Soft tissue pain in the thoracic region is more likely to be postural or associated with somatic dysfunction than to be traumatic in nature. The physical examination should include observation for signs of trauma.

## ■ SCOLIOSIS

*Scoliosis* is an abnormal lateral curvature of the spine lying in the coronal plane. The thoracic spine is especially prone to development of scoliosis or *kyphoscoliosis* (side-bending of the spine with an excessive flexion of the spine). Scoliosis can be generally classified into two major types:

1. *Structural scoliosis,* sometimes called *idiopathic scoliosis*
2. Functional scoliosis

### Structural Scoliosis

Structural scoliosis is often referred to as idiopathic scoliosis because the cause of the condition was not well understood. It is certainly often the result of a genetic predisposition. There is often a family history of structural scoliosis. It is more common in females and can generally be diagnosed in the preteen or early teen-age years.

The scoliosis is named for the side of the convexity of the curve. A spine that side-bends toward the right and is thus convex on the left is called a *levoscoliosis* and one that has the convexity on the right is termed a *dextroscoliosis.*

On physical examination, the spinous processes may be palpated and a lateral curve noted. The best diagnostic finding is the *rib hump*, which can be noted on forward bending. The ribs on the side of the convexity will be found to be posterior to those on the concave side as the vertebrae rotate toward the convexity, carrying the ribs with them. This provides a good screening test that can be used in schools to determine which students might need further evaluation.

The extent of the curve can be measured on a standing x-ray of the involved spine. This measurement is known as the *Cobb angle*. A line is drawn across the superior surface of the body of the vertebra at the top of the curve and another across the inferior surface of the body of the one at the bottom of the curve. Perpendicular lines are drawn from each of the former lines and the angle where they intersect is measured. This angle, the Cobb angle, determines the degree of severity; the greater the angle, the more severe the scoliosis. On the x-ray, it will also be noted that the ribs on the convex side are more widely separated and on the concave side they are pressed closer together.

The curve may be C-shaped or S-shaped. An S-shaped curve, a double curve with a convexity changing from one direction to another, is generally less deforming because the individual appears to be standing up straight. With the double curve, the lumbar spine is often involved as well. The C-shaped curve can cause a more misshapen appearance. In severe cases of thoracic scoliosis, the heart and lungs may become compromised.

The condition is often progressive with spurts of angle increase during puberty and during pregnancy. It must, therefore, be monitored especially closely in young women.

Bracing, casting, or surgical treatment may be necessary to prevent severe deformity. Osteopathic manipulative treatment is helpful in keeping the patient comfortable and in slowing the progress of the curvature. Patients with scoliosis are at risk for the herniation of the intervertebral disks, so they should be instructed in the care of the back. Exercises to strengthen the muscles of spinal support should be given along with exercises to stretch the muscles on the concave side of the curve.

## Functional Scoliosis

Functional scoliosis is usually a correctible condition that is caused by postural or biomechanical factors. However, if it is not diagnosed and treated while it is still flexible, it can progress to a structural problem.

Some causes of functional scoliosis include:

1. *Muscle hypertonicity.* A long muscle on one side of the spine that is hypertonic can have a bowstring effect on the spine. Relaxing and stretching that muscle will allow the spine to straighten. This may be caused by a type I somatic dysfunction.
2. *Short leg syndrome.* If one lower extremity is shorter than the other, the sacrum and pelvis will tilt toward the lower side. This will cause the spine to curve back as it attempts to keep the head (and eyes) level. This condition is discussed in more detail in Chapter 68.
3. *Compensation.* An area of the spine adjacent to a scoliotic curve often curves in the opposite direction. The thoracic spine may curve to compensate for a curve in the lumbar spine or, occasionally, one in the cervical spine. It is even possible that a cranial side-bending dysfunction of long-standing may be the key to the problem, with compensatory curves developing in the spine below it. The basic cause of the curvature must be eliminated to allow straightening of the compensatory curve.
4. *Weak Musculature.* If the paravertebral muscle on one side of the spine is weaker than its opposing muscle, the stronger normal muscle may also create a bowstring effect on the spine. Exercise should help this condition if it is postural or functional. If the muscle has been weakened or paralyzed, as by poliomyelitis, the condition is not correctible and can be considered structural.

All functional scolioses are benefited by osteopathic manipulation once the cause has been eliminated or corrected. Myofascial techniques, muscle energy, and exercises are most helpful when working on the muscles.

## ■ KYPHOSIS

Kyphosis is an abnormal forward bending of the thoracic spine. It can be postural or structural.

An x-ray is helpful in determining any structural cause such as arthritis or spondylosis. Postural kyphosis may be caused by a habitual slouching posture, occupation, or weakness of supporting muscles. If the condition is postural, the patient must be instructed on correct posture and given exercises to stretch and strengthen involved muscles.

Osteopathic manipulation is useful to correct associated somatic dysfunctions. A slouching posture most often gives rise to flexion dysfunctions, which cause discomfort with correct posture and prevent the patient from trying to sit and stand correctly. Correcting these somatic dysfunctions relieves such discomfort.

## ■ FLAT BACK

The condition of "flat back" in the thoracic spine may be caused by an exaggerated "military" type of posture or may be caused by bilateral paravertebral muscle hypertonicity or spasm. Extension somatic dysfunctions may cause the individual to keep the back in an unusually straight posture because of discomfort or pain on flexing. The cause of the problem must be determined. Most of the causes are responsive to osteopathic manipulation.

## ■ CASE 1

A 15-year-old girl was brought to the clinic with a symptom of upper back pain for the past month. She asked to be excused from physical education class because of the pain. The pain was worse in the afternoons and evenings. Rest relieved the pain as did acetaminophen. Stress and activities involving use of the arms aggravated the pain.

She had had no significant injuries or surgeries. Her medical history was positive only for chicken pox at the age of 6. A review of systems revealed only occasional headaches, mild dysmenorrhea, and the symptom of upper back pain.

Physical examination was normal except for the musculoskeletal system. On observation, the upper back appeared normal; however, with forward bending, a significant rib hump was seen on the right. Palpation of the spine revealed a dextroscoliosis from T4 to T10. There was signif-

icant muscle tension in the area, most apparent on the left. A somatic dysfunction was found at T4–(T4FS$_L$R$_L$) and another at T8–(T8FS$_L$R$_L$).

A thoracic spine x-ray showed a dextroscoliosis with a Cobb angle of 15 degrees.

On further questioning, it was reported that two aunts had scoliosis, for which one had surgical treatment with the placement of a Harrington rod.

Treatment consisted of stretching of the paravertebral muscles on the left and muscle energy techniques to help stretch those muscles. The two somatic dysfunctions were treated with muscle energy and high-velocity, low-amplitude (HVLA) thrusting technique with resolution.

The patient was taught exercises to stretch the left-sided muscles and strengthen the right-sided muscles. She was given a series of flexibility exercises for the thoracic, cervical, and lumbar spine. She was given instructions on proper care of the back: how to lift, posture when seated and standing, and ergonomic use of a computer that she used for schoolwork.

At the next visit, 1 week later, she was having less discomfort in the thoracic spine. The dysfunction at T4 had not returned. The one at T8 was present but responded easily to a facilitated positional release technique. The left muscles were less hypertonic. She was instructed to continue the exercise program and to return for a follow-up x-ray in 6 months, unless the pain and discomfort recurred.

### Discussion

This case demonstrates the typical presentation of idiopathic scoliosis. In a young person, the discomfort present in association with scoliosis is usually caused by soft tissue dysfunction and somatic dysfunction of the vertebrae. Scoliosis is not usually painful in and of itself in younger persons, whose bodies are able to tolerate the stresses created better than older persons. An exercise program will assist in preventing discomfort and allow reasonably normal activities. Careful monitoring is important during this time to watch for rapid progression that might lead to deformity.

## ■ CASE 2

A 72-year-old woman was seen in the clinic with a symptom of mid-thoracic pain of several months' duration. She had slipped on a wet spot on the floor and fallen into a sitting position. She had a sharp pain in the thoracic region for approximately 1 week. It gradually diminished to a dull, aching pain that had persisted.

Her medical history was positive for high blood pressure, asthma that was usually only bothersome when around dust, molds, or strong odors, and a hysterectomy and oophorectomy at age 38 for endometriosis. She had previously had a fractured wrist at age 68 after a fall when she tripped going up the stairs. Medications she was using included atenolol, a salmeterol xinafoate inhaler twice daily, and occasional courses of prednisone when the asthma was more severe. She had used hormone replacement therapy for 4 years after the gynecologic surgery, but none since then.

Physical examination revealed a blood pressure of 138/86, with heart sounds and rhythm normal. A few crackles on exhalation were noted scattered throughout the lung fields. The thoracic spine was mildly kyphotic. There were several somatic dysfunctions found: $T1FS_RR_R$, $T4FS_LR_L$, and $T10ES_LR_L$. The paravertebral muscles were hypertonic and tender throughout the thoracic region.

Because of her age and the history of steroid use, she was sent for a dexascan, which showed osteoporosis of the spine and hip. An x-ray of the thoracic spine showed a healed fracture of T9.

She was treated with gentle myofascial, soft-tissue techniques to the paravertebral muscles and all tender points were treated with counterstrain techniques. She was given gentle stretching and flexibility exercises. She was given instructions on care of the back, especially how and what she could lift, and how to prevent falls. She was given a prescription for alendronate. She was treated with osteopathic manipulation weekly for 3 weeks, then every 2 weeks for 2 months. The somatic dysfunctions resolved and she had less back pain.

## Discussion

Osteoporosis is a thinning of the bones that occurs when osteoclastic activity is greater than osteoblastic. There is a failure of calcium deposition into the bony matrix leaving a thin, fragile structure. Bone mass density decreases significantly in women during and after menopause as estrogen levels decrease. The poorer the bone mass prior to menopause, the more severe the osteoporosis will be later in life. Early menopause, such as this lady had as a result of surgery, is a strong risk factor for osteoporosis. Prolonged use of steroids leads to osteoporosis and should raise a suspicion of its presence. This patient had two risk factors, other than age alone, leading to the necessity of evaluating her for osteoporosis before manipulative treatment.

A significant concern in treating osteoporotic patients with osteopathic manipulation is that bones may fracture. While this is certainly a concern, it does not indicate that a patient with osteoporosis should not receive manipulation. Gentleness is the key. No significant force should be exerted on fragile bone, especially the ribs. Gentle stretching of soft tissues, positioning techniques such as counterstrain, and proper exercises are very helpful in decreasing back pain. Often the pain experienced is not the result of the osteoporosis, but rather from tense soft tissues. Somatic dysfunctions can be treated with balanced ligamentous tension techniques or counterstrain. Osteopathy in the cranial field is nontraumatic to these patients.

In the presence of new compression fractures, no manipulation should be performed in the area, but manipulation of distant areas is still possible. Once the fracture heals, the manipulation can be performed near that vertebra.

Older individuals, especially menopausal women, should be carefully screened before the use of any type of compressive force.

### REFERENCES

DiGiovanna EL. *An Encyclopedia of Osteopathy*. Indianapolis, IN: American Academy of Osteopathy, 2003.

DiGiovanna EL, Schiowitz S. *An Osteopathic Approach to Diagnosis and Treatment*. Philadelphia: Lippincott-Raven, 1997.

Ward RC. *Foundations for Osteopathic Medicine*. Baltimore: William & Wilkins, 1997.

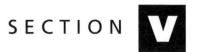

# Lumbar Spine

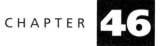

# Lumbar Anatomic Considerations

*Stanley Schiowitz*

The five lumbar vertebrae are separated from one another by intervertebral disks. The combined unit of the vertebrae and disks, in the upright position, forms the anteroposterior lordotic lumbar spinal curve between the thoracic spine and the sacral base.

## ■ OSTEOLOGY

The lumbar vertebral bodies are larger than the thoracic vertebral bodies. They are wider transversely than in the anteroposterior dimension and are higher in front than in back, creating a posterior body wedge. In conjunction with a similar intervertebral disk shape, the wedge shape of the lumbar vertebral bodies helps maintain lumbar lordosis.

The spinous processes of the lumbar vertebrae are large, quadrangular, and directed dorsally in a horizontal plane. The transverse processes are long, thin, and directed laterally in a horizontal plane. In contrast to the different planar relationships of the thoracic vertebral structures, the spinous process, transverse processes, and vertebral body all lie at the same spinal level.

The fifth lumbar vertebra differs from those above it by having a larger body, thicker and shorter transverse processes, and a smaller spinous process. It is also markedly higher in its anterior aspect. The largest number of spinal congenital defects occur at the level of the fifth lumbar vertebra.

The superior articular facets of the lumbar vertebrae are concave and face primarily medially and backward. They are rotated 45 degrees from the sagittal plane toward the frontal plane. The inferior articular facets are convex and face laterally and forward. The superior and inferior articular facets of the contiguous lumbar vertebrae fit into each other, forming *zygophyseal joints*.

Many variations of articular facets occur in the lumbar region, notably at the lumbosacral articulation. These variations include sagittal plane rotations of 0 to 90 degrees, a horizontal planar orientation, and facet asymmetries. These variants contribute to low back instability, disk disease, and somatic dysfunction.

## ■ INTERVERTEBRAL MOTION

All individual vertebral motions follow the rules of coupled motions:

1. Flexion and extension are coupled with a anterior–posterior translatory slide in the sagittal plane.
2. Lateral flexion is coupled with a contralateral translatory slide in the frontal plane.
3. Rotation is coupled with disk compression in the horizontal plane.

The motions of flexion and extension are greatest at all levels, as influenced by the vertical sagittal orientation of the facets. There is a small degree of lateral flexion present that is always accompanied by very limited rotation. The convex–concave articular shapes mandate the combined roll-and-slide motion.

## ■ SOMATIC DYSFUNCTION

Group lateral curves are common in the lumbar region and are usually secondary to thoracic scoliosis or to sacral base unleveling. Single-segment vertebral somatic dysfunctions involve restricted motion in all three planes; however, rotation is the primary motion most commonly restricted. This rotation restriction is accompanied by ipsilateral lateral flexion.

Somatic dysfunctions are commonly diagnosed by monitoring the rotary motions of the lumbar transverse processes.

## ■ INTERVERTEBRAL DISKS

A healthy disk consists of a jelly-like substance, the *nucleus pulposus*, surrounded by a fibrotic ring, the *annulus fibrosis*. The annulus comprises a series of collagen fibers that are firmly attached to their superior and inferior vertebral endplates. The fibroelastic mesh is formed by concentric circumferential lamellae. The collagen fibers of the lamellae lie at a 65-degree angle from the vertical, and their vertical orientation alternates in successive lamellae. This anatomical arrangement allows the disk to undergo rotary motions and shearing forces while still maintaining a restrictive stability. The nucleus moves in a direction opposite to vertebral motion, creating pressure on the annulus and a normalizing force distribution mechanism.

The lumbar intervertebral disks sustain the most degenerative changes and dysfunctions of all the spinal disks, with the possible exception of the C5–C6 disk. It is thought that sitting postures in which the lumbar spine is flexed cause more fluid to be expressed from the lumbar disks than do erect postures. This motion, by extensive standing, fusion, degenerative arthritis, or spinal motion restriction of any cause is postulated to reduce nutrient flow to the disks and hasten lumbar disk degeneration. Degenerative changes result in loss of tissue elasticity, loss of restrictive stability, depressed feedback mechanisms, and loss of disk height. The relationships of the superior to inferior articular facets become abnormal. The ligaments connecting the vertebrae and disks become lax, and there is a greater tendency toward dysfunction.

Herniated disks are most common in the lower lumbar region because of narrowing of the posterior longitudinal ligament, the increased incidence of degenerative disk disease, ligament laxity, and excessive stress placed on the disks in this location.

## ■ NEUROLOGY

The lumbar plexus lies within the posterior part of the psoas major muscle and in front of the transverse processes of the lumbar vertebrae. It consists of the ventral rami of the first, second, third, and part of the fourth lumbar nerves.

The spinal cord ends at about the level of the second lumbar vertebra. Lower nerve roots run caudally and laterally to exit from the intervertebral foramina. This termination of the cord into a spray of nerve roots is known as the *cauda equina*. Disk herniation disturbs the nerve root of the lower of the vertebrae involved. Therefore, an L5–S1 herniated disk will cause dysfunction of the first sacral nerve root.

At a minimum, the clinician should be able to recognize the symptoms of L4, L5, and S1 nerve root dysfunctions. Dysfunction of the L4 nerve causes diminution in the patellar reflex, reduction of strength in the quadriceps and anterior tibialis muscles, and cutaneous sensation changes on the medial aspect of the leg and foot. Dysfunction of the L5 nerve does not affect a reflex but does impose a loss of strength of the first toe in dorsiflexion, loss of strength of the extensor hallucis muscle, and cutaneous sensation changes on the side of the leg and top of the foot. Dysfunction of the S1 nerve causes diminution in the Achilles reflex, a reduction of strength in the peroneus longus and brevis muscles, and sensation changes on the lateral aspect of the foot.

## ■ MYOLOGY

The erector spinae are large muscle groups lying at each side of the vertebral column. It originates at the sacrum and continues through to the cervical region. At the lumbar region they are divided, medially to laterally, into the spinalis, longissimus, and iliocostalis muscles. Bilateral muscle contraction causes extension of the vertebral column. Unilateral contraction causes ipsilateral extension and side-bending.

The multifidus and rotatores muscles are small muscles of the back lying deep to the erector spinae. They function primarily as postural muscles, with control of individual vertebral motions. Bilateral contraction creates local extension, and unilateral contraction causes lateral flexion with contralateral rotation.

The quadratus lumborum is a lateral muscle attached to the twelfth rib, iliac crest, and vertebral column. Its rib attachment allows it to function with respiration by fixing the last rib and assisting in stabilizing the origin of the diaphragm. Bilateral contraction creates extension; unilateral contraction causes extension with ipsilateral side-bending.

The synergistic action of the abdominal muscles creates forward bending. External oblique contraction creates rotation to the opposite side; internal oblique contraction creates rotation to the same side. The combined actions of the abdominal muscles provide a coordinated mechanism for controlling extreme torque, bending, and shear stresses in the lumbar spine. Their normal functioning is essential to the maintenance of the spinal mechanism.

The iliopsoas muscle plays an important role in the function and stability of the lumbar region. It is composed of two muscles. The psoas major originates from the anterior surfaces and lower borders of the transverse processes of all the lumbar vertebrae by five digitations, each extending from the body of the two vertebrae and their intersegmental disks, starting from the twelfth thoracic vertebra and ending at the fifth lumbar vertebra. The muscle descends along the pelvic brim, passes behind the inguinal ligament and in front of the capsule of the hip joint, and ends in a tendon that receives, on its lateral side, nearly the whole of the fibers of the iliacus. The psoas major inserts into the lesser trochanter of the femur.

The iliacus muscle originates from the superior two thirds of the concavity of the iliac fossa, from the inner lip of the iliac crest, from the ventral sacroiliac and iliolumbar ligaments, and from the upper, lateral surface of the sacrum. In front, it reaches as far as the anterosuperior and anteroinferior iliac spines, and receives some fibers from the upper part of the capsule of the hip joint. It inserts into the lateral side of the tendon of the psoas major, which inserts into the lesser trochanter of the femur.

From above, the iliopsoas flexes the thigh on the pelvis; from below, it flexes the trunk forward by bilateral contraction. Unilateral contraction creates lateral trunk flexion with a pelvic shift to that side.

The iliopsoas remains in constant activity in the erect posture and prevents hyperextension of the hip joint in a standing subject. An increase in lumbar lordosis while standing erect causes increased activity of the psoas and low back instability and dysfunction.

The cardinal signs of iliopsoatic dysfunction in the standing and supine positions are as follows:

1. Standing: hip and knee flexion and pelvic tilt on the side of the dysfunction, a positive Trendelenburg sign, and a typical psoatic stance and gait.
2. Supine: exaggerated lumber lordosis and a positive Thomas test.

Somatic dysfunction of the lumbar region that is related to iliopsoas contracture usually occurs at the upper lumbar vertebral levels.

In the pelvis, these muscles create a supportive mechanism for the abdominal viscera, the psoas shelf, as they traverse the pubic bones in their descent to the lesser trochanters. Any somatic dysfunction that changes this structural relationship can cause visceral symptoms and pathology. Anterior sacral or pelvic tilt, psoas contracture, abdominal muscle weakness, pregnancy, wearing of high-heel shoes, poor posture, and somatic reflexes can all increase the stress of the viscera onto the abdominal wall, which in turn can lead to diaphragmatic hernia, inguinal and femoral hernias, retroverted uterus, renal and visceral ptosis, and syndromes such as dysmenorrhea, menorrhagia, polyuria, constipation, and colitis.

The iliopsoas muscle also plays an important role in the synergistic activities of the muscles of the low back in maintaining a normal lumbosacral angle and proper postural balance.

## ■ LUMBOSACRAL ANGLE (FERGUSON'S ANGLE)

The lumbosacral angle is the angle formed in the upright position, from a side view, by extending the line of inclination of the sacrum as it meets a line parallel to the ground. This angle is normally between 25 and 35 degrees. A major portion of low back pain is attributable to an increased lumbosacral angle. The greater the angle, the greater is the inclination and the higher the shear stress placed on the lumbosacral joint and its attachments. In addition, the increased angle increases lumbar lordosis.

Factors that can influence the lumbosacral angle are obesity, pregnancy, abdominal muscle weakness, wearing of high-heel shoes, foot pronation. Achilles valgus, atypical lumbosacral facets, spondylolisthesis, diminished disk height, ligamentous weakness, organic kyphoscoliosis, poor posture, occupation, somatotype, heredity, psoatic dysfunction, anterior sacral/pelvic tilt, and somatic dysfunction.

An increased lumbosacral angle changes the articular relationships, because the inferior lumbar facets slide caudally on their matched superior sacral facets.

## ■ SYNERGISTIC ACTION OF THE MUSCLES IN MAINTAINING LUMBAR CURVATURES

The abdominal muscles support and assist in the flattening of the lumbar lordosis. The psoas muscles pull on the vertebrae and anterior pelvis, increasing the lumbar lordosis. The gluteus maximus and hamstrings pull on the posterior pelvis, decreasing the lumbar lordosis. The erector spinae muscles and the abdominal muscles assist in flattening the lumbar lordosis.

## ■ LUMBAR–PELVIC RHYTHM

When a subject bends forward to touch the floor, combined motions of the lumbar vertebrae, pelvis, and hip joints are put into play. The individual vertebrae flex on each other, straightening the lumbar lordosis and sometimes causing a mild reversal of that curve. Simultaneously, a secondary pelvic rotation motion occurs around the axis of the hip joints as the hip joints move posteriorly in the horizontal plane. These are smooth, interrelated motions, both in total forward bending and in its reversal, straightening up.

In evaluating gross body movement, the physician must examine all three aspects of lumbosacral rhythm. It is common to relate all forward-bending restrictions to lumbar dysfunction. This assumption is not correct. Hip joint or pelvic dysfunctions are often at fault.

### REFERENCES

Adams MA, Hutton HC. The effect of posture on the fluid content of lumbar intervertebral discs. *Spine* 1983;8: 665–671.

Basmajian JV. *Muscles Alive*. Baltimore: Williams & Wilkins, 1978.

Bogduk N, Twomey T. *Clinical Anatomy of the Lumbar Spine*. Edinburgh: Churchill Livingstone, 1987.

Cailliet R. *Low Back Syndrome*, 2nd ed. Philadelphia: F.A. Davis, 1968.

DiGiovanna EL, Schiowitz S. *An Osteopathic Approach to Diagnosis and Treatment*, 2nd ed. Philadelphia: Lippincott-Raven, 1997.

Farfan HF, Sullivan JD. The relation of facet orientation to intervertebral disc failure. *Can J Surg* 1967;10:179–185.

Farfan HF. Muscular mechanism of the lumbar spine and the position of power and efficiency. *Orthop Clin North Am* 1975;6:135–144.

Jayson IV. *The Lumbar Spine and Back Pain*, 3rd ed. Edinburgh: Churchill Livingstone, 1976.

Jones L. *The Postural Complex*. St. Louis: Charles C Thomas, 1955.

Kapanji IA. *The Physiology of the Joints, vol 3. The Trunk and the Vertebral Column*. Edinburgh: Churchill Livingstone, 1974.

Warwick R, Williams PL. *Gray's Anatomy*, 35th British ed. Philadelphia: W.B. Saunders, 1973.

Weisel SW, Bernini P, Rothman RH. *The Aging Lumbar Spine*. Philadelphia: W.B. Saunders, 1982.

White AA, Panjabi MM. *Biomechanics of the Spine*. Philadelphia: J.B. Lippincott, 1978.

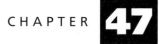

# Evaluation of the Lumbar Spine

*Eileen L. DiGiovanna*

The lumbar spine consists of five vertebrae, the largest in size is the spinal column. Most congenital anomalies occur to the fifth lumbar vertebra. Both the thoracic spine and the sacrum and pelvis have significant effects on the posture and function of the lumbar spine. When performing an evaluation of the lumbar spine, it is necessary to include these areas in the examination.

## ■ HISTORY

As in every region of the body, a thorough history is valuable in determining the cause of the problem. Low back pain may be centered in the lumbar spine or in the sacral region, thus requiring that the patient identify the exact location of any pain as nearly as possible. The interviewer should seek any known association of low back pain with an activity, because it may be related to sports, occupation, posture, lifting heavy weights, bending, or stretching. Of course, a visceral or other cause must be considered.

## ■ PHYSICAL EXAMINATION

### Observation

The skin should be inspected for areas of unusual redness, skin discoloration, blemishes, or hairy patches. Some hairy patches ("faun's beard") are indicative of a congenital anomaly (typically spina bifida) of the bone. Birthmarks over the lumbar spine may also indicate some bony pathology. The region should be inspected for evidence of injury or past surgery. Any masses such as lipomata should be noted.

Gait and standing posture should be observed. The spine is viewed from the side for an increase in the lumbar lordosis or a flattening of the curve. Then it is viewed from the back for a lateral curve (scoliosis).

### Gross Motion Testing

Gross motion of the lumbar spine is generally evaluated in conjunction with that of the thoracic spine. The patient is standing with his weight evenly distributed and his two feet are spaced 4 to 6 inches apart. The physician kneels or squats directly behind the patient; his eyes are level with the lumbar spine.

1. The physician places his hands flat on the top if the patient's iliac crests with his fingers monitoring the anterior superior iliac spines (ASIS) and his thumbs monitoring the posterior superior iliac spines (PSIS).
2. The physician will note any limitation of motion, the fluidity with which the motion is achieved, and the symmetry or asymmetry created.
3. Most of the rotation will occur in the thoracic spine because of the fact that the lumbar vertebrae are limited to approximately 5 degrees of rotation in each direction.
4. The pelvis will rotate during the evaluation of rotation; however, monitoring the ASIS can minimize this.
5. Forward Bending (Flexion):
   a. The patient is instructed to bend forward beginning with the head and neck as if to

touch the toes, keeping the knees straight (Fig. 47-1).

b. The physician observes the fluidity with which the thoracic and lumbar spine moves and notes any areas of restricted motion. The angle of flexion should approximate 160 degrees.

c. The patient then returns to an upright, neutral position.

6. Backward Bending (Extension):

a. The patient is instructed to slowly bend backwards toward the physician (Fig. 47-2). Most of the motion will occur above the waist.

b. Once the physician feels motion at the ASIS, the patient is instructed to stop motion.

c. The fluidity and amount of the motion is noted. The angle of extension should approximate 60 degrees.

d. The patient is instructed to return to an upright, neutral position.

7. Side-Bending

a. The patient is instructed to slide one hand down the lateral aspect of the ipsilateral thigh without deviating into either flexion or extension while keeping the knees straight (Fig. 47-3).

b. The physician monitors the iliac crests. When he feels motion of the contralateral

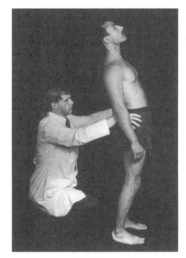

■ **FIG. 47-2** Thoracolumbar regional motion testing: backward bending.

crest, he instructs the patient to stop bending.

c. The fluidity and amount of motion is noted. The angle of side-bending should approximate 40 degrees.

d. The patient is instructed to return to an upright, neutral position.

e. The process is repeated for the contralateral side. Right side-bending is compared to the left for symmetry of motion.

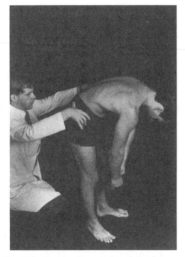

■ **FIG. 47-1** Thoracolumbar regional motion testing: forward bending.

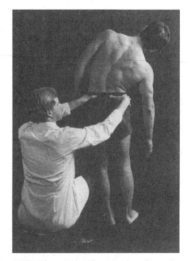

■ **FIG. 47-3** Thoracolumbar regional motion testing: side-bending.

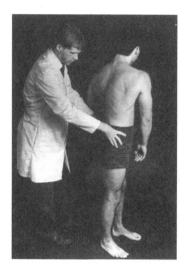

■ **FIG. 47-4** Thoracolumbar regional motion testing: rotation.

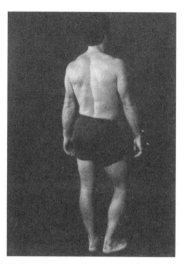

■ **FIG. 47-5** Hip drop test: side-bending.

8. Rotation:
   a. The patient is instructed to turn his body, from the waist up, to one side, while keeping his feet firmly on the ground with the knees straight (Fig. 47-4).
   b. The physician is monitoring motion at the anterior superior iliac spines. When he feels the pelvis beginning to rotate, the patient is instructed to stop moving.
   c. The physician observes the fluidity and amount of motion.
   d. The patient is then instructed to return to a neutral position.
   e. The above steps are repeated in the contralateral direction.
   f. The physician then compares the right and left rotation for symmetry and any restriction is noted. The angle of rotation should approximate 40 degrees.

## Lateral Lumbar Flexion: Hip Drop Test

Another method for assessing the ability of the lumbar spine to side-bend without a significant contribution from the thoracic spine is the *hip drop test*. The patient is standing with his weight equally distributed and his feet 4 to 6 inches apart. The physician stands behind the patient with his eyes relatively level with the lumbar region. He may kneel or squat to do so.

1. The patient is instructed to bend one knee, keeping both feet flat on the ground and the opposite knee straight (Fig. 47-5).
2. The patient should allow the compensatory shift in body weight distribution.
3. The physician notes the fluidity and amount of motion as the lumbar spine curves laterally to compensate for the drop in the pelvis on the side of the bent knee. The amount of drop in the iliac crest is noted.
4. The process is repeated to the contralateral side.
5. The right and left side-bending of the lumbar spine are compared. The iliac crest that drops the greatest amount is the side opposite that to which the lumbar spine side-bends the most, or, stated another way, the side of greatest drop is the side of restricted side-bending. The spinal curve should be smooth and unimpeded.

## Palpation

Palpation is best performed with the patient prone on a table and the physician standing at the side of the table facing the patient. The *erythema test* may be performed at this time, as may the *skin drag test*. When these tests are positive they are indicators or somatic dysfunction as explained in Chapter 8.

The deeper layers of tissue are palpated next, including the subcutaneous tissues and the fascia. Occasionally *fibro-lipomata* may be palpated around the lumbosacral junction and the sacrum. These are firm, benign masses that occur in these areas.

The physician then palpates deeper into the muscle tissue. The paraspinal muscles lie parallel to the spinal column. They are larger in the lumbar region than in other regions of the spine. The quadratus lumborum attaches to the twelfth rib, the spinal column, and the crest of the ilium. These muscles are frequently the source of low back pain and should be evaluated for hypertonicity, spasm, bogginess, and other tissue texture changes.

Once the soft tissues have been palpated, the bony structures should be evaluated. The spinous processes and transverse processes are palpated and their symmetry compared. The tops of the iliac crests are in a line with the L4–L5 interspace. From this site it is possible to identify the other lumbar vertebrae. Another method for identifying the vertebrae is to find the twelfth rib and follow it to its attachment to T12. The first vertebra below T12 is L1, and the spinous processes can be counted down from there. The transverse processes lie at the same level as the vertebral body and are usually quite long in the lumbar region. They may be palpated deep to the erector spinae muscles.

## Intersegmental Motion Testing

To test the individual vertebral motions, the patient will lie on the table, prone for testing rotation, and side-lying for testing flexion, extension, and side-bending. The physician stands at the side of the table facing the patient.

1. Rotation Testing
   a. With the patient prone, the physician places a monitoring finger or thumb on each transverse process of the vertebra being evaluated.
   b. The physician applies a firm downward pressure on one of the transverse processes and, releasing that, to the contralateral transverse process.
   c. The ease of ventral motion indicates the ability of the vertebral body to rotate to the contralateral direction. The two sides are compared to determine if there is any restriction to rotation.
   d. *Example:* If the right transverse process moves ventrally more easily, then the vertebra is rotating to the left more easily and there is a restriction in right rotation.
   e. This procedure is repeated at each lumbar level.
2. Side-bending/Rotation
   a. The patient is lying on one side with the physician facing him.
   b. The physician places one finger on the spinous process or transverse process of the vertebra being evaluated.
   c. The patient's hips and knees are flexed until the physician feels motion at the monitoring finger.
   d. The physician leans onto the patient's knees, and then using the knees as a fulcrum, the physician lifts the patient's ankles upward toward the ceiling until motion is again felt at the monitoring finger (Fig. 47-6). This creates side-bending of the lumbar spine with the convexity of the curve nearest the table.
   e. The physician notes the ease with which the vertebra side-bends. He also notes any posterior rotation of the transverse process of the vertebra being monitored. A posterior rotation indicates a type II somatic dysfunction at that level. Ventral rotation indicates a type I somatic dysfunction at that vertebra.

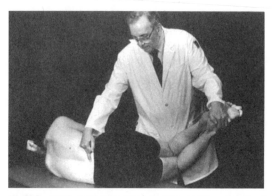

■ **FIG. 47-6** Intersegmental motion testing: rotation/side-bending.

f. The procedure is repeated at each vertebral level and the motion of each is compared with the others.

3. Flexion/Extension

a. With the patient in the position described, the physician flexes and extends the lumbar spine. One finger is monitoring the spinous process of the vertebra being evaluated.

b. Moving the flexed knees towards the patient's abdomen creates flexion. Flexion continues only until motion is felt at the monitoring finger.

c. The physician induces extension by moving the patient's legs and knees away from the abdomen and applying axial compression through the patient's femurs. Motion is created until it is felt at the monitoring fingers.

d. The physician compares the ability of each vertebra to flex and extend.

e. Ease of flexion with a barrier to extension indicates a flexion somatic dysfunction. Ease of extension with a barrier to flexion indicates an extension somatic dysfunction.

## Rotoscoliosis Motion Testing

Rotoscoliosis motion testing provides another method to identify somatic dysfunction of a lumbar vertebra. This technique uses the principle that a type II somatic dysfunction will have a restriction to motion in all three planes of its ability to move. If a barrier is reached in flexion or extension, the vertebra will tend to rotate and side-bend towards its ease of motion.

**Patient Position:** prone on the table
**Physician Position:** standing on one side of the table, facing the patient.
**Technique:**

a. The physician will place his fingers on the transverse processes of the vertebra being evaluated.

b. Each vertebra is evaluated in all three positions before the next vertebra is examined. The physician's fingers maintain firm con-

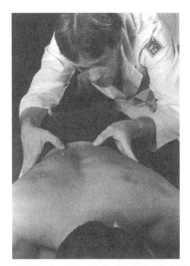

■ **FIG. 47-7** Lumbar rotoscoliosis testing in initial prone position.

tact with the transverse processes until all three positions have been examined.

c. *Neutral:* With the patient prone, the physician determines the anteroposterior symmetry or asymmetry of a vertebra by comparing the corresponding right and left transverse processes (Fig. 47-7).

d. *Hyperextension:* The patient is instructed to hyperextend the spine by lifting his upper body off the table, leaning on his hands or his elbows (Fig. 47-8). Extension is continued until the monitoring fingers feel motion. The physician compares the transverse processes for symmetry or asymmetry of position.

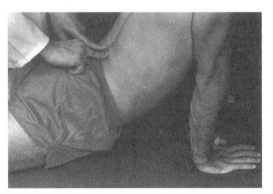

■ **FIG. 47-8** Lumbar rotoscoliosis testing in extension.

e. *Flexion:* The patient is seated with his feet firmly and equally supported and is instructed to forward-bend, allowing the arms to fall between the knees (Fig. 47-9). Flexion continues until the physician

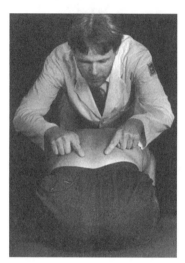

■ **FIG. 47-9** Lumbar rotoscoliosis testing in flexion.

feels motion at the monitoring fingers. The physician compares the transverse processes for symmetry or asymmetry of position.

f. Asymmetry of the transverse processes in flexion indicates an extension somatic dysfunction with rotation and side-bending to the side of the posterior displacement of one transverse process.

g. *Example:* If the right transverse process moves more posteriorly than the left when the patient is hyperextending, the diagnosis is a flexion somatic dysfunction with right side-bending and rotation.

### REFERENCES

DiGiovanna EL, Schiowitz S. *An Osteopathic Approach to Diagnosis and Treatment.* Philadelphia: Lippincott-Raven, 1997.

Hoppenfeld S. *Physical Examination of the Spine and Extremities.* Norwalk, CT: Appleton & Lange, Norwalk, 1976.

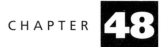

# Myofascial Techniques

*Eileen L. DiGiovanna and Toni Spinaris*

This chapter describes the application of passive, active direct, and active indirect myofascial or soft tissue techniques to the lumbar region. These techniques may be used as the main part of the treatment or in preparation for the use of other osteopathic techniques.

## ■ PASSIVE TECHNIQUES
### Prone Technique

1. **Patient position:** prone.
2. **Physician position:** standing at the side of the table, opposite the side to be treated.
3. **Technique:**
   a. The physician places the thumb of one hand parallel to the paravertebral muscle on the side opposite where she is standing, between the muscle and spinous processes. The thumb is reinforced by placing the thenar eminence of her other hand on top of it (see Figs. 37-1 and 37-2).
   b. The muscle is pushed away from the spinous processes by keeping her elbows straight and using body weight to move the muscle.
   c. The stretch is held a few seconds, allowing the muscle to relax, and then slowly released.
   d. The stretch is repeated several times. The thumb and reinforcing hand may be moved up and down the spine to stretch various portions of the muscle.

### Alternate Prone Technique

1. **Patient and physician positions** remain the same.

2. **Technique:**
   a. The stretch is made using the heel of the cephalad hand, which is pushing the muscle away from the spinous processes.
   b. The caudad hand grasps the anterior superior iliac spine (ASIS) on the far side and rotates the pelvis by pulling the ASIS up and toward the physician. This provides an additional stretch on the lumbar muscles.

### Lateral Recumbent Technique

1. **Patient position:** Lying on side with muscles to be treated uppermost and knees and hips slightly flexed for balance.
2. **Physician position:** Standing at the side of the table facing the patient.
3. **Technique:**
   a. The physician grasps the upper paravertebral muscles with the fingers of both hands.
   b. Keeping the elbows straight, the physician leans back and stretches the muscles by pulling them perpendicularly away from the spinous processes (Fig. 48-1).
   c. This stretch is held for several seconds and then slowly released.
   d. This may be repeated several times, with the physician moving the hands up and down the spine to stretch various parts of the muscle.

### Alternate Lateral Recumbent Technique

This technique will add a longitudinal stretch to the perpendicular technique described.

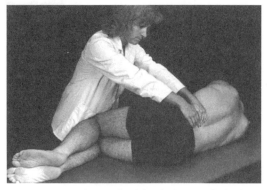

■ **FIG. 48-1** Passive myofascial technique applied to lumbar spine, patient recumbent.

1. Patient and physician positions: remain the same.
2. **Technique:**
   a. The physician grasps the muscle as described. She then places her cephalad forearm on the patient's shoulder and her caudad forearm on the patient's iliac crest.
   b. As she pulls the muscle perpendicularly, she adds a longitudinal stretch by pushing the shoulder and iliac crests with her forearms to separate them.

## ■ ACTIVE DIRECT TECHNIQUE

### Lateral Recumbent Technique

1. **Patient position:** Recumbent on his side, with the affected muscles down.
2. **Physician position:** Standing at the side of the table facing the patient.

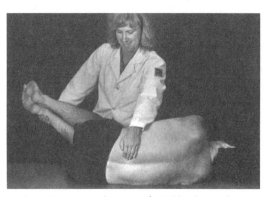

■ **FIG. 48-2** Active, direct myofascial lumbar technique, patient recumbent.

3. **Technique:**
   a. The physician grasps the patient's ankles and raises them off the table, stretching the involved muscles (those closer to the table) (Fig. 48-2).
   b. The patient is instructed to push his ankles down toward the table and to hold this contraction for several seconds.
   c. The physician exerts a resistive force equal to the patient's contraction, causing an isometric contraction.
   d. The patient relaxes and the physician induces further side-bending by raising the ankles further.
   e. The process may be repeated several times to relax the muscles.
   f. The physician may localize the area being treated by flexing the patient's hips. Approximately 90 degrees of hip flexion will bring maximum contraction to the lower lumbar spine. Greater flexion will bring maximum contraction further up the lumbar spine.

## Alternate Lateral Recumbent Technique

1. **Patient position:** recumbent on his side with the affected muscles up away from the table. Hips and knees are flexed.

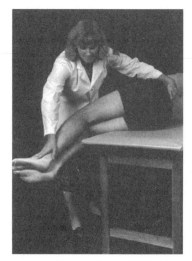

■ **FIG. 48-3** Modified active direct myofascial lumbar technique.

2. **Physician position:** standing at the side of the table facing the patient.
3. **Technique:**
   a. The physician grasps the patient's ankles and lowers his legs below the level of the tabletop (Fig. 48-3).
   b. The patient is asked to push his ankles toward the ceiling. This causes contraction of the uppermost muscles.
   c. The physician provides an isometric resistive force for several seconds; then the patient is allowed to relax.
   d. The technique is repeated several times.

## ■ ACTIVE INDIRECT TECHNIQUES

### Lateral Recumbent Technique

1. **Patient position:** recumbent on his side with affected muscles down toward the table. Hips and knees are flexed for balance.
2. **Physician position:** standing at the side of the table facing the patient.
3. **Technique:**
   a. The physician grasps the patient's ankles and lowers them off the table below the level of the tabletop.

   b. The patient is instructed to push his ankles up toward the ceiling. This causes contraction of the uppermost muscles (those antagonistic to the involved muscle).
   c. The physician provides an isokinetic resistance (resistive force that allows the ankles to move against that resistance).
   d. This process may be repeated several times. This procedure uses contraction of the antagonist muscles to relax the agonist muscle by reciprocal inhibition.

### Alternate Lateral Recumbent Technique

The aforementioned technique may be modified to treat the uppermost muscles by raising the ankles toward the ceiling and having the patient push down toward the floor. The legs are allowed to move against an isokinetic resistance. The patient is now contracting the muscles closest to the table to relax the uppermost muscles by reciprocal inhibition. A passive stretch may be added at the end of either of these techniques.

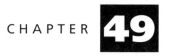

# Muscle Energy Techniques For The Lumbar Spine

*Sandra D. Yale, Nancy Brous, and Dennis J. Dowling*

This chapter describes the application of muscle energy techniques to group curves and single-segment somatic dysfunctions in the lumbar spine. For the described techniques, the patient lies on his side on the table or in a modified *Sims position*. The transverse processes of the segment to be treated are oriented either upwards or downwards, according to the precise technique.

## ■ TYPE I NEUTRAL (GROUP) CURVES

1. **Patient position:** Side-lying with concavity of the curve toward the table; the posteriorly rotated transverse processes are up.
2. **Physician position:** standing at the side of the table facing the patient.
3. **Technique:**
   a. The physician monitors the apex of the curve with the hand that is closer to the patient's head.
   b. The physician flexes the patient's hips and knees to approximately 90 degrees.
   c. The physician side-bends the lumbar spine to the apex by elevating the patient's ankles with the nonmonitoring hand (Fig. 49-1).
   d. The patient is instructed to push his feet toward the floor for 3 to 5 seconds.
   e. The physician provides isometric resistance, producing a static contraction.
   f. The patient is directed to relax for 3 to 5 seconds typically, but may be slightly longer if necessary.
   g. The physician further elevates the pa-

tient's feet and lower legs until motion is felt at the new barrier.
   h. The procedure is repeated at least three times.
   i. A passive stretch is added after the last repetition.

## ■ TYPE II FLEXED SOMATIC DYSFUNCTION

1. **Patient position:** Side-lying on the table. The posteriorly rotated transverse process to be treated is downward, toward the table. The patient will be placed into a lateral recumbent position (the mnemonic "FDR" may be used to indicate *F*lexion, posterior facets *D*ownward, and *R*ecumbent position).
2. **Physician position:** standing at the side of the table facing the patient.
3. **Technique:**
   a. The physician monitors at the level of the somatic dysfunction with his cephalad hand.
   b. With his other hand, the physician flexes the patient's hips and knees until motion is localized at the level below the dysfunction (i.e., at L2 on L3).
   c. The patient is directed to straighten his lower leg and the physician further extends it until motion is felt at the same level.
   d. The flexed top leg is "locked" in place with the dorsum of the foot placed in the

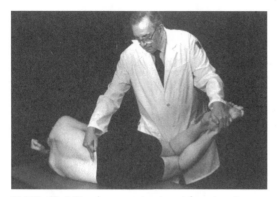

■ **FIG. 49-1** Muscle energy treatment for a type I curve, convex right.

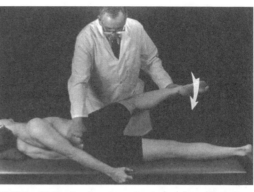

■ **FIG. 49-2** Muscle energy treatment for a flexed somatic dysfunction.

popliteal space of the lower leg by the physician. This places the somatic dysfunction into an extension barrier.

e. The physician temporarily switches monitoring hands so that the caudad (with respect to the patient) hand is now monitoring the involved segment.

f. With his other hand, the physician grasps the patient's lower arm and pulls it forward and upward, until motion is felt at the level of the restriction. This brings the patient into the lateral recumbent position and creates rotation of the dysfunction into the barrier direction.

g. Further rotation and localization can be achieved by directing the patient to grasp the table edge behind his back with his other hand.

h. The physician places his cephalad hand on the patient's shoulder.

i. The patient is instructed to take a deep breath and then exhale completely. The physician resists the motion that occurs during inhalation and then follows the shoulder into backwards rotation during exhalation. The patient is directed to reach further down the table edge with his hand.

j. The physician again switches hands and uses his cephalad hand to monitor the level of the restriction.

k. The physician grasps the ankle of the patient's top leg and elevates it until the lumbar spine side-bends to the motion barrier.

l. The patient is directed to push his elevated foot down toward the table for 3 to 5 seconds.

m. The physician provides isometric resistance, producing a static contraction.

n. The patient is directed to relax for 3 to 5 seconds typically, but this may be slightly longer if necessary

o. The physician further elevates the patient's upper foot and leg until motion is felt at the new barrier (Fig. 49-2).

p. The physician then increases extension, side-bending, and rotation into the new motion barriers by again elevating the patient's upper ankle.

q. The procedure is repeated at least three times or until the somatic dysfunction is improved.

r. A passive stretch is given after the last repetition.

## ■ TYPE II EXTENDED SOMATIC DYSFUNCTION

1. **Patient position:** Side-lying on the table. The posteriorly rotated transverse process to be treated faces upward. The patient is placed into a modified Sims position (the mnemonic "SUE" to indicate *S*ims, posterior facets *U*pward, and *E*xtension dysfunction may be used).

2. **Physician position:** standing at the side of the table facing the patient.

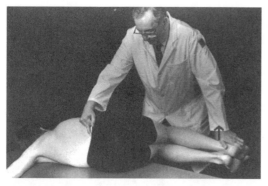

■ **FIG. 49-3A** Muscle energy treatment for an extended somatic dysfunction. Physician standing.

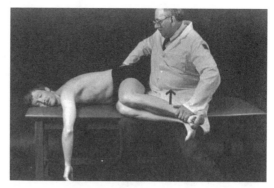

■ **FIG. 49-3B** Physician seated.

3. **Technique:**
   a. The physician faces the patient and monitors the somatic dysfunction with his cephalad hand.
   b. With his other hand, the physician flexes the patient's hips and knees until motion is localized at the level below the dysfunction (i.e., at L2 on L3).
   c. The physician switches monitoring hands so that the caudad hand is then on the somatic dysfunction.
   d. The patient is directed to bring the arm that is on the table behind him and rotate his chest towards the table. This rotation creates a modified Sims position.
   e. The physician places his cephalad hand on the patient's shoulder.
   f. Additional rotation is induced by having the patient inhale and then exhale completely while simultaneously reaching toward the floor.
   g. The physician pushes down on the patient's shoulder toward the table with his cephalad hand until the torso is rotated down to the monitored segment, exaggerating the modified Sims position.
   h. The physician again switches monitoring hands with now the cephalad becoming and remaining the monitoring one.
   i. The physician lowers the patient's legs off the side of the table to create lumbar sidebending up to the restricted area (Fig. 49-3A).
   j. Because this position may be uncomfortable for the patient, the physician may either place a pillow under the patient's lower knee or sit behind the patient and put his thigh between the patient's legs and the table (Fig. 49-3B). (This position requires the physician to change the hand monitoring.)
   k. The patient is directed to push his feet toward the ceiling for 3 to 5 seconds.
   l. The physician provides isometric resistance, creating a static contraction.
   m. The patient is directed to relax for 3 to 5 seconds typically, but may be slightly longer if necessary
   n. The physician engages a new motion barrier by further lowering the patient's legs toward the floor.
   o. The procedure is repeated at least three times or until the somatic dysfunction is improved.
   p. A passive stretch is given after the last repetition.

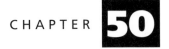

# Counterstrain Techniques

*Eileen L. DiGiovanna*

The counterstrain tender points of the lumbar spine are named for the dysfunctional lumbar vertebrae. Anterior tender points are treated with the patient supine and posterior tender points are treated with the patient prone. Many of the counterstrain techniques for lumbar somatic dysfunctions are facilitated by slight rotation of the patient's thighs and pelvis, and by resting some part of the patient's leg on the physician's thigh or knee.

## ■ ANTERIOR TENDER POINTS

Figure 50-1 shows the locations of the anterior lumbar tender points. Anterior tender points will generally require a position of flexion. The positioning is accomplished by using the lower extremities as levers to move the lumbar spine.

### L1 Anterior Tender Point (Medial to Anterior Superior Iliac Spines)

1. **Patient position:** supine, with upper body propped up on pillows.
2. **Physician position:** standing next to the table on the side of the tender point.
3. **Technique:**
   a. Both knees are flexed and rotated toward the tender point. Because the lower body is rotated, this position is equivalent to upper body rotation away from the tender point (Fig. 50-2).
   b. The hips are side-bent toward the tender point.
   c. The patient's legs may be supported on the physician's thigh if desired.

d. The position is held for 90 seconds, legs returned to neutral, and the tender point is reassessed.

*Note: The L1 tender point is treated in the same manner as the tender points corresponding to vertebrae T9–T12.*

## L2 Anterior Tender Point Technique

1. **Patient position:** supine.
2. **Physician position:** standing at the side of the table opposite the tender point, which is located on the inferior medial surface of the anterior inferior iliac spine.
3. Both thighs are rotated 60 degrees away from the tender point, with side-bending away (Fig. 50-3).
4. The position is held for 90 seconds, legs returned to neutral and tender point is reassessed.

## Abdominal L2 Tender Point

The abdominal L2 tender point is an additional tender point for the second lumbar vertebra and is found 2 inches lateral to the umbilicus. The treatment is the same as for the anterior inferior iliac spine tender point except that the thighs are rotated toward the tender point (the equivalent of rotation away from the tender point at the vertebral level) (Fig. 50-4).

## L3, L4 Anterior Tender Points

1. **Patient position:** supine.
2. **Physician position:** standing at the side of

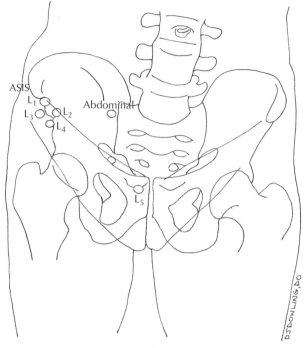

**■ FIG. 50-1** Anterior lumbar tender points.

the table on the side of the tender point, with one foot on the table.

3. **Technique:**
   a. The patient's hips and knees are flexed. His legs rest on the physician's thighs.
   b. The spine is side-bent away from the tender point with slight rotation toward the tender point.
   c. The position is held 90 seconds, legs returned to neutral, and tender point reassessed.

## L5 Anterior Tender Point

1. **Patient position:** supine.
2. **Physician position:** standing at the side of

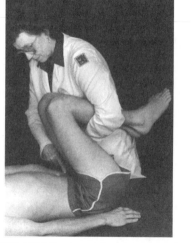

**■ FIG. 50-2** Treatment for L1 tender point.

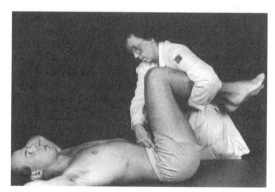

**■ FIG. 50-3** Treatment for L2 tender point.

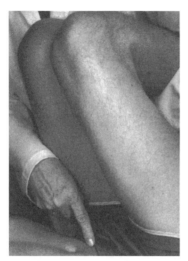

■ **FIG. 50-4** Treatment for abdominal lumbar tender point.

the table next to the tender point, which is on the pubic ramus. Her foot is on the table.

3. **Technique:**
   a. The patient's hips and knees are flexed. His legs rest on the physician's thighs.
   b. The far ankle is crossed over the one closer to the physician. The knees are dropped slightly apart (Fig. 50-5).
   c. There is side-bending away from the tender point and slight rotation toward it.
   d. The position is held for 90 seconds, legs

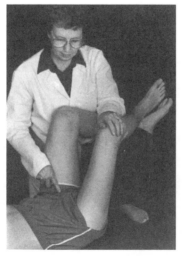

■ **FIG. 50-5** Treatment for L5 tender point.

returned to neutral, and the tender point is reassessed.

## ■ POSTERIOR TENDER POINTS

Posterior lumbar tender points are generally located on the spinous process, between the spinous processes, or over a transverse process. There are some points located in the buttocks or, for lower pole L5, on the sacrum. Figure 50-6 shows the locations of the posterior tender points.

The posterior tender points generally require extension. Lower pole L5 is an exception in that it requires flexion as the main component of treatment. In each technique, the position is held for 90 seconds, then the legs are returned to a neutral position and the tender point is reassessed to assure resolution.

### L1–L5 Tender Points (Spinous or Transverse Process)

1. **Patient position:** prone.
2. **Physician position:** standing at the side of the table. If the tender point is in the midline, it is best if the physician stands on the same side as the leg being elevated (Fig. 50-7). If the point is over a transverse process, it is best if the physician stands opposite the tender point.
3. **Technique:**
   a. The extended leg is elevated, extending the lumber spine. Both legs may be used.
   b. If the tender point is near the midline, this position may be sufficient.
   c. If the tender point is over the transverse process, some rotation may be necessary. This is best performed with the physician standing at the side opposite the tender point. The leg is elevated and adducted over the other leg enough to cause rotation at the vertebral level being treated. External rotation of the thigh assists this process (Fig. 50-8).

### Alternative Technique

If the patient is unable to lie prone, the above technique may be performed with the patient in a lateral recumbent position, with the physician

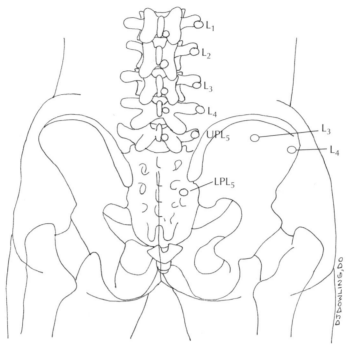

■ **FIG. 50-6** Posterior lumbar tender points.

standing behind him. The leg positioning is the same.

### ■ L3, L4, L5 UPPER POLE TENDER POINTS

The L3 to L5 vertebrae also have tender points in the lateral buttock muscles (gluteals). The lower pole L5 tender point is superior and slightly medial to the posterior inferior iliac spines. L3 and L4 tender points are treated in a manner similar to that described for tender points on the transverse processes. The leg of the prone patient is elevated and adducted. It may rest on the operator's knee, which is placed on the table.

### Lower Pole L5 Tender Point

1. **Patient position:** prone.
2. **Physician position:** seated on a stool at the side of the table next to the tender point.

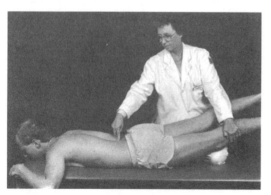

■ **FIG. 50-7** Treatment for spinous process tender point.

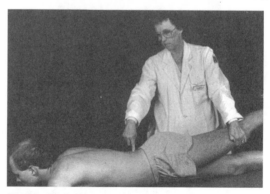

■ **FIG. 50-8** Treatment for transverse process tender point with induced rotation.

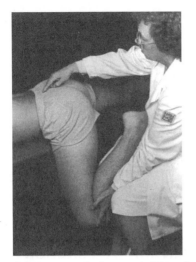

■ **FIG. 50-9** Treatment for lower pole L5 tender point.

3. **Technique:**
   a. The patient's leg is dropped off the table with the knee and hip flexed. The hip is slightly rotated internally.
   b. While supporting the patient's leg, the physician pushes the knee toward the table, adducting the thigh (Fig. 50-9).
   c. Treatment is monitored at the tender point just medial to the posterior inferior iliac spine and just inferior to it.

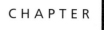

# Facilitated Positional Release

*Stanley Schiowitz*

## ■ SUPERFICIAL MUSCLE HYPERTONICITY (LEFT LOW BACK)

1. **Patient position:** prone, with a pillow under the abdomen. The pillow should be large enough to cause flattening of the lumbar lordosis.
2. **Physician position:** standing at the left side of the table of the muscle hypertenicity (left).
3. **Technique:**
   a. The physician monitors the area of hypertonicity with his index finger.
   b. The physician places his left knee on the table beside the patient's left ilium.
   c. With his right hand, the physician slides the patient's legs toward the left side of the table, producing side-bending of the patient's lumbar spine with the physician's left knee as a fulcrum. Side-bending is continued until tissue motion is felt by the left (monitoring) index finger (Fig.51-1).
   d. The physician releases the patient's legs, crosses the patient's right leg over the left at the ankle, and then places his right hand under the patient's right thigh. The physician grasps the patient's right thigh medially, extends it posteriorly, and externally rotates it until motion is felt by the left (monitoring) index finger in the area of tissue tension. A torsional motion is created up to the monitoring finger.
   e. This position is held for 3 seconds, and then released; the dysfunction is reevaluated.

## ■ SOMATIC DYSFUNCTION— EXTENSION DYSFUNCTION (L4 ES$_L$R$_L$)

1. **Patient position:** prone, with a pillow under the abdomen. A second pillow is placed between the patient's left thigh and the table. This protects the patient's thigh and acts as a fulcrum for motion.
2. **Physician position:** standing at the left side of the table.
3. **Technique:**
   a. The physician monitors the left transverse process of the L4 vertebra with his left index finger.
   b. The physician grasps the patient's left lower leg or ankle with his right hand.
   c. The patient's left leg is brought into abduction until motion is felt at the monitoring finger; then internal rotation up to the monitoring finger is added.
   d. The patient's left leg is then pressed down toward the floor until motion is felt by the physician's monitoring finger (Fig. 51-2).
   e. The position is held until the physician feels articular release. This usually occurs in 3 to 4 seconds.
   f. The position is released and the patient is returned to a neutral position. The dysfunction is reevaluated.

## ■ SOMATIC DYSFUNCTION— EXTENSION (L4 ES$_L$R$_L$)

### Alternate Technique

1. **Patient position:** Lying on the right side, with both legs in full extension on the table.

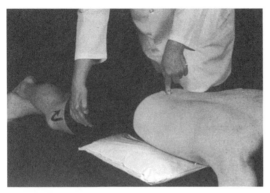

■ **FIG. 51-1** Facilitated positional release treatment for the left low back, superficial muscle hypertonicity.

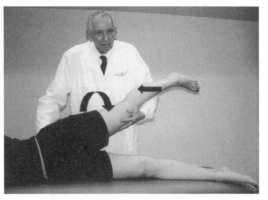

■ **FIG. 51-3** Facilitated positonal release alternate treatment for a lumbar extension somatic dysfunction.

2. **Physician position:** Standing at the side of the table, behind the patient.
3. **Technique:**
   a. The physician places one finger of his right hand on the posteriorly rotated left transverse process of L4.
   b. The physician grasps the patient's left knee with his left hand and has the patient's left foot resting on his left forearm.
   c. The physician brings the patient's left hip into abduction until the motion is felt at the monitoring finger. Internal rotation of that hip is added by turning the patient's foot internally, using a rotating motion of the physicians left forearm.
   d. The patient's left leg is now brought into extension by the physician stepping back slowly until the motion is felt at the monitoring finger (Fig. 51-3).

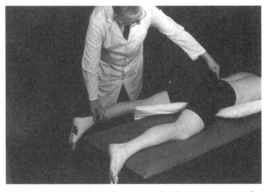

■ **FIG. 51-2** Facilitated positional release treatment for a lumbar extension somatic dysfunction.

   e. The position is held until the physician feels articular release, usually 3 to 5 seconds.
   f. The position is released. The patient is returned to a neutral position and the dysfunction is reevaluated.

■ **SOMATIC DYSFUNCTION— FLEXION DYSFUNCTION (L4 F $S_R R_R$)**

1. **Patient position:** prone, with a pillow placed under the abdomen.
2. **Physician position:** sitting at the right side of the table, facing the patient's head. The physician's left lateral thigh and knee are beside the table.
3. **Technique:**
   a. The physician monitors the transverse process of L4 on the right side with one finger of the left hand.
   b. The physician drops the patient's flexed right knee and thigh off the table over his left thigh.
   c. The physician grasps the patient's knee with the right hand and flexes the patient's hip until motion is felt at the monitored transverse process.
   d. The physician pushes the patient's right knee toward the table, into adduction, using his knee and thigh as a fulcrum, until motion is felt at the monitored transverse process.
   e. With his right hand, the physician uses the

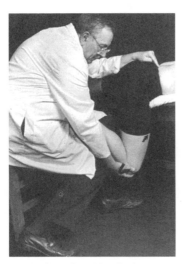

■ **FIG. 51-4** Facilitated positional release treatment for a lumbar flexion somatic dysfunction.

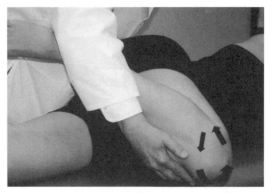

■ **FIG. 51-5** Facilitated positional release alternate treatment for a lumbar flexion somatic dysfunction.

patient's knee to rotate the thigh, creating internal rotation of the hip (Fig. 51-4).

f. This position is held until the physician feels articular release.

g. This position is held for 3 seconds and then released; the dysfunction is reevaluated.

## ■ SOMATIC DYSFUNCTION— FLEXION DYSFUNCTION (L4 F S_RR_R)

### Alternate Technique

1. **Patient position:** Lying on his left side on the table with both hips and knees flexed.
2. **Physician position:** Standing at side of table. The physician's left index finger monitors the posteriorly rotated transverse process.
3. **Technique:**
   a. The physician places one finger of his left hand on the right posteriorly rotated transverse process.
   b. The physician grasps the patient's right knee with his right hand.
   c. The physician flexes the patient's left hip and knee until motion is felt at the monitoring finger.
   d. The physician adducts and internally rotates the patient's right hip.
   e. The physician adds a compressive force by

using his right hand to push the patient's right femur toward the physician's monitoring finger (Fig. 51-5).

f. The position is held until articular release is felt, usually 3 to 5 seconds. The position is then released and the dysfunction is reevaluated.

## ■ LUMBAR TECHNIQUE FOR DISKOGENIC PAIN SYNDROME

This technique is useful for patients with radicular pain, bulging disks, stenosis, or disk herniation, or for patients with residual pain after laminectomy. Treatment is described for a right-sided dysfunction.

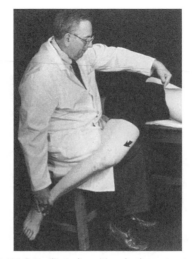

■ **FIG. 51-6** Facilitated positional release treatment for sciatic radiation of pain caused by herniated lumbar disc.

1. **Patient position:** prone, with a pillow placed under the abdomen.
2. **Physician position:** seated at the right side of the table, facing the patient's head. The physician's thighs and knees are parallel to the table.
3. **Technique:**
   a. The physician monitors the area at the site of the disk herniation with his index finger.
   b. The patient's right hip and thigh are flexed and the thigh is placed over both of the physician's legs, allowing the knee to flex down toward the floor.
   c. The physician places his right hand on the patient's right ankle.
   d. The physician raises his right heel off the floor, lifting the patient's thigh, until motion is felt at the monitoring finger.
   e. The physician pushes his right knee laterally against the back of the patient's knee, creating a traction force that is monitored by his finger.
   f. With his right hand, the physician turns the patient's right leg down toward the floor, creating a rotary motion of the thigh and hip, with the knee acting as the fulcrum (Fig. 51-6).
   g. Mild tension is maintained at the monitoring finger until motion is felt. The physician will feel a release of tissue tension in 3 to 5 seconds.
   h. The physician releases the position, returns the leg to the table, and reevaluates the dysfunction.

*Note:* This treatment may be applied to both sides for optimum results.

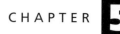

# Still Techniques

*Dennis J. Dowling*

This chapter describes Still techniques for treating somatic dysfunctions of the lumbar spine. The lumbar region has type I (regional) and type II (segmental, single) somatic dysfunctions and is treated by positioning into the directions of ease. The lumbar region may be treated in much the same manner as the typical thoracic vertebral somatic dysfunctions. Although the primary position of application is with the patient supine, the patient may also be treated in the seated position with the thoracic techniques. Compression is most typically used. Occasionally, the portion of the treatment involving movement toward the barriers may result in an articulatory "pop." The descriptions are for the specific side-bending and rotation components with flexion and extension as modifications into the appropriate directions.

## ■ LUMBAR TYPE II EXTENDED SOMATIC DYSFUNCTION (L3 E S$_R$ R$_R$)—PATIENT SUPINE

1. **Patient position:** supine.
2. **Physician position:** standing at the side of the patient on the side of the somatic dysfunction.
3. **Technique:**
   a. The physician places the pad of the index or middle finger of his monitoring cephalad hand on the posterior transverse process on the side of the side-bending/rotation component of the somatic dysfunction (the left finger contacts the patient's L3 right transverse process in this example).

b. The physician uses his other hand to grasp the patient's leg on the dysfunctional side and flex the patient's hip and knee until motion is felt at the monitoring finger (the physician's right hand grasps and flexes the patient's right leg in this example).

c. The physician abducts the patient's knee of the affected side and externally rotates the leg until motion and soft tissue relaxation is felt at the monitoring finger. This creates relative extension, rotation, and side-bending of the somatic dysfunction (Fig. 52-1A).

d. A modification is for the physician to insert the forearm of his caudad arm from lateral to medial beneath the patient's knee and places his hand on the patient's anterior thigh. This can add torsion to the modifying and localizing forces (Fig. 52-1B).

e. The physician puts downward compression with his caudad (right) arm or shoulder from the patient's knee through his femur, toward the pelvis and hip, and directed toward the lumbar somatic dysfunction until further softening of the tissue is noted at the monitoring finger.

f. While maintaining the compression, the patient's leg is gently carried through adduction across the midline and slightly increased hip flexion, thus engaging the extension barrier, then through neutral position and into the barrier directions (side-bending left and rotating left in this case).

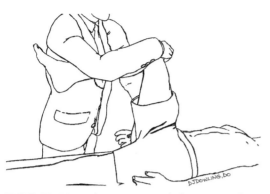

■ **FIG. 52-1A** Lumbar type II extended somatic dysfunction (L3 E S$_R$ R$_R$), patient supine.

g. The patient's hip and knee are brought back to the neutral position by extending both, and then the lumbar somatic dysfunction is reassessed.

## ■ LUMBAR TYPE II FLEXED SOMATIC DYSFUNCTION (L3 F S$_R$ R$_R$)— PATIENT SUPINE

1. **Patient position:** supine.
2. **Physician position:** standing at the side of the table, typically on the side of the dysfunction.
3. **Technique:**
   a. The physician places the pad of the index or middle finger of his monitoring cephalad hand on the posterior transverse process on the side of the side-bending/rotation component of the so-

matic dysfunction (the left finger contacts the patient's L3 right transverse process in this example).
b. The physician uses his other hand to grasp the patient's leg on the dysfunctional side and flex the patient's hip and knee until motion and soft tissue relaxation is felt at the monitoring finger (the physician's right hand grasps and flexes the patient's right leg in this example).
c. The physician adducts the patient's ipsilateral knee and internally rotates the leg until motion and soft tissue relaxation is felt at the monitoring finger. This creates relative extension, rotation, and side-bending to the somatic dysfunction (Fig. 52-2A).
d. A modification is for the physician to insert the forearm of his caudad arm beneath the patient's knee from medial to lateral and place his hand on the patient's lateral thigh. This can add torsion to the modifying and localizing forces (Fig. 52-2B).
e. The physician puts downward compression with his caudad (right) arm or shoulder from the patient's knee through his femur, toward the pelvis and hip, and directed toward the lumbar somatic dysfunction until further soft tissue is noted at the monitoring finger.
f. While maintaining the compression, the patient's leg is gently carried through abduction and external rotation across and slightly decreased hip flexion by engaging

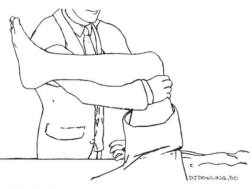

■ **FIG. 52-1B** Lumbar type II extended somatic dysfunction (L3 E S$_R$ R$_R$), patient supine. (Modification of physician hand/arm position.)

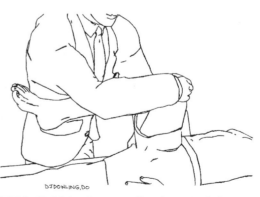

■ **FIG. 52-2A** Lumbar type II flexed somatic dysfunction (L3 F S$_R$ R$_R$), patient supine.

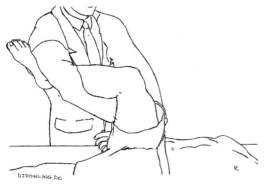

■ **FIG. 52-2B** Lumbar type II flexed somatic dysfunction (L3 F $S_R$ $R_R$), patient supine. (Modification of physician hand/arm position.)

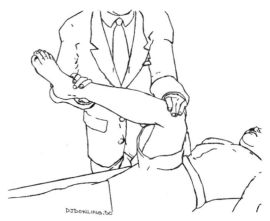

■ **FIG. 52-3** Lumbar type I group curve somatic dysfunction (L1–5 N $S_R$ $R_L$), patient supine.

the extension barrier, then through neutral position and into the barrier directions (side-bending left and rotating left in this case).

g. The patient's hip and knee are brought back to the neutral position by extending both, and then the lumbar somatic dysfunction is reassessed.

## ■ LUMBAR TYPE I GROUP CURVE SOMATIC DYSFUNCTION (L1–5 N $S_R$ $R_L$)—PATIENT SUPINE

1. **Patient position:** supine.
2. **Physician position:** standing facing the table on the side of the concavity of the group curve.
3. **Technique:**
   a. The physician places the pad of the index or middle finger of his monitoring hand at the apex of the curve on the concave side of the group curve by passing the monitoring hand beneath the patient's back (the left finger contacts the patient's right L3 transverse process in this example). The palm of that hand contours to and supports the patient's back in this region.
   b. The physician grasps the patient's knee on the side of the side-bending and flexes the hip and knee to approximately right angles (the physician's right hand holds the patient's right leg in this example) or until motion is localized to the monitoring finger and there is soft tissue relaxation.

c. The physician then holds the leg above the ankle and takes the monitoring finger out to hold the knee (right hand holds the right lower leg; left hand holds the right knee).

d. The physician rotates the leg internally by pulling the lower leg laterally and also adducts the knee by pushing the knee medially. This side-bends the patient's body toward the group curve concavity and rotates the lumbar towards the opposite side for further tissue relaxation.

e. The physician puts approximately 5 pounds of downward pressure toward the table with the hand on top of the patient's knee through the femur and toward where the monitoring finger had been (Fig. 52-3).

f. While maintaining the compression, the knee is gently carried through the neutral position abduction while simultaneously bringing the foot toward the midline creating full leg external rotation.

g. The patient's leg is brought back to the neutral position and the lumbar group curve is reassessed.

## ■ ALTERNATIVE LUMBAR TYPE I GROUP CURVE SOMATIC DYSFUNCTION (L1–5 N $S_R$ $R_L$)—PATIENT SUPINE

1. **Patient position:** supine.
2. **Physician position:** standing facing the pa-

tient on the side of the side-bending component of the group curve.

3. **Technique:**

a. The physician places the pad of the index or middle finger of his monitoring hand at the apex of the curve on the concave side of the group curve by passing the monitoring hand beneath the patient's back (the left finger contacts the patient's right L3 transverse process in this example). The palm of that hand contours to and supports the patient's back in this region.

b. The physician grasps the patient's knee on the side of the side-bending and flexes the hip and knee to approximately 90 degrees (the physician's right hand holds the patient's right leg in this example) or until motion is localized to the monitoring finger and there is soft tissue relaxation.

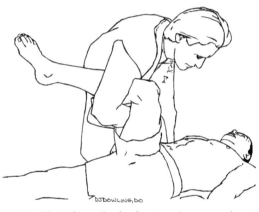

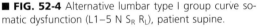

**■ FIG. 52-4** Alternative lumbar type I group curve somatic dysfunction (L1–5 N $S_R$ $R_L$), patient supine.

c. The physician then places his arm beneath the patient's bent knee from medial to lateral, holds the patients thigh with that hand, and places his shoulder against the patient's knee (right arm beneath the patient's right knee; right shoulder against the right knee).

d. The physician rotates the leg internally by pushing the knee medially and directing the lower leg laterally. This side-bends the patient's body toward the group curve's concavity and rotates the lumbar vertebrae toward the opposite side for further tissue relaxation.

e. The physician puts approximately 5 pounds of downward pressure toward the floor with the shoulder on top of the patient's knee through the femur and toward the monitoring finger (Fig. 52-4).

f. While maintaining the compression, the knee is gently carried through the neutral position abduction while simultaneously bringing the leg into external rotation by the physician rotating his arm in the patient's popliteal region.

g. The patient's leg is brought back to the neutral position and the lumbar group curve is reassessed.

## REFERENCES

Van Buskirk RL. A manipulative technique of Andrew Taylor Still. *J Am Osteopath Assoc* 1996;96:597–602.

Van Buskirk RL. *The Still Technique Manual*. Indianapolis, IN: American Academy of Osteopathy, 1999.

Van Buskirk RL. Treatment of somatic dysfunction with an osteopathic manipulative method of Dr. Andrew Taylor Still. In Ward RC, ed. *Foundations for Osteopathic Medicine*. Philadelphia: Lippincott Williams & Wilkins, 2003: 1094–1114.

# PINS Techniques

*Dennis J. Dowling*

This chapter describes PINS technique for treating somatic dysfunctions of the lumbar region. The examples provided are not the only ones that are possible (Fig. 53-1); however, they are fairly common. Occasionally, patterns in the lumbar region may continue into or from adjacent regions. The patient is most commonly treated in the prone position but could be treated seated. The physician should be positioned comfortably facing the region to be treated or alongside the table. The principles and methods of PINS can be applied:

1. Locate a sensitive point in the region of the symptoms.
2. Analyze the structures that are deep to that point
3. Locate another sensitive point at the other end of a connecting structure (i.e., muscle, ligament, nerve, etc.). The more sensitive point is the primary point and the lesser sensitive point is the endpoint.
4. Apply inhibitory pressure to both points for 30 seconds or more. The soft tissue at the more sensitive point will typically lessen in tension.
5. Beginning at the more sensitive of the two points, locate another sensitive point approximately 2 to 3 centimeters toward the lesser sensitive point.
6. Repeat the procedure progressively toward the endpoint.
7. Reassess the status of the dysfunction. Determine if additional treatment or the application of other modalities is necessary.

## ■ QUADRATUS LUMBORUM

1. **Technique:**
   a. The physician places the pad of his index or middle finger on the iliac crest of in the mid-axillary line. A finger of the physician's other hand locates a sensitive point superior at the inferior edge of the common costal cartilage in the mid to posterior axillary line. Another common pattern involves a sensitive point near L5 (possibly involving the iliolumbar ligament) medially and extending toward the lateral rib cage.
   b. The pattern of intervening points is usually straight, but the depth of pressure may indicate the muscles involved (the iliolumbar ligament is fairly deep but the sensitivity is usually very high).
2. **Clinical Correlation:**
   a. Hip pain
   b. Rib inhalation dysfunction
   c. Low back pain

## ■ LATISSIMUS DORSI

1. **Technique:**
   a. The physician places the pad of his index or middle finger on a point in the mid to upper lumbar region lateral to the transverse processes. A lateral sensitive point may be found at the inferior angle of the scapula, in the posterior axillary fold, or in the bicipital groove of the humerus.
   b. The pattern of intervening points is generally straight (muscle pattern) but may be slightly variable, because the muscle extends over a fairly great distance and in-

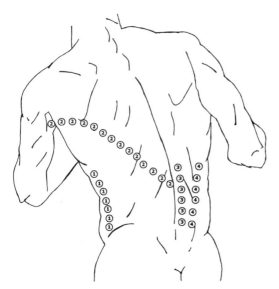

■ **FIG. 53-1** PINS lumbar point patterns; *1, quadratus lumborum; 2, latissimus dorsi; 3, paravertebral muscles; 4, iliocostalis.*

volves the lumbar, thoracic, and upper extremity regions.

2. **Clinical Correlation:**
   a. Back pain
   b. Rib pain
   c. Shoulder pain
   d. Shoulder restriction

## ■ PARAVERTEBRAL MUSCLES

1. **Technique:**
   a. The physician places the pad of his index or middle finger lateral to spinous processes. A finger of the physician's other hand locates a sensitive point either cephalad or caudad. The point may be at the level as low as the PSIS.
   b. The pattern of intervening points is generally slightly curved or straight (muscle pattern).

2. **Clinical Correlation:**
   a. Back pain
   b. Lumbar disc herniation
   c. Flank pain
   d. Nephrolithiasis (can mimic or be related to renal calculi)

## ■ ILIOCOSTALIS

1. **Technique:**
   a. The physician places the pad of his index or middle finger near the medial iliac crest. A finger of the physician's other hand locates a sensitive point laterally on the twelfth rib.
   b. The pattern of intervening points generally follows the lateral border of the iliocostalis muscles but may be more medial.

2. **Clinical Correlation:**
   a. Back pain
   b. Rib pain

### REFERENCES

Dowling DJ. Progressive inhibition of neuromuscular structures (PINS) technique. *J Am Osteopath Assoc* 2000;100: 285–286, 289–298.

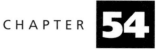

# CHAPTER 54

# Thrusting Techniques For The Lumbar Spine

*Eileen L. DiGiovanna, Barry S. Erner, and Paula D. Scariati*

This chapter describes high-velocity, low-amplitude thrusting techniques for treating somatic dysfunctions of the lumbar spine. The soft tissues in the region should be prepared with myofascial techniques or muscle energy before a thrust being performed.

## ■ LUMBAR SOMATIC DYSFUNCITON

1. **Patient position:** lateral recumbent, with the posteriorly rotated transverse process up.
2. **Physician position:** standing facing the front of the patient.
3. **Technique:**
   a. The physician uses one hand to monitor the posteriorly rotated transverse process at all times while positioning and treating the patient.
   b. The physician flexes the patient's hips and knees until motion just above the dysfunctional vertebra is felt by his monitoring hand.
   c. The patient is asked to straighten the lower leg while the physician maintains the flexion of the upper leg.
   d. The toes of the upper foot are hooked behind the popliteal fossa of the inferior leg, which is resting on the table in an extended position.
   e. The physician rotates the patient's torso in the same direction as the posteriorly rotated transverse process by pulling on the patient's lower arm. Rotation is in-

duced down to, but not including, the vertebral segment of the somatic dysfunction.
   f. The physician places the forearm of his thrusting arm over the patient's superior iliac crest and maintains finger monitoring of the dysfunction.
   g. The physician places his other arm beneath the patient's upper arm and stabilizes the patient's lateral torso and rib cage. The fingers of this hand now replace the fingers of the thrusting arm to monitor the segment being treated.
   h. A slight springing force is exerted by introducing a very slight lower body rotation toward the physician to determine that localization is correct.
   i. The patient is instructed to inhale deeply and then exhale fully.
   j. At the end of exhalation, the physician exerts a rapid rotary thrust. This is achieved by rotating the patient's pelvis forward and toward the table (Fig. 54-1).

## ■ LEG OFF TABLE

1. **Patient position:** lateral recumbent position with the posteriorly rotated transverse process up.
2. **Physician position:** standing facing the front of the patient.
3. **Technique:**
   a. The method is the same as in the technique just described, except that the pa-

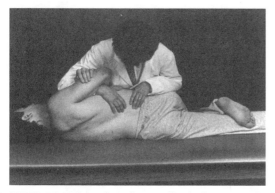

■ **FIG. 54-1** High-velocity low-amplitude thrusting technique for the lumbar spine.

tient's superior leg is dropped off the table into full hip flexion. This leg is then locked between the physician's legs and maintained in full hip flexion.
   b. Localization and thrust are the same as in the first technique.

## ■ POSTERIOR TRANSVERSE PROCESS DOWN

1. **Patient position:** lateral recumbent with posterior transverse process down.
2. **Physician position:** standing at the side of the table facing the front of the patient.
3. **Technique:**
   a. The physician uses one hand to monitor the posteriorly rotated transverse process at all times while positioning and treating the patient.

   b. The physician flexes the patient's hips and knees until motion is felt just caudad to the posteriorly rotated transverse process at his monitoring finger.
   c. The patient is instructed to straighten his lower leg and the physician hooks the toes of the upper foot behind the popliteal fossa while maintaining the flexion of the upper hip and knee.
   d. The physician rotates the patient's upper torso in the same direction as the posteriorly rotated transverse process by pulling on the patient's lower arm. Rotation is induced down to and including the vertebral segment of the somatic dysfunction.
   e. The physician places the forearm of his thrusting arm over the patient's superior iliac crest and maintains finger monitoring of the dysfunction. The lower body is rotated toward the physician until motion is localized to the level of the posterior transverse process.
   f. The physician's other arm is placed against the patient's shoulder to maintain the upper body rotation.
   g. The patient is instructed to inhale deeply and then exhale fully.
   h. At the end of exhalation, the physician rapidly thrusts by rotating the patient's pelvis forward and toward the table.

*Note:* Many schools teach this as the typical method. Each technique is equally effective and the physician should use the one with which he or she is most comfortable.

CHAPTER 55

# Exercise Therapy

*Stanley Schiowitz and Albert R. DeRubertis*

Low back pain is the single most common cause of work absenteeism in the United States. Approximately 70% to 80% of adults experience low back pain at some time in their lives. It is important that primary care physicians understand low back structural biomechanics because they will regularly encounter patients with low back pain.

A comprehensive therapeutic approach includes exercises designed to establish and maintain musculoskeletal structural integrity. A simple approach is to evaluate the lumbar lordosis, the structures involved in its formation, and the muscles that act synergistically to maintain it.

The three questions to be answered are:

1. Is the anteroposterior lumbar curve flattened or exaggerated?
2. Do the individual vertebrae move freely?
3. Do the muscles involved require stretching (extensibility) or strengthening (contractility)?

The muscles involved in creating low back pain are usually the erector spinae, the gluteus maximus, the hamstrings, the iliopsoas, and the abdominals. With the exception of the abdominals and occasionally the back extensors, these muscles require stretching. Regional motion testing may demonstrate restriction caused by muscle contraction. Specific testing for motion, stretch, and strength should be used.

The exercises described in this chapter are based on the aforementioned approach. Many serve more than one function.

## ■ ABDOMINAL MUSCLES
### Upper Abdominal Strengthening Exercise

1. **Patient position:** supine, hips and knees flexed, feet on floor, arms extended.
2. **Instructions:**
   a. Roll your head, neck, and upper back off the floor.
   b. Try to touch your knees with your hands (Fig. 55-1).
   c. Hold this position for 5 to 15 seconds. Slowly lower your body to the floor.
   d. Relax, rest, and repeat.

### Rotary Abdominal Strengthening Exercise

1. **Patient position:** supine, hips and knees flexed, feet on floor, arms extended.
2. **Instructions:**
   a. Roll your head, neck, and upper back off the floor.
   b. Try to touch your left knee only with both hands, creating a body twist (Fig. 55-2).
   c. Hold this position for 5 to 15 seconds. Slowly lower your body back to floor.
   d. Relax and rest.
   e. Repeat by trying to touch your right knee.

### Lower Abdominal Strengthening Exercises
*Exercise 1*

1. **Patient position:** supine on floor, both knees slightly bent, heels on floor.

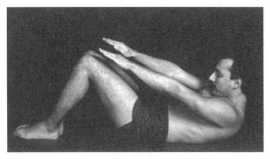

■ **FIG. 55-1** Upper abdominal strengthening exercise.

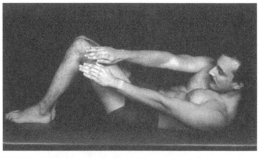

■ **FIG. 55-2** Rotary abdominal strengthening exercise.

2. **Instructions:**
   a. Tighten your abdominal muscles and maintain your back flat against the floor.
   b. Raise your left leg off the floor 6 to 8 inches. Maintain both knees in their slightly flexed position (Fig. 55-3).
   c. Hold this position for 5 to 15 seconds.
   d. Slowly lower the left leg to the floor.
   e. Relax, rest, and repeat by raising your right leg.

### Exercise 2

1. **Patient position:** supine on floor, both hands over the head and firmly holding onto a solid structure.
2. **Instructions:**
   a. Tighten your abdominal muscles, keeping your back flat against the floor.
   b. Flex both knees to 45 degrees. Now raise both feet 6 to 8 inches off the floor (Fig. 55-4).
   c. Hold this position for 5 to 15 seconds.
   d. Slowly lower both feet to the floor.

   e. Relax, rest, and repeat.

## ■ LOWER BACK MUSCLES STRETCH

### Exercise 1

1. **Patient position:** seated on edge of chair, both feet flat on floor.
2. **Instructions:**
   a. Cross both arms in front of your chest.
   b. Let your body bend forward between your legs. Let the body weight create low back stretch (Fig. 55-5).
   c. Hold for 5 to 15 seconds.
   d. Return slowly to the upright position. Relax, rest, and repeat.

*Caution: Discontinue if dizziness or lightheadedness occurs.*

### Exercise 2

1. **Patient position:** seated on the floor or a table with both legs extended.

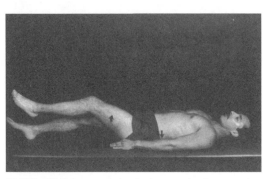

■ **FIG. 55-3** Lower abdominal strengthening exercise, one leg raised.

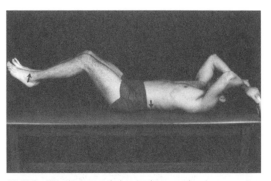

■ **FIG. 55-4** Lower abdominal strengthening exercise, both legs raised.

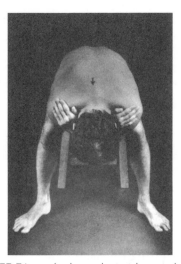

■ **FIG. 55-5** Lower back muscle stretch, seated on chair.

2. **Instructions:**
   a. Lean forward and grasp your shins with each hand.
   b. Pull your trunk into further forward bending by bringing your hands down your legs (Fig. 55-6).
   c. Feel stretch in the lower back. Hold for 5 to 15 seconds. Slowly return to the starting position.
   d. Relax, rest, and repeat.

## Rotary Stretch

### Exercise 1

1. **Patient position:** supine, arms and legs extended.

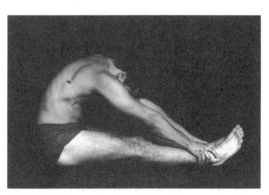

■ **FIG. 55-6** Lower back muscle stretch, seated on floor.

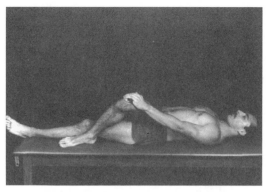

■ **FIG. 55-7** Lower back muscle rotary stretch, legs extended.

2. **Instructions:**
   a. Bend your right knee up, cross it over your left leg, and place the right foot flat on the floor, close to the left knee.
   b. Grasp your right knee with your left hand and slowly pull it toward the left side of the floor. Keep your shoulders flat on the floor (Fig. 55-7).
   c. This will create a right low back rotary stretch. Hold for 5 to 15 seconds.
   d. Release right knee, relax, and repeat.
   e. For left low back rotary stretch, reverse the knee and hand instructions.

### Exercise 2

1. **Patient position:** supine, both hips and knees bent, feet together and flat on the floor.

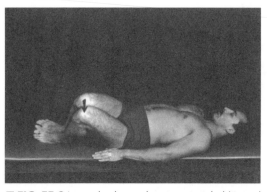

■ **FIG. 55-8** Lower back muscle rotary stretch, hips and knees bent.

2. **Instructions:**
   a. Using your left foot as a fulcrum, pivot both knees to the left. Allow the weight of the legs to create a right low back rotary stretch (Fig. 55-8).
   b. Keep your shoulders flat on the floor. Do not use muscular contraction to increase stretch.
   c. Hold at maximum relaxed stretch for 5 to 15 seconds. Return knees to starting position.
   d. Relax, rest, and repeat.
   e. For left rotary stretch, reverse the instructions.

## ■ GLUTEUS MAXIMUS MUSCLES

### Active Stretch

1. **Patient position:** supine, both knees bent, feet on floor.
2. **Instructions:**
   a. Bring your right knee up to your chest as far as possible and grasp with both hands. At the same time fully extend your left leg (Fig. 55-9).
   b. Hold for 5 to 15 seconds.
   c. Reverse the procedure by bringing your left knee up to your chest and fully extending your right leg.
   d. Hold this position for 5 to 15 seconds. Return to starting position.
   e. Relax, rest, and repeat.

### Passive Stretch

1. **Patient position:** supine, arms at sides, knees bent, feet on floor.

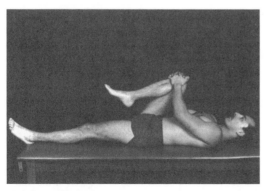

■ **FIG. 55-9** Gluteus maximus active muscle stretch.

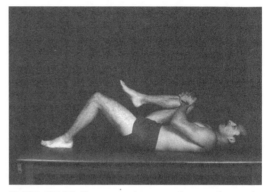

■ **FIG. 55-10** Gluteus maximus passive muscle stretch.

2. **Instructions:**
   a. Bring your right knee to your chest. Clasp both your hands over that knee.
   b. Passively and slowly, pull your right knee to your chest (Fig. 55-10). Hold this position for 5 to 15 seconds.
   c. Return to starting position; repeat with other knee.
   d. Repeat, flexing both hip and knees to chest at one time.

*Note:* If you have knee dysfunction, clasp both hands on the posterior thigh near the popliteal region.

## ■ LUMBAR SPINE

### Lumbar Flattening (Pelvic Tilt to Decrease Lordosis)

1. **Patient position:** supine, arms above head, both knees bent, feet on floor.
2. **Instructions:**
   a. Tighten your abdominal muscles and your buttocks at the same time.
   b. Flatten your back firmly against the floor. Roll your pelvis backward if necessary to achieve full flattening (Fig. 55-11).
   c. Hold this position for 5 to 15 seconds.
   d. Relax, rest, and repeat.

### Cat Back—Lumbar Flexibility

1. **Patient position:** hands and knees on the floor, back up, fully lengthened and straight.

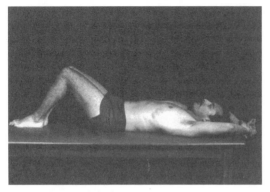

■ **FIG. 55-11** Pelvic tilt.

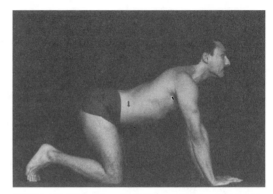

■ **FIG. 55-13** Lumbar flexibility—extension (cat back).

2. **Instructions:**
   a. **Flexion:**
      (1) Drop your head down between your arms, looking toward your thighs.
      (2) Arch your back upward and try to bring your pelvis toward your head (Fig. 55-12).
      (3) Try to achieve full back flexion with reversal of lumbar lordosis.
      (4) Hold this position for 5 to 15 seconds, return to starting position.
      (5) Relax, rest, and then perform the following extension exercise.
   b. **Extension:**
      (1) Bring your head back into full head and neck extension.
      (2) Arch your back down toward the floor. Try to bring your buttocks toward your head.
      (3) Try to achieve full back extension, ex-

aggerating the lumbar lordosis (Fig. 55-13).
      (4) Hold this position for 5 to 15 seconds. Return to starting position.
      (5) Relax, rest, and repeat the entire exercise.

*Note:* Try to maintain your abdominal muscles in a flattened, mildly contracted position throughout the exercise.

### Lumbar Flattening

1. **Patient position:** kneeling, buttocks resting on heels.
2. **Instructions:**
   a. Bring both fully extended arms forward. Touch both palms to floor, bringing your chest parallel to floor.
   b. Contract your abdominal muscles while pushing both arms forward. This should bring your chest against your knees (Fig. 55-14).

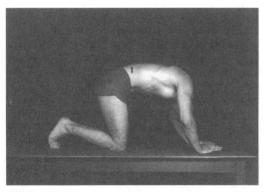

■ **FIG. 55-12** Lumbar flexibility—flexion (cat back).

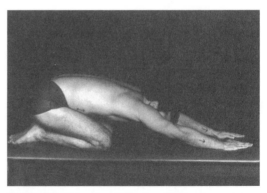

■ **FIG. 55-14** Lumbar flattening stretch.

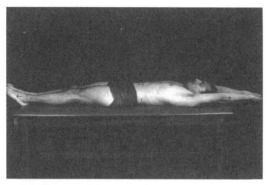

■ **FIG. 55-15** Full body stretch.

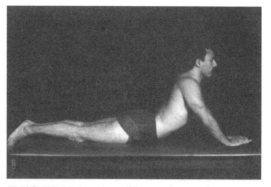

■ **FIG. 55-16** Anterior pelvic muscle stretch.

c. Maintain maximum stretch for 5 to 15 seconds. Return to starting position.
d. Relax, rest, and repeat.

## Full Body Stretch (Flatten All Curves)

1. **Patient position:** supine, arms fully extended overhead, legs fully extended downward.
2. **Instructions:**
   a. Stretch your arms overhead and your legs downward. Point your toes into plantar flexion.
   b. Tighten your abdominal muscles and flatten your lumbar spine.
   c. Tuck in your chin and flatten your cervical spine (Fig. 55-15).
   d. Hold this position for 5 to 15 seconds.
   e. Relax, rest, and repeat.

## ■ ANTERIOR PELVIC MUSCLE STRETCH

1. **Patient position:** prone, legs extended, arms at sides.
2. **Instructions:**
   a. Place both hands, palms down, on the floor at shoulder level.
   b. Raise your upper body off the floor by fully extending your arms. Keep your upper thighs on the floor (Fig. 55-16).
   c. Allow your abdomen and pelvis to sag (stretch) toward the floor. Your body weight will perform the necessary stretch.
   d. Hold this position for 5 to 15 seconds. Lower your body to the floor.
   e. Relax, rest, and repeat.

## ■ BACK EXTENSOR MUSCLE STRENGTHENING

1. **Patient position:** prone, arms fully extended upward, legs fully extended downward. Two pillows are placed under the abdomen.
2. **Instructions:**
   a. Raise your left arm and right leg up off the floor, fully extended (Fig. 55-17). Hold for 5 seconds. Lower and repeat with your left arm and right leg.
   b. Raise your right arm and right leg off the floor, fully extended (Fig. 55-18). Hold for 5 seconds. Lower and repeat with your left arm and left leg.
   c. Raise both arms, fully extended, off the floor (Fig. 55-19). Hold for 5 seconds. Lower. Now raise both legs fully extended off the floor (Fig. 55-20).

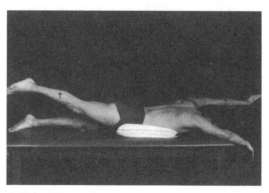

■ **FIG. 55-17** Back extensor muscle strengthening, left arm and right leg raised.

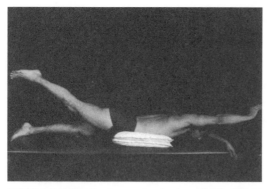

■ **FIG. 55-18** Back extensor muscle strengthening, right arm and right leg raised.

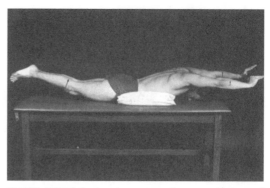

■ **FIG. 55-21** Back extensor muscle strengthening, all extremities raised.

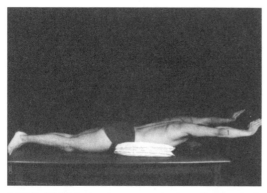

■ **FIG. 55-19** Back extensor muscle strengthening, both arms raised.

d. Raise all four fully extended extremities off the floor simultaneously (Fig. 55-21). Hold for 5 seconds. Lower.

e. Relax, rest, and repeat the entire exercise.

## ■ HIP FLEXOR STRETCH

### Psoas Stretch—Assisted

1. **Patient position:** supine on edge of table or bed, so that side to be stretched can drop off toward the floor (right side).

2. **Instructions:**
   a. Bend your left hip and knee to chest and hold them with both hands. Keep your low back flat on the table.
   b. Drop your right leg off the table toward floor.
   c. The assistant holds the left hip and knee in full flexion, while gently pushing down on the right thigh, creating stretch (Fig. 55-22).

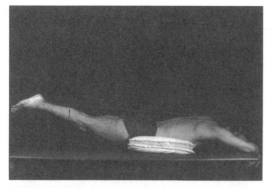

■ **FIG. 55-20** Back extensor muscle strengthening, both legs raised.

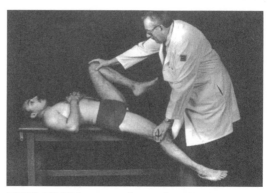

■ **FIG. 55-22** Psoas muscle stretch, assisted.

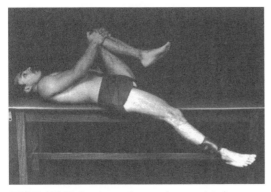

■ **FIG. 55-23** Psoas muscle stretch, unassisted.

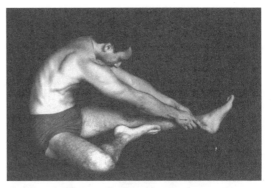

■ **FIG. 55-24** Hamstring muscle stretch, seated.

d. Hold maximum painless stretch for 5 to 15 seconds. Return both legs to the table in full extension.
e. Relax, rest, and repeat.

## Psoas Stretch—Unassisted

1. **Patient position:** supine on edge of table or bed, so that side to be stretched can drop off toward the floor (right side).
2. **Instructions:**
   a. Bend your left hip and knee to chest. Hold them firmly against your chest. Keep your low back flat on the table.
   b. Drop your right leg off the table toward the floor. Allow its weight to create stretch.
   c. For additional stretch, a 3- to 5-pound weight can be added at the ankle (Fig. 55-23).
   d. Hold the maximum painless stretch for 5 to 15 seconds. Return both legs to the table in full extension.
   e. Relax, rest, and repeat.

## ■ HAMSTRING STRETCH

### Seated Stretch

1. **Patient position:** seated with the back upright and the left leg in full extension. The right leg is bent so that the right foot is touching the left thigh.
2. **Instructions:**
   a. Bend forward from your hips. Place both hands on your left leg until you feel stretch (left-sided).
   b. Hold this position; then, walk your hands

farther down the left leg to increase the stretch to maximum (Fig. 55-24).
   c. Hold this position for 5 to 15 seconds. Return to the upright position.
   d. Relax, rest, and repeat.
   e. To stretch the right side, reverse instructions.

## Supine Stretch

1. **Patient position:** supine, hips and knees flexed, both feet flat on the floor.
2. **Instructions:**
   a. Flex the hip to be stretched toward your chest. Then extend that leg fully toward the ceiling. Bend your toes down toward your body. Hold in maximum painless stretch.
   b. Bring both hands or a towel around and behind the extended knee or thigh. Slowly

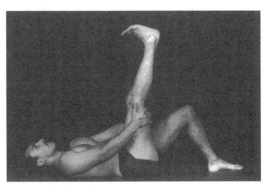

■ **FIG. 55-25** Hamstring muscle stretch, supine.

pull your thigh toward your chest. Maintain full leg extension (Fig. 55-25).

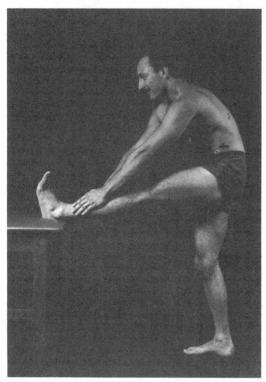

■ **FIG. 55-26** Hamstring muscle stretch, standing.

c. Hold this position for 5 to 15 seconds. Return to the original position.

d. Relax, rest, and repeat.

e. To stretch the other side, reverse instructions.

## Standing Stretch

1. **Patient position:** standing near a table or other firm support. Support must be of sufficient height to allow stretch.

2. **Instructions:**

   a. Place the heel of the foot to be exercised on the support. Keep the knee fully extended.

   b. With both hands on your leg, slowly bend forward from your hips until you feel maximum painless stretch in the back of your raised leg (Fig. 55-26).

   c. Hold for 5 to 15 seconds, increasing the painless stretch as tolerated. Return leg to floor.

   d. Relax, rest, and repeat.

   e. To stretch the other side, reverse instructions.

### REFERENCES

Mitchell FL Jr, Moran PS, Pruzzo NT. *An Evaluation and Treatment Manual of Osteopathic Muscle Energy Procedures.* Valley Park, MO: Mitchell, Moran, and Pruzzo, 1979.

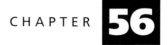

# CHAPTER 56

# Practical Applications and Case Histories

*Stanley Schiowitz and Eileen L. DiGiovanna*

Pain in the low back region is one of the major symptoms that the primary care physician will encounter. It is a major cause of lost time at work. Although musculoskeletal somatic dysfunctions are by far the most common cause of these symptoms, they do not cause all of them. Low back pain can be visceral, vascular, neurologic, biomechanic, or psychogenic in origin.

The most common visceral systems that create back pain are the renal, gynecologic, and gastrointestinal systems. Vascular system involvement most frequently includes aneurysms or occlusions of the descending aorta and should be included, when appropriate, as considerations in the cause of low back pain.

Any pathology that affects the spinal cord or its nerve roots can create low back pain. Common problems are herniation of an intervertebral disc, degenerative arthritis, congenital osseous changes, or neoplasm. When the nerve root becomes involved, as in a herniated disc, the symptoms may include pain and loss of function of the muscles of the extremity involved.

Often, the most difficult diagnosis to make is when the pain is of psychogenic cause. Among these are *tension myositis* and possibly *fibromyalgia*. The treatment of either of these conditions is usually very daunting. Osteopathic manipulative treatment (OMT) is helpful, along with exercise, in playing a significant role in the treatment of these conditions. Contributing psychological factors should be sought and treated. The importance of always obtaining a comprehensive history and performing a thorough physical examination on any patient with a chief complaint of low back pain cannot be overstated.

Dysfunctions of a musculoskeletal cause are the ones commonly treated by the primary care physician in the ambulatory setting. As mentioned, a comprehensive history and physical examination must always be obtained to differentiate those caused by trauma from those caused by infection, neoplasm, or rheumatic diseases.

A trauma that will cause low back pain can be an abnormal amount of stress applied to the normal back, a normal stress applied to the normal back that is unprepared for the stress, or a normal stress applied to the abnormal back. The physician can determine by obtaining a comprehensive history which of these applies.

The commonly seen *"chronic low back syndrome"* falls into the third of these categories, normal stress on an abnormal back. Somatic dysfunctions are always found in these patients. Resolving these dysfunctions will relieve the symptoms but the physician must seek the cause of the abnormality, and treat it, to achieve a lasting result.

## ■ POSTURAL IMBALANCE

Good posture is almost effortless, nonfatiguing, painless, and esthetically acceptable. The common causes of back pain related to postural imbalance are lumbar scoliosis with or without a leg length discrepancy and an increased lumbar lordosis. A standing x-ray of both the anterior–posterior and lateral views of the lumbar spine are of great value in arriving at a diagnosis. The findings of a short leg are discussed in Section VI, Chapter 58. Correction of this finding will assist in the correction of a functional lumbar scoliosis.

The effect of an increased lumbosacral angle as well as possible causes has been discussed previously. Of great importance in the treatment of this condition is the prescription of proper exercises. These must include abdominal strengthening, paravertebral muscle stretching, lumbar flattening, and psoas and hamstring stretching.

The patient's physical fitness will play a dominant role in postural imbalance as a cause of back pain as well as in the treatment of it. This nation's epidemic of obesity has recently received a great deal of publicity, including children as a population. Obesity should be treated vigorously. In addition, America has become a nation of "couch potatoes," few of whom participate in proper exercise programs. The prescription of specific exercises for the back as well as general fitness exercises is a must.

The patient's occupation, present and former, must be considered. Poor ergonomics in the workplace can affect the patient's posture negatively.

## ■ HERNIATION OF INTERVERTEBRAL DISC

The intervertebral disc acts as a shock absorber for the vertebrae. One is located between each pair of vertebrae. The disc consists of a fibrous annulus of concentric rings with a gelatinous mucopolysaccharide *nucleus pulposus*. As forces are transmitted through the spinal column, the discs act to distribute the force evenly. It facilitates vertebral motion. The *annulus fibrosus* attaches to the edges of the hyaline cartilage of adjacent vertebral endplates. Microtrauma, in the form of rotational stresses, predisposes the disc to damage. A sudden compressive and/or rotation force may then cause a tear in the weakened annulus, through which the nucleus pulposus may bulge or an actual herniation may occur. The released nuclear material may impinge on adjacent nerve roots or on the spinal cord itself.

In addition, other elements such as epineuriem and supportive fat may be directly affected by protruded disc and in turn directly affect the contents of the intervertebral foramina. Besides the segmental nerve, arteries and veins may likewise be compressed, bringing about vascular stasis. The loss of shock absorption, inflammation, and edema may lead to back pain. Impingement on a nerve root may lead to a radiculopathy into an extremity.

A posterolateral herniation is most common. In the lumbar region, the most common disc herniations occur at L5-S1 or L4–L5. These account for approximately 95% of all lumbar disc herniations. Most serious is the impingement of the cauda equina in the lower spinal canal or the spinal cord at a higher level leading to *cauda equina syndrome*. Bowel and/or bladder dysfunction, paresis, or paralysis may result.

Patients may experience a sudden onset of low back pain with bending or lifting an object or a more gradual onset of low back pain. The pain may radiate into a lower extremity, frequently following the course of the sciatic nerve. Depending on the nerve root involved and the severity of the herniation, there may be sensory or reflex changes or motor weakness. Neurologic deficit helps differentiate radiculopathy from referred pain.

Magnetic resonance imaging (MRI) is probably the clinical test of choice to confirm the herniation, although the herniation may also be seen on computerized tomography (CT scan). However, asymptomatic herniated discs have been shown by CT and myelography to occur in 25% to 60% of the general population.

Most patients with disc herniation may be treated conservatively. Bed rest for no more than a few days, ice followed by moist heat, and nonsteroidal antiinflammatory medication or a short course of steroids is generally sufficient during the acute phase. Prolonged bed rest may reduce aggravating movements but may also contribute to decompensation of muscles. Also, braces could add a false sense of confidence and may, likewise, reduce dependence on muscular competence while switching dependency to the stiffness of the brace. Osteopathic manipulation with an exercise program or physical therapy provides relief for many once the acute phase has subsided. Somatic dysfunction is a common occurrence with disc herniation and responds well to manipulation. The facilitated positional release technique for discogenic pain is useful for many patients in relieving sciatic radiation of pain caused by disc herniation. It appears to ease the impingement on the nerve root from the nucleus pulposus fragment. A major goal of manipulation is the relaxation of regional muscles that may be contributing to compression of the vertebra on the disc.

Surgery may be indicated in the presence of intractable pain, progressive, or moderate to severe neurologic deficit. These may include foot drop, paralysis, or bowel or bladder dysfunction. Surgical intervention may offer only a short-term solution, particularly in cases involving psychological or legal factors.

## ■ SPINAL STENOSIS

Spinal stenosis refers to a narrowing of the spinal canal. A variety of causes exists for stenosing the canal. These include:

1. Herniated or bulging intervertebral disc
2. Tumor
3. Osteophytes from osteoarthritis or other bony infringement into the canal (spondylosis)
4. Scar tissue from previous surgery

The patient will experience back pain, frequently with radiculopathy. This condition is generally diagnosed by MRI, with or without contrast. The stenosis may be either lateral or central. The lateral type generally occurs in the region of L4 to S1. Manipulation was shown by Kirkaldy-Willis and Cassidy to offer relief of symptoms in approximately 50% of patients. Severe cases require surgery.

Central stenosis may result in *neurogenic claudication* described as a burning or numbness in the low back and buttocks, aggravated by walking up an incline and relieved by a few minutes of rest. It must be differentiated from vascular claudication. Kirkaldy-Willis and Cassidy found that high-velocity-low amplitude thrusting technique brought significant relief in five of eleven patients with central stenosis. Relief of muscle spasm is a major goal of treatment, so that soft tissue myofascial techniques are useful as well.

## ■ SPONDYLOLISTHESIS AND SPONDYLOLYSIS

Spondylolisthesis is a forward slippage of one vertebral body on the one below it. A backward slippage is generally referred to as *retrolisthesis*. Spondylolisthesis is commonly associated with *spondylolysis;* 20% to 70% of persons with spondylolisthesis also have a spondylolysis. Spondylolysis represents a fracture and separation of the pars interarticularis of the vertebral arch. (See Figures 56-1 and 56-2.)

*Dysplastic spondylolisthesis* is a congenital abnormality most typically of the first sacral or fifth lumbar neural arch. This defect generally becomes apparent during childhood or adolescence. This can be diagnosed on lateral view x-rays of the lumbar spine.

*Degenerative spondylolisthesis* is the result of degenerative changes in the posterior facet joints and disc that permit forward slippage of the vertebra, commonly of L4 on L5. It is most often seen in persons older than age 50.

Trauma may play a role in any of these or may be the primary cause of a spondylolisthesis when a fracture of the neural arch occurs.

Children and adolescents seldom report pain or do not have enough symptoms to seek medi-

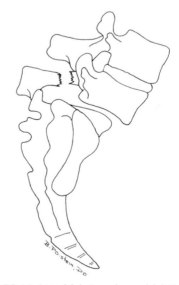

■ **FIG. 56-1A** Spondylolysis and spondylolisthesis of L5 on S1. (Adapted from: Rothman R, Simeone AF. *The Spine*, 2nd ed, vol. 1. Philadelphia: Saunders, 1982: 263–284.)

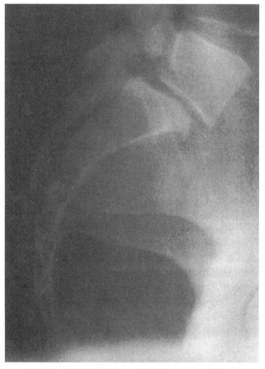

■ **FIG. 56-1B** Radiograph of same condition.

cal care until the early twenties. The usual report is of low back pain, with or without radiculopathy into the buttocks, posterior thigh, or down the leg to the foot. Hamstring muscle spasm and pain is a fairly common finding when there are symptoms. This spasm may cause abnormal posture or gait. Certain physical and sports activities, such as gymnastics, football, wrestling, or hyperextension injuries may give a clinical clue as to the presence of spondylolysis.

Because of the instability caused by the slippage, there is often degeneration of the facet joints and/or the disc. There may be herniation of one of the involved discs caused by the stresses placed on it.

Oblique lumbar spine x-rays taken in the upright position are used to diagnose spondylolysis and spondylolisthesis. The defect in the pars is seen typically as the collar around the neck of a *Scottie dog* (Fig. 56-3).

Treatment is generally conservative and may include an exercise program, a nutritional program to assist in any necessary weight loss, and osteopathic manipulative treatment. Although OMT does not correct the lesion, it is helpful in relieving other problems, such as muscle spasm, which accompany the condition.

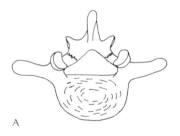

A

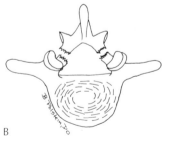

B

■ **FIG. 56-2** Cross-sectional view of bilateral spondylolysis at the pars interarticularis. (Adapted, with permission, from Rosse K. *The Musculoskeletal System in Health and Disease*. New York: Harper & Row, 1980:132.)

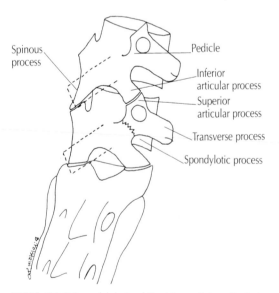

Spinous process
Pedicle
Inferior articular process
Superior articular process
Transverse process
Spondylotic process

■ **FIG. 56-3** Spondylolysis of the L5 pars interarticularis, oblique view. Note the appearance of a collar around the neck of a Scottie dog. (Adapted from McGee D. *Orthopedic Physical Assessment*. Philadelphia: W.B. Saunders 1987:112.)

## ■ CASE 1

A 17-year-old boy was seen in the clinic with a chief symptom of recurrent low back pain of 2 months' duration.

The patient denied any previous history of back pain or an incident of acute trauma to the back. The patient had joined his high school football team approximately 3 months previously and had been participating in their practices and games whenever he felt physically able to do so. He found that the pain worsened after a strenuous practice session but was relieved with a few days of rest. He denied the presence of any radicular symptoms.

He is the only child and there was no history of back pain in his immediate family. His medical history was otherwise noncontributory, as was the review all his systems.

A total physical examination was performed, which elicited no changes from the normal except for the low back area. Examination of the low back resulted in the following findings. He was a well-developed young male who, in the upright position, revealed no observable postural deficits, except for a moderately increased lumbar lordosis. His iliac crests appeared level and there was no restriction in forward bending, but the patient reported mild localized pain in the low back with extreme extension of the low back. His standing flexion test was normal. In the prone position, palpation of the patient's spine revealed a step-down depression of the spinous process at the fifth lumbar vertebra. There was tenderness bilaterally over the transverse processes in that area, and bilateral muscle hypertonicity. The straight leg-raising test was normal, as were all the deep tendon reflexes of the lower extremity. There was no evidence of cutaneous skin sensory changes or muscle weakness. There was marked limitation of motion at the fifth lumbar on the sacrum as well as somatic dysfunctions found at L2–L3 and T8–T9.

X-rays were taken of the lumbar region: anterior–posterior, lateral, and oblique views. They revealed that the patient had a first-degree spondylolisthesis of L5 on S1.

The patient was treated using facilitated positional release techniques for the hypertonic muscles as well as the somatic dysfunctions that were found at L2–L3 and T8–T9, with good results. He was placed on bed rest for the next 48 hours and an exercise program was introduced to strengthen his abdominal muscles and reduce the lordosis.

The nature of the condition was explained to him, as well as to his mother, with the admonition that playing football or any other activity that could result in low back trauma would create a return and worsening of the condition.

The patient was seen once more in a month's time, at which visit he stated that his symptoms were gone and had not returned. He had continued to perform his exercises and had been attending school regularly. He felt that he could perform all his usual physical activities except those as discussed previously.

Examination revealed that the previous areas of muscle hypertonicity were no longer present, nor were the previously found somatic dysfunctions.

He was told to continue his exercises and gradually increase his physical activities, but not to participate in any activity that could create trauma to his back.

### Discussion

Spondylolisthesis is defined as forward slippage of one vertebra on its subadjacent vertebra. Most commonly, it is associated with a defect of the pars interarticularis (spondylolysis). Spondylolysis is usually not seen until the age of 5 or 6. The slippage will usually occur by the twentieth year. Symptoms may not be created by the slippage and may not be present until trauma is introduced to that region. It is not unusual to find the condition as an incidental finding on x-ray of that area for other reasons. Generally, most cases of spondylosis are not symptomatic until they exceed a grade II (>50%). Once found, it is best to explain the condition to the patient and prescribe weight control, if needed, and exercises as preventative measures.

## ■ CASE 2

A 41-year-old woman was seen in the clinic with a chief symptom of acute, severe pain in her left buttock with radiation down her left leg. This pain had been present for the previous 3 days.

She denied having any history of radiating leg pain but had had recurrent attacks of low back pains. She treated these attacks with bed rest and aspirin for 3 to 4 days with good results. The present symptoms were different from those that accompanied her previous backaches in that she had never had pain down the leg previously.

She denied any history of acute trauma, nor had she performed any new or strenuous activities. She was a secretary whose duties kept her sitting almost all day. In addition, she had the responsibilities for the care of her home. She was married with three teenaged children who were all very cooperative and assisted in the shopping and household chores.

She had been able to obtain mild relief from the pain with bed rest and lying on her left side in a fetal position. She stated that there were no cutaneous skin changes or weakness of either leg present. On further questioning, the patient was able to localize the pain as being primarily in the left buttock, the left side of her leg, and the dorsum of her left foot.

With the exception of the chief symptom, all other histories were noncontributory.

A total physical examination was performed that elicited no changes from the normal in any other system than the low back region. Observation of the patient in the upright position revealed that she stood with the lumbar spine in slight flexion and shifted to the left. The patient had restriction of motion in all directions, but attempts at extension exaggerated the pain. Her lumbar lordotic curve was flattened. When the patient was asked to try to squat, stand on her toes, and then stand on her heels, she had difficulty performing all of these maneuvers because of motion restriction of her back.

With the patient in the sitting position, her lower extremity muscle strength, cutaneous sensation, and deep tendon reflexes were evaluated. There was a slight diminution of the left Achilles reflex present. The seated straight leg-raising test was positive.

With the patient in the prone position, the previously seen lateral lumbar shift was diminished. There was marked hypertonicity of the left low back muscles, with a tender point at the left buttock and tenderness and restriction of motion of the left sacroiliac articulation. An extension somatic dysfunction was found at L5–S1 and a flexion somatic dysfunction at L1–L2. There was hypertonicity and point tenderness of the left piriformis muscle and tensor fascia lata, as well as tenderness at the left sciatic notch. There was no evidence of muscle weakness or atrophy of the lower extremities; however, the left Achilles deep tendon reflex was again slightly diminished.

With the patient in the supine position, the straight leg-raising test was positive at 45 degrees.

A tentative diagnosis of a herniation of the disc between L5 and S1 was made. Magnetic resonance imaging (MRI) was performed, which confirmed this diagnosis. It was reported as a bulging disc with mild left lateral extrusion present between L5 and S1.

The patient was treated using facilitated positional release techniques for relief of the muscle hypertonicity as well as the restrictions and somatic dysfunctions found. Special attention was given to the treatment of the piriformis and tensor fascia lata muscles. A prescription was given for nonsteroidal antiinflammatory (NSAID) medication.

The patient was seen again in 3 days and reported partial relief of symptoms. Re-evaluation found that the muscle hypertonicity had partially returned in all areas. The lumbar lateral shift had lessened, and the restriction of the left sacroiliac articulation and the extension somatic dysfunction at L5–S1 had returned. Osteopathic manipulative treatment was repeated, as needed. The bed rest and NSAIDs were continued for an additional week. Mild exercises were prescribed.

The patient was next seen a week later; at which time, she reported that her symptoms were gone and that she felt much improved. The NSAIDs were gradually reduced in dosage, and the exercises were increased, with special emphasis being placed on strengthening the abdominal muscles and stretching the muscles of the lower back.

The patient's posture at work was discussed with her. This included the type of chair being used. A recommendation was made regarding the chair needed, and she was told that she had to stand at least for 1 minute every hour and that she should perform pelvic rock exercises while she was standing. She was allowed to return to work and an appointment for further evaluation was made for 1 month.

## Discussion

A herniated disc, with concurrent radicular pain, usually occurs in adults ages 30 to 50. However, it can occur at any age. The fourth or fifth lumbar disc is most often involved. There may be a history of acute trauma as the immediate cause, but more often the history is one of recurrent low back pain with a sudden onset of radicular pain after no or minor trauma. In these cases, it is necessary to seek the underlying causes that created the predilection for the recurrent back pains as well as the radicular pain. In the case discussed, the patient sat for too many hours in a chair that was not ergonomically suited for her body or the work that she was doing. In addition, she had neglected doing any exercise, which allowed her back muscles to tighten with shortening of her hamstrings and weakening of the abdominal muscles.

Physicians have the added benefit of the information that is available from an MRI test. One must be aware that most of these syndrome complexes are caused by local inflammation of the nerve root and not by direct discal pressure. Therefore, conservative therapy will often alleviate the symptom complex. It is then mandatory that the underlying causes are sought and a complete plan for removing them developed. This must include diet and instructions on how to lift, bend, and perform their prescribed job.

The symptoms and physical findings presented in this case are typical for a herniated disc that follows a history of recurrent low back pain. The patient responded well to antiinflammatory medication and osteopathic manipulative treatment.

She will require further followup care for a period of time to insure that the prescribed program is followed and that there are no recurrences of the findings.

In addition to what was prescribed, after a few months she should start aerobic exercises. Walking daily is a simple and effective means of doing this.

Surgery, for the reduction of discal pressure, is indicated in patients when the neurological findings start to worsen, that is, further diminishing of the reflex and weakness of the muscles involved.

### REFERENCES

Bernard TN Jr, Kirkaldy-Willis WH. Recognizing specific characteristics of non-specific low back pain. *Clin Orthop* 1987;217:266–280.

Braunwald E, Fauci AS, Isselbacher KJ, et al. *Harrison's Principles of Internal Medicine, thirteenth ed.* New York: McGraw Hill 1994.

Cailliet R. *Low Back Pain Syndrome.* Philadelphia: F. A. Davis 1995.

D'Ambrosia RD. *Musculoskeletal Disorders.* Philadelphia: J. B. Lippincott Co, 1977.

DiGiovanna EL. Schiowitz S. *An Osteopathic Approach to Diagnosis and Treatment, 2nd ed.* Philadelphia: Lippincott-Raven, 1997.

Hoppenfeld S. *Physical Examination of the Spine and Extremities.* Norwalk, CT: Appelton and Lange, 1978.

Kirkaldy-Willis WH. Five common back disorders: how to diagnose and treat them. *Geriatrics* 1978;33:32–33, 37–41.

Kirkaldy-Willis WH, Hill RJ. A more precise diagnosis for low back pain. *Spine* 1979;4:102–109.

Kirkaldy-Willis WH. Musculoskeletal disorders: a three article symposium. *Postgrad Med* 1981;70:166.

Kirkaldy-Willis WH. *Managing low back pain, 2nd ed.* Edinburgh: Churchill-Livingstone, 1988.

Porter RW, Miller CG. Neurologic claudication and root claudication treated with calcitonin. A double blind trial. *Spine* 1988;13:1061.

Turek SL. *Orthopedics Principles and Applications.* Philadelphia: J. B. Lippincott, 1994.

Yong-Hing K, Kirkaldy-Willis WH. Pathophysiology of degenerative disease of the lumbar spine. *Orthop Clin North Am* 1983;14:491–504.

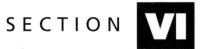
# Pelvis and Sacrum

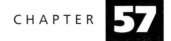

# CHAPTER 57

# Pelvic and Sacral Anatomic Considerations

*Stanley Schiowitz*

## ■ BONES

The pelvis consists of two innominate bones that meet at the midline anteriorly at the pubic symphysis and end posteriorly in a wedge-shaped opening that is filled by the sacrum. The sacrum completes the ring-like shape of the pelvis.

Each innominate consists of three bones, the ilium, ischium, and pube, which fuse in late adolescence to form one bone. On the lateral surface of the innominate is the acetabulum, which articulates with the head of the femur to create the hip joint.

The sacrum is a large bone in the shape of an inverted triangle that is formed by the fusion of the five sacral vertebrae. It is inserted between the two innominates in the upper, posterior aspect of the pelvic cavity. The upper aspect of the sacrum—the base of the triangle—articulates with the fifth lumbar vertebra, creating, with the L5 intervertebral disk, the lumbosacral articulation. The weight of the upper body is transmitted through the sacrum, innominate bones, and acetabulum to the femurs, then down to the feet and the supporting surface.

In the upright position, the sacrum lies in an oblique plane, running from above downward in an anteroposterior direction. Its anterior surface is concave. Its posterior surface is convex and contains the palpable spinous tubercles. The sacrum contains the sacral canal, in which are located the cauda equina and four sacral foramina. These apertures provide passageway for the ventral and dorsal rami of the first four sacral spinal nerves. Bilaterally, the sacrum has auricular surfaces that articulate with the innominate bones to form the sacroiliac joints.

## ■ JOINTS

The sacroiliac articulations are kidney-shaped and convex ventrally. The sacral and iliac articulations seem to match in a crescent-shaped, convex–concave arrangement, but this is not true for the joints' entire bony relationship. Horizontal sections from various levels of the sacroiliac articulation show that the convex–concave relationship exists only at the upper and middle portions. In the lower portion, the relationship is variously described as a flattened, planar joint or a reverse, concave–convex relationship (Fig. 57-1); anatomists differ in their descriptions of the sacroiliac articulations.

Occasionally, the right and left sacroiliac articulations do not mirror each other in the same body. It is generally agreed that the mid-articulation has the greatest convex–concave relationship, promoting joint stability and flexion–extension motions. This is usually found at the level of the second sacral vertebra.

The multiple forms and contours found at any sacroiliac articulation account for the diversity of motions of this joint. Its ligaments hold the joint together. There are no direct muscular attachments from the sacrum to the ilium.

## ■ PELVIC MOTIONS

The pelvis moves as a single unit whose gross motions are initiated by the motions of other

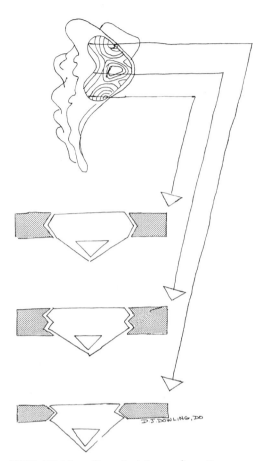

■ **FIG. 57-1** Sacroiliac articulation configurations as seen at different sacral levels.

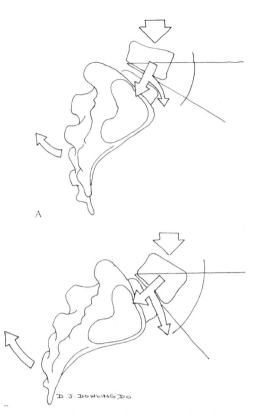

■ **FIG. 57-2** An increase in the lumbosacral angle creates a greater anterior vector force, which increases the lumbosacral strain.

body segments. Rotation, side-bending, and forward and backward bending are all related to the hip or trunk motions. In addition, there are patterns of movement between the sacrum and the ilium, and there are patterns of movement at the pubic articulation.

Review of some everyday activities demonstrate their effect on the pelvic structures. In the standing position, body weight is transmitted through the fifth lumbar vertebra to the sacrum, where the force vector splits in two. One force vector drives the sacrum into its articulation, and the other rotates the sacrum anteriorly. The greater the lumbosacral angle, the greater is the anterior vector force, which in turn increases the lumbosacral strain (Fig. 57-2).

During the act of walking, the ilium on the side of the stance leg is elevated, while the ilium on the swing side is tilted down, and rotated toward the stance leg. This creates pubic shear and torsion (Fig. 57-3, *top*). The stance leg, from heel strike to toe-off, is associated with a close-packed hip joint articulation and causes anterior rotation of the ilium (Fig. 57-3, *bottom*). The body weight shifts to the side of the stance leg, creating lateral flexion stress of the sacrum. The one-legged weight stress produces unilateral stance leg sacroiliac joint locking, allowing the creation of the oblique axis. This in turn permits sacral torsional motion.

Respiratory motions create sacral flexion/extension. Flexion and extension of the sacrum create pressure on the ilia, which is transmitted to the pubic articulation.

The three principal kinds of motions that occur in the pelvis are sacral motions on the ilium, ilial motions on the sacrum, and pubic motions.

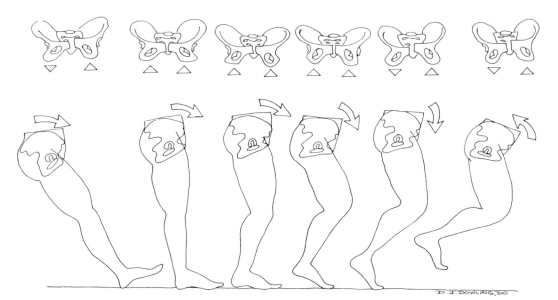

■ **FIG. 57-3** Pubic shear and torsion in walking (*top*), corresponding to the position of the weight-bearing ilium as the stance leg moves from heel strike to toe-off (*bottom*).

## Sacral Motion of the Ilium

The sacral motions on the ilium and the axes on which they occur are as follows:

1. Sacral flexion and extension are caused by respiratory motion and occur on a superior transverse axis, also known as the respiratory axis, that is located at the level of the articular processes of the second sacral segment.
2. Sacral flexion and extension are transmitted as force vectors through the lumbar spine to the middle transverse axis, located at the level of the second sacral body.
3. Rotation of the sacrum occurs on a theoretical vertical axis.
4. Lateral flexion of the sacrum occurs on a theoretical anteroposterior axis.
5. Torsional motions of the sacrum occur on a right or left oblique axis, located from the superior end of the articular surface of one side to the inferior end of the articular surface of the other side.

The axes of sacral motion on the ilium are shown in Figure 57-4.

The coupled motions of rotation and lateral bending of the sacrum are variable, depending somewhat on how those movements are initi-

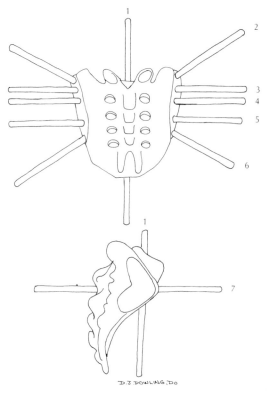

■ **FIG. 57-4** Axes of motion of the sacrum on the ilia. *1*, vertical axis; *2*, right oblique axis; *3*, respiratory axis; *4*, sacroiliac axis; *5*, iliosacral axis; *6*, left oblique axis; *7*, anteroposterior axis.

ated. According to Kappler, sacral rotation induced by lumbar spinal rotation occurs in the same direction as the lumbar spinal rotation, but lateral flexion of the sacrum occurs to the opposite side. When lateral sacral flexion is induced by lateral flexion of the lumbar spine, sacral rotation may occur to either side.

## Ilial Motions on the Sacrum

The motions of the ilia on the sacrum, and the axes on which these movements occur, are as follows.

1. Anteroposterior rotation of the ilium on the sacrum occurs on the inferior transverse axis,

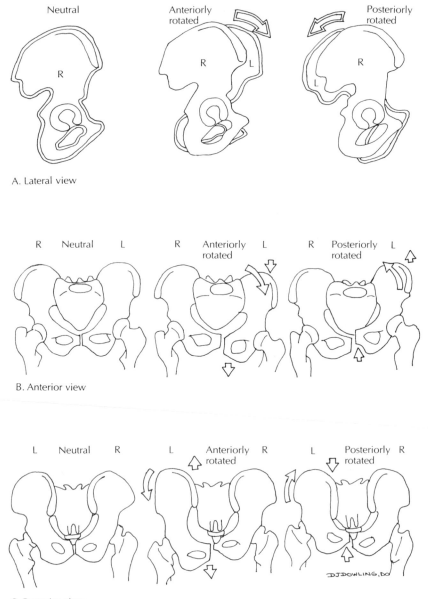

■ **FIG. 57-5** Anteroposterior rotation of the innominate on the sacrum. The directions are named for left-sided movement in this illustration.

located at the inferior pole of the lower sacral articulation (Fig. 57-5).

2. Ilial translatory motions on the sacrum occur in a superoinferior direction (Fig. 57-6).
3. Ilial translatory motions on the sacrum occur in an anteroposterior direction (Fig. 57-7).

## Pubic Motions

The pubic motions are as follows:

1. Caliper motion (with flexion–extension of sacrum) (Fig. 57-8A).
2. Torsional motion (with swing-tilt of swing leg) (Fig. 57-8B).
3. Superoinferior translatory motion (with one-legged weight-bearing) (Fig. 57-8C).

## ■ THE PELVIS DURING PREGNANCY

During vaginal delivery, the sacrum undergoes a process called *nutation* (nodding) that facilitates

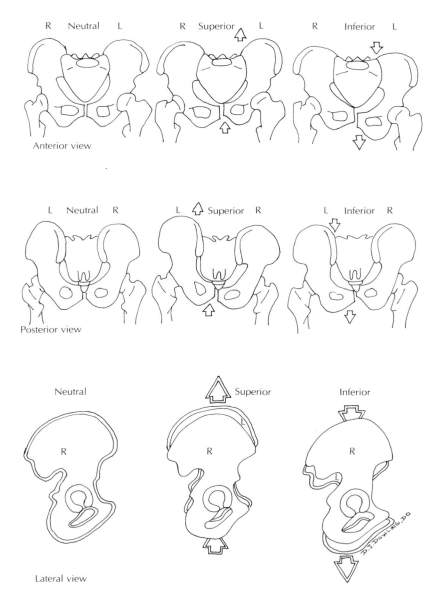

■ **FIG. 57-6** Superoinferior translatory motion of the innominate on the sacrum. The directions are named for the left-sided movement.

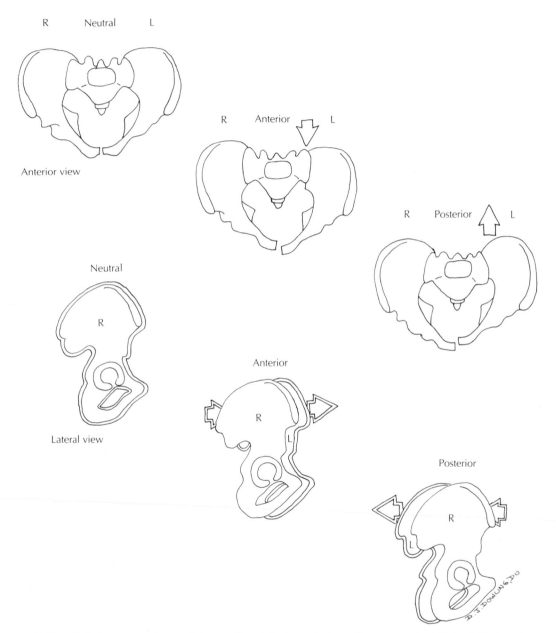

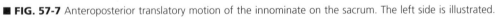

■ **FIG. 57-7** Anteroposterior translatory motion of the innominate on the sacrum. The left side is illustrated.

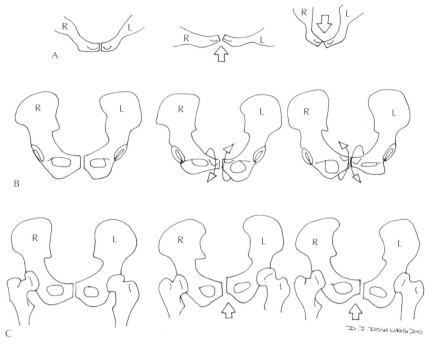

■ **FIG. 57-8** Pubic motions. **(A)** Caliper motion. **(B)** Torsional motion. **(C)** Superoinferior translatory motion.

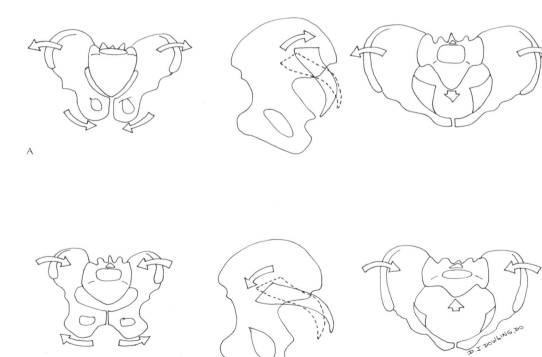

■ **FIG. 57-9** Sacral movements during vaginal delivery. **(A)** Counternutation. **(B)** Nutation.

delivery. In nutation, the sacrum flexes at its middle transverse axis. This diminishes the anteroposterior diameter of the pelvic brim. At the same time the iliac bones approximate, narrowing the transverse diameter of the pelvic brim, and the ischial tuberosities separate, widening the pelvic outlet (Fig. 57-9).

The patient's position and the stress involved, when added to the laxity of the ligaments at delivery, can create sacroiliac dysfunctions. These dysfunctions worsen and are locked into malposition as the ligaments regain their normal tensile strength postpostum. Dysfunction can be prevented after delivery by holding the hip in internal rotation as each leg is removed from the lithotomy position and extended onto the table.

## ■ PELVIC SOMATIC DYSFUNCTIONS

Pelvic somatic dysfunctions are of the following types:

1. Primary pubic dysfunctions are superior–inferior or abducted–adducted dysfunctions.
2. Dysfunctions of motion created by the sacrum moving on the ilium are commonly unilateral anterior or posterior sacral dysfunctions, a unilateral shear of the sacrum along the articulation or oblique rotational sacral dysfunctions. If the fifth lumbar vertebra is not involved in the oblique rotation, the dysfunction is described as a *sacral rotation dysfunction*. If the fifth lumbar vertebra rotates in a direction opposite that of the sacrum, it is described as a *sacral torsion*.
3. Dysfunction created by the ilium moving on

the sacrum usually involves anteroposterior ilial rotation or superoinferior ilial shear along the articulation.

These dysfunctions may be difficult to diagnose individually because many of the motion functions and diagnostic findings overlap. Specific treatment of a specific dysfunction is most effective. However, because of the firm ligamentous attachments of this articulation, nonspecific treatment may be equally as effective.

### REFERENCES

DiGiovanna EL. Schiowitz S. *An Osteopathic Approach to Diagnosis and Treatment*. Philadelphia: Lippincott-Raven, 1997.

Kapandji IA. *The Physiology of the Joints, vol III. The Trunk and Vertebral Column*. New York: Churchill Livingstone, 1974.

Kappler R. Lecture notes. Chicago: College of Osteopathic Medicine, 1975.

Larson NJ. *Physiologic Movement of the Sacrum*. Read before the Chicago College of Osteopathic Medicine, February 1984.

Mitchell FL. Structural pelvic function. In: Barnes M, ed. *1965 Year Book of Selected Osteopathic Papers, vol II*. Carmel, CA: Academy of Applied Osteopathy, 1965: 178–199.

Mitchell FL Jr, Moran PS, Pruzzo NT. *An Evaluation and Treatment Manual of Osteopathic Muscle Energy Procedures*. Valley Park, MO: Mitchell, Moran, and Pruzzo Associates, 1979.

Moore KL. *Clinically Oriented Anatomy*. Baltimore: Williams & Wilkins, 1980.

Sutherland WG. *The Cranial Bowl*. Mankato, MN: Free Press, 1936.

Warwick R, Williams PL. *Gray's Anatomy*, 35th British edition. Philadelphia: W. B. Saunders, 1973.

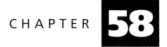

# Gait and Postural Considerations

*Stanley Schiowitz, Eileen L. DiGiovanna, and Joseph A. DiGiovanna*

Hippocrates and Aristotle probably made the first scientific observations of gait. As clinicians, we continue that tradition by observing patients walking every day and by selecting certain characteristics for assessment.

The examiner focuses on asymmetric movement while viewing the patient from the front, side, or back. Asymmetric movements are characterized by reduced or excessive displacements or by a change in the speed of movement during parts of the gait cycle. Asynchronous movement in the sagittal plane is best observed from the side, and coronal plane dysfunction is best observed from the front or back.

To use gait fully as a diagnostic tool, the clinician should be aware of the normal gait parameters—the usual speed, step length, and step rate. A variation in any one of these parameters will affect the others.

## ■ KINEMATICS OF GAIT

Physiologic, efficient locomotion entails translation of the body's center of gravity through space along a path requiring the least expenditure of energy. The center of gravity is constantly being displaced beyond the body's base of support. The resulting potential loss of balance is corrected by moving one lower extremity forward to change the base of support. Repetition of this pattern on alternating legs creates the walking cycle.

The normal walking cycle is divided into two phases—stance phase, when the foot is on the ground, and swing phase, when it is moving forward. Sixty percent of the normal cycle is spent in stance phase. Of this 60%, 25% is in double stance. The remaining 40% of the walking cycle is in swing phase.

Stance phase is divided into the following segments: heel strike, foot flat, mid-stance, and push- or toe-off. Swing phase is divided into acceleration, mid-swing, and deceleration.

The average width of the base of gait, as measured from heel to heel, is between 2 and 4 inches. The average length of a step is 15 inches, with a cadence of 90 to 120 steps per minute. The feet are usually in slight abduction.

The forces acting in gait are gravity, muscle contraction, and momentum. Muscle contraction generally initiates motion; gravity and momentum then add their contributions. According to Winter and Robertson, during swing phase, gravity, muscle contraction, and knee acceleration cause the shank to rotate. In the first half of the swing, gravity and momentum contribute 80% of the force, whereas in the second half of the swing, muscles contribute 80% of the force.

The counterpressure of the ground against the feet is the force that propels the body. We are not usually aware of the earth's thrust. However, in soft snow, sand, or mud, this thrust is reduced, necessitating increased muscular activity and energy used to maintain forward locomotion. Friction between the foot and the ground is essential for transmission of the ground's pressure. The friction must be sufficient to counterbalance the horizontal vector component of force. The greater the horizontal force, the greater is the dependence on friction. The corollary holds true: on icy streets, small, almost vertical steps are taken.

Walking is initiated through the complex interplay of neural mechanisms, muscular activity, and biomechanical forces. The triceps surae relaxes, permitting forward inclination of the body ahead of the center of gravity. The line of the center of gravity, which is midway between the feet and anterior to the ankle joint, moves toward the swing limb in a posteroanterior direction. As the swing limb prepares for toe-off, the center of gravity shifts to the stance side. The weight is balanced on the stance leg to allow forward propulsion of the swing limb.

Both phases of gait are in operation simultaneously, alternating sides at the completion of each cycle. The swing phase leg rotates the pelvis toward the stance side, with concomitant rotation of the spine to the swing side. The hip joint flexes with this swing action. The knee joint flexes during the first half and extends during the second half of the swing, while the ankle and foot are dorsiflexed.

On the stance side, the hip joint extends, accompanied by muscular contraction that prevents dropping of the pelvis toward the swing side. The knee joint is in slight flexion at the moment of foot contact, or heel strike, after which the knee is extended.

The foot and ankle in this segment, from heel strike to full weight-bearing, is in plantar flexion of the ankle. The foot then converts to a rigid lever for transferring the body weight to the forefoot for push-off. At this time, the heel rises rapidly and the foot everts, causing increased external rotation of the leg with hyperextension of the metatarsophalangeal joints at the end of the propulsive phase. The clinical significance of the mechanics of the subtalar joint (as used in the stance phase) cannot be overemphasized. The slightest disturbance will cause noticeable dysfunction.

A definite sequence is observed in weight-bearing on the osseous tripod of the foot: the weight passes from the heel to the fifth metatarsal head and then across the metatarsal heads to the big toe. Any change in pressure on one of these points will be accompanied by a change in the normal sequence of motion and weight-bearing at other points. Calluses usually develop at these sites.

The normal walking cycle in the lower extremities is accompanied by regular motions of the shoulders, arms, and head. Their actions are part of any clinical evaluation. When the pelvis on the swing side moves forward, the shoulder on that side drops back. Therefore, the opposite arms and legs swing in tandem.

The action of the arm in the anteroposterior plane reduces rotation of the shoulders, which directly aids in keeping the head forward. Arm swing balances the rotation of the pelvis. These motions are in direct proportion to each other. If the arms do not swing, the upper trunk will rotate in the same direction as the pelvis.

## ■ GAIT EFFICIENCY

Efficiency of gait can be considered in terms of the translatory movement of the body's center of gravity through a smooth undulating pathway of low amplitude. The center of gravity in the erect, motionless human is just anterior to the second sacral vertebra. In walking, it is displaced both vertically and horizontally, describing a sinusoidal curve.

Vertical displacement of the center of gravity occurs twice during the cycle from heel strike to heel strike of the same foot. The total amount of vertical displacement is approximately 1.8 inches. The summits occur at 25% and 75% of the cycle. At the midpoint of the gait cycle (double weight-bearing), the center of gravity is at its lowest point.

Saunders, Inman, and Eberhart have proposed six major determinants of gait for the maintenance of mechanical efficiency:

1. **Pelvic rotation.** The pelvis rotates on the swing side, approximately 4 degrees on either side of the central axis. Because the pelvis is a semi-rigid structure, this rotation occurs alternately at each hip joint as the hip passes from relative internal rotation to external rotation during stance phase.
2. **Downward pelvic tilt.** The pelvis tilts downward in the coronal plane on the swing side. The alternate angular displacement is 5 degrees at the stance hip joint, creating relative adduction of the extremity in stance and relative abduction in swing.

3. **Knee flexion of the swing leg.** These three determinants of gait—pelvic rotation, pelvic tilt, and swing knee flexion—all act by flattening the vertical arc through which the center of gravity is moving. Pelvic rotation elevates the extremities of the arc, while pelvic tilt and knee flexion depress its summit.

4. and 5. **The combined actions of the foot, ankle, and knee of the stance leg** constitute the fourth and fifth determinants of gait. These actions help maintain a smooth pathway for the translatory motion of the center of gravity. A first arc occurs at heel strike when the ankle rotates from dorsi-flexion to plantar flexion, with the heel functioning as the fulcrum. A second arc occurs with rotation of the foot, with the forepart of the foot functioning as the fulcrum. This occurs with heel rise. Both arcs are accompanied by stance knee flexion, which maintains a level center of gravity.

6. **Displacement of center of gravity.** Displacement of the center of gravity over the weight-bearing extremity aids in maintaining body balance as the swing leg is lifted from the ground. The relative adduction of that hip, along with the tibio-femoral angle, reduces the amount of lateral displacement necessary for balance. The center of gravity deviates laterally approximately 1.75 inches. Thus, deviation of the center of gravity is almost equivalent in horizontal and vertical planes.

## ■ PELVIC MOTION

The pelvis is not a rigid structure. It has an anterior articulation at the symphysis pubis and two articulations with the sacrum.

As the pelvis rotates and tilts, a torsional effect develops at the symphysis pubis. This is created because every part of the pelvis is moving at a different linear velocity. Measuring the displacement of rotation and tilt of the lateral edge of the right innominate from the fixed left hip will show that the angular velocity is constant from every part of the left and right innominates, but the linear velocity, and therefore the distance traveled, increases from left to right. Thus, the combined motions of rotation and tilt occur at different speeds of linear displacement for different parts of the pelvis and create a torsion at the symphysis pubis with every step taken.

The sacrum moves with the innominate and undergoes the same rotation, tilt, and lateral shift as does the innominate, but not at the same speed. When swing of the right leg initiates rotation of the right innominate toward the left, with right innominate tilt and left lateral shift, the sacrum will move on its vertical axis and rotate to the left, with right sacral flexion. Simultaneously, the center of gravity in the horizontal plane shifts to the left, producing left sacral lateral flexion. The vertical center of gravity moves to the superior pole of the left sacroiliac, locking the articulation into a mechanical position that establishes movement of the sacrum on the left oblique axis. This sets the pattern so the sacrum can torsionally turn to the left (Mitchell, 1965). Walking creates the mechanics of oblique sacral motion without dysfunction, or, in the aforementioned example, a left-on-left sacral rotational motion (Fig. 58-1).

During these motions, the lumbar spine rotates to the right and flexes laterally to the left, compensating for the right sacral flexion created by pelvic rotation toward the left with right pelvic tilt. The relationship of the rotated right L5 to the left-on-left sacral rotation completes the picture

This left-on-left sacral torsional pattern. It is not pathological or dysfunctional because it is temporary and instantaneous and the adaptive motion of the lumbar region is for the side-bending and rotation to occur in opposite directions.

## ■ ASYMMETRIC MOTION

In the perfectly balanced, symmetric human, the joint motions of gait have little or no effect on the body's structural integrity. However, asymmetry develops in virtually everyone and causes constant small structural stress situations that can lead to somatic dysfunctions.

What happens to symmetry of gait in short leg syndrome? What happens to the comparative reversals of motions of lumbar rotation and lateral flexion if scoliosis is present? Radiographs of patients with low back problems often show lateral flexion, rotation deformity of one lumbar

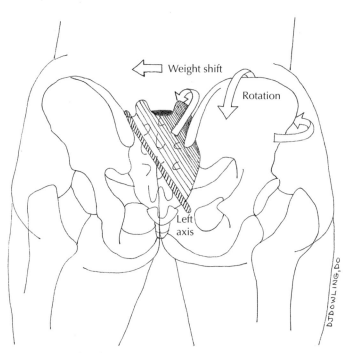

■ **FIG. 58-1** Pelvic determinates of normal gait, posterior view. Shown as left on left sacral torsional motions.

vertebra on the one below it. Disk wedging and intervertebral spondylytic changes can be present even if the site has not sustained previous specific trauma. This condition is very likely produced by the constant stress of gait on a localized somatic dysfunction.

Structural deformities should be treated, even if asymptomatic, while the subject is young. This will prevent some of the constant microtraumas that occur with daily locomotion and will prevent symptomatic dysfunction in later life.

■ **NEUROLOGIC GAIT PATTERNS**

Analysis of gait is the most important test in neurology and one of the least performed. The following points should be noted in this evaluation: the position of the body, movement of the legs, position and movement of the arms, distance between the feet, both in forward direction (stride) and in lateral direction (width), regularity of movements, ability to walk in a straight line, ease of turning, and ease of stopping. Along with these observations, the examiner should note any changes in the six major determinants of gait.

Following are descriptions of several neurologic gait patterns.

*Hemiplegic gait.* In hemiplegic gait, the affected leg is usually stiff, with loss of flexion at the hip and knee joints. The patient leans to the affected side and throws the whole leg outward from the body before bringing it back toward the trunk, producing a circumduction movement. The shoe is dragged against the floor, and there is usually an accompanying affected arm that does not swing but is held in fixed position against the abdomen with the elbow flexed.

*High steppage gait.* High steppage gait can be divided into two characteristic patterns. In the first pattern, the toe touches the floor first, with a foot drop caused by paralysis of pretibial or peroneal muscles. The leg is raised high by abnormal knee and hip flexion. The toe touches the ground first, followed by a slapping noise as the foot strikes the floor.

In the second pattern, the heel touches the floor first because of loss of sense of position. The high steppage gait is bilateral, with ataxia and side-to-side reeling. The heel touches the floor first and a stomp of the foot is heard. Romberg's sign is present, caused by a dysfunction of the afferent portion of peripheral nerves or posterior roots.

Carcinoma, diabetic neuropathy, tabes dorsalis, Friedreich's ataxia, subacute combined degeneration of the cord, compression lesions of the posterior columns, and multiple sclerosis that affects the posterior columns may all produce a high steppage gait.

*Shuffling gait.* Shuffling gait can be described as small, flat-footed shuffling steps; the foot does not clear the ground. In Parkinsonism, rigidity, tremor, paucity of movement, shuffling with haste, and difficulty in starting, stopping, or turning are noted. The patient is in truncal flexion, with lack of extension movements at the hips, knees, and elbows. The thorax and pelvis rotate in the same direction in swing phase. The amplitude of vertical excursions of the head is lessened in forward motion. The first noticeable motor signs in Parkinsonism may be a nonrhythmic pattern with random or poorly timed activity of the arms in gait.

The shuffling gait seen in arteriosclerosis is due to loss of confidence and equilibrium. The patient stands erect, takes small shuffling steps with a wide base, and seems to stare at a distant point. Turning is achieved through a series of small steps made by one foot, the other foot acting as a pivot.

*Ataxic gait.* Ataxic gait is a reeling, unsteady gait with a wide base and a tendency to fall toward the side of the lesion. Vertigo may accompany ataxia. It may be found in cerebellar disease, multiple sclerosis, and sometimes myxedema. Ataxic gait must be differentiated from drunken and staggering gait, in which the subject reels, totters, tips forward and backward, and may lose balance and fall. This gait is seen in alcohol or barbiturate poisoning, drug reaction, polyneuritis, or general paresis.

*Scissors gait.* In scissors gait, the legs are adducted, crossing alternately in front of one another. Both lower limbs are spastic, and there is spasm of the adductor muscles at the hip joints, often accompanied by pronounced compensatory motions of the trunk and upper extremities. Bilateral upper motor neuron lesions, advanced cervical spondylosis, or multiple sclerosis may produce this gait pattern.

*Waddling gait.* Waddling gait can be described as rolling from side to side. The pelvic rotation and tilt on the swing side are increased (penguin walk). Muscular dystrophy with weakness of hips, exaggerated lordosis, and pot-bellied posture can produce this gait.

*Hysterical gait.* Hysterical gait may simulate any paralysis or may be bizarre. There may be inability to walk, but in bed the subject may lose the characteristic spasticity.

When outlining therapy for the neurologic patient, the clinician must discuss all problems with him. Many of these patients hope that osteopathic manipulation will cure their problems, and they must be advised of the limitations of the expected results. Some have, as a secondary symptom, severe pain and dysfunction of the low back area. These symptoms can be greatly relieved. Some have asymptomatic somatic dysfunctions of the upper cervical vertebrae, which should be treated.

## ■ MUSCULOSKELETAL GAIT PATTERNS

Several musculoskeletal gait patterns are described.

*Antalgic gait.* Antalgic gait is characterized by a short stance phase and a rapidly executed swing phase: the patient tries to avoid standing on a painful extremity. Most musculoskeletal dysfunctions of gait are antalgic. The physician must evaluate where the pain is located. A simple question such as, "When you put your weight on that foot, where does it hurt?" may assist in accurate diagnosis.

*Gluteus medius gait.* A gluteus medius gait is characterized by a shift of the body toward the deficient side, indicating a weakness of that gluteus medius muscle. It can be evaluated by finding a Trendelenburg sign in the upright position.

*Gluteus maximus gait.* In gluteus maximus deficiency, the trunk and pelvis are hyperextended backward over both hips to maintain the center of gravity behind the involved hip joint.

*Short lower extremity.* In short lower extremity, the pelvis and trunk depress in stance phase.

*Elevated pelvis gait.* In elevated pelvis gait, there is a hiking or elevation of the pelvis on the swing side if that hip or knee joint has motion limitation from any cause.

*Congenital hip dislocation.* Congenital dislocation of the hip creates a waddling gait.

*Osteoarthrosis gait.* Severe osteoarthrosis of the hip or knee joints will produce the scissors gait.

*Foot problems.* Any dysfunction of the foot may alter normal mechanics. These could include Morton's foot (neuroma), corns, calluses, bunions, hallux rigidus, plantar warts, or poorly fitting shoes. If plantar flexion is absent, there is no push-off and the heel and forefoot come off the floor together.

## ■ PEDIATRIC GAIT PATTERNS

Pediatric musculoskeletal problems should be evaluated and treatment instituted before the onset of weight-bearing. Equinus, calcaneus valgus, pronation, flatfoot, tibial torsion, metatarsal varus, clubfoot, and congenital dislocation of the hips should all be diagnosed and treated properly before the child begins to walk.

In one study, 64% of limping children with no history of gait dysfunction or trauma had primary involvement of the hip joint. Most cases were caused by transient synovitis and resolved with rest. Many children with hip-related gait dysfunction have had a recent upper respiratory tract infection. Other causes include osteitis, rheumatic fever, rheumatoid arthritis, and Perthes disease.

## ■ GAIT PATTERNS IN LOW BACK DYSFUNCTION

An initial diagnosis of somatic dysfunction may often be made by evaluating the patient's gait. The most obvious problems are those relating to low back dysfunction.

A psoas dysfunction secondary to lumbar vertebral osteopathic somatic dysfunctions will produce the typical psoatic limp. The patient bends forward and toward the side of the dysfunction, and that hip will be in abduction. The somatic dysfunction is usually found in the upper lumbar area. Neglecting this site and treating the lower back or sacroiliac articulation is usually a futile effort.

Persons with psoas spasm that is severe enough to affect their stance or gait generally will show stiffness and even push against their thighs with their hands to support and slowly stretch the psoas and iliacus muscles when arising from sitting to standing.

Unilateral erector spinae contraction will cause lateral flexion to the side of contraction, scoliosis with convexity to the opposite side, and extension of the spine. The patient walks with a stiff back, with no lumbar rotation or flexion. The spinal areas involved are usually at the fourth or fifth lumbar and first sacral segments. An acute anterior sacrum dysfunction on the same side may also be present. If findings include a raised iliac crest height, lumbar scoliotic convexity, and sciatic pain distribution, all on the same side, the prognosis for a speedy recovery is often good. If the pain is on the other side, the cause may be a prolapsed disk or some other serious pathologic condition, and both physician and patient may be in for a difficult time.

## ■ GAIT PATTERNS IN LOWER EXTREMITY DYSFUNCTION

Sciatica is associated with an antalgic, erector spinae gait pattern as the patient tries to avoid weight-bearing on the affected side. A common somatic dysfunction pattern in these patients comprises unilateral sacral flexion and flexion of the fifth lumbar vertebra, with rotation and side-bending to the painful side, accompanied by trigger points at the piriformis, gluteus maximus, and gluteus medius muscles.

Observation of an asymmetric pelvic swing or tilt noted should be followed by a hip drop test. The findings on this test often concur with the gait observations, pointing toward lumbar lateral flexion restriction.

Somatic dysfunctions involving the lower extremity usually manifest with an antalgic gait. The clinician can use observation to determine the area involved but then must depend on palpation and motion testing to establish the diagnosis.

The skill of observation can be improved if the physician is aware of the alterations of motion commonly produced by localized somatic dysfunction. At the hip joint, look for limitation in internal and external rotation in the swinging lower extremity. In the knee joint, there will be a restriction of femoral medial rotation on the tibia when attempting a close-packed position in extension of the stance lower extremity. At the ankle, the subtalar joint will be limited in eversion–inversion as the leg rotates internally–externally in stance phase. Lateral weight-bearing of the foot will shift toward the medial arch, with cuboid dysfunction during stance phase.

## Postural Balance

Human bipedal posture has made balance extremely important to musculoskeletal function. In the erect human, gravity pulls on all parts of the body. Although a column of vertebrae stacked evenly on top of each other would have been well-balanced given little motion, antero-posterior curves developed in the spine to promote flexibility and increase strength. The transitions between spinal curves are well-suited to meet the force of gravity. Correct posture is essential to keep the force of gravity centered on those vertebrae designed for this function.

Few persons are totally symmetric, and therefore postural imbalance is a significant source of musculoskeletal problems.

The body has certain automatic compensatory mechanisms that tend to right the body and maintain it in a state of equilibrium. For example, if while standing, the left leg is lifted off the ground, the body's center of gravity will automatically move to the right, and the spine will shift and curve in the frontal plane to maintain the body in balance. Similarly, if the arms are held in front of the body, the spine will shift and curve in the sagittal plane, increasing lumbar lordosis to maintain balance. If a weight is held in the outstretched hands, the lordosis will exaggerate further to maintain body equilibrium. Thus, the body will make any adjustments necessary to maintain its balance and upright posture. Numerous conditions can produce asymmetry in body mechanics and lead to functional postural imbalance. They include:

1. Trauma
2. Degenerative processes
3. Habit or occupation
4. Genetic tendencies
5. Mental status
6. Pregnancy
7. Obesity
8. Loss of muscle tone
9. Disease processes such as osteoporosis or polio
10. Congenital anomalies

## Kyphosis

Kyphosis is a curvature of the spine in the sagittal plane with the convexity posteriorly. A moderate degree is normal in the thoracic spine. However, an exaggeration of the curve is abnormal. Poor posture with weakened musculature is the most common cause. In this case, the shoulders slouch forward, the head drops down and forward, and the thoracic spinal curve is increased. The abdomen tends to protrude. Habit and occupation are the main offenders.

Pathologically the thoracic spine may curve because of osteoporosis, in which the anterior part of the vertebral body undergoes microfractures with collapse and loss of height. Eventually the loss of height is enough to cause a forward bowing of the thoracic spine with the typical *dowager's hump* of osteoporosis. Arthritic changes may cause forward bending of the thoracic spine as well.

The thoracic kyphosis may increase as a compensation for increased lordosis in the cervical or lumbar spine. Kyphosis is often associated with a structural scoliosis, *kyphoscoliosis*.

## Thoracic Flattening

Localized thoracic flattening is most often caused by areas of posterior muscular tension and/or somatic dysfunction. It can also be habitual in nature as in a *military posture*, with the shoulders held back and the spine straightened. Flattening can also be compensatory because of flattening in other regions of the spine, cervical or lumbar.

## Lordosis

Normally there is a lordosis of the cervical and lumbar spinal regions. The term, *lordosis*, is also used to express an abnormal exaggeration of the curve in one or both of these areas.

## Cervical Lordosis

An increase in the lordosis of the cervical spine is most often caused by postural changes with the head carried forward of the line of gravity through the body. The head tilts back to keep the eyes level, thus increasing the cervical lordosis. Cervical lordosis may occur as the result of compensation for an increase in the thoracic kyphosis.

## Lumbar Lordosis

An increased lumbar lordosis, frequently referred to as *sway back,* is generally a postural problem usually involving weakened abdominal muscles and a slouched posture. It will increase with obesity as the abdomen enlarges and normally during pregnancy. Wearing high-heel shoes will cause an increase in the lumbar lordosis.

As the curvature increases, the weight of the body from above is shifted off the T12–L1 transitional vertebrae and the sacral base. More stress is placed on the muscles for support, and thus lordosis becomes a cause of low back pain.

## Lumbar Flattening

Flattening of the lumbar lordosis is often caused by muscle spasm and may be a part of a herniated disc syndrome. The flattening associated with a herniated disc generally is seen with a listing of the patient away from the side toward which the disc has herniated. The flattening may also be compensatory to flattening of the kyphosis in the thoracic spine.

## ■ SCOLIOSIS

Scoliosis is a lateral curvature of the spine, occurring in the coronal plane. Scoliosis may be either:

1. Structural
2. Functional

Structural scoliosis is discussed in Section IV, Chapter 45. Functional scoliosis is usually a correctible problem that may be due to tense muscles on one side of the body, causing a "bowstring" effect on the spine. A frequent cause in the "normal" population is *short leg syndrome.*

## Short Leg Syndrome

Short leg syndrome occurs when one leg is shorter or longer than the other. The frequency of the occurrence of a short leg is higher in persons with low back pain than in persons without low back pain, and the patients tend to be older.

## Diagnosis

### History

The patient commonly reports bending over and feeling pain in the back, or feeling as though the back had locked. He may notice that he wears out one shoe faster than the other or that one pant leg or shirtsleeve seems longer than the other.

Screening for scoliosis is often required by the school system and may allow early recognition of a postural problem.

### Physical Examination

Scoliosis is often discovered during a routine physical examination. It must be determined if the scoliosis is caused by a short leg (functional) or is developmental in origin (structural). A structural examination for asymmetry may yield important clues to solving the problem. A difference in leg length is estimated by measuring with a tape measure from the anterior superior iliac spine to the medial malleolus of each leg. This method is less accurate than a standing postural x-ray.

### Radiologic Assessment

Once the diagnosis of short leg syndrome is suspected, the patient may be further evaluated with standing postural radiographs of the low back and femoral heads. These films are made with the patient standing erect, toes pointing forward, and the feet approximately 6 inches apart. Equilibrium must be maintained as much as possible. A level floor is essential.

The iliac crests, sacral base, and femoral heads are measured bilaterally. This may be performed with use of a specially gridded film or by use of a T-square to draw horizontal lines. A standard vertical line can be established by using radio-opaque fishing line and a plumb or by placing a carpenter's level on the x-ray film cartridge. The most important measurement is the sacral base (Fig. 58-2).

Normally, the lumbar spine is convex on the side of the short leg as the spine side-bends back toward the midline. Occasionally, a compensatory curve will develop in the thoracic spine in the opposite direction from that in the lumbar spine. Sacral base leveling with straightening of the spinal curvature is the goal of therapy.

Various types of unleveling of the femoral heads and sacral base may be found as follows:

1. Parallel unleveling: sacral base unleveling equal and on the same side as the low femoral head.
2. Femoral head unleveling greater than sacral base unleveling: both low on the same side.
3. Sacral base unleveling greater than femoral head unleveling: both low on the same side.
4. Femoral head unleveling without sacral tilt
5. Sacral base tilt without a short leg.

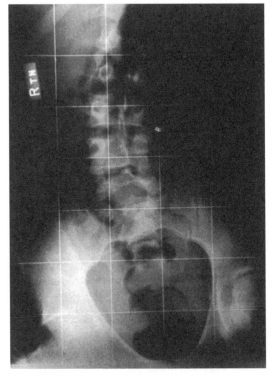

■ **FIG. 58-2** Postural radiograph showing short right leg with marked sacral base unleveling. Note spinal convexity on the side of the short leg.

6. Sacral base low on one side with short leg on the opposite side.
7. Sacral base low on one side, lumbar spine convex on the side of the short leg.

## Physical Manifestations

A short leg has numerous effects on the body. Usually, the sacral base tilts toward the side of the short leg. The iliac crest is generally low on the short leg side. Occasionally, the innominate on the shorter side will rotate forward or the opposite side posteriorly as a means of compensating for the leg length discrepancy. The lumbar spine develops a convexity toward the side of the short leg, and once the problem has existed for sufficient time, a compensatory curve will develop in the thoracic spine. The shoulder will be low on one side, depending on whether a secondary thoracic curve is present: the scapula will be low on the same side as the shoulder. The cervical angle will be more acute as the head tilts toward the midline to keep the eyes level.

Asymmetric tensions are palpable in the paravertebral muscles. The muscles on the side of the convexity are stretched and those on the side of the concavity are shortened. There is usually a gapping of the medial knee compartment on the side of the longer leg. Stress is also created in the hip and ankle joints of the longer leg.

## Treatment

1. Osteopathic manipulative treatment:
   a. Relaxes and stretches contracted muscles
   b. Corrects somatic dysfunctions
   c. Increases mobility
   d. Normalizes tissues
2. Exercises: Exercises should be designed to stretch and tone the asymmetric muscles.
3. Lift therapy: A lift is placed in the heel of the shoe on the side of the short leg lifts the leg, pelvis, and sacrum to correct the lateral imbalance. The lift should be made of a firm, comfortable substance such as leather, cork, or hard rubber. Foam rubber is not satisfactory because it flattens during weight-bearing and the prescribed height is not maintained.

When a heel lift is prescribed, the patient must be informed of the need to wear the lift at all times when walking or standing. Once he is out of bed for the day, he must wear shoes or slippers with the lift in place. The strain on the back is too great if the lift is worn only occasionally. The only exception is when walking on sand, where the surface is soft and giving and already uneven.

When considering whether to prescribe a heel lift, several factors must be considered:

1. **Sacral base unleveling:** determined by radiographic assessment. Sacral base unleveling rather than femoral head heights has been deemed most significant. Most osteopathic physicians are of the opinion that anything more than one quarter of an inch should be lifted. In certain cases, even an eighth of an inch should be treated.
2. **Length of time present:** The period may be short, as in the case of a fractured lower extremity, or longer, as in the case of a developmental shortening.
3. **Amount of compensation:** includes such factors as the degree of side-bending and rotation of the spine, wedging of the vertebrae, and alteration of facets. Generally, the longer the condition has been present, the more compensation will have occurred.

David Heilig developed a formula useful for determining the height of the lift to be used:

$$\text{Lift height} = \frac{\text{Sacral base unleveling}}{\text{Duration} + \text{Compensation}}$$

$$L = \frac{SBU}{D + C}$$

Duration is graded on a scale of 1 to 3:

1 = 1–10 years
2 = 10–30 years
3 = more than 30 years

Compensation is graded on a scale of 0 to 2:

0 = side-bending without rotation
1 = rotation toward the convexity
2 = wedging, alteration of facets

Except in the very young or in cases of acute shortening, it is best to begin lift therapy by adding half the total difference in leg length. In older persons or in cases of greater compensation, it is best to start with no more than one-eighth of an inch. The lift is slowly increased over time, with manipulative treatment used to aid in adaptation to the lift. After the lift has been worn for a period of time and the patient is comfortable with it, the postural x-ray study should be repeated with the lift in place to determine if the correction is adequate.

If the lift is more than one-quarter of an inch in thickness, it will have to be put on the outside of the heel of the shoe. Lifts may also be added as part of an orthotic device. If the total lift required is greater than one-half of an inch, half the height of the heel lift will have to be added to the sole of the shoe as well.

Before adding a lift to the patient's shoe, it is important to ascertain that the shortening of the leg is not caused by pronation of one foot. In this case, an orthotic device to correct the pronation will probably correct the shortening of the leg.

Correcting a shortened extremity will correct many other postural problems, because it is the key to many musculoskeletal abnormalities. Besides correction of the postural deficits mentioned in the structural evaluation, a whole shift of body weight will occur. The pelvis will shift back to the midline, realigning the center of gravity and the weight-bearing portions of the body. The new position will affect the biomechanics of the entire musculoskeletal system.

## REFERENCES

Adams RD, Victor M. *Principles of Neurology.* New York: McGraw-Hill, 1985.

Basmajian JV. *Muscles Alive, 4th ed.* Baltimore: Williams & Wilkins, 1987.

Bickerstaff RE. Gait. *Neurological Examination in Clinical Practice, 2nd ed.* Oxford: Blackwell Scientific Publications, 1968.

Cailliet R. *Foot and Ankle Pain.* Philadelphia: F.A. Davis, 1968.

Cailliet R. *Low Back Pain Syndrome,* 3rd ed. Philadelphia: F.A. Davis, 1981.

Forssberg H, Grillner S, Rossignol S. Phasic gain control of reflexes from the dorsum of the paw during spinal locomotion. *Brain Res* 1977;132:121–139.

Henszinger RN. Limp. *Pediatr Clin North Am* 1977;24: 723–730.

Hoppenfeld S. *Physical Examination of the Spine and Extremities.* New York: Appleton-Century-Crofts, 1976.

Illingworth CM. 128 limping children with no fracture, sprain, or obvious cause. *Clin Pediatr* 1978;17:139–142.

Kappler RE. Role of psoas mechanism in low-back complaints. *J Am Osteopath Assoc* 1973;72:794–801.

Kappler RE. Postural balance and motion patterns. *J Am Osteopath Assoc* 1982;81:598–606.

Mann RA, Hagy JL, White V, et al. The initiation of gait. *J Bone Joint Surg* [Am] 1979;61:232–239.

Merrifield HH. Female gait patterns in shoes with different heel heights. *Ergonomics* 1971;14:411–417.

Michelle AA. *Iliopsoas.* St. Louis: Charles C Thomas, 1962.

Mitchell FL. *Structural pelvic function.* Academy of Applied Osteopathy. 1965 Year Book, vol II. Colorado Springs, CO: Academy of Applied Osteopathy, 1965.

Morris JM. Biomechanics of the foot and ankle. *Clin Orthop* 1977;122:10–17.

Murray MP, Sepoc SB, Gardner GM, et al. Walking patterns of men with parkinsonism. *Am J Phys Med* 1978;57: 278–294.

Rasch PJ, Burke RK. *Kinesiology and Applied Anatomy, 6th ed.* Philadelphia: Lea & Febiger, 1978.

Saunders JB, Inman VT, Eberhart HD. The major determinants in normal and pathological gait. *J Bone Joint Surg* [Am] 1953;35:543–558.

Schwartz RP, Heath AL, Misiek W, et al. *Kinetics of Human Gait.* Rochester, NY: University of Rochester Medical Society, 1933.

Simon RB. A neurologic screening exam in six minutes. *Diagnosis* 1979;1:44–58.

Smidt GL. Methods of studying gait. *Phys Ther* 1974;54: 13–17.

Soderberg GL, Dostal WF. Electromyographic study of three parts of the gluteus medius muscle during functional activities. *Phys Ther* 1978;58:691–696.

Wells KF, Luttgens K. *Kinesiology, 6th ed.* Philadelphia: W.B. Saunders, 1976.

Winter DA, Robertson DGE. Joint torque and energy patterns in normal gait. *Biol Cybernet* 1978;29:137–142.

Zarrugh MY, Radcliff CW. Computer generation of human gait kinematics. *J Biomech* 1979;12:99–111.

Zohn DA, Mennell JMcM. *Musculoskeletal Pain: Diagnosis and Physical Treatment.* Boston: Little, Brown, 1987.

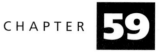

# Evaluation of the Pelvis

*Dennis J. Dowling*

The diagnosis of pelvic dysfunction concentrates on two aspects of the innominate: the ilium and the pubic components. Generally, the landmarks of the posterior superior iliac spine (PSIS), anterior superior iliac spine (ASIS), pubic rami, and their other relative structures can give some static findings as to the diagnosis. As with other regions of the body, motion testing indicates the side of the dysfunction.

## ■ STATIC EXAMINATION

### Patient Standing (Fig. 59-1)

1. **Patient position**: standing, barefoot, with the feet parallel and 6 to 8 inches apart.
2. **Physician position**: kneeling or squatting behind the patient with his eyes approximately at the level of the iliac crests and the posterior superior iliac spines (PSIS).
3. **Technique**:
   a. **Iliac crests**: The physician places his hands on the patient's iliac crests and evaluates the symmetry of heights of the two crests.
      (1) The physician should begin by placing the edges of his index fingers lateral and below the actual iliac crests.
      (2) Then the physician slides these fingers upward and medially to come into contact with the superior aspect of the iliac crests.
      (3) A false appreciation of height may occur if the crests are approached from above as skin, muscle, and fat may intervene.

   b. **Posterior superior iliac spines (PSIS)**: A landmark for the PSIS is usually visible as a skin dimple indicating the location of attachment of the deep fascia. The physician places his thumbs at these locations, hooks his thumbs beneath the PSIS, and compares heights.
   c. **Gluteal folds**: The physician directly observes these folds, which delineate the lower border of the gluteus maximus muscle, and compares heights.
      (1) A flatter, higher fold may indicate an anterior rotation of the innominate on the same side.
      (2) A more defined, lower fold may indicate a posterior rotation of the innominate on the same side.
      (3) When the configuration of the buttocks are the same but there is a difference in the height of the folds, then there is a possibility of a superior or inferior shear or the influence of a leg length discrepancy.
      (4) A variation in height may indicate the influence of habitual patterns, postural imbalances, leg length differences, neurological dysfunction, or other factors.
   d. **Greater trochanters**: The physician directly palpates these outermost components of the femurs and compares heights. A variation in height may indicate leg length differences, asymmetrical genu varus or valgus, asymmetrical calcaneal varus or valgus, asymmetrical plantar arch patterns, or other components.

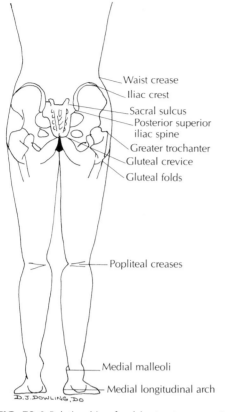

Waist crease
Iliac crest
Sacral sulcus
Posterior superior iliac spine
Greater trochanter
Gluteal crevice
Gluteal folds

Popliteal creases

Medial malleoli
Medial longitudinal arch

D.J.DOWLING,DO

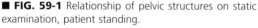

■ **FIG. 59-1** Relationship of pelvic structures on static examination, patient standing.

e. **Ischial tuberosities**: The physician directly palpates these lowermost components of the innominates near the gluteal folds and compares heights.
   (1) A higher ischial tuberosity may indicate an anterior rotation or superior shear of the innominate on the same side.
   (2) A lower ischial tuberosity may indicate a posterior rotation or inferior shear of the innominate on the same side.
   f. A variation in height may indicate leg length differences, asymmetrical genu varus or valgus, asymmetrical calcaneal varus or valgus, asymmetrical plantar arch patterns, or other components.
2. **Other findings**: The physician may also examine asymmetry of the popliteal creases, the medial malleoli, and the medial longitudinal arches of the feet.

## ■ MOTION TESTING (STANDING FLEXION TEST)

### Patient Standing

1. **Patient position**: standing, barefoot, with the feet parallel and 6 to 8 inches apart.
2. **Physician position**: kneeling or squatting behind the patient with his eyes approximately at the level of the iliac crests and the posterior superior iliac spines (PSIS).
3. **Technique**:
   a. The physician places his thumbs at the inferior aspect of the PSIS bilaterally.
   b. The patient is directed to bend forward from the waist and reach with his hands toward his toes without bending his knees (Fig. 59-2). A more sensitive variation that has been used and that has been effective is to have the patient rise up halfway, the physician repositions his thumbs beneath the PSIS bilaterally, and then have the patient attempt to bend downwards again.
   c. As the patient is flexing forward, the physician observes the movement of the PSIS as the ilium moves on the sacrum.
   d. Flexion of the spine carries the base of the sacrum anteriorly and motion is introduced into the sacroiliac joint. A certain amount of play occurs before the movement of the sacrum carries the ilium into anterior rotation, which in turn causes the PSIS to rise superiorly.
   e. Restriction on one side causes the iliosacral joint to lock prematurely on that side,

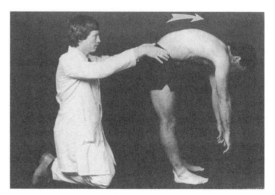

■ **FIG. 59-2** Static examination, standing flexion test.

causing the PSIS to elevate sooner and probably farther than the PSIS on the other side. This is considered a positive test result. Generally, if there is a discrepancy between the side that moves first and that which moves furthest, the preference is to go with the side that moves first.

f. A positive test indicates iliosacral somatic dysfunction on the ipsilateral side.

2. **Variations:**
   a. The PSIS may initially be at different heights. Asymmetry may indicate somatic dysfunction but does not determine which side is involved.
   b. Placement of a wooden shim under the foot on the same side as the lower PSIS, until both of the PSIS are at the same level, may facilitate diagnosis if the physician is distracted by the asymmetry. Although some sources indicate that a shim be placed beneath a foot if there is initial asymmetry in PSIS heights, there is no indication that this increases the sensitivity or specificity of the test.
   c. Proceed with test as outlined.

### ■ MOTION TESTING (STORK TEST)

1. **Patient position:** standing, barefoot, with the feet parallel and 6 to 8 inches apart.
2. **Physician position:** kneeling or squatting behind the patient with his eyes approximately at the level of the iliac crests and the posterior superior iliac spines (PSIS).
3. **Technique:**
   a. The physician places his thumb on the side to be tested at the inferior aspect of the PSIS on the side to be tested. The thumb of the other hand is placed on the sacral crest and the rest of the hand is on the iliac crest of the nonexamined side.
   b. The patient is directed to flex the hip and knee and raise the foot on the side to be tested. The other stance leg remains positioned and the physician's hands can aid in steadying the patient.
   c. The physician notes the change in position of the PSIS relative to the monitored location of the thumb at the sacral crest.
   d. The patient is directed to lower his leg, the physician repositions his hands to assess the other side, and the patient raises the other leg
   e. Motion of the PSIS relative to the sacrum in an inferior direction is normal. Restriction or superior motion of the PSIS is positive for a same-sided iliac restriction. Comparison can also be made as to the direction and amount of motion between the testing of the two sides.

### ■ STATIC EXAMINATION

1. **Patient position:** supine.
2. **Physician position:** varies according to the region examined.
3. **Technique:**
   a. **Pubic tubercles**
      (1) The pubic tubercles are located on the anterior superior aspects of the pubic bones (Fig.59-4). The pubic symphysis is located medially.
      (2) The patient is more comfortable if he voids before the examination.
      (3) The physician places the palm of one hand flat on the patient's lower abdomen.
      (4) The physician gently slides this hand downward until the pubic bones are located.
      (5) The tubercle positions are located bilaterally by placing the pads of the index fingers gently on the cephalad aspect.
      (6) The physician brings his eyes directly over the pubic region and evaluates the relative position of his index fingers relative to each other.
      (7) Asymmetry of position indicates a pubic dysfunction. The diagnosis is

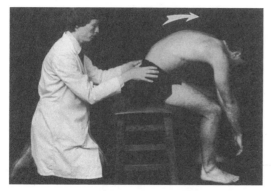

■ **FIG. 59-3** Motion testing, seated flexion test.

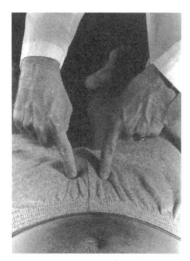

■ **FIG. 59-4** Location of pubic tubercles.

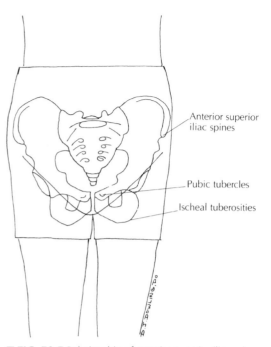

■ **FIG. 59-5** Relationship of anterior superior iliac spines to other pelvic structures.

named according to the side on which the standing flexion test is positive and according to the relative position of the pubic tubercle involved.

b. **Anterior superior iliac spines (ASIS)**
   (1) The ASIS is a bony protuberance on the anterior portion of the ilium (Fig. 59-5).
   (2) The physician places the pads of his thumbs under the ASIS bilaterally.
   (3) With his eyes directly over the pelvic region, the physician evaluates the relative position of the ASIS (superior/inferior, ventral/dorsal) to each other.
   (4) Asymmetry of position may indicate ilial dysfunction. The diagnosis is named according to the side on which the standing flexion test is positive

c. **Medial malleoli**
   (1) The physician stands at the foot of the table and places his thumbs under the distal edges (styloid processes) of the medial malleoli (Fig. 59-6).
   (2) The physician evaluates the relative positions of the malleoli (caudal/cephalad).
   (3) The side of the positive standing flexion test determines the side of the dysfunction.
      a. A malleolus that is more cephalad on the side of the positive standing

flexion test may indicate a shorter leg, a superior innominate shear, or a posteriorly rotated ilium on that side.
      b. A malleolus that is more pedad on the side of the positive standing flexion test may indicate a longer

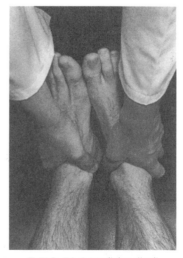

■ **FIG. 59-6** Medial malleoli.

leg, an inferior innominate shear, or an anteriorly rotated ilium on that side.

## ■ MOTION TESTING

1. **Patient position**: supine
2. **Physician position**: The physician stands on the side of the table, facing toward the patient's head.
3. **Innominate/ilial/pelvic rocking**
   a. The physician places his thenar and hypothenar eminences against the ASIS on either side.
   b. A gentle but firm rocking motion against the ASIS is directed along planes that are approximately para-sagittal (Fig. 59-7). Each ASIS should be examined alternately
   c. The physician allows the ilia to recoil anteriorly against gentle pressure.
   d. Resistance to motion in posterior rocking or in slow and resistant recoil indicates the side and direction of restriction. Often a clue of an inferior or superior ASIS is present. An inferior ASIS on one side may indicate an anteriorly rotated ilium on that side or a posterior rotation on the opposite side. Ease of motion in anterior and posterior directions is noted as the innominates are rocked.
   e. The diagnosis is made by noting the resistance to motion.

4. **Supine iliosacral test or dynamic leg lengthening or shortening test**
   a. The physician stands towards the foot of the table initially.
   b. The patient flexes both of his knees and places his feet flat on the table.
   c. The patient elevates his buttocks off the table then lowers them back onto the table.
   d. The physician extends the patient's legs to their full length and notes the relative position of the medial malleoli.
   e. The physician then:
      (1) Fully flexes one of the patient's hips and knees.
      (2) Externally rotates and abducts the hip (Fig. 59-8).
      (3) Firmly extends the patient's leg while maintaining the external rotation.
      (4) Compares the change in position of the ipsilateral medial malleolus relative to its original position and to the other side.
      (5) Fully flexes the ipsilateral hip and knee.
      (6) Internally rotates and adducts the hip (Fig. 59-9).
      (7) Firmly extends the patient's leg while maintaining the internal rotation.
      (8) Compares the change in position of the ipsilateral medial malleolus rela-

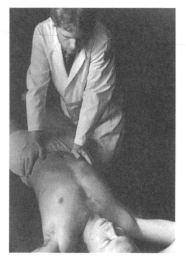

■ **FIG. 59-7** Innominate rocking.

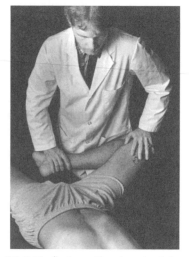

■ **FIG. 59-8** Hip flexion with external rotation, abduction, and extension of the hip and knee.

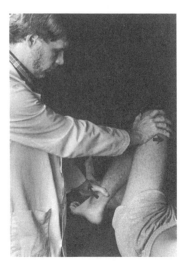

**■ FIG. 59-9** Hip flexion with internal rotation, abduction, and extension of the hip and knee.

tive to its original position and to the other side.

(9) Repeats the procedure for the other leg.

f. The physician notes the total excursion each medial malleolus appeared to have undergone during the procedure

g. A smaller amplitude of malleolar excursion on one side indicates dysfunction of the iliosacral joint on that side.

h. Note: The physician should flex both sides equally. Inequality of motion testing may produce erroneous results.

i. The action of flexion, along with internal or external rotation, changes the orientation of the ilium relative to the sacrum if there is no restriction. The subsequent extension of the leg maintains this change in relationship. If the iliosacral joint is restricted, hip flexion induces posterior rotation of the ilium, which causes posterior movement of the sacral base. Little or no change occurs at the joint, as indicated by the small total excursion of the medial malleolus.

## ■ STATIC EXAMINATION—PATIENT PRONE

1. **Patient position**: prone.
2. **Physician position**: varies according to the region examined

3. **Posterior superior iliac spines**
   a. The physician stands at the side of the table and faces toward the patient's head.
   b. The physician places his thumbs on the inferior slope of each PSIS and, viewing them directly from above, notes their relative orientation (superior/inferior, ventral/dorsal).
   c. The finding is named according to the side on which the standing flexion test is positive.

4. **Sacral sulci**
   a. The physician stands at the side of the table and faces toward the patient's head.
   b. The physician places his thumbs on each PSIS.
   c. The physician hooks his thumbs medially along the PSIS and brings his pads into the sacral sulci bilaterally (Fig.59-10).
   d. The physician evaluates the relative depth of the sulci by two means:
      (1) By palpating the depth of each sulcus by thumb position.
      (2) By lowering his eyes to the level of the sulci for visual evaluation of depth.

5. **Ischial tuberosities**
   a. The physician directly palpates these lowermost components of the innominates near the gluteal folds and compares heights.
      (1) A cephalad ischial tuberosity may indicate an anterior rotation or superior shear of the innominate on the same side.

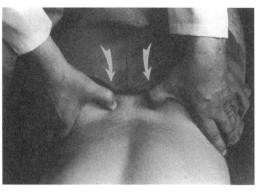

**■ FIG. 59-10** Position for evaluating sacral sulci.

(2) A pedad ischial tuberosity may indicate a posterior rotation or inferior shear of the innominate on the same side.

## ■ INTERPRETATION

The tests for pelvic dysfunctions have fair specificity and variable sensitivity. The presence of a sacral dysfunction can obscure or exaggerate the findings for pelvic dysfunction. The standing flexion test can be falsely positive if there is an overwhelmingly positive seated flexion test and sacroiliac dysfunction. The depth of the sacral sulcus is not specific to pelvic dysfunction because a deep sulcus can also indicate a forward sacral torsion with the axis opposite to the deep sulcus, a unilateral sacral shear, as well as a posteriorly rotated ilium on the same side. A shallow sulcus can also indicate sacral dysfunction in addition to an anterior rotated ilium on that side.

The presence of asymmetrical positioning of the ASIS, PSIS, ischial tuberosities, and pubic rami indicate the very probable presence of some sort of pelvic dysfunction. One or more positive findings with the motion tests can confirm as well as indicate the side of the dysfunction. Determining the diagnosis depends to a great extent on understanding the basic "wobbly wheel" construction of the pelvic bones at the iliosacral joints. The pelvic bones are wheel-like, with an eccentric axle or axis at the superior–posterior portion of the wheel. The ASIS is anterior and the PSIS is posterior to this axis. Anterior rotation of the ilium results in the ASIS going downward and the PSIS on the same side moving upward. Posterior rotation of the ilium results in the direct opposite findings of the ASIS and PSIS. The acetabulum, because it is on the anterior–inferior portion of the innominate, typically follows the position of the ASIS. An inferior ASIS will accompany an inferior acetabulum. This will in turn appear to lengthen the leg. A superior ASIS will likewise raise and appear to shorten the same-sided leg. The actual measurement at the medial malleoli may vary. A posterior rotation of the ilium may be an adaptation to a same-sided longer leg and the compensation may be excessive, adequate, or inadequate. The anteriorly rotated ilium with its superior PSIS and inferior ASIS may compensate fully for a short leg, fail to approximate the medial malleoli, or overcompensate. These anterior and posterior innominate motions occur naturally as part of the gait cycle. However, when there is a locking of the iliosacral joint, the positioning persists and there is a preferential direction of pelvic movement, as indicated by the positive test of laterality.

The anterior and posterior rotations are by

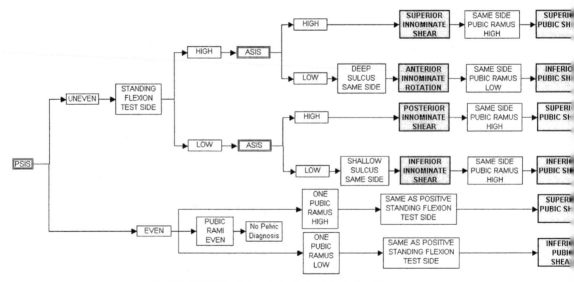

■ **FIG. 59-11** Typical and atypical pelvic dysfunctions.

# TABLE 59-1 TYPICAL AND ATYPICAL PELVIC DYSFUNCTIONS

| TESTS | | | STATIC FINDINGS | | | | | | DIAGNOSIS |
|---|---|---|---|---|---|---|---|---|---|
| Standing Flexion | Stork Test | Iliosacral Rock | ASIS Higher | ASIS Lower | Deep Sulcus | PSIS Higher | PSIS Lower | Pubic Rumus | |
| Right | Right | Right | Right | Left | Right | Left | Right | | Right posteriorly rotated innominate |
| Left | Left | Left | Left | Right | Left | Right | Left | | Left posteriorly rotated innominate |
| Right | Right | Right | Left | Right | Left | Right | Left | | Right anteriorly rotated innominate |
| Left | Left | Left | Right | Left | Right | Left | Right | | Left anteriorly rotated innominate |
| Right | Right | Right | Right | Left | | Right | Left | | Right superior shear |
| Left | Left | Left | Left | Right | | Left | Right | | Left superior shear |
| Right | Right | Right | Left | Right | | Left | Right | | Right inferior shear |
| Left | Left | Left | Right | Left | | Right | Left | | Left inferior shear |
| Right | | | | | | | | Right higher | Right superior pubic shear |
| Left | | | | | | | | Left higher | Left superior pubic shear |
| Right | | | | | | | | Right lower | Right inferior pubic shear |
| Left | | | | | | | | Left lower | Left superior pubic shear |

far the most common type of iliosacral dysfunctions. There is also the possibility of upslipped (superior innominate shear) and downslipped (inferior innominate shear). These will also be named as per the findings of the motion tests. The ASIS and PSIS will be oriented in the same direction in these dysfunctions as opposed to in opposite directions of the iliac rotations. A superior ASIS and PSIS indicates a superior shear. A PSIS and ASIS that are inferior indicate an inferior innominate shear. The mechanism of injury may give some clue as to the expected finding. A hard landing onto a straightened leg or falling on a buttock could cause a superior shear. A situation whereby the leg is suddenly tugged or dragged may lead to an inferior shear.

Other fairly rare diagnoses of inflare and outflare pelvic bones may also be more dependent on the clinical cause of the condition. Pregnancy, with its many physical changes, may cause an enlargement that persists and limits functioning. Compression from a trauma may cause the ASIS on both sides to approximate and remain abnormally so.

Pubic dysfunctions are likewise named for the positive motion tests. The pubic ramus typically follows the position of the ASIS, but this is not always the case. The plasticity of bone may allow for some warping, opposite to the ASIS finding. Before drawing a conclusion, examination must be performed. A superior pubic shear and an inferior pubic shear may occur in the expected ASIS direction. They can be opposite. There are also torsions possible, as well as adducted and abducted pubes. Childbirth, wherein cartilage is softened by relaxin, is probably the greatest predisposing factor for abducted pubic dysfunction. Adducted pubes may be trauma or rebound related. Sometimes the only indications that there is a dysfunction when the pubic rami appear symmetrical are the symptoms of the patient. Aseptic cystitis, pubic pain, prostatitis, pelvic paresthesias, enuresis, or other symptoms may also be better indicators of pubic dysfunction.

Figure 59-11 and Table 59-1 demonstrate the typical and atypical pelvic dysfunctions.

## REFERENCES

Bourdilion JF. A torsion free approach to the pelvis. *Manual Med* 1987;3:20–23.

DiGiovanna EL. Schiowitz S. *An Osteopathic Approach to Diagnosis and Treatment, 2nd ed.* Philadelphia: Lippincott-Raven, 1997.

Dowling DJ. *An Illustrated Guide to OMT of the Neck and Trunk.* Self-published, 1985.

Fryette HH. *Principles of Osteopathic Technique.* Carmel, CA: Academy of Applied Osteopathy, 1959.

Greenman PE. Innominate shear dysfunction in the sacroiliac syndrome. *Manual Med* 1986;2:114–121.

Kapandji IA. *The Physiology of the Joints, vol. III. The Trunk and Vertebral Column.* New York: Churchill Livingstone, 1974.

Kappler R. Lecture notes. Chicago: College of Osteopathic Medicine, 1975.

Kennedy H. Unilateral sacroiliac dysfunction.1975 Yearbook of Selected Osteopathic Papers. In: Hewitt R, ed. Colorado Springs: American Academy of Osteopathy, 1975.

Kidd R. Pain localization with the innominate upslip dysfunction. *Manual Med* 1988;3:103–105.

Larson NJ. Physiologic movement of the sacrum. Read before the Chicago College of Osteopathic Medicine, February 1984.

Mitchell FL. *Structural pelvic function. 1965 Year Book of Selected Osteopathic Papers, vol. II.* In: Barnes M, ed. Carmel, CA: Academy of Applied Osteopathy, 1965:178–199.

Mitchell FL Jr, Moran PS, Pruzzo NT. *An Evaluation and Treatment Manual of Osteopathic Muscle Energy Procedures.* Valley Park, MO: Mitchell, Moran, and Pruzzo Associates, 1979.

Mitchell FL Jr, Mitchell PGK. *The Muscle Energy Manual, volume III: Evaluation and Treatment of the Pelvis and Sacrum.* East Lansing, MI: MET Press, 1999.

Moore KL. *Clinically Oriented Anatomy.* Baltimore: Williams & Wilkins, 1980.

Northup TL. Sacroiliac lesions primary & secondary. *Academy of Applied Osteopathy Year Book, 1943–1944.* Ann Arbor: Academy of Applied Osteopathy, 1943:53–54.

Schwab WA. Principles of manipulative treatment: The low back problems. *Academy of Applied Osteopathy 1965 Yearbook of Selected Osteopathic Papers, vol. II.* In: Barnes M, ed. Carmel, CA: Academy of Applied Osteopathy, 1965: 65–69.

Sutherland WG. *The Cranial Bowl.* Mankato, MN: Free Press, 1936.

Warwick R, Williams PL. *Gray's Anatomy*, 35th British Edition. Philadelphia: W.B. Saunders, 1973.

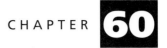
# Evaluation of the Sacrum

*Dennis J. Dowling*

The diagnosis of sacral dysfunction may appear to be very complex. However, with attention to the combined findings of positional and motion examination, it is possible to discern a specific diagnosis. The system that is used is based on the Mitchell model and not on the Strachan sacral model. Both systems are valid, but the more specific application of muscle energy technique requires the findings described.

## ■ STATIC EXAMINATION

### Patient Prone (Fig. 60-1)

1. **Patient position**: prone.
2. **Physician position**: varies according to the region examined
3. **Sacral sulci**
   a. The physician stands at the side of the table and faces toward the patient's head.
   b. The physician places his thumbs on each PSIS.
   c. The physician hooks his thumbs medially along the PSIS and brings his finger pads into the sacral sulci bilaterally (Fig.60-2).
   d. The physician evaluates the relative depth of the sulci by two means:
      (1) By palpating the depth of each sulcus by thumb position.
      (2) By lowering his eyes to the level of the sulci for visual evaluation of depth.
3. **Sacral crest**
   a. The physician stands at the side of the table and faces the patient.
   b. The physician locates each PSIS.
   c. Drawing a line between the PSIS of each

ilium and then halving the distance will give the location of the sacral crest.
   d. The crest will be a series of bumps and will lead to the sacral hiatus.
   e. An absence of a crest portion may indicate a spina bifida. Deviations or asymmetries may indicate the presence of somatic dysfunction or congenital malformations.
4. **Sacral Hiatus and Sacral Cornu**
   a. The sacral hiatus is frequently located in the gluteal crevice and is a depression at the end of the sacral crest.
   b. It may be barely wide enough for the placement of the tip of the fifth finger
   c. The sacral cornu, slight bumps, are located to either side of the hiatus and are oriented towards the patient's coccyx
   d. The sacral hiatus is a site of injecting anesthetic to administer a "saddle" block.
4. **Inferior lateral angles**
   a. The inferior lateral angles are bony protuberances located lateral to the sacral hiatus and sacral cornu. They outline the inferior lateral aspect of the sacrum and represent what is the fusion of the transverse processes of S4 and S5.
   b. The physician may locate the inferior lateral angles by palpating down the length of the sacral crest to the hiatus and then moving his thumbs laterally to the inferior lateral angles (Fig. 60-3). Alternatively, palpating the lateral edges of the sacrum and then locating the angle where the edge is more directed medially can locate the ILA.

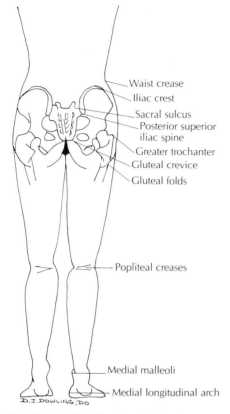

Waist crease
Iliac crest
Sacral sulcus
Posterior superior
iliac spine
Greater trochanter
Gluteal crevice
Gluteal folds

Popliteal creases

Medial malleoli
Medial longitudinal arch

D.J.DOWLING,DO

■ **FIG. 60-1** Relationship of pelvic structures on static examination, patient standing.

c. The position of the inferior lateral angles may be evaluated in two orientations:

(1) Posterior/anterior

The physician places his thumbs on the surface of the sacrum at posterior aspects of the ILAs

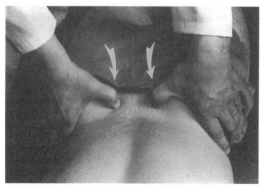

■ **FIG. 60-2** Position for evaluating sacral sulci.

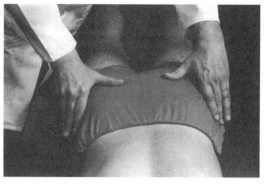

■ **FIG. 60-3** Positioning for evaluating inferior lateral angles.

He lowers his eyes to the level of the sacrum to note if there is asymmetry and if one side is more posterior than the other.

The relative positions of inferior lateral angles are described as anterior or posterior

(2) Superior/inferior

The physician places his thumbs along the lower edges of the inferior lateral angles.

He views the sacrum from above.

The positions are described as superior or inferior.

Note: Because of sacral structure and the types of movement available, the inferior lateral angles exhibit pairing in these positions: posterior/inferior and anterior/superior are coupled positions.

5. Coccyx
   a. The coccyx is located in the gluteal crevice.
   b. The coccygeal cornu are oriented in an opposite direction to the sacral cornu.
   c. The coccyx can be oriented backwards or forwards. These positions may be natural, congenital, or the result of trauma. Trauma can also cause a twisting that can place a strain on the ligaments and muscles of the region.
   d. Coccygodynia is a painful condition that results most commonly from injury. It can be aggravated by pressure, especially sitting.
6. Observation and palpation
   a. The presence of a patch of hair or "faun's beard" may indicate the presence of a

spina bifida, sacralization, or other congenital malformation.

b. Sacral lipomas are fairly common and may be of no clinical significance.

c. Skin changes (café au lait, hemangiomas, etc.) may indicate congenital malformations of the sacrum.

## ■ MOTION TESTING (SEATED FLEXION TEST)

### Patient Seated–Seated Flexion Test

1. **Patient position**: seated on a stool, both feet flat on the floor and the arms resting comfortably on the thighs.
2. **Physician position**: kneeling or squatting behind the patient with his eyes at the level of the iliac crests.
3. **Technique**:
   a. The physician places his thumbs at the inferior aspect of the posterior superior iliac spine (PSIS) bilaterally.
   b. The patient is directed to bend forward from the waist and reach toward the floor (Fig. 60-4).
   c. As the patient bends forward, the physician observes the movement of the PSIS, indicating movement of the sacrum on the ilium.
   d. In the seated position, the innominate is initially locked in place via the ischial tuberosity resting upon the surface of the stool. The sacroiliac portion of the joint becomes involved as the sacrum engages the ilium, which rotates anteriorly with

sacral flexion, elevating the PSIS bilaterally.

e. Restriction on one side causes the sacroiliac joint to lock prematurely as compared to the non-restricted side. The ilium and PSIS begin and carry through excursion sooner and probably farther than on the contralateral side. This is considered a positive test result.

f. A positive test indicates sacroiliac somatic dysfunction on the ipsilateral side.

2. **Variations**:

An uneven PSIS level may be related to such factors as wallets, clothing restriction, twisting of the torso, or other influences. A magazine or book can be placed beneath the buttock on one side to make the initial positions of the PSIS more symmetrical.

## ■ MOTION TESTING (OTHER TESTS OF SACROILIAC JOINT DYSFUNCTION LATERALITY)

1. **Patient position**: prone.
2. **Physician position**: varies according to the region examined
3. **Sacral mobility** (Sacral rock test)
   a. The physician stands at the side of the table and faces toward the patient's head.
   b. The physician places his palms on the patient's inferior lateral angles and the fingertips at the sacral sulci (Fig. 60-5).

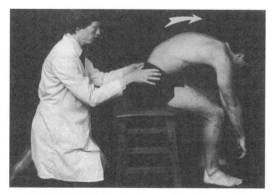

■ **FIG. 60-4** Motion testing—seated flexion test.

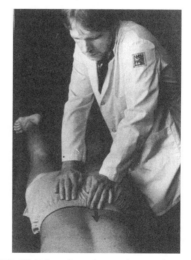

■ **FIG. 60-5** Sacral motion testing, patient prone.

c. The physician directs a force cephalad from the inferior lateral angles into the sacroiliac joint on the same side. Force should not be directed obliquely because this may give erroneous findings.

d. A positive test indicating dysfunction consists of a decrease in joint play on one or both sides and restriction of sacral motion.

4. **Spring test**

   a. The physician stands at the side of the table facing across the patient's body.

   b. The physician places his hands transversely across the patient's lumbar spine.

   c. Gentle pressure is exerted downward through the lumbar spine (Fig. 60-6).

   d. In a normal response, some play is transmitted through the spine. A positive test consists of a steel-like resistance to the exerted force. This indicates locking of the sacrum posteriorly with the fifth lumbar vertebral facets. A positive test indicates either a bilateral sacral extension or a backwards sacral torsion.

5. **Sacral mobility**—respiratory motion

   a. The physician stands at the side of the table facing across the table.

   b. The physician's cephalad hand is placed over the sacrum with the thenar and hypothenar eminences at the sacral base and the fingertips at the apex. The other hand is placed over the first hand in the opposite direction (fingertips above the sacral base). The physician should stand comfortably with elbows flexed (Fig. 60-7).

   c. The patient takes a deep breath. The sacral

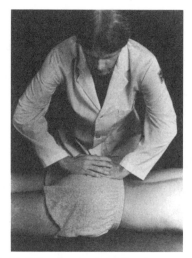

■ **FIG. 60-7** Test for sacral mobility during respiration.

base moves posteriorly during inhalation and anteriorly during exhalation.

   d. The physician monitors sacral motion during inhalation and exhalation, with attention to asymmetric movement.

6. **Sphinx test**

   a. The physician stands to one side of the patient and places his thumbs on the inferior lateral angles (ILAs) on both sides

   b. The physician should position himself so that his dominant eye is closer to the table and patient and is over the patient's midline and distal to the sacrum.

   c. The physician notes the relative position of the ILAs.

   d. The patient is instructed to raise his upper body onto his elbows and rest his chin on the palms of both hands.

   e. It may be necessary to increase the lumbar extension by having the patient put the palms of his hands on the table and then straighten his arms (Fig. 60-8).

   f. Asymmetrical positioning of the ILAs that is maintained or worsened indicates a backward sacral torsion. With a forward sacral torsion, the asymmetry lessens or disappears.

## ■ MOTION TESTING—L5 DIAGNOSIS

The findings for L5 affect the specific diagnosis of a sacral dysfunction. Patient and physician positions vary as to the test applied.

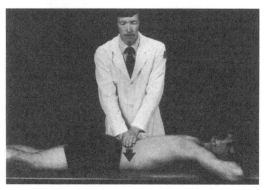

■ **FIG. 60-6** Spring test, patient prone.

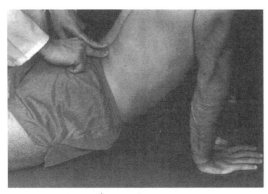

■ **FIG. 60-8** Sphinx test.

1. **Rotoscoliosis testing**
   a. Flexion component
      (1) The patient sits with his feet either flat on the floor or supported on stool rungs.
      (2) The physician kneels or squats behind the patient with eyes at the approximate level of the lumbar region
      (3) The physician places his thumbs on the skin overlying the transverse processes of the L5 vertebra.
      (4) The physician notes the posterior transverse process.
      (5) The patient is instructed to bend forward slowly.
      (6) The physician notes the change that occurs in the relative position of the transverse processes:

   If the posterior transverse process becomes more so (increase in asymmetry), then flexion is the barrier. If the transverse processes become more symmetrical, then flexion is the freedom. The side-bending and rotation of the diagnosis is to the side of the posterior transverse process.

   b. Extension component
      (1) The patient lies prone.
      (2) The physician stands at the side of the table facing the patient's head with his dominant eye closer to the patient and over the L5 vertebra.
      (3) The physician places his thumbs on the skin overlying the transverse processes of the L5 vertebra.
      (4) The physician notes the posterior transverse process.
      (5) The patient is instructed to raise his upper body upwards from the table and either supports himself on his elbows or, if necessary, on his hands with his arms straight.
      (6) The physician notes the change that occurs in the relative position of the transverse processes.

If the posterior transverse process becomes more so (increase in asymmetry), then extension is the barrier. If the transverse processes become more symmetrical, then extension is the freedom. The sidebending and rotation of the diagnosis is to the side of the posterior transverse process.

**Motion Testing**
   a. The patient lies prone.
   b. The physician stands at the side of the table facing the patient's head with his dominant eye closer to the patient and over the L5 vertebra.
   c. The physician places his thumbs on the skin overlying the transverse processes of the L5 vertebra.
   d. The physician notes the posterior transverse process.
   e. The physician alternately presses the transverse processes anteriorly and notes freedom and resistance. A transverse process that resists anterior movement is rotated opposite to the direction introduced and freer in rotation on the side of the posterior transverse process.
   f. The physician alternately pushes the transverse processes toward the patient's head and notes freedom and resistance. A transverse process that resists cephalad movement is sidebent opposite to the direction introduced and freer in sidebending on the side of the posterior transverse process.
   g. The physician shifts his thumbs to the upper edges of the transverse processes and pushes both anteriorly and towards the patient's head and notes freedom and resistance. Resistance of this movement indicates flexion is a barrier and extension the freedom. Then the physician shifts his thumbs to the lower edges of the trans-

verse processes and pushes both anteriorly and toward the patient's sacrum and notes freedom and resistance. Resistance of this movement indicates extension is a barrier and flexion the freedom.

## ■ INTERPRETATION

Most of the tests for sacral dysfunctions have lower than optimum specificity and sensitivity. The presence of a concomitant pelvic dysfunction can obscure or exaggerate the findings for sacral dysfunction. The *seated flexion test* can be falsely positive if there is an overwhelmingly positive standing flexion test and iliosacral dysfunction. The depth of the sacral sulcus is not specific to sacral dysfunction. A deep sulcus can indicate a forward sacral torsion with the axis opposite to the deep sulcus, a unilateral sacral shear, or a posteriorly rotated ilium on the same side. A shallow sulcus can indicate a backward sacral torsion with the axis opposite to the shallow sulcus or an anteriorly rotated ilium on the same side. Bilateral sacral flexions (Figure 60-9A) and extensions (Figure 60-9B) may have equivocal results. Chronic decrease in lumbar lordosis may give a false-positive lumbar spring test result whereas a lordotic posture may result in a false-negative result of the same test. Using the mechanism of injury, all of the findings, as well as clinical experience will help refine the diagnosis.

The sacrum has fairly complicated motions that result in shifting of the axis of movement. Ambulation typically results in alternating oblique axes (Fig. 60-10) being established. These create physiological forward rotation motions of right-on-right (R on R) or left-on-left (L

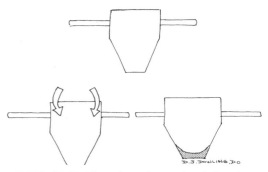
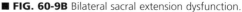

■ **FIG. 60-9B** Bilateral sacral extension dysfunction.

on L) rotations with a normal compensation of L5 rotating in the opposite direction. However, the difference between these occurrences and somatic dysfunctions of the sacrum is that these are instantaneous and easily reversible, whereas the latter persist. By convention, written sacral diagnoses that occur about oblique axes are written as ____ (ROTATION) on ____ (AXIS) or ____ on ____ for short. Somatic dysfunctions are pathological. Other typical findings are always pathological. Backward sacral rotations, which consist of right-on-left (R on L) and left-on-right (L on R), typically occur with full or extreme forward bending accompanied by a twisting motion. Again, as with the forward torsions, the axis is oblique and torsions occur with the compensatory rotation of the L5 in the opposite direction. The key of the L5 is important to the maintenance of the dysfunction and is also related to the application of muscle energy technique. This accounts for the similarity of positioning between flexion lumbar dysfunctions and backward sacral torsions and extension lumbar dysfunctions and forward sacral torsions. Each of these diagnoses has a deep sulcus on the

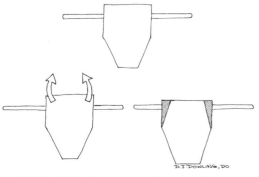
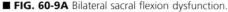

■ **FIG. 60-9A** Bilateral sacral flexion dysfunction.

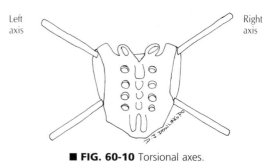

Left axis

Right axis

■ **FIG. 60-10** Torsional axes.

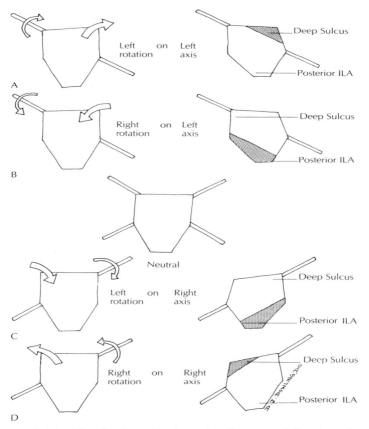

■ **FIG. 60-11** Sacral torsion. **(A)** Left rotation of sacrum on left oblique axis. **(B)** Right rotation of sacrum on left oblique axis. **(C)** Sacrum on left oblique axis. **(D)** Right rotation of sacrum on right oblique axis.

side opposite to the posterior ILA. The forward torsions have an axis that has a superior portion that is located opposite to deep sulcus. The backward torsions have the axis that appears to go through the deep sulcus. In either case, the axis is actually physiological and remains functioning because of the existing restriction on the opposite side. The positive seated flexion test, or other tests of laterality (sacral mobility or rock), occurs opposite to the axis (Fig. 60-11).

Unilateral sacral shears, also known as unilateral sacral flexions, have complicated axes that are still undergoing debate. However, the findings of deep sulcus and posterior ILA on the same side are quite typical (Fig. 60-12). The seated flexion test also occurs to the same side and the sacroiliac dysfunction is ipsilateral.

Clinically, there are typical findings that occur. There are some common counterstrain

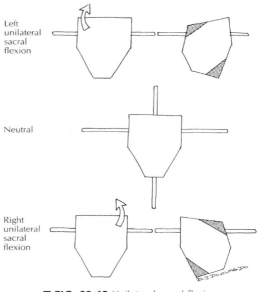
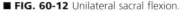

■ **FIG. 60-12** Unilateral sacral flexion.

## TABLE 60-1

| STATIC FINDINGS | | | | TESTS | | | DIAGNOSIS | AXIS |
|---|---|---|---|---|---|---|---|---|
| ILA Posterior | Deep Sulcus | Shallow Sulcus | L5 Rotation | Seated Flexion | Lumbar Spring | Sphinx Test | | |
| Right | Right | Left | | Right | Negative | Negative | Right Unilateral Shear | |
| Left | Left | Right | | Left | Negative | Negative | Left Unilateral Shear | |
| Right | Left | Right | Right | Left | Negative | Negative | Right on Right (R on R) Rotation | Right Oblique |
| Right | Left | Right | Left | Left | Negative | Negative | Right on Right (R on R) Torsion | Right Oblique |
| Left | Right | Left | Left | Right | Negative | Negative | Left on Left (L on L) Rotation | Left Oblique |
| Left | Right | Left | Right | Right | Negative | Negative | Left on Left (L on L) Torsion | Left Oblique |
| Right | Left | Right | Right | Right | Positive | Positive | Right on Left (R on L) Rotation | Left Oblique |
| Right | Left | Right | Left | Right | Positive | Positive | Right on Left (R on L) Torsion | Left Oblique |
| Left | Right | Left | Left | Left | Positive | Positive | Left on Right (L on R) Rotation | Right Oblique |
| Left | Right | Left | Right | Left | Positive | Positive | Left on Right (L on R) Torsion | Right Oblique |
| Even | Bilateral | | | Equivocal | Negative | Negative | Bilateral Sacral Flexion | Transverse |
| Even | | Bilateral | | Equivocal | Equivocal | Negative | Bilateral Sacral Extension | Transverse |

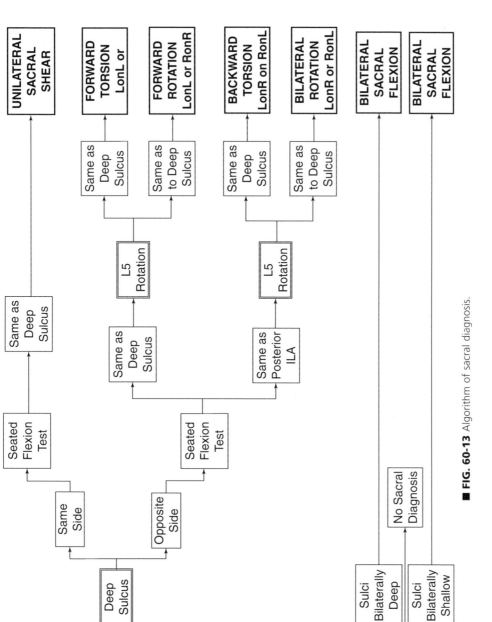

■ **FIG. 60-13** Algorithm of sacral diagnosis.

tenderpoints that occur, but a lower pole L5 (LPL5) probably is one of the most frequent and found on the side of a deep sulcus with forward torsions and unilateral sacral shears. The tenderpoint may actually be a reflection of an anterior sacroiliac joint dysfunction. The piriformis muscle is also frequently found to be in spasm on the side of the posterior ILA. Whether this is a cause or an effect is not as crucial as the need to address the finding. The related tenderpoints of piriformis, mid-pole sacroiliac, and lateral trochanteric are commonly found. Other musculoskeletal findings may include paravertebral spasm, iliopsoas spasm, and gluteal and hamstring spasm, which may need to be addressed, as well as other regional and even distal components.

Bilateral sacral flexions and extensions are not as common as the other findings. The report of symptoms in the apparent absence of positive tests of laterality and asymmetry may be more indicative. Observation of the decrease of movement with respiration and clinical experience may be the best indications as to the presence of these bilateral diagnoses.

The key factor to sacral diagnosis for most conditions is the presence of an asymmetry of the ILAs. If the ILA is on the same side as the deep sulcus, then a unilateral sacral shear is present on that side. A positive seated flexion test on that side confirms the diagnosis. When the ILA is on the side opposite to the deep sulcus, there is at least a sacral rotation occurring. A positive seated flexion test on the side of the deep sulcus indicates a forward sacral rotation. A negative spring test and an increase in symmetry of the ILAs during the stork test confirm this. An L5 rotated to the side of the deep sulcus indicates a forward sacral torsion. A positive seated flexion test on the side opposite to the deep sulcus indicates a backward sacral rotation. A positive spring test and an increase in asymmetry of the ILAs during the stork test confirm this. An L5 rotated to the side of the deep sulcus indicates a forward sacral torsion.

An algorithm as to a process as well as a chart of the sacral diagnoses is presented in Table 60-1 and Figure 60-13.

## REFERENCES

Bourdilion JF. A torsion free approach to the pelvis. *Manual Med* 1987;3:20–23.

Dowling DJ. *An Illustrated Guide to OMT of the Neck and Trunk.* Self-published, 1985.

Fryette HH. *Principles of Osteopathic Technique.* Carmel, CA: Academy of Applied Osteopathy, 1960.

Greenman PE. Innominate shear dysfunction in the sacroiliac syndrome. *Manual Med* 1986;2:114–121.

Jones LH. Personal communication, 1992.

Kapandji IA. *The Physiology of the Joints, Vol. III The Trunk and Vertebral Column.* New York: Churchill Livingstone, 1974.

Kappler R. Lecture notes. Chicago: College of Osteopathic Medicine, 1975.

Kennedy H. Unilateral sacroiliac dysfunction. In: Hewitt R, ed. *1975 Yearbook of Selected Osteopathic Papers.* Colorado Springs: American Academy of Osteopathy, 1975.

Kidd R. Pain localization with the innominate upslip dysfunction. *Manual Med* 1988;3:103–105.

Larson NJ. Physiologic movement of the sacrum. Read before the Chicago College of Osteopathic Medicine, February 1984.

Mitchell FL. Structural pelvic function. *1965 Year Book of Selected Osteopathic Papers, vol. II.* In: Barnes M, ed. Carmel, CA: Academy of Applied Osteopathy, 1965:178–199.

Mitchell FL Jr, Moran PS, Pruzzo NT. *An Evaluation and Treatment Manual of Osteopathic Muscle Energy Procedures.* Valley Park, MO: Mitchell, Moran, and Pruzzo Associates, 1979.

Mitchell FL Jr, Mitchell PGK. *The Muscle Energy Manual, volume III: Evaluation and Treatment of the Pelvis and Sacrum.* East Lansing, MI: MET Press, 1999.

Moore KL. *Clinically Oriented Anatomy.* Baltimore: Williams & Wilkins, 1980.

Northup TL. Sacroiliac lesions primary & secondary. *Academy of Applied Osteopathy Year Book, 1943–1944.* Ann Arbor: Academy of Applied Osteopathy, 1943:53–54.

Schiowitz S, DiGiovanna EL, Ausman PJ. *An Osteopathic Approach to Diagnosis and Treatment.* Old Westbury, NY: New York College of Osteopathic Medicine, 1983.

Schwab WA. Principles of manipulative treatment: The low back problems. *Academy of Applied Osteopathy 1965 Yearbook of Selected Osteopathic Papers, vol. II.* In: Barnes M, ed. Carmel, CA: Academy of Applied Osteopathy, 1965:65–69.

Sutherland WG. *The Cranial Bowl.* Mankato, MN: Free Press, 1936.

Warwick R, Williams PL. *Gray's Anatomy,* 35th British Edition. Philadelphia: W.B. Saunders, 1973.

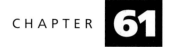

# Muscle Energy

*Dennis J. Dowling and Lisa R. Chun*

This section describes muscle energy techniques for sacrum and pelvic somatic dysfunctions.

## ■ PELVIC DYSFUNCTIONS

### Anterior Iliac-Innominate-Pelvic Dysfunction

1. **Patient position:** prone; near the edge of the table on the side of the dysfunction. The patient's hip can be slightly off the table and can be angled towards the opposite side for stability
2. **Physician position:** standing on the same side of the table as the dysfunction, facing the patient's head.
3. **Technique:**
   a. The physician's hand that is closer to the table monitors medial to the PSIS on the side of the dysfunction to determine motion of the iliosacral joint.
   b. With his other hand, the physician flexes both the hip and the leg on the side of the dysfunction until motion is felt at the iliosacral joint.
   c. The physician places the patient's foot against physician's shin or thigh to maintain this position.
   d. The physician's non-monitoring hand grasps and supports the patient's flexed knee.
   e. The patient is instructed to attempt to straighten the flexed leg by pushing the sole of the foot against the physician's extended leg for 3 to 5 seconds.

f. The physician resists this motion, causing an isometric contraction (Fig. 61-1).
g. After 3 to 5 seconds, the patient is instructed to relax.
h. After the patient relaxes, the physician engages the new motion barrier by further flexing the patient's hip and knee on the dysfunctional side until motion is felt at the involved iliosacral joint.
i. The procedure is repeated at least three times or until improvement of the somatic dysfunction.
j. A passive stretch is introduced after the last attempt.

### Posterior Iliac-Innominate-Pelvic Dysfunction

1. **Patient position:** prone
2. **Physician position:** standing on the opposite side of the table as the dysfunction, facing the patient's head.
3. **Technique:**
   a. The physician's hand that is farther from the table monitors medial to the PSIS on the side of the dysfunction to determine motion of the iliosacral joint.
   b. With his other hand, the physician places his hand medial and anterior to the patient's thigh of the leg on the side of the dysfunction.
   c. The physician lifts the patient's leg, creating hip extension, until motion is felt at the iliosacral joint with his non-monitoring hand.

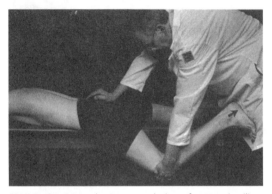

■ **FIG. 61-1** Muscle energy technique for anterior iliac-innominate-pelvic dysfunction, patient prone.

d. The physician may place a pillow or his bent knee between the patient's leg and the table to assist in maintaining this position.
e. The patient is instructed to attempt to push his leg downwards towards the table for 3 to 5 seconds.
f. The physician resists this motion, causing an isometric contraction (Fig. 61-2).
g. After 3 to 5 seconds, the patient is instructed to relax.
h. After the patient relaxes, the physician engages the new motion barrier by further lifting the patient's leg on the dysfunctional side until motion is felt at the involved iliosacral joint. The position of the physician's leg or the pillow can be adjusted to support the position of the patient's leg.

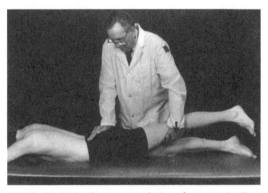

■ **FIG. 61-2** Muscle energy technique for posterior iliac-innominate-pelvic dysfunction, patient prone.

i. The procedure is repeated at least three times or until improvement of the somatic dysfunction.
j. A passive stretch is introduced after the last attempt.

## Superior Iliac-Innominate-Pelvic Shear

1. **Patient position:** supine, with lower extremities extended and resting on the table. The patient may be instructed to hold onto the table with both hands to keep from sliding on the surface. The technique may also be performed with the patient prone. It also has an articulatory component.
2. **Physician position:** standing at the foot of the table, facing the patient and more to the side of the superior innominate.
3. **Technique:**
   a. The physician grasps the distal portions of the tibia and fibula on the side of the dysfunction proximal to the ankle joint with both hands.
   b. The physician abducts, flexes (if patient supine), or extends (if patient prone) at the patient's hip and then internally rotates the involved leg until the loose-packed position of the sacroiliac joint is identified.
   c. The physician applies continuous long axis traction on the involved lower limb while maintaining the lower limb in flexion or extension, abduction, and internal rotation (Fig. 61-3).
   d. The patient is instructed to pull his leg away for 3 to 5 seconds and then relax for 3 to 5 seconds. The effort is primarily exerted by the glutei and quadrata muscles.
   e. The physician then maintains traction on the lower limb position.
   f. The patient is directed to inhale deeply and then to cough sharply.
   g. Simultaneous to the cough, the physician engages the final barrier by further tractioning the patient's leg and then sharply tugging the patient's leg.
   h. The procedure may be repeated if necessary.

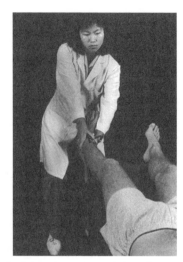

■ **FIG. 61-3** Muscle energy technique for superior iliac-innominate-pelvic shear.

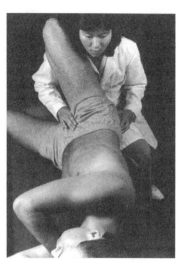

■ **FIG. 61-4** Muscle energy technique for inferior iliac-innominate-pelvic shear.

## Inferior Iliac-Innominate-Pelvic Shear

1. **Patient position:** lateral recumbent, with dysfunctional side up. The leg on the side of the dysfunction is up and away from the table and is flexed and placed on the physician's shoulder.
2. **Physician position:** sitting on the table behind the patient.
3. **Technique:**
   a. The physician places one hand placed on both the pubic and ischial rami of the dysfunctional side, with the other hand placed on both the ischial tuberosity and the posterior superior iliac spine of the dysfunctional side.
   b. With the patient relaxed, the physician laterally distracts the innominate bone.
   c. Maintaining this position, the physician then applies a cephalad force on the pubic and ischial rami, ischial tuberosity, and posterior inferior iliac spine of the dysfunctional side (Fig. 61-4).
   d. The physician then instructs the patient to inhale deeply and exhale completely.
   e. The physician maintains the cephalad force on the distracted innominate during the inspiratory phase of the patient's inhalatory respiratory cycle.
   f. During the expiratory phase of the patient's respiratory cycle, the physician in-

creases the cephalad force on the distracted innominate.
   g. The steps may be repeated.

## ■ PUBIC DYSFUNCTIONS

## Inferior Pubic Dysfunction

1. **Patient position:** supine.
2. **Physician position:** sitting on or standing at the same side of the table as the dysfunction, facing the patient.
3. **Technique:**
   a. The physician places the monitoring finger of the cephalad hand on the anterior superior iliac spine of the dysfunctional side
   b. With his non-monitoring hand, the physician flexes the patient's involved hip until motion is felt at the monitoring finger.
   c. The physician's non-monitoring hand is placed in a fist (palm up) against the ischial tuberosity of the dysfunctional side. The fist also rests on the table.
   d. The physician places the patient's flexed knee against the anterior aspect of his shoulder.
   e. The patient is instructed to attempt to straighten the flexed hip The amount of force should be sufficient and localized to the monitoring finger.

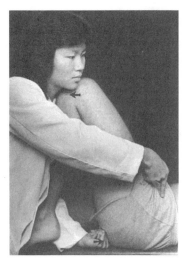

■ **FIG. 61-5** Muscle energy technique for inferior pubic dysfunction.

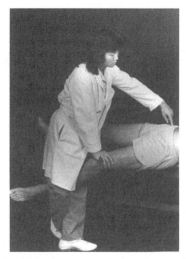

■ **FIG. 61-6** Muscle energy technique for superior pubic dysfunction.

f. The physician resists this with isometric force, creating static contraction, while applying a cephalad force on the involved ischial tuberosity with the fist (Fig. 61-5).

g. After 3 to 5 seconds, the patient is instructed to discontinue the attempt and to relax.

h. The physician instructs the patient to relax for 3 to 5 seconds, while maintaining both hip flexion and the cephalad force at the ischial tuberosity.

i. The physician engages the new restricted motion barrier by repositioning the involved hip into further flexion until motion is felt under the monitoring finger.

j. The procedure is repeated at least three times or until improvement of the somatic dysfunction.

## Superior Pubic Dysfunction

1. **Patient position:** supine.
2. **Physician position:** standing on the same side of the table as the dysfunction, facing the patient.
3. **Technique:**
   a. The physician's monitoring finger of the hand that is closer to the table monitors on the anterior superior iliac spine contralateral to the dysfunctional side

b. The physician's other hand lowers the patient's leg off the edge of the table on the dysfunctional side until motion is felt at the monitoring hand.

c. The physician supports the patient's hanging extended leg with his own leg.

d. The physician places the palm of his nonmonitoring hand on the anterior thigh of the patient's hanging leg.

e. The patient is instructed to attempt to raise the extended leg upward with sufficient force to maintain localization.

f. The physician resists using isometric force, creating a static contraction for 3 to 5 seconds (Fig. 61-6).

g. The patient is instructed to relax for 3 to 5 seconds.

h. The physician engages the new motion barrier by repositioning the involved hip into further extension until motion is felt under the monitoring finger.

i. The procedure is repeated at least three times or until improvement of the somatic dysfunction.

## Abduction (Open) Pubic Dysfunction

1. **Patient position:** supine, hips flexed and knees flexed to 90 degrees; lying closer to one side of the table than the other.

2. **Physician position:** standing at the side of the table to which patient is closest and facing the patient.
3. **Technique:**
   a. The physician wraps his arms around the patient's flexed knees and draws them against himself.
   b. The patient is instructed to attempt to spread his knees apart with maximal force.
   c. The physician resists this effort with isometric force, creating static contraction.
   d. After 3 to 5 seconds, the patient is instructed to relax.
   e. The physician allows the patient to relax for 3 to 5 seconds, while maintaining the position attained.
   f. The steps are repeated three or more times.
   g. The physician reevaluates the status of the dysfunction.
   h. Treatment may be repeated if indicated.

## Adduction (Closed) Pubic Dysfunction

1. **Patient position:** supine, hips flexed, and knees flexed to 90 degrees.
2. **Physician position:** standing at the side of the table facing the patient.
3. **Technique:**
   a. The physician's forearm is placed between the patient's knees. One hand is on the medial aspect of one of the patient's knees, with the elbow joint on the medial aspect of the other knee.
   b. The patient is instructed to attempt to bring his knees together with a maximal force.
   c. The physician's forearm resists this attempt by acting as a solid bar.
   d. After 3 to 5 seconds, the patient is instructed to relax.
   e. The physician allows the patient to relax for 3 to 5 seconds while maintaining the position attained.
   f. A new abduction barrier is engaged. The physician may add a fist or maintain position with both of the physician's hands.
   g. The procedure is repeated at least three times or until improvement of the somatic dysfunction.

h. The physician reevaluates the status of the dysfunction.
i. Treatment may be repeated if indicated.

## ■ SACRAL DYSFUNCTIONS

### Unilateral Sacral Flexion Dysfunction

1. **Patient position:** prone, arms hanging off the sides of the table.
2. **Physician position:** standing at the same side of the table as the dysfunction.
3. **Technique:**
   a. The physician places the heel of his cephalad hand on the lower and outer edge of the inferior lateral angle (ILA) of the sacrum on the side to be treated. The middle or index finger of that hand is placed in the sacral sulcus.
   b. The physician abducts the lower extremity of the involved side with his other hand until motion is localized at the monitored sacral sulcus.
   c. The physician maintains the abduction while introducing internal rotation until motion is felt at the sacral sulcus being monitored. This position of abduction and internal rotation is maintained.
   d. Using the hand on the patient's sacrum and an extended elbow, the physician applies a constant force at the posterior inferior lateral angle down toward the table and cephalad (Fig. 61-7). The force applied is more cephalad.
   e. The patient is instructed to inhale deeply and to hold his breath.

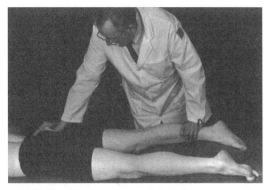

■ **FIG. 61-7** Muscle energy technique for treating unilateral sacral flexion dysfunction.

f. The physician increases the pressure on the inferior lateral angle during the inhalatory phase.

g. The patient is instructed to exhale completely.

h. The physician maintains the cephalad force on and resists the backwards tendency of movement of the posterior inferior lateral angle during the exhalatory phase.

i. The procedure is repeated at least three times or until improvement of the somatic dysfunction.

j. At the end of the last exhalatory phase, an additional cephalad thrust may be provided by the physician on the posterior inferior lateral angle.

k. The physician places the abducted and internally rotated leg into a neutral midline position.

l. Treatment may be repeated if indicated.

## Forward Sacral Torsion Dysfunction

1. **Patient position:** Sims position (patient's chest with upper torso prone and hips and knees flexed), with the axis of the dysfunction down toward the table. The patient's arms hang off the sides of the table.

2. **Physician position:** standing at the side of the table facing the patient.

3. **Technique:**

   a. The physician faces the patient and monitors the somatic dysfunction with his cephalad hand.

   b. With his other hand the physician flexes the patient's hips and knees until motion is localized at the sacroiliac joint on the deep sulcus side (medial to the PSIS).

   c. The physician switches monitoring hands so that the caudad hand is then on the somatic dysfunction.

   d. The patient is directed to bring the arm that is on the table behind him and rotate his chest towards the table. This rotation creates a modified Sims position.

   e. The physician places his cephalad hand on the patient's shoulder.

   f. Additional rotation is induced by having the patient inhale, then exhale com-

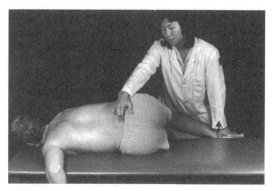

■ **FIG. 61-8** Muscle energy technique for treating forward sacral torsion dysfunction.

pletely while simultaneously reaching towards the floor.

g. The physician pushes down on the patient's shoulder toward the table with his cephalad hand until the torso is rotated down to the monitored segment, exaggerating the modified Sims position.

h. The physician again switches monitoring hands with now the cephalad becoming and remaining the monitoring one.

i. The physician lowers the patient's legs off the side of the table to create lumbar sidebending up to the restricted area (Fig. 61-8).

j. Because this position may be uncomfortable for the patient, the physician may either place a pillow under the patient's lower knee or sit behind the patient and put his thigh between the patient's legs and the table (Fig. 61-9). (This position

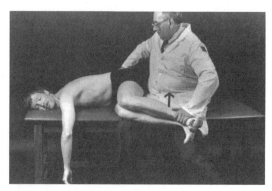

■ **FIG. 61-9** Alternative position for Muscle energy technique for treating forward sacral torsion dysfunction.

requires the physician to change the hand monitoring.)

k. The patient is directed to push his feet towards the ceiling for 3 to 5 seconds.

l. The physician provides isometric resistance, creating a static contraction.

m. The patient is directed to relax. This is maintained for 3 to 5 seconds typically but may be slightly longer if necessary

n. The physician engages a new motion barrier by further lowering the patient's legs toward the floor.

o. The procedure is repeated at least three times.

p. A passive stretch is given after the last repetition.

## Backward Sacral Torsion Dysfunction

1. **Patient position:** lateral recumbent position with the axis of the dysfunction down toward the table; knees flexed.

2. **Physician position:** standing at the side of the table facing the patient's anterior.

3. **Technique:**
   a. The physician monitors at the lumbosacral junction.
   b. The physician's non-monitoring hand is used to engage the restricted motion barriers.
   c. To facilitate engagement of the restricted motion barriers, the hand monitoring the lumbosacral junction is switched during the procedure.
   d. The physician flexes the patient's hips and knees until motion is felt at the monitoring finger(s).
   e. The physician maintains this position by leaning into the patient's upper knee.
   f. The patient is instructed to straighten the leg that is on the table.
   g. The physician hooks the foot of the patient's leg that is closer to the ceiling onto the straightened lower leg.
   h. While still leaning on the patient's upper knee, the physician moves the patient's knee into extension and drops the leg toward the floor.

i. Hip flexion is continued until motion is felt at the lumbosacral junction.

j. The physician maintains this position by placing the forearm of his monitoring hand on the patient's hip.

k. The physician grasps the patient's arm that is on the table and pulls directly forward and toward the ceiling, thereby rotating the patient's torso backward.

l. The patient is then instructed to reach his top arm behind him and grasp the edge of the table.

m. The patient is instructed to inhale deeply.

n. The patient is instructed to exhale completely and simultaneously to reach down the edge of the table. At the end of the exhalation, the patient grasps the edge of the table.

o. The physician may facilitate this motion by pressing the patient's upper shoulder back toward the table and caudad while the patient is exhaling.

p. For this rotation motion to be localized at the lumbosacral junction, this may have to be repeated. This is continued only until motion is felt at the monitoring fingers. Once motion is felt, the position is maintained.

q. The physician lowers the patient's upper leg below the table until motion is felt at the lumbosacral junction.

r. Once motion is felt, this position is maintained.

s. The patient is instructed to attempt to bring the ankle of the leg that is hanging off the table toward the ceiling. An alternative can be to have the patient push the thigh of that leg upward toward the ceiling.

t. The physician isometrically resists this attempt, creating static contraction.

u. After 3 to 5 seconds, the patient is instructed to stop the attempt and to relax.

v. The physician allows the patient to relax for 3 to 5 seconds.

w. The physician reengages the restricted motion barriers by repeating the previous steps.

x. The procedure is repeated at least three

times or until improvement of the somatic dysfunction.
y. The physician places the patient into a
neutral position.
z. The physician reevaluates the status of
the dysfunction.

## REFERENCES

Greenman PE. Innominate shear dysfunction in the sacroiliac syndrome. *Manual Med* 1986;2:114–121.

Mitchell FL, Mitchell P-KG. *The Muscle Energy manual*: Volume Three Examination of the Pelvis and Sacrum. East Lansing, MI: MET Press, 1995.

Moran PS, Pruzzo NA, et al. *An Evaluation and Treatment Manual of Osteopathic Manipulative Procedures, vol I. The Postural Structural Model.* Kansas City: Institute for Continuing Education in Osteopathic Principles, 1973.

Schiowitz S, DiGiovanna E, Ausman P. *An Osteopathic Approach to Diagnosis and Treatment.* Old Westbury, NY: New York College of Osteopathic Medicine of the New York Institute of Technology 1983.

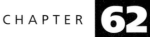

# Counterstrain Techniques for the Sacrum and Pelvis

*Eileen L. DiGiovanna*

## ■ ANTERIOR TENDER POINTS

There are three significant tender points generally related to the pelvis or sacrum: the low ilium anterior sacral tender point, located on the superior surface of the pubes; the iliacus tender point, located in the lower quadrant of the abdomen and deep in the fossa (often a tender point of concern in dysmenorrhea); and the inguinal ligament tender point, located on the inguinal ligament at its attachment to the pubes (Fig. 62-1). Techniques for treating each of these tender points are described.

### Low Ilium Sacroiliac/Anterior Sacral Tender Point

1. **Patient position:** supine
2. **Physician position:** standing at either side of the table
3. **Technique:**
   a. The thigh is flexed to approximately 40 degrees or both thighs may be flexed as in the treatment of the lumbar tender point.
   b. One finger of the hand closest to the patient's head is used to monitor the tender point (Fig. 62-2).
   c. This position is held for 90 seconds and then the legs are moved passively by the physician back to the table and the ankles uncrossed.
   d. The tender point is re-evaluated for tenderness.

### Iliacus Tender Point

1. **Patient position:** supine
2. **Physician position:** standing at the side of the table near the tender point, with one foot on the table.
3. **Technique:**
   a. Both of the patient's legs are flexed with the legs resting on the physician's thigh.
   b. The physician monitors the tender point with the hand nearest the patient's head.
   c. The ankles are crossed and the knees are dropped apart. This motion externally rotates the patient's thighs (Fig. 62-3).
   d. This position is held for 90 seconds and then the physician passively moves the legs back to the table and uncrosses the ankles.
   e. The tender point is reassessed for tenderness.

### Inguinal Ligament Tender Point

1. **Patient position:** supine
2. **Physician position:** standing at the side of the table opposite the tender point with her foot on the table.
3. **Technique:**
   a. The patient's legs are flexed and rested on the physician's thigh.
   b. The leg nearest the physician is crossed at the knee over the further leg.
   c. The lower leg is internally rotated by the physician pushing laterally on the ankle (Fig. 62-4).

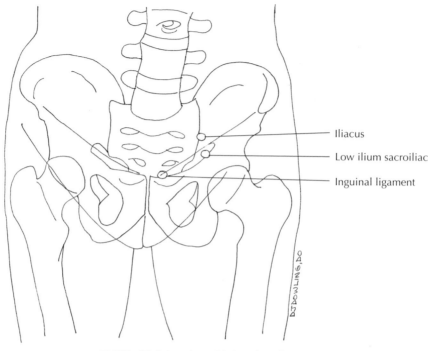

Iliacus

Low ilium sacroiliac

Inguinal ligament

■ **FIG. 62-1** Anterior pelvic/sacral tender points.

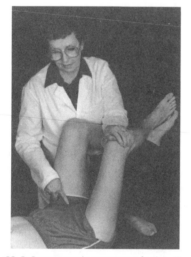

■ **FIG. 62-2** Counterstrain treatment for low ilium/anterior sacral tender point.

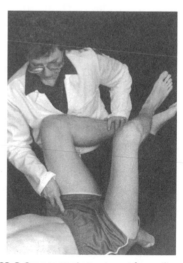

■ **FIG. 62-3** Counterstrain treatment for an iliacus tender point.

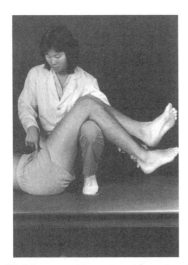

**■ FIG. 62-4** Counterstrain treatment for an inguinal ligament tender point.

## ■ POSTERIOR TENDER POINTS

The location of the posterior tender points are shown in Figure 62-5.

### Piriformis Tender Point

This is a tender point most commonly associated with sacral dysfunctions and is frequently involved in sciatica pain because of its close association with the sciatic nerve. It is located in the belly of the muscle.

1. **Patient position:** prone, with the leg on the involved side off the edge of the table.
2. **Physician position:** seated at the side of the dysfunction, facing the patient's head.
3. **Technique:**
   a. The physician monitors the tender point with one finger of the hand closer to the table.
   b. The patient's hip and knee are flexed.
   c. The leg is externally rotated and abducted and may be rested on the physician's lap (Fig. 62-6).
   d. The movement of flexion and external rotation may be modified to achieve maximal softening of the piriformis.
   e. The position is held for 90 seconds and then the leg is returned passively by the physician to the table.
   f. The tender point is reassessed for tenderness.

### Midpole Sacral Tender Point

This tender point is palpated by pushing the monitoring finger medially on the lateral edge of the sacrum at the midpoint between the posterior superior iliac spine (PSIS) and the sacral apex. This is at the site of the piriformis attachment to the sacrum and probably represents a second piriformis tender point. It is often found in association with the tender point in the belly of the muscle.

1. **Patient position:** prone
2. **Physician position:** standing or sitting at the side of the table next to the tender point.
3. **Technique:**
   a. The physician monitors the tender point with one finger of the hand nearer the patient's head.
   b. The leg is abducted straight laterally until the tender point softens and is no longer tender (Fig. 62-7). External rotation may assist.
   c. With some patients, there may be a report of stretching the medial thigh muscles. In this case, the leg should be abducted as far as is comfortable and then pressure put against the pelvis by the physician with the heel of the monitoring hand, moving the pelvis away from the physician slightly.
   d. This position is held for 90 seconds and then the physician passively returns the leg to the table.
   e. The tender point is reassessed for tenderness.

### High Flare-out Sacroiliac Tender Point

This tender point is located on the posterior surface of the sacrum. It is one and three-fourths inches inferior and one-half of an inch medial to the lower surface of the PSIS. It is frequently associated with coccygodynia.

1. **Patient position:** prone
2. **Physician position:** standing at the side of the table
3. **Technique:**
   a. The physician monitors the tender point with one finger.
   b. The patient's leg is extended (Fig. 62-8)

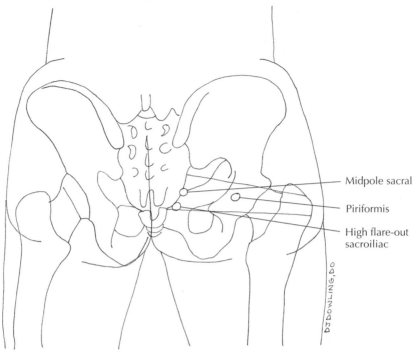

**■ FIG. 62-5** Posterior pelvic/sacral tender point.

Midpole sacral

Piriformis

High flare-out sacroiliac

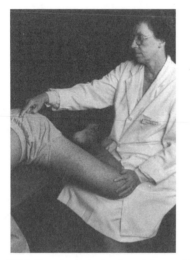

**■ FIG. 62-6** Counterstrain treatment for a piriformis tender point.

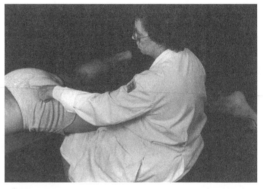

**■ FIG. 62-7** Counterstrain treatment for a midpole sacral tender point.

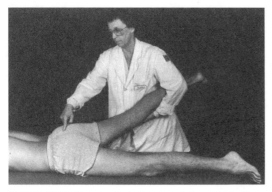

■ **FIG. 62-8** Counterstrain treatment for a high flare-out sacroiliac tender point.

c. Some adduction and external rotation may be needed. In these cases it is easier to stand on the side of the table opposite the tender point. The leg can then be pulled toward the physician to adduct it and then externally rotated.

d. The position is held for 90 seconds and then the leg is passively returned to the table.

e. The tender point is reassessed for tenderness.

## REFERENCES

DiGiovanna EL, Schiowitz S. *An Osteopathic Approach to Diagnosis and Treatment*. Philadelphia: Lippincott-Raven, Philadelphia, 1997.

Jones LH, Kusunose R, Goering E. Strain-Counterstrain. Boise, ID: Jones' Strain-Counterstrain, Inc., 1995.

Yates HA, Glover JC. *Counterstrain, Handbook of Osteopathic Technique*. Tulsa, OK: Y Knot Pub, 1995.

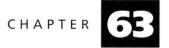

# Facilitated Positional Release Techniques for the Sacrum and Pelvis

*Stanley Schiowitz*

This chapter describes facilitated positional release (FPR) techniques for the sacrum and pelvis. The principles of FPR apply: the lumbosacral spine is flattened by placing a pillow under the abdomen of the prone patient, the involved area is placed into the freedoms of motion of the involved joint or the muscles being treated are shortened, and a facilitating force is added, either compresson or torsion.

## ■ PELVIC SUPERFICIAL MUSCLE HYPERTONICITY

### Piriformis Muscle (Right)

1. **Patient position**: prone, with a pillow placed under the abdomen.
2. **Physician position**: sitting beside the table on the side of the dysfunction (right), facing toward the patient's head. The physician's left thigh and knee are alongside the table.
3. **Technique**:
   a. The physician monitors the tissue to be treated with one finger of the left hand.
   b. The physician drops the patient's flexed right knee and thigh off the table over his left thigh and between both of his knees.
   c. The physician holds the patient's right knee with his right hand, gently flexing the patient's hip until motion is felt at the monitoring finger.
   d. The physician pushes the patient's right

knee towards the table (adduction), using his left knee and thigh as a fulcrum, until motion is felt at the monitoring finger
   e. With his right hand, the physician turns the patient's right knee cephalad and medially, producing internal rotation of the hip, until motion is felt at the monitoring finger.
   f. With his right hand the physician pushes the patient's right knee up (dorsally) toward his monitoring finger producing a mild compressive force. There should be an immediate release of the tissue hypertonocity felt by the monitoring finger. (Fig. 63-1)
   g. Hold the position for 3 to 5 seconds, release and reassess the somatic dysfunction.

### Gluteus Maximus Muscle (Right)

1. **Patient position**: prone with pillow placed under the abdomen.
2. **Physician position**: sitting beside the table on the side of the dysfunction (right), facing toward the patient's head. The physician's left thigh and knee are alongside the table.
3. **Technique**:
   a. The physician monitors the tissue to be treated with one finger of the left hand. (Note that the hypertonic tissue is usually

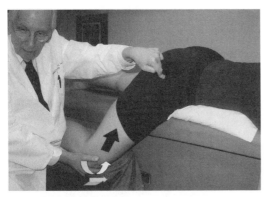

■ **FIG. 63-1** Facilitated positional release treatment for hypertonicity of the right piriformis muscle.

palpable in the middle and directly inferior to the crest of the ilium.)

b. The physician brings the patient's right hip and knee off the table into full abduction and rests the knee upon his outside thigh, with the knee flexed at 90 degrees.

c. The physician raises his outside foot (right) off the floor by raising his heel, thus elevating his thigh, until he feels motion at the monitoring finger.

d. The physician, using the patient's right knee as a fulcrum on his thigh, pushes the patient's knee externally, creating external rotation of the patient's hip joint. There should be an immediate release of the tissue felt by the monitoring finger (Fig. 63-2).

e. Hold the position 3 to 5 seconds. Release and reevaluate.

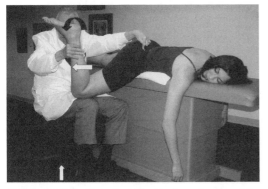

■ **FIG. 63-2** Facilitated positional release treatment for hypertonicity of the right gluteus maximus muscle.

## Tensor Fascia Lata (Right)

The muscle tissue of the tensor fascia lata is palpated starting at the anterior superior iliac spine (ASIS) and descending downwards for approximately 4 to 6 inches. It will feel like a firm rope and be tender to the touch when hypertonic.

1. **Patient position**: prone with a pillow placed under the abdomen. The patient's pelvis should be slightly off the table to the right.

2. **Physician position**: sitting beside the table at the side of the dysfunction (right) facing toward the patient's head. The physician's left thigh and knee are alongside the table. A pillow is placed between the physician's knees.

3. **Technique**:

   a. The patient's right knee is dropped off the table and placed between the physician's knees, with the pillow that is present at the medial aspect of the patient's knee and the physician's left knee.

   b. The physician monitors the tissue to be treated with one finger of his (right) hand. The physician pushes the patient's right knee towards the table, into adduction under the physician's left knee until the monitoring finger feels motion. The physician's left knee acts as a fulcrum, and both the physicians' thigh and the pillow cushion the patient's knee.

   c. With his left hand the physician pushes the patient's right knee towards his monitoring finger producing a mild compression force. There should be immediate release of the tissue hypertonicity felt by the monitoring finger (Fig.63-3).

   d. Hold the position for 3 to 5 seconds, release and reevaluate.

## ■ SACRUM

There are no muscles that directly insert into both the sacrum and the ilium exclusively. Therefore, the usual facilitated positional release techniques do not apply. What will be described is a method for diagnosing sacral motion restriction on the ilium and a biomechanical technique to normalize the joint motion, if needed.

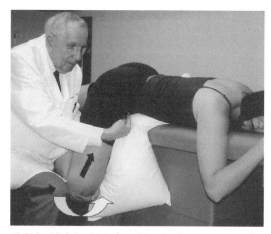

■ **FIG. 63-3** Facilitated positional release treatment for hypertonicity of the right tensor fascia lata.

## Sacral Motion Restriction

### Diagnosis

1. **Patient position**: prone with a pillow placed under the abdomen.
2. **Physician position**: Standing alongside the table, on the side of his dominant eye, and facing the patient's head.
3. **Technique**:
   a. The physician places the heels of both hands inferior to the patient's inferior lateral angles (ILA) of the sacrum. The physician's right hand under the patient's right ILA, and left hand under the left ILA.
   b. The physician directs a force with both hands cephalad (toward the patient's head), parallel to the table and as directly in the horizontal plane as he is able. The force can be induced simultaneously, testing both sides at once, or one time at a time and comparing results (Fig. 63-4).
   c. Motion of the sacrum will be created on its articulation with the ilium. If there is one-sided restriction present, the physician will feel that one side does not move as far as the other side. It might feel as if the restricted side is acting as a fulcrum around which the other side is moving freely. To judge bilateral restriction of motion, the physician will have to be acquainted with the normal expected motion usually found at these articulations.

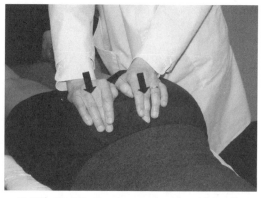

■ **FIG. 63-4** Testing for sacral motion, bilaterally.

## Restriction of Right Sacral Motion on the Ilium

1. **Patient position**: Prone with pillow placed under the abdomen and a second pillow placed under the patient's right upper thigh, just below the hip joint. The firmer and higher this second pillow is, the better the results obtained, because this pillow will act as a fulcrum as well as a cushion.
2. **Physician's position**: Standing alongside the right side of the table. Facing towards the patient's head.
3. **Technique**
   a. The physician places the middle finger of his left hand, at the right sacroiliac articulation, and uses it as a monitor. The rest of his hand lies flat on the sacrum, with the heel of his hand under the Inferior Lateral Angle (ILA).
   b. With his right hand, the physician brings the patient's right leg off the table into abduction of the hip, until he feels motion at the monitoring finger.
   c. The physician pushes the right leg straight down toward the floor. The second pillow acts as a fulcrum and the physician should feel that the ILA has tilted upwards, toward the ceiling. The physician now repositions his left hand so that the heel of that hand is placed inferior and against the bottom of the ILA.
   d. The patient is asked to take a deep breath and then exhale slowly.
   e. As the breath is released, the physician pushes against the ILA of the sacrum in a

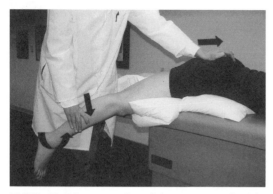

■ **FIG. 63-5** Demonstration of the treatment of a right sacral motion restriction.

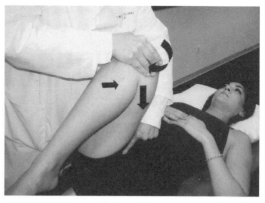

■ **FIG. 63-6** Demonstration of the treatment of the right pubes, restricted superiorly.

direction that is parallel to the table and up toward the patient's head. The physician will feel the sacrum move in that direction (Fig. 63-5).

f. Release and reevaluate.

## Pubic Symphysis Restriction

1. **Patient position**: supine
2. **Physician position**: Standing alongside either side of the table, facing toward the patient's head.
3. **Technique**:
   a. If the physician is standing on the right side of the patient, the physician places one finger of his right hand at the pubic symphysis to monitor motion and, using his left hand, bends the patient's right hip and knee at 90 degrees to the table.
   b. The physician leans on the patient's knee, causing a force downward toward the table with compression of that hip joint.
   c. The physician pushes the right knee and hip joint into adduction, until motion is felt at the monitoring finger.
   d. The physician turns the patient's knee into internal rotation, which will cause inferior motion of the right pubes. Turning the patient's knee in a external rotation direction will cause the right pubes to move in a superior direction (Fig. 63-6).
   e. Hold in the position you wish to accomplish for 3 to 5 seconds.
   f. Release and reevaluate.

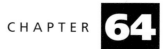

# Still Techniques

*Dennis J. Dowling*

This chapter describes Still techniques for treating somatic dysfunctions of the sacrum and pelvis. There are several systems of diagnosis, but the techniques described in this chapter are related to the systems that are used in this textbook. There are also seated techniques described, albeit less effective than the supine ones described. Because of the complexity, interested students should refer to Dr. Van Buskirk's more thorough book and chapters for other techniques and diagnoses.

## ■ ILIAC/INNOMINATE DYSFUNCTIONS

### Anterior Ilium/Anterior Innominate (Right)—Patient Supine

1. **Patient position:** supine.
2. **Physician position:** standing at the side of the patient on the side of the dysfunction, facing the patient.
3. **Technique:**
   a. The physician places the pad of his index or middle finger of his monitoring cephalad hand medial to the posterior superior iliac spine (PSIS) as a means of following the iliosacral motion (the left finger contacts the area medial to PSIS on the right).
   b. The physician uses his other hand to grasp the patient's leg on the dysfunctional side and flexes the patient's hip and knee until motion is felt at the monitoring finger (the physician's right hand grasps and flexes the patient's right leg in this example) (Fig. 64-1A).
   c. The physician abducts the patient's knee that knee and externally rotates the leg

until motion and soft tissue relaxation are felt at the monitoring finger (Fig. 64-1B). A modification is for the physician to insert the forearm of his caudad arm from lateral to medial beneath the patient's knee and place his hand on the patient's anterior thigh. This can add torsion to the modifying and localizing forces.
   d. The physician puts downward compression with his caudad (right) arm or shoulder onto the patient's knee through his femur, toward the pelvis and hip and directed toward the sacroiliac joint until further softening of the tissue is noted at the monitoring finger.
   e. While maintaining the compression, the patient's leg is gently carried through adduction in an arc across the midline and with increased hip flexion by engaging the sacroiliac barrier (rotating the innominate/ilum posteriorly).
   f. The patient's hip and knee are brought back to the neutral position by extending both the hip and knee.
   g. The iliosacral somatic dysfunction is reassessed.

### Posterior Innominate/Posterior Ilium (Right)—Patient Supine

1. **Patient position:** supine.
2. **Physician position:** standing at the side of the patient on the side of the somatic dysfunction, facing the patient.
3. **Technique:**
   a. The physician places the pad of the index or middle finger of his monitoring cepha-

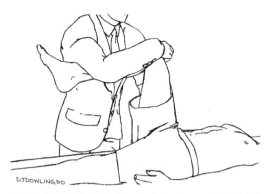

■ **FIG. 64-1A** Anterior ilium/anterior innominate (right), patient supine.

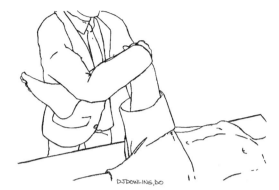

■ **FIG. 64-1B** Anterior ilium/anterior innominate (right), patient supine.

lad hand medial to the posterior superior iliac spine (PSIS) as a means of following the iliosacral motion (the left finger contacts the area medial to PSIS on the right).

b. The physician uses his other hand to grasp the patient's leg on the dysfunctional side and fully flexes the patient's hip (more than 90 degrees) and knee until motion is felt at the monitoring finger. The knee is adducted (the physician's right hand grasps and flexes the patient's right leg in this example).

c. The physician puts downward compression with his caudad (right) arm or shoulder onto the patient's knee through his femur, toward the pelvis and hip, and directed toward the sacroiliac joint until further soft tissue is noted at the monitoring finger (Fig. 64-2A).

d. The physician abducts the knee and externally rotates the leg until motion and soft tissue relaxation is felt at the monitoring finger.

e. The physician then uses his abdomen or hip to maintain compression through the femur (Fig. 64-2B).

f. While maintaining the compression and external rotation, the patient's leg is gently carried through extension and to the neutral position.

g. The iliosacral somatic dysfunction is reassessed.

## Upslipped Innominate (Right)—Patient Supine

1. **Patient position:** supine.
2. **Physician position:** initially standing at the foot of the table.

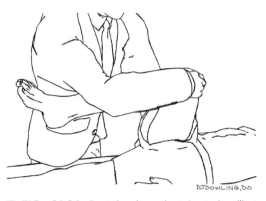

■ **FIG. 64-2A** Posterior innominate/posterior ilium (right), patient supine.

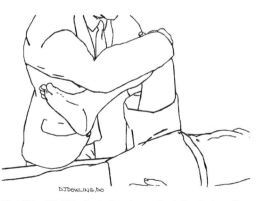

■ **FIG. 64-2B** Posterior innominate/posterior ilium (right), patient supine.

3. **Technique:**
   a. The physician grasps the ankle on the dysfunctional side with both hands and externally rotates and compresses the leg towards the hip and iliosacral joint (Fig. 64-3).
   b. The physician then internally rotates the patient's leg on the involved side until just before the ASIS lifts upwards.
   c. The physician then progressively reduces the compression and transitions to traction until localized to the involved joint (occasionally, a slighter sharper long axis tug can be placed to encourage downslip of the somatic dysfunction).
   d. The Still technique for a posteriorly rotated innominate/ilium is applied; followed by the Still technique applied for an anteriorly rotated innominate/ilium.
   e. This series is designed to "ratchet" the upslipped innominate/ilium into place.
   f. The dysfunction is reassessed.

## Downslipped Innominate (Right)—Patient Supine

1. **Patient position:** supine.
2. **Physician position:** initially standing at the foot of the table.
3. **Technique:**
   a. The physician grasps the ankle on the dysfunctional side with both hands and externally rotates and tractions the leg toward the physician by pulling parallel to the table.

   b. The physician then internally rotates the patient's leg on the involved side until just before the ASIS lifts upwards.
   c. The physician then progressively reduces the traction and transitions to compression until localized to the involved joint
   d. The Still technique for an anteriorly rotated innominate/ilium is applied, followed by the Still technique applied for a posteriorly rotated innominate/ilium.
   e. This series is designed to "ratchet" the downslipped innominate/ilium into place.
   f. The dysfunction is reassessed.

## ■ PUBIC DYSFUNCTIONS

### Pubic Ramus Dysfunction

1. **Patient position:** supine.
2. **Physician position:** standing at the foot of the table.
3. **Technique:**
   a. The physician grasps the patient's ankles and flexes the hips and knees and then places the patient's feet upon the table. The knees are bent approximately 90 degrees and the feet placed together.
   b. The physician places both palms of his hands on the anterior inferior knees and introduces long axis compression through the femurs toward the pubic bones.
   c. While maintaining the compression, the physician symmetrically separates the patient's knees laterally creating thigh external rotation to the approximate soft tissue barrier (Fig. 64-4).

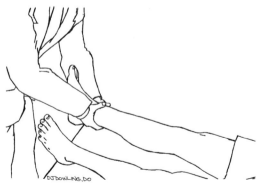

■ **FIG. 64-3** Upslipped innominate (right), patient supine.

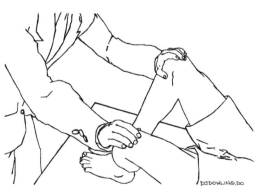

■ **FIG. 64-4** Pubic ramus dysfunction (L1-5 N $S_R$ $R_L$), patient supine.

d. The physician then releases the knees and grasps the ankles. The position of the knees is maintained by gravity and the patient's passive compliance.

e. The physician then pulls the patient's ankles towards himself by straightening the patient's legs until the hips and knees are in a neutral position.

f. The pubic dysfunctions are reassessed.

## ■ SACRAL DYSFUNCTIONS

### Unilateral Sacral Shear/Flexion Dysfunction (Right)

1. **Patient position:** supine.
2. **Physician position:** standing at the side of the table facing the patient on the side of the dysfunction.
3. **Technique:**
   a. The physician places the pad of the index or middle finger of his monitoring caudad hand under the patient and monitors just medial to the posterior superior iliac spine (PSIS) on the involved side (left).
   b. The physician's cephalad hand (left) reaches across and down from the patient's body and grasps the patient's opposite (left) knee and flexes that hip and knee to approximately 90 degrees or to the point where motion is noted at the monitoring finger (Fig. 64-5A).
   c. The opposite (left) knee is abducted and adducted in an alternating sequence until relaxation is noted at the monitoring finger. The position is temporarily main-

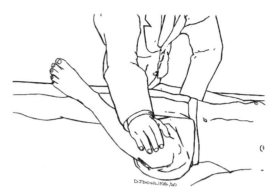

■ **FIG. 64-5B** Unilateral sacral shear/flexion dysfunction (right).

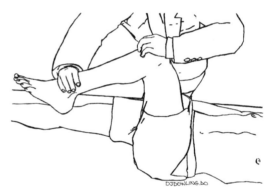

■ **FIG. 64-5C** Unilateral sacral shear/flexion dysfunction (right).

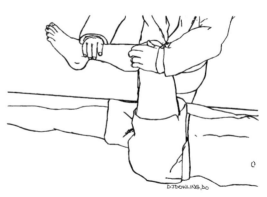

■ **FIG. 64-5D** Unilateral sacral shear/flexion dysfunction (right).

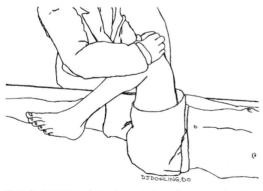

■ **FIG. 64-5A** Unilateral sacral shear/flexion dysfunction (right).

tained and compression is introduced from that knee downwards through the femur towards the sacroiliac joint. (Fig. 64-5*B*)

d. The physician moves the monitoring hand from beneath the patient to the knee of the opposite (left) leg.

e. While maintaining the compression with the cephalad (left) hand, the physician then pushes the patient's (left) leg laterally.

f. The patient's (left) knee is then adducted past the midline. The left side of the pelvis may lift slightly from the table (Fig. 64-5*C*).

g. The patient's (left) ankle is then brought towards and past the midline (toward the physician) (Fig. 64-5*D*).

h. The compression is maintained and the patient's (left) leg is gradually straightened.

i. The sacroiliac dysfunction is reexamined.

## Sacral Rotations and Torsions (Left on Left)

1. **Patient position:** supine.
2. **Physician position:** standing at the side of the table facing the patient on the side of the dysfunction.
3. **Technique:**

a. The physician places the pad of his index or middle finger of his monitoring cephalad hand under the patient and monitors just medial to the posterior superior iliac spine (PSIS) on the deep sacral sulcus side (right)

b. The physician's other (caudad) hand scoops both of the patient's legs from under the knees and lifts both and bends the knees 90 degrees or more until motion is felt at the monitoring finger (Fig. 64-6*A*).

c. The physician then shifts the monitoring (cephalad) hand from beneath the patient and transfers it to the patient's knees. The other (caudad) hand is transferred to the patient's ankles (Fig. 64-6*B*).

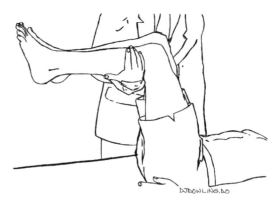

■ **FIG. 64-6A** Sacral rotations and torsions (left-on-left).

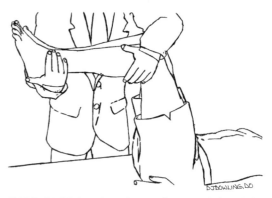

■ **FIG. 64-6B** Sacral rotations and torsions (left-on-left).

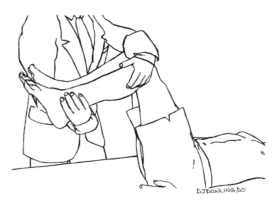

■ **FIG. 64-6C** Sacral rotations and torsions (left-o-left).

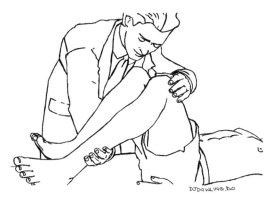

**■ FIG. 64-6D** Sacral rotations and torsions (left-on-left).

d. The patient's knees are rotated toward the side opposite the deep sulcus (left) (toward the physician).
e. The patient's feet are moved toward the same side as the knees (left) (Fig. 64-6C).

f. The physician then simultaneously shifts the patient's knees and ankles toward the opposite direction (right) across the midline (away from the physician) (Fig. 64-6D).
g. At approximately 45 degrees from the vertical, the physician gradually begins to extend the patient's legs.
h. Once the legs are back on the table the somatic dysfunction can be reassessed.

## REFERENCES

Van Buskirk RL. A manipulative technique of Andrew Taylor Still. *J Am Osteopath Assoc* 1996;96:597–602.

Van Buskirk RL. *The Still Technique Manual*. Indianapolis, IN: American Academy of Osteopathy, 1999.

Van Buskirk RL. Treatment of somatic dysfunction with an osteopathic manipulative method of Dr. Andrew Taylor Still. In Ward RC, ed. *Foundations for Osteopathic Medicine*. Philadelphia: Lippincott Williams & Wilkins, 2003; 1094–1114.

# PINS Techniques

*Dennis J. Dowling*

This chapter describes PINS technique for treating somatic dysfunctions of the sacral and pelvic region (Figs. 65-1 and 65-2). The examples provided are not the only ones that are possible (Figure 53-1); however, they are fairly common. Occasionally, patterns in the sacral and pelvic region may continue into or from adjacent regions. The patient is most commonly treated in the supine and prone positions but could be treated side-lying if necessary. The physician should be positioned comfortably facing the region to be treated or alongside the table. The principles and methods of PINS can be applied:

1. Locate a sensitive point in the region of the symptoms.
2. Analyze the structures that are deep to that point.
3. Locate another sensitive point at the other end of a connecting structure (i.e., muscle, ligament, nerve, etc.). The more sensitive point is the primary point and the less sensitive point is the endpoint.
4. Apply inhibitory pressure to both points for 30 or more seconds. The soft tissue at the more sensitive point will typically lessen in tension.
5. Beginning at the more sensitive of the two points, locate another sensitive point approximately 2 to 3 centimeters toward the less sensitive endpoint.
6. Repeat the procedure progressively toward the endpoint.
7. Reassess the status of the dysfunction. Determine if additional treatment or the application of other modalities is necessary.

## ■ PIRIFORMIS

1. **Technique:**
   a. The physician places the pad of his index or middle finger on the lateral border of the sacrum approximately halfway between the PSIS and the ILA. A finger of the physician's other hand locates a sensitive point superior at greater trochanter.
   b. The pattern of intervening points is usually straight but the depth of pressure may indicate other muscles involved (gemmeli or obturator).
2. **Clinical Correlation:**
   a. Hip pain
   b. Sacral dysfunction
   c. Sciatica

## ■ ILIOTIBIAL BAND

1. **Technique:**
   a. The physician places the pad of his index or middle finger on a point on the greater trochanter. An inferior sensitive point may be found at the fibular head or lateral condyle of the femur.
   b. The pattern of intervening points is generally straight (muscle pattern) but may be slightly variable. There may also be a typical continuation of the pattern to the lateral malleolus or anterior portion of the talus.
2. **Clinical Correlation:**
   a. Hip pain
   b. Knee pain

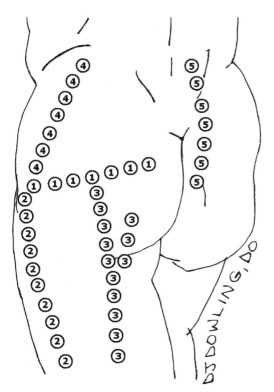

■ **FIG. 65-1** PINS sacrum and pelvis point patterns. Posterior: *1, piriformis muscle; 2, iliotibial band; 3, sciatic nerve/ posterior femoral cutaneous nerve/hamstring muscles; 4, gluteal muscles; 5, sacroiliac.*

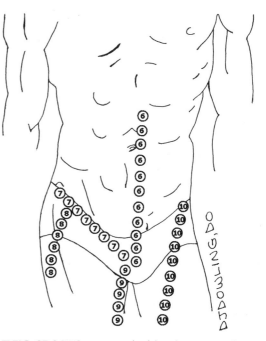

■ **FIG. 65-2** PINS sacrum and pelvis point patterns. Anterior: *6, rectus abdominus muscle/pubic; 7, inguinal ligament; 8, lateral femoral cutaneous nerve; 9, adductor (gracilis) muscle; 10, sartorius.*

## ■ SCIATIC NERVE/POSTERIOR FEMORAL CUTANEOUS NERVE/ HAMSTRING MUSCLE

1. **Technique:**
   a. The physician places the pad of his index or middle finger in the middle of the gluteal region. An alternative may be found at the ischial tuberosity. A finger of the physician's other hand locates a sensitive point distally. The point may be as low as the knee in the popliteal region and may be medial, in the middle, or lateral.
   b. The pattern of intervening points is generally slightly curved or straight (muscle pattern) or zigzag when involving a nerve.
2. **Clinical Correlation:**
   a. Rectal symptoms
   b. Pelvic pain
   c. Sciatica

## ■ GLUTEAL MUSCLES

1. **Technique:**
   a. The physician places the pad of his index or middle finger near and inferior to the medial iliac crest. A finger of the physician's other hand locates a sensitive point laterally on the upper portion of the femur, possibly at the greater trochanter.
   b. The pattern of intervening points generally follows the origins and insertions of glutei maximus, medius, and minimus.
2. **Clinical Correlation:**
   a. Buttock pain
   b. Hip pain

## ■ SACROILIAC

1. **Technique:**
   a. The physician places the pad of his index or middle finger medial and inferior to the PSIS. A finger of the physician's other hand locates a sensitive point in the gluteal crevice near the coccyx.

b. The pattern of intervening points generally follows the edge of the sacrum.

2. **Clinical Correlation:**
   a. Sacroiliac pain
   b. Coccygodynia

# ■ RECTUS ABDOMINUS MUSCLE/ PUBI

1. **Technique:**
   a. The physician places the pad of his index or middle finger lateral to the xiphoid process on the medial aspect of the seventh rib anteriorly. A finger of the physician's other hand locates a sensitive point on the pubic ramus.
   b. The pattern of intervening points generally follows the origins and insertions of rectus abdominus.

2. **Clinical Correlation:**
   a. Abdominal pain
   b. Dysuria, cystitis, prostatitis

# ■ INGUINAL LIGAMENT

1. **Technique:**
   a. The physician places the pad of his index or middle finger medial and inferior to the ASIS. A finger of the physician's other hand locates a sensitive point on the pubic ramus.
   b. The pattern of intervening points generally follows the origins and insertions of the inguinal ligament.

2. **Clinical Correlation:**
   a. Abdominal pain
   b. Dysuria
   c. Dysmenorrhea
   d. Meralgia paresthetica

# ■ LATERAL FEMORAL CUTANEOUS NERVE

1. **Technique:**
   a. The physician places the pad of his index or middle finger one third of the distance medially from the ASIS and slightly inferior to the inguinal ligament. A finger of the physician's other hand locates a sensitive point on the lateral thigh.
   b. The pattern of intervening points generally follows a slightly zigzag pattern of the nerve.

2. **Clinical Correlation:**
   a. Meralgia paresthetica
   b. Hip pain

# ■ ADDUCTOR (GRACILIS) MUSCLE

1. **Technique:**
   a. The physician places the pad of his index or middle finger on the pubic ramus. A finger of the physician's other hand locates a sensitive point on the medial knee or pes anserine.
   b. The pattern of intervening points generally follows a slightly zigzag pattern of the nerve.

2. **Clinical Correlation:**
   a. Inguinal pain
   b. Medial knee pain

# ■ SARTORIUS

1. **Technique:**
   a. The physician places the pad of his index or middle finger medial to the ASIS. A finger of the physician's other hand locates a sensitive point on the medial knee or pes anserine.
   b. The pattern of intervening points generally follows a curved or straight pattern of the muscle.

2. **Clinical Correlation:**
   a. Inguinal pain
   b. Medial knee pain

## REFERENCES

Dowling DJ. Progressive inhibition of neuromuscular structures (PINS) technique. *J Am Osteopath Assoc* 2000;100: 285–286, 289–298.

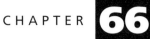

# Thrusting Techniques

*Eileen L. DiGiovanna, Dennis J. Dowling, and Barry S. Erner*

High-velocity, low-amplitude thrusting techniques may be applied to the pelvic and sacral articulations. There should be soft tissue preparation as for any other area.

## ■ INNOMINATE AND SACRAL SOMATIC DYSFUNCTIONS

### Posterior Iliac Somatic Dysfunction/ Unilateral Sacral Shear/Forward Sacral Rotations and Torsions

1. **Patient position:** lateral recumbent with somatic dysfunctional side up.
2. **Physician position:** standing, facing the front of the patient.
3. **Technique:**
   a. The physician uses one hand to monitor the iliosacral/sacroiliac joint medial to the posterior superior iliac spine (PSIS) at all times while positioning and treating the patient.
   b. The physician flexes the patient's hips and knees until motion is felt at the monitoring hand.
   c. The patient is asked to straighten the lower leg while the physician maintains the flexion of the upper leg. The physician then hooks the foot of the flexed leg in the popliteal fossa of the inferior leg.
   d. Grasping the patient's arm that is in contact with the table, the physician rotates the patient's upper torso forward until motion is felt at the monitoring hand.
   e. The physician places his thrusting forearm over the patient's iliac crest and moni-

tors the segment with the fingers of his other hand. The lower body is rotated toward the physician until motion is localized at the sacroiliac joint.
   f. He then places his other arm against the patient's shoulder. This maintains the upper body rotation during the rest of the treatment.
   g. Sufficient rotation is engaged to localize motion to the somatic dysfunction level. The position is firmly maintained.
   h. A slight springing force is exerted by introducing a very slight anterior lower body rotation towards the floor to determine that localization is correct.
   i. The patient is asked to inhale and then exhale fully.
   j. Taking up all the slack, the physician exerts a rapid rotational forward thrust through the dysfunctional ilium at the end of the patient's exhalation (Fig. 66-1).
   k. The dysfunction is then reassessed.

### Anterior Iliac Somatic Dysfunction/ Backward Sacral Rotation or Torsion

1. **Patient position:** lateral recumbent position with somatic dysfunction side up.
2. **Physician position:** standing, facing the front of the patient.
3. **Technique:**
   a. The physician uses one hand to monitor the iliosacral/sacroiliac joint medial to the posterior superior iliac spine (PSIS) at all times while positioning and treating the patient.

**349**

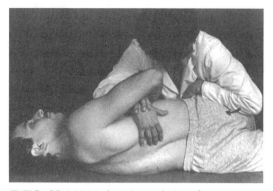

■ **FIG. 66-1** HVLA thrusting technique for a posterior iliac somatic dysfunction.

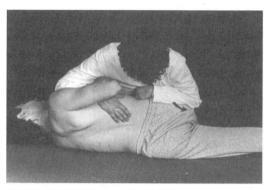

■ **FIG. 66-2** HVLA thrusting technique for an anterior iliac somatic dysfunction.

b. The physician flexes the patient's hips and knees until motion is felt at the monitoring hand.

c. The patient is asked to straighten the lower leg while the physician maintains the flexion of the upper leg.

d. The upper leg is then dropped off the table and held between the physician's knees.

e. Grasping the patient's arm that is in contact with the table, the physician rotates the patient's upper torso forward away from the table until motion is felt at the monitoring hand.

f. The physician places his thrusting arm on the patient's inferior iliac crest.

g. With his other arm he maintains the upper body rotation.

h. A slight springing force is exerted to assure that localization is correct.

i. The patient is instructed in inhale deeply and then exhale fully.

j. The physician exerts a quick, rotational, slightly downward thrust posteriorly through the iliac crest following the long axis of the patient's lower leg (Fig. 66-2).

k. The dysfunction is then reassessed.

## ■ PUBIC SOMATIC DYSFUNCTION
### Inferior Pubes

1. **Patient position:** supine.
2. **Physician position:** seated on the side of the table, on the same side as the dysfunction.
3. **Technique:**
   a. The physician flexes the patient's knee/hip on the side of the dysfunction and rests the patient's ankle/calf on his shoulder.

b. The physician makes a tight fist with his treating hand.

c. The physician places his fist against the ischial tuberosity on the side of the pubic dysfunction.

d. The patient is directed to inhale deeply and the physician resists the movement of the patient's ischial tuberosity against his hand. The patient is then directed to exhale completely.

e. At the end of exhalation, the physician exerts a rapid cephalad/forward thrust through the ischium (Fig. 66-3).

f. The somatic dysfunction is then reassessed.

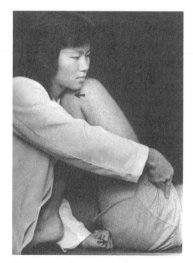

■ **FIG. 66-3** HVLA thrusting technique for an inferior pubic somatic dysfunction.

## Alternative Technique to Treat Pubic Restrictions

1. **Patient position:** supine, with hips and knees bent and feet together and flat on the table.
2. **Physician position:** standing at the side of the table.
3. **Technique:**
   a. The physician abducts and externally rotates the patient's legs bilaterally into a "frog-leg" position until the motion is resisted by the muscle tension.
   b. The patient is instructed to push both knees medially against the physician's isometric resistance for 3 to 5 seconds. At the end of the effort, the patient's knees are further abducted and the legs externally rotated. This is repeated three or more times.
   c. The patient is instructed to inhale deeply and exhale fully.
   d. At the end of exhalation, the physician exerts a quick downward and outward thrust through the patient's knees bilaterally, symmetrically, and simultaneously, which gaps the pubic symphysis (Fig. 66-4).
   e. The patient's legs are extended and the somatic dysfunction is reassessed.

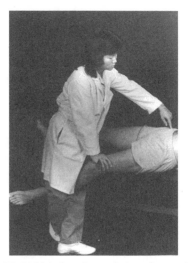

■ **FIG. 66-4** HVLA thrusting technique for restriction of pubic symphysis.

## ■ SACRUM

The sacrum frequently becomes restricted in its motion at the sacroiliac articulation. Thrusting techniques may be used to create motion at this articulation.

### Anterior Sacral Flexion

1. **Patient position:** prone.
2. **Physician position:** standing at the same side of the table as the side of the dysfunction.
3. **Technique:**
   a. The physician places the thenar eminence of his treating hand over the inferior lateral angle of the restricted side of the sacrum, maintaining firm contact and monitors the sacroiliac joint medially to the PSIS with the finer of the same hand.
   b. The physician extends and internally rotates the patient's leg on the side of the dysfunction with his other hand. The leg is then abducted until the palpating fingers of the monitoring hand feel motion.
   c. The patient is instructed to inhale deeply and hold it.
   d. The physician exerts a downward and cephalad pressure over the sacrum at the inferior lateral angle (ILA), creating relative extension.
   e. The patient is instructed to exhale fully and the physician resists the backward motion of the ILA. This is repeated.
   f. At the end of the final exhalation, the physician exerts a quick downward and cephalad thrust with his thenar eminence over the inferior lateral angle(Fig. 66-5).
   f. The somatic dysfunction is reassessed.

### Anterior Sacral Flexion/Unilateral Sacral Shear/Sacral Rotations orTorsions

1. **Patient position:** supine; the patient should be lying closer to the edge of the table on the side of the deeper sacral sulcus.
2. **Physician position:** standing on the same side as the deeper sacral sulcus.
3. **Technique:**
   a. The physician side-bends the patient's legs away from the side of the deeper sulcus.

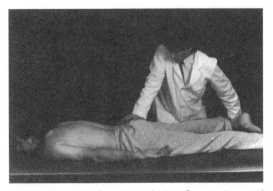

**■ FIG. 66-5** HVLA thrusting technique for anterior sacral flexion dysfunction.

b. The physician side-bends the patient's torso away from the side of the deeper sulcus. (The patient is now in a "C" position. Both the physician and the deep sulcus are on the side of the convexity and at the apex.)

c. The patient is instructed to clasp his hands behind his neck.

d. The physician places the thenar eminence of his caudad hand on the patient's anterior superior iliac spine (ASIS) on the side opposite to the deep sulcus.

e. The physician places his cephalad hand over the patient's opposite shoulder. (The hand can be placed over this arm and then between the forearm and upper arm with the back of the physician's hand resting on the patient's sternum.)

f. To help stabilize the patient in the next step, the physician may place his cephalad knee next to the patient's shoulder.

g. The physician uses his cephalad hand/arm to rotate the patient's upper torso toward the physician as far as possible while maintaining comfort and stability.

h. The physician's hand holds the patient's opposite ASIS and resists its tendency to lift from the table during the rotation.

i. The patient is instructed to inhale deeply and exhale completely.

j. A rotational thrust of the patient's upper body is introduced by the physician's cephalad arm at the end of exhalation.

k. The patient is brought back to neutral and the dysfunction is reassessed.

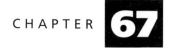

# Exercise

*Stanley Schiowitz*

$W$hen prescribing an exercise program for dysfunctions of the muscles in the pelvic region, consideration must be given to the fact that its gross motions involve other body regions. Dysfunctions will often involve pelvic tilt and lateral muscle hyper/hypotonicity

## ■ LATERAL ROTATOR MUSCLE STRENGTHENING

The lateral rotator muscles of the hip include the piriformis and the obturater internus. The piriformis muscle has its medial attachment to the lateral border of the sacrum and is often involved in sacral dysfunctions.

1. **Patient position**: Prone on table with head under arms, big toes together, and heels separated laterally.
2. **Instructions**:
   a. Slowly bring your heels together by contracting your hip muscles while maintaining the position of your toes.
   b. Hold heels firmly against each other for a count of 10 seconds.
   c. Slowly rotate heels laterally to their fullest spread position.
   d. Relax, rest, and repeat. (Fig. 67-1)

Note: An assistant creating an isokinetic resistive force against the medial aspect of the heels will increase the effectiveness of the exercise.

## ■ PIRIFORMIS STRETCH

1. **Patient position**: Supine on table, arms at the side of the body.

2. **Instructions**:
   a. Bend knee and hip of extremity involved and plant its heel firmly on the table alongside the lateral aspect of the other knee joint (Fig. 67-2A)
   b. Maintaining this position, pivot on the heel rotating the extremity toward the other extremity as far as it can go (Fig. 67-2B).
   c. Hold in this position allowing the weight of the extremity to create a stretching force.
   d. Slowly pivot the extremity back to its original position.
   e. Relax, rest, and repeat.

Note: An assistant creating an isometric resistive force against the lateral aspect of the knee as the extremity is being pivoted laterally back to its original position will increase the effectiveness of the exercise.

## ■ LATERAL ROTATOR MUSCLE STRETCHES

### Technique 1

1. **Patient position**: Supine on table, lower extremities extended, with heels 6 inches apart and ankle dorsiflexed at 90 degrees (Fig. 67-3A).
2. **Instructions**:
   a. Slowly bring the big toes together by contracting the muscles of the hips.
   b. Hold the toes firmly together for a count of 10 seconds (Fig. 67-3B).

**353**

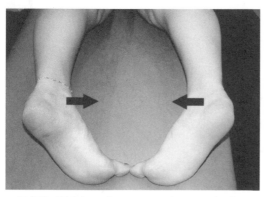

■ **FIG. 67-1** Lateral rotator muscle strengthening.

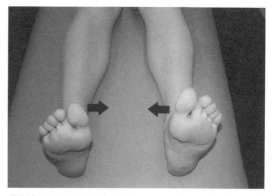

■ **FIG. 67-3A** Lateral rotator muscle stretch starting position.

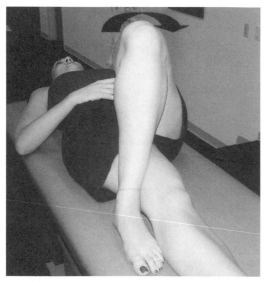

■ **FIG. 67-2A** Piriformis stretch starting position.

c. Slowly rotate the feet back to its original position
d. Relax, rest, and repeat.

Note: An assistant creating an isometric resistant force against the medial aspect of the big toes as the feet are rotated inwards will increase the effectiveness of the exercise.

## Technique 2

1. **Patient position**: Seated firmly at the edge of a table with both legs hanging downward.
2. **Instructions:**
   a. Grasp the sides of the table to maintain stability.
   b. Slowly rotate the involved leg laterally as far as it can go without moving the thigh or knee from their positions on the table (Fig. 67-4).

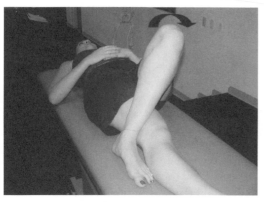

■ **FIG. 67-2B** Priiformis stretch ending position.

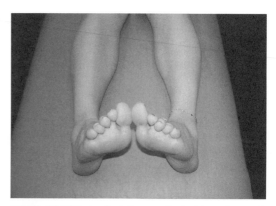

■ **FIG. 67-3B** Lateral rotator muscle stretch ending position.

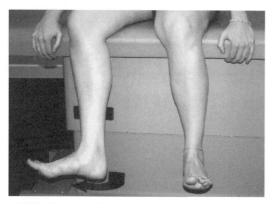

**■ FIG. 67-4** Lateral rotator muscle stretch, technique 2.

c. Hold firmly for a count of 10 seconds.

d. Slowly rotate the leg back to its original position.

e. Relax, rest, and repeat.

Note: An assistant creating an isometric force against the leg as it is trying to rotate will increase the effectiveness of the exercise.

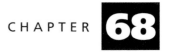

# CHAPTER 68

# Practical Applications and Case Histories of the Sacrum and Pelvis

*Eileen L. DiGiovanna*

The sacrum forms a vital link between the spinal column and the ring-shaped pelvis and the lower extremities. Dysfunctions of the sacral–pelvic complex can affect normal function of the spinal column, gait, childbearing, pelvic viscera, and can be involved in a host of localized painful conditions. The lower fibers of the parasympathetic nervous system exit from the spinal canal through the sacral foramina along with motor and sensory nerves. Sacral dysfunctions can therefore be involved in widespread effects on tissues and organs innervated by these nerves.

## ■ SACROILITIS (ANKYLOSING SPONDYLITIS)

Sacroiliitis is an inflammatory condition of the sacroiliac joint. This is most often associated with *ankylosing spondylitis*. Mechanical dysfunctions of this joint will be painful with motion; the pain of sacroiliitis is usually present more persistently. In males, ankylosing spondylitis first manifests as a sacroiliitis and then moves up the spine. In females, ankylosing spondylitis may begin in any joint and follows no specific pattern. Ankylosing spondylitis is a seronegative *spondyloarthritis* beginning in young adulthood and affects multiple joints. It appears to be genetic (HLAB27) in origin. After the initial sacroiliitis, the joint will eventually ossify, as do the facet joints of the spine and extremity joints as the disease progresses.

Osteopathic manipulation begun early enough in the disease may help maintain joint function for a longer period of time. Exercise of all joints is essential for the maintenance of motion.

## ■ PIRIFORMIS SYNDROME

The piriformis muscle lies deep to the gluteal muscles. It originates on the anteriolateral surface of the sacrum, joint capsule, and anterior sacrotuberous ligament and attaches to the superomedial surface of the greater trochanter of the femur. It is an external rotator and abductor of the thigh. This muscle has an intimate relationship to the sciatic nerve, which passes just beneath it, or, sometimes, through the muscle belly or between two tendinous origins of the piriformis.

Hypertonicity or spasm of the piriformis muscle may cause irritation of the sciatic nerve, sometimes to the point of causing neuritis. Although the sciatic nerve most typically passes inferior to the piriformis, normal variants exist with its passage through or posterior to the piriformis muscle. The sciatic involvement often causes confusion between piriformis syndrome and a disc herniation.

Piriformis syndrome is manifested as pain in the buttocks or hip with radiation into the calf or foot. It can be severe enough to result in the patient becoming bedridden. More rarely, there is low back pain as well, especially around the sacroiliac joint. Examination demonstrates decreased internal rotation and adduction of the hip with pain accompanying these motions.

Muscle strength in external rotation and abduction is generally normal but may exhibit some decrease. The muscle and its attachments are tender to palpation. There are three counterstrain tender points associated with piriformis syndrome: mid-pole sacrum, piriformis muscle, and the posteromedial trochanteric point.

Clinically, a hypertonic piriformis is correlated with a posterior inferior lateral angle (ILA) on the same side. The muscle could be significant in causing or maintaining sacral somatic dysfunctions.

Counterstrain and facilitated positional release techniques are most useful. Each of the three tender points must be treated, if they are present, to be effective. Any dysfunction of sacral motion should also be corrected. A piriformis stretching exercise should be prescribed for use at home.

## ■ CONGENITAL ABNORMALITIES OF THE SACRUM

The sacrum is subject to abnormalities in association with the fifth lumbar vertebra, including partial or complete fusion of the fifth lumbar and the first sacral segment, *sacralization* of L5. Fusion may also occur between one or both transverse processes of L5 with the sacral base. The first sacral segment may not fuse to form a normal sacrum, but remain as a sixth lumbar vertebra, *lumbarization* of the first sacral segment.

*Spina bifida* may affect the sacrum as well as the lumbar vertebrae and results from failure of the two components of the spinous process fusing in the midline. This may be *occulta* and covered with skin and other soft tissues or open to the external environment as a more problematic form. The spina bifida occulta may often be asymptomatic or may cause localized low back pain.

Although osteopathic manipulation will not correct congenital abnormalities, it may be used to keep adjacent joints mobile and tissues in a relaxed, non-tense condition to allow as much normal function as possible in the region.

## ■ COCCYGODYNIA

Pain in the coccyx is known as *coccygodynia*. The most common cause is trauma to the coccyx, generally with associated inflammation of soft tissues in the area. It may also be caused by infection, fracture, dislocation, or soft tissue injuries. The condition may be acute or chronic.

Pain is most noticeable with sitting, straining with a bowel movement, or during sexual intercourse. On examination, the coccyx is tender to palpation. There may be pain in the levator ani or coccygeus muscles. A rectal examination may help localize the tenderness to the coccyx.

Coccygodynia responds well to osteopathic manipulation. The sacrococcygeal joint may be mobilized through the rectum, pushing the tip of the coccyx anteriorly if it is posterior or pushing it posteriorly if it is anterior. A counterstrain tender point (high flare-out sacroiliac) is found caudad and medial to the posterior superior iliac spine on the posterior surface of the sacrum. It is frequently involved in coccygodynia and should be treated in such cases. Myofascial release of the pelvic diaphragm may be done from an external approach to relieve fascial tension on the coccyx.

## ■ SOMATIC DYSFUNCTION OF SACRUM AND PELVIS

Somatic dysfunctions of the sacrum and pelvis are common and are among the most common causes of low back and pelvic pain. The articulation of L5–S1, the sacroiliac joints, and the pubic articulation are all sources of pain resulting from dysfunctions. These are described in detail in previous chapters.

Proper sacral and pelvic joint motion should be achieved in all gait, posture, and spinal motion problems. Because the sacrum is closely associated with cranial motion, the sacrum must be evaluated as part of the cranial motion evaluation. Lower extremity dysfunction often results from or may cause pelvic dysfunctions.

### Case 1

R.T. was a 32-year-old woman who was seen in the clinic with a report of low back and left buttocks pain with some radiation into the posterior thigh and calf of the left leg for approximately 10 days. She gave a history of stepping sideways over a gate she had placed in a doorway to protect her young child several times per day. A day or two later, she noticed pain in her left buttocks and by that evening it was radiating down the back of her thigh and calf. Over-the-counter anti-inflammatory medication gave her temporary relief. She had been shopping the previous day and the pain had worsened and the radiating pain was reaching to her foot.

She had had a similar pain after the birth of her first child 6 years previously, but the birth of her youngest child 1 year previously had been without event. With the first child, she had experienced low back pain throughout the third trimester and had experienced the buttocks pain with radiation into the calf of her left leg for approximately 1 week after the baby was delivered. It had resolved spontaneously.

Her past medical history was without significance. She had had no falls or accidents. She used only birth control medication and a vitamin. She had no allergies. The review of systems was non-contributory.

On examination, the left buttocks was tender to palpation and there were tender points at the mid-pole of the sacrum on the lateral border and one deep to the gluteus maximus, where a tense piriformis could be palpated. There was a unilateral sacral flexion (sacral shear) present on the left. No lumbar somatic dysfunctions were present. There was mild tenderness at the sciatic notch of the ischium. Deep tendon reflexes were normal and muscle strength of the thigh was normal. There was some pain on internal rotation and adduction of the left hip.

Left piriformis syndrome was diagnosed and was treated with osteopathic manipulation. The sacral shear was treated with a muscle energy technique and the tender points were treated with counterstrain. She was given a piriformis stretch to perform at home three time daily. She experienced immediate improvement after the treatment.

She was seen 1 week later and most of the symptoms were gone. The sacral shear had not returned. The mid-pole tender point had not returned but the piriformis tender point was still present. This was treated with relief of tenderness. She did not need to return for further treatments.

## Discussion

This case is typical of piriformis syndrome. An overstretch of the muscle had caused it to con-

tract. The spasm in the muscle impinged the sciatic nerve giving the patient radiating pain down the course of the nerve. Once the spasm of the muscle was released and the accompanying sacral dysfunction corrected, the pain ceased.

If a patient does not respond after several treatments, it is important to search for some activity the patient is doing that is either aggravating the piriformis muscle or causing a sacral dysfunction that puts abnormal tension on the muscle. Rarely, the obturator muscle is involved and mimics piriformis syndrome. This may need to be ruled out in obstinate cases.

## Case 2

J.G. was a 48-year-old woman who came to the clinic reporting pain in the coccyx on sitting for the past 2 weeks. She had begun an exercise program, which included stationary bicycle riding each day for approximately 20 minutes. After exercising for 1 week she began to experience the pain. It had gradually gotten worse until she had had to stop riding the bicycle approximately 4 days previously. Stopping the bike riding had not relieved the pain. An over-the-counter anti-inflammatory had given minimal relief. She could not sit comfortably. There was no history of a fall or a blow to the area. Her past medical history was noncontributory. She had one child who was 17 years old. She had undergone a hysterectomy 5 years previously.

Physical examination revealed a slightly obese woman in obvious discomfort. She preferred to stand rather than sit on the examination table. The sacrum was freely movable and no somatic dysfunctions of the lumbar spine were noted. The coccyx was markedly tender to palpation and the soft tissues around it were tense and tender. There was a high flare-out tender point on the posterior surface of the sacrum. Rectal examination confirmed tenderness of the coccyx, but it was not severe enough to indicate a fracture and the coccyx was not dislocated.

She was treated with mobilization of the coccyx during the rectal examination and the tender point was treated with counterstrain. She was advised to get a "doughnut" cushion to keep weight off the coccyx when sitting.

She was seen and treated on three more occasions with complete relief of the coccygodynia. She was cautioned to obtain a wider bicycle seat and perhaps cushion it so that she could continue her exercise program.

## Discussion

Coccygodynia can be caused by constant pressure, especially a moving pressure as in bicycle riding, on the coccyx. The pain can be quite severe and is aggravated by the pressure of sitting as the ischial tuberosities are spread. Osteopathic manipulative treatment assists in restoring normal motion to the coccyx and relieves tension of the soft tissues attached to the coccyx. An air cushion with a central opening makes sitting more comfortable during the treatment process, until the pain is gone.

A history of a fall or blow to the coccyx should prompt the physician to obtain x-rays to rule out fracture or dislocation.

## REFERENCES

DiGiovanna EL, Schiowitz S. *An Osteopathic Approach to Diagnosis and Treatment*, 2nd ed. Philadelphia: Lippincott-Raven, 1997.

Hoppenfeld S. *Physical Examination of the Spine and Extremities*. Norwalk, CT: Appleton & Lange, 1976.

Salter RB. *Textbook of Disorders and Injuries of the Musculoskeletal System*, 3rd ed. Baltimore: Williams & Wilkins, 1999.

Wadsworth CT. *Manual Examination and Treatment of the Spine and Extremities*. Baltimore: Williams & Wilkins, 1988.

Ward RC. *Foundations for Osteopathic Medicine*. Philadelphia: Lippincott Williams & Wilkins, 2003.

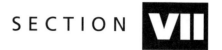

# Thoracic Cage

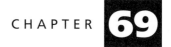

# Anatomic Considerations of the Thoracic Cage

*Dennis J. Dowling*

## ■ LANDMARKS

On palpation, several landmarks may be noted and their relations to specific ribs established. The first rib is attached to the manubrium of the sternum just inferior to the clavicle anteriorly; posteriorly, it is cephalad to the superior border of the scapula. The second rib articulates with both the manubrium and the body of the sternum at the sternal angle anteriorly. Posteriorly, the third rib is located at approximately the median aspect of the spine of the scapula. The costal cartilage of the seventh rib attaches to the sternal body and xiphoid process ventrally, and the angle of the rib rests near the tip of the scapula's inferior angle. The cartilage of the tenth rib is palpated at the lowest aspect of the thoracic cage in the mid-clavicular line. The twelfth rib is almost horizontal and is found by palpating in the soft tissues posteriorly above the iliac crests.

## Structure of Ribs

The ribs are often classified as *true* or *false*. "True" ribs are ribs one through seven, whereas ten through twelve are "false." The cartilage of the true ribs, the first through seventh ribs, attaches to the sternum. The false ribs, ribs eight through twelve, are further divided into *vertebrochondral ribs* (eighth through tenth ribs) and *floating ribs* (eleven and twelve). The cartilage of the vertebrochondral ribs unites with the cartilage of the seventh ribs. The floating ribs lack cartilage and float freely.

### Typical Ribs

The third through ninth ribs are typical ribs. The round, knob-like rib head is followed by the neck and tubercle, a body that arcs at the region of the rib angle, and a distal concavity where the cartilage attaches. The body of a typical rib is thin and flat, with interior and exterior surfaces and a costal groove on the inferior edge.

Each rib head has two facets for articulation with the body of the next superior vertebra and the same-numbered vertebral body. These articulations jointly constitute the costovertebral articulation. The tubercle articulates with the transverse process of the same vertebra via a facet and is known as the costotransverse articulation.

### Atypical Ribs

The first, second, tenth, eleventh, and twelfth ribs are considered atypical ribs. The first rib is flat, has the greatest curvature and the shortest length of all the ribs, and has no angle or costal groove. Its superior surface has grooves for passage of the subclavian vessels and elevations for the attachment of the anterior and middle scalene muscles. The single facet of the head articulates with the body of the T1 vertebra.

The second rib is similar to the 1st but longer and not as flat. The two demifacets on the rib head articulate with the T1 and T2 vertebrae.

The tenth rib is typical in every respect expect its costovertebral articulation. The single articular facet on the head forms a joint with the facet on the body of the T10 vertebra.

The eleventh and twelfth ribs have neither neck nor tubercles. As in the tenth rib, the heads have single facets corresponding to facets on the same-numbered vertebral bodies. The ventral ends float freely. The twelfth rib does not possess a costal groove.

# ■ SUPPORTING STRUCTURES

The other bony structures supporting the thoracic cage consist of the clavicle and the sternum. Posteriorly, support is provided by the vertebral column.

The *clavicle* is located at the anterosuperior aspect of the thoracic cage. Its medial end articulates with the manubrium and the cartilage of the first rib. Even though the clavicle and its component joints are considered a part of the shoulder in function, it is important during respiration. As the occiput can be considered $C_0$, the clavicle can be thought of as $Rib_0$. It must remain mobile during each phase of respiration for the rib cage, especially the first rib, to function properly.

The *sternum* is composed of three parts: the xiphoid, body, and manubrium. The lateral edges of the sternum are scalloped for the attachment of costal cartilage.

The shape of the *thoracic vertebrae* defines the posterior portion of the thoracic cage and much of its motion. The bodies of the thoracic vertebrae have costal facets for articulation with the heads of the ribs. The long, thick, transverse processes have facets on their bulbous tips for articulation with the rib tubercles.

## Articulations

The *sternoclavicular joint*, one of the true joints of the shoulder girdle, may affect rib cage motion either primarily, via the manubrium and ligamentous attachments to the costal cartilage, or secondarily, because of the position of the upper extremity.

The *costovertebral joint* is the articulation of the rib head with the bodies of one or two vertebrae. For a typical rib, the costovertebral joint includes the bodies of the vertebra at the same level and the vertebra immediately above, the annulus fibrosis of the intervening disk, and the costal facets. It is a synovial joint with a single capsule. The facets of the costovertebral joint are slightly convex and form an angle that fits into the depression formed by the vertebral facets and the disk. Several ligaments are associated with the costovertebral joint, including the interosseous ligament and the superior, intermediate, and inferior bands of the radiate ligament.

The *costotransverse articulation* is likewise a simple synovial joint surrounded by a capsule. Three ligaments—the superior, posterior, and interosseous costotransverse ligaments—connect the transverse process to the neck of the tubercle. The superior costotransverse ligament also connects the transverse process to the neck of the next lower rib.

Together, the costotransverse and costovertebral joints form a complex coupled joint. An imaginary line drawn between the two articulations is the axis that defines the direction of rib motion (Fig. 69-1).

The *costochondral region* of a rib consists of a concave pit on the end of the bony portion, to which is attached the cone-shaped cartilage.

The *sternochondral articulation* is formed by the costal cartilage and the triangular notches of the sternum. Small synovial joints are present. The apex of each notch faces medially, with an anteroposterior axis that allows freedom of motion along the coronal plane. Radiate ligaments support the joints.

# ■ MUSCLES

The major muscle of inspiration is the *thoracic diaphragm*, which is responsible for at least sixty percent of the generated thoracic cage pressure change. The muscular portion inserts onto the xiphoid process, the lower six ribs, and the upper lumbar vertebrae. All of these muscular portions converge on the aponeurotic *central tendon* (Fig. 69-2).

The diaphragm is a dome-shaped muscle with two lateral hemi-diaphragms whose shape is influenced by the viscera. In addition to inspiration and expiration, the diaphragm is important in micturition, defecation, parturition, circulation of blood, lymphatic pumping, and speech.

Other *inspiratory muscles* include the external intercostals, the levator costarum, and the so-called secondary or accessory muscles. In truth, these muscles are used whenever inhalation oc-

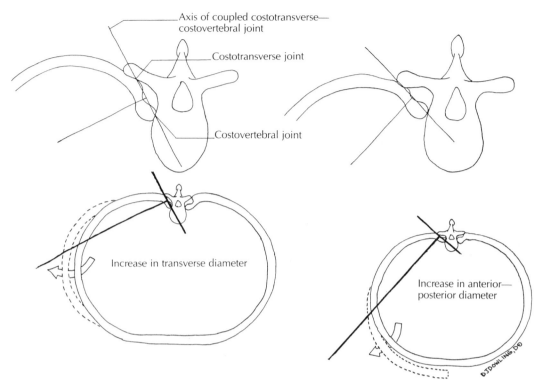

**FIG. 69-1** Axes of the costotransverse-costovertebral joints.

curs. In conditions such as asthma or emphysema, they become more pronounced as their percentage of inhalation increases. The accessory muscles are called into action for forced inspiration, such as is needed during exercise, or in pathologic states, including attacks of asthma. These *auxillary inspiratory muscles* include the sternocleidomastoid, the scalenes, the serratus posterior superior, the pectoralis, the inferior fibers of the serratus anterior, the latissimus dorsi, and the superior fibers of iliocostalis muscles.

*Expiration* is primarily produced by recoil of the diaphragm and the energy stored in the costal cartilage. The sternocostalis and internal intercostalis muscles are also involved. The *accessory expiratory muscles* include the rectus abdominis, external oblique, internal oblique, transversus abdominis, serratus posterior inferior, transversus thoracic, pyramidalis, subcostalis, quadratus lumborum, iliocostalis, longissimus, and latissimus dorsi muscles (the latissimus may play a role in either expiration or inspiration, depending on the fixed position of the arm).

## Innervation

The vertebral region is supplied primarily by dorsal rami, and the ventral rami form the eleven pairs of intercostal nerves and the pair of subcostal nerves. They begin in the intercostal space and then enter the costal groove of the first through eleventh ribs at the level of the angle. The intercostals connect to the sympathetic chain via the *rami communicantes*. The sympathetic trunks are located anterior to the heads of the ribs.

The diaphragm is innervated by the *phrenic nerve*, which consists of the ventral rami of the third, fourth, and fifth cervical nerves. Sensory input is also conducted through the phrenic nerve, with contributions from the intercostals.

## Biomechanics of the Thoracic Cage

During inspiration, the diaphragm descends as it contracts. Movement is checked by the stretching of the mediastinal contents and by resistance of the abdominal organs. Simultaneous descent and contraction of the diaphragm decreases intrathoracic pressure and thereby increases the

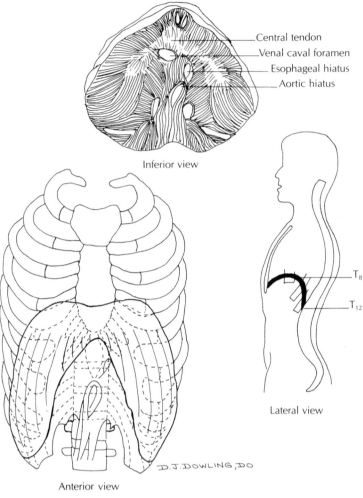

Central tendon

Venal caval foramen

Esophageal hiatus

Aortic hiatus

Inferior view

$T_8$

$T_{12}$

Lateral view

D.J.DOWLING, DO

Anterior view

■ **FIG. 69-2** The thoracic diaphragm.

volume of the thoracic cavity. As the central tendon becomes fixed, continued contraction of the muscular fibers causes elevation of the lower ribs. Elevation of the upper ribs is assisted by the sternum.

Diaphragmatic movement increases the thoracic volume in three dimensions. Depression of the central tendon alters the vertical dimension, elevation of the ribs increases the transverse dimension, and elevation of the sternum and upper ribs changes the anteroposterior dimension (Fig. 69-3). Both the external intercostals and the levator costarum assist in inspiration by elevating the ribs.

The sternocostalis and internal costalis muscles depress the ribs during expiration. The ac-

cessory expiratory muscles can be divided into abdominal muscles, thoracic cage muscles, and thoracolumbar muscles. The abdominal muscles strongly depress the thoracic floor and increase intra-abdominal pressure. Thoracic cage muscles such as the serratus posterior inferior act directly on rib attachments to draw the ribs downward. The thoracolumbar muscles also depress the ribs and possibly the scapula.

## ■ RIB MOTION

The axis formed by the coupled costovertebral and costotransverse joints determines the primary direction of rib movement. This is influenced by the angle between the vertebral body and the transverse process and by the distance

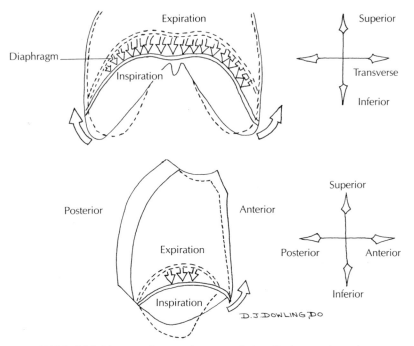

■ **FIG. 69-3** Diameter changes that occur during diaphragmatic motion.

between the costal articulations with the vertebra. The axes of the ribs permit three basic types of motion: *bucket handle, pump handle,* and *caliper* motion (Fig. 69-4).

### Bucket Handle Motion

The handle on a bucket is fixed at both ends. The axis is closer to a sagittal plane in the lower ribs. With one end of the bucket handle fixed at the vertebral end, the majority of the rib elevation occurs through upward excursion of the lateral portion. This motion increases the transverse diameter of the rib cage.

### Pump Handle Motion

The term *pump handle motion* is derived from the similarity between the rib motion and that of an old-fashioned water pump. One end is fixed, and the free end describes an arc. The costovertebral–costotransverse axis of the upper ribs lies close to the coronal plane. As the ribs move about this axis, they increase the anteroposterior diameter of that portion of the rib cage.

### Mixed Pump and Bucket Handle Motion

The costovertebral-costotransverse axis for the middle ribs lies at an approximately 45-degree angle to the sagittal and coronal planes. The motion of these ribs is of a mixed pump and bucket handle type with an increase in both the transverse and anteroposterior dimensions.

### Caliper Motion

The eleventh and twelfth ribs have only costovertebral articulations. Because there are no transverse process limitations, the motion of these ribs is caliper-like along a horizontal plane. This motion produces slight changes in both the anteroposterior and the transverse dimensions.

## Anteroposterior Thoracic Cage Shape Changes

During inhalation, the first through tenth ribs elevate. The sternum moves upward and forward. The small amount of motion possible at the sternal angle—because it is usually a symphysis—allows the angle to flatten. The upper ribs move farther forward than the lower ribs

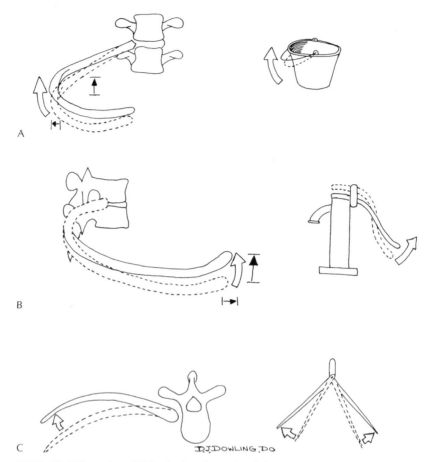

■ **FIG. 69-4** Rib motions. **(A)** Bucket handle motion. **(B)** Pump handle motion. **(C)** Caliper motion.

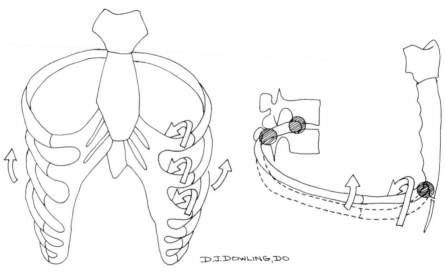

■ **FIG. 69-5** Elasticity of the costal cartilage.

because of the greater pump handle motion that occurs in this region.

## Costal Cartilage Elasticity

The costal cartilage is hyaline. It is basically unossified embryonic cartilaginous rib and contributes significantly to thoracic cage mobility. During inspiration, the sternum has a greater superior excursion than the ribs. The ribs initially move inferiorly relative to the sternum. Because the cartilage is basically fixed at the sternal end, it twists along the long axis and behaves as a torsion rod and stores potential energy. As the diaphragm relaxes and ascends, this energy is released as the cartilage recoils (Fig. 69-5).

## ■ OSTEOPATHIC DIAGNOSIS

Palpation and visual observation are used during osteopathic examination. Knowledge of the structure and biomechanics of the area under evaluation is integral to this process. Somatic dysfunctions restrict motion of the thoracic cage and its components. The bucket handle and pump handle movements may be limited when examined at the greatest extent of inspiration and expiration. Asymmetric excursion and difficulty in movement imply restriction of the region examined.

### REFERENCES

Castilio Y, Ferris-Swift L. The effect of direct splenic stimulation on the cells and the antibody content of the blood stream in acute infectious diseases. The College Journal, Kansas City College of Osteopathy and Surgery 1934; 18(7).

Castilio Y, Ferris-Swift L. Effects of splenic stimulation in normal individuals on the actual and differential blood cell count and the opsonic index. Kansas City College of Osteopathy and Surgery Bulletin 1932;16:10–16.

Cathie AG. Physiologic motions of the spine as related to respiratory activity. Academy of Applied Osteopathy—1965 Yearbook. Carmel, CA: Academy of Applied Osteopathy, 1965.

Chiles HL. Editorial: a new survey of public health. *J Am Osteopath Assoc* 1:227–230.

DiGiovanna EL, Schiowitz S. *An Osteopathic Approach to Diagnosis and Treatment, 2nd ed.* Philadelphia: Lippincott-Raven, 1997.

Galewaler JE. Motion, the lymphatics and manipulation. *J Am Osteopath Assoc* 1969;69:247–254.

Guyton AC. *Textbook of Medical Physiology,* 7th ed. Philadelphia: W.B. Saunders, 1986.

Kapandji IA. *The Physiology of the Joints, vol III.* Edinburgh: Churchill Livingstone, 1974.

Kohn GC. *Encyclopedia of Plague and Pestilence.* New York: Facts on File, 1995.

Langley L, Telford IR, Christensen JB. Dynamic *Anatomy and Physiology,* 5th ed. New York: McGraw-Hill, 1980.

Measel JW. The effect of the lymphatic pump on the immune response: I. Preliminary studies on the antibody response to pneumococcal polysaccharide assayed by bacterial agglutination and passive hemaglutination. *J Am Osteopath Assoc* 1982;82:28–31.

Measel JW. Introduction: thoughts on osteopathic practice and infectious diseases. *Osteopath Ann* 1982;10:92–94.

Moore KL. Clinically Oriented Anatomy, 2nd ed. Baltimore: Williams & Wilkins, 1985.

Moore KL. *The Developing Human: Clinically Oriented Embryology,* 4th ed. Philadelphia: W.B. Saunders, 1988.

Pansky B. *Review of Gross Anatomy,* 5th ed. New York: Macmillan, 1984.

Robbins SL. *Pathologic Basis of Disease, 3rd ed.* Philadelphia: W.B. Saunders, 1984.

Sabiston DC. *Textbook of Surgery: The Biological Basis of Modern Surgical Practice.* Philadelphia: W.B. Saunders, 1986.

Tucker EE. Spanish influenza—what and why? *J Am Osteopath Assoc* 1919;18:270–273.

Watson JO, Percival EN. Pneumonia research in children at Los Angeles County Osteopathic Hospital. *J Am Osteopath Assoc* 1939;39:153–159.

Webster GV. Subdiaphragmatic drainage. *J Am Osteopath Assoc* 1928;28:145.

Williams G. *Virus Hunters.* New York: Alfred A. Knopf, 1960.

Zink JG, Lawson WB. The role of pectoral traction in the treatment of lymphatic flow disturbance. *Osteopath Ann* 1978;6:439–496.

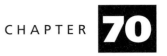

# Evaluation of the Thoracic Cage

*Eileen L. DiGiovanna*

There are several reasons for evaluating the thorax during a structural examination. The status of the rib cage is an important clue to the status of the respiratory mechanism. Free motion of the ribs is necessary for full expansion of the lungs. Conversely, pulmonary diseases cause secondary changes in rib motion and function.

The ribs may also be a source of chest wall or upper back pain. Rib dysfunction may result in shoulder, arm, or neck pain. Finally, rib dysfunctions may be primary or secondary to thoracic spine dysfunction.

## ■ OBSERVATION

Observation of the chest wall will reveal any asymmetry of its structures. One should note the typical *barrel chest* of chronic pulmonary diseases. Retraction of the intercostal muscles or use of the accessory muscles of respiration (scalenes, sternocleidomastoids) can indicate the severity of respiratory difficulty, especially in status asthmaticus. The rate of respiration and the degree to which the patient uses abdominal versus thoracic breathing should be noted. The physician should inspect for any signs of trauma to the thoracic cage, as well as any surgical scars.

## ■ PALPATION

The thorax is palpated to detect static asymmetries as well as asymmetries or restrictions of rib motion. Static asymmetries represent anterior or posterior ribs. Palpation for static asymmetries is particularly helpful when localized pain is caused by rib dysfunction. Ribs may be palpated along the posterior thorax at the angle of the ribs with the patient prone. A *posterior rib* on palpation appears to lie more posteriorly than the rib above or below it. Posterior ribs are frequently caused by posterior rotation of the transverse process with which the rib articulates. As with any somatic dysfunction, there will be associated tissue changes in the area of the rib head.

Palpation along the sternal border anteriorly will reveal ribs that have moved anteriorly (*anterior ribs*), a common cause of anterior chest wall pain. The patient may mistake rib dysfunction on the left side for cardiac pain. Tenderness and tissue changes may be palpated along the sternal border and at the costochondral junction in the case of somatic dysfunction.

Palpation of the anterior chest wall may disclose elevated or depressed ribs. In the case of a depressed rib, the space between it and the rib below will be narrowed, while the space between it and the rib above will be widened. These differences are reversed for an elevated rib: the space between it and the rib above will be narrowed, while the space between it and the rib below is widened. A single rib or a group of ribs may be elevated or depressed. Motion testing is necessary for diagnosis, as the findings on static palpation may be misleading. Generally, a depressed rib will restrict the motion of the ribs below and when inhalation occurs and an elevated rib will restrict the motion of the ribs above it when exhalation occurs.

### Diagnostic Terminology

Various authors use different terms to describe rib dysfunctions. In reading the literature, it is important to understand these terms. Some common terms are:

1. Anterior or posterior ribs
2. Elevated or depressed ribs
3. Ribs in a position of inspiration or expiration (inhalation or exhalation dysfunctions)
4. Ribs restricted in inspiration or expiration (inhalation or exhalation restrictions)

When reading a diagnosis, note whether the author states that a rib is in a *position of inspiration* (elevated) or *restricted* in inspiration (depressed). An inspiration restriction denotes a rib that does not move into a position of inspiration but is held in a depressed or expiratory position. Inspiratory and expiratory restrictions are restrictions of motion of the rib on its respiratory axis; that is, during inspiration the anterior portion of the rib is elevated and during expiration the rib is depressed.

## ■ EVALUATION OF RIB MOTION

Ribs may be evaluated for motion as groups of ribs or may be evaluated individually.

### Evaluation of the First Rib

The first rib is unlike the other ribs because of its attachments to the scalene muscles and its functional relationship to the clavicle. It is customarily palpated at three sites:

1. The posterior superior surface, deep to the trapezius
2. The anterior superior surface, in the depression superior to and behind the clavicle
3. The anterior articulation just below the clavicle at the sternal border

The technique for motion testing of the first rib is described.

1. **Patient position:** supine.
2. **Physician position:** seated at the head of the table.
3. **Technique:**
   a. The physician places her thumbs or finger pads on the anterior surface in the supraclavicular depression and evaluates the static position of the first ribs. Is one rib higher than the other?
   b. Tissue texture and muscle tone over the rib are examined for changes from normal.
   c. The physician places her thumbs on the posterior surface just anterior to the trapezius and springs the ribs lightly, evaluating

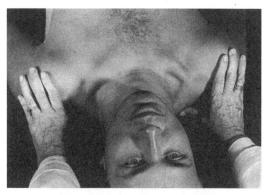

■ **FIG. 70-1** Position for evaluating the first rib.

the resistance of the ribs (Fig. 70-1). If resistance is felt when the rib is sprung, that rib is dysfunctional.
   d. The physician evaluates rib motion by placing her thumbs or finger pads on the anterosuperior surface of the first ribs and asking the patient to make a full inspiratory and expiratory effort.
   e. **Significance:**
      (1) If one rib stops moving before the other rib during inspiration, that rib has an *inspiratory restriction.*
      (2) If one rib stops moving before the other rib during exhalation, that rib has an *expiratory restriction.*

### Gross Motion Testing of the Ribs

This section describes a general screening test for evaluating motion of groups of ribs.

1. **Patient position:** supine.
2. **Physician position:** standing at the side of the table, facing the patient's head.
3. **Technique:**
   a. **Upper ribs (one to three)**
      (1) Pump handle motion
         (a) The physician places her fingers flat along the sternal border bilaterally, with the fingertips touching the inferior surface of the clavicle (Fig. 70-2).
         (b) Motion is evaluated as the patient inhales and exhales deeply.
      (2) Bucket handle motion
         (a) The physician places her fingers flat on the upper chest wall and

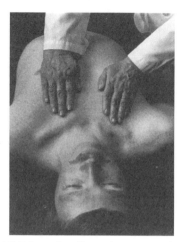

**FIG. 70-2** Pump handle motion testing of the upper ribs.

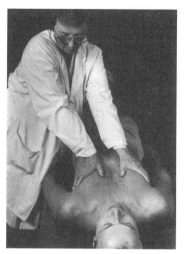

**FIG. 70-4** Gross motion testing of the middle ribs.

at a 45-degree angle to the sternal border, with the index finger lying just below clavicle (Fig. 70-3).

(b) Motion is evaluated in full inhalation and exhalation.

b. **Middle ribs (four to seven)**

(1) The physician places her thumbs along the sternal border with the tips toward the patient's head.

(2) The fingers are placed laterally along the middle ribs, each finger covering one rib (Fig. 70-4).

(3) As the patient inhales and exhales fully:

(a) Evaluate pump handle motion with the thumbs.

(b) Evaluate bucket handle motion with the fingers.

(4) In a female patient, it may be preferable to evaluate pump handle and bucket handle motions individually by placing the fingers along the sternal border first and then along the ribs at the mid-axillary area.

c. **Lower ribs (eight to ten)**

(1) The physician places her thumbs along the costochondral border and spreads the fingers along the ribs laterally (Fig. 70-5).

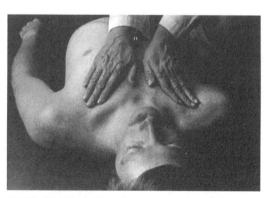

**FIG. 70-3** Bucket handle motion testing of the upper ribs.

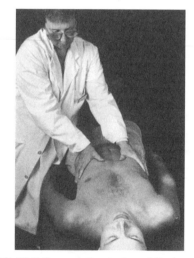

**FIG. 70-5** Gross motion testing of the lower ribs.

(2) The evaluation of the lower ribs follows that for the middle ribs.

d. **Ribs eleven and twelve**

(1) These ribs are evaluated with the patient prone. Their caliper-type motion is evaluated.

(2) The physician forms a C with her thumb and second and third fingers. The thumb is placed at the area of the rib heads and the fingers along the ribs (Fig. 70-6).

(3) Rib motion is evaluated in full inhalation and exhalation.

4. **Significance:**

a. If a group of ribs stops moving on one side before the other during inhalation, one or more ribs in that group have an inhalation restriction. The restriction may be of pump handle motion, bucket handle motion, or both.

b. If a group of ribs stops moving on one side before the other during exhalation, one or more ribs in that group have an exhalation restriction. The restriction may be of pump handle motion or bucket handle motion.

c. Occasionally bilateral restrictions may be present. Their identification requires knowledge of normal rib excursions, which comes with experience and concentration on full ranges of motion.

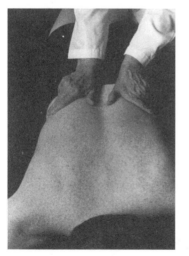

■ **FIG. 70-6** Gross motion testing of ribs 11 and 12.

## Individual Rib Motion Testing

The individual ribs are tested in the manner just described for each level of ribs, but only one rib on each side is tested and compared. Individual ribs may be tested if one rib is painful or if restriction of motion is found on gross motion testing. If a group inhalation restriction has been found, usually the top rib in the group is responsible for the restriction. If a group exhalation restriction has been found, usually the lowest rib in the group is responsible.

## ■ EVALUATION OF THE STERNUM

Because of the close association of the sternum with the ribs, the sternum must be evaluated when respiratory excursion appears limited. The sternum is evaluated by placing the thumb of one hand on the manubrium and the other thumb on the body of the sternum (Fig. 70-7). By applying pressure with each thumb alternately, the physician can determine if sternal motion is free at the angle of Louis. The hinge motion can also be evaluated by studying the change during each of the respiratory phases.

## ■ EVALUATION OF THE CLAVICLE

Evaluation of the clavicle is discussed in Chapter 80 (Evaluation of the Shoulder). Because of the close relationship between the clavicle and the first rib, when first or second rib restriction is found, the clavicle must be evaluated. Its normal position, structure, and motions are all significant to normal functioning of the thoracic cage.

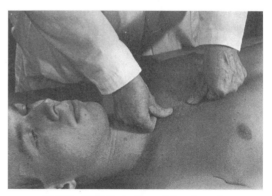

■ **FIG. 70-7** Evaluation of the sternum.

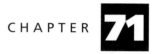

# Muscle Energy Techniques for the Ribs

*Eileen L. DiGiovanna*

Muscle energy treatment of the ribs is used to correct inhalation and exhalation restrictions of the ribs. Each treatment entails the following general principles: *pump handle* and *bucket handle* restrictions are treated with slight modifications to the given technique.

1. Patient contracting a muscle to move a rib
2. Patient providing respiratory assistance
3. Force applied by physician to resist motion into the direction of relative freedom and assist motion into the barrier direction.

Techniques are described separately for the first rib, the second through tenth ribs, and the eleventh and twelfth ribs. Each rib group indicated can be treated in the same manner.

## ■ EXHALATION DYSFUNCTIONS (INHALATION RESTRICTIONS)

When a rib is restricted in its ability to move into inhalation and is held in a depressed, exhaltion position, the following techniques are useful:

### First Rib: Pump Handle Motion

1. **Patient position:** supine.
2. **Physician position:** standing at the side of the table, facing the patient's head.
3. **Technique:**
   a. The patient places his hand, palm up, on his forehead.
   b. The physician reaches under the patient with her near hand and grasps the poster-osuperior surface of the first rib with her fingers.
   c. The physician places her other hand, palm down, on top of the patient's hand on the side of the dysfunction.
   d. The patient is asked to raise his head off the table while simultaneously inhaling deeply.
   e. As the patient lifts his head, the physician resists motion by pressing down on the patient's hand providing isometric resistance. The physician simultaneously pulls in a caudad direction on the back of the rib (Fig. 71-1). This is maintained for 3 to 5 seconds.
   f. Repeat these steps at least three times.
   g. The dysfunction is reassessed.
4. Three mechanisms have aided in assisting the rib to free its inhalation, pump handle motion:
   a. Patient's contraction of the anterior scalene muscle assists in elevating the rib, because the head is fixed.
   b. The deep inhalation assists the rib into an elevated position.
   c. The physician's pull on the posterior part of the rib results in the reciprocal motion of the anterior part of the rib moving upward.

### First Rib: Bucket Handle Motion

1. **Patient position:** supine
2. **Physician position:** standing at the side of the table, facing the patient's head.

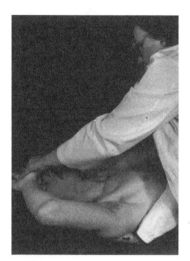

■ **FIG. 71-1** Muscle energy technique for treatment of inhalation restriction of first rib pump handle motion.

3. **Technique:**
   a. The patient places his hand, palm up, on his forehead with his head turned 40 degrees from the midline, toward the rib being treated.
   b. The physician reaches under the patient with her hand that is closer to the table and grasps the posterosuperior surface of the first rib with her fingers.
   c. The physician places her other hand, palm down, on top of the patient's hand on the dysfunction side.
   d. The patient is asked to push his head off the table into the direction that he is facing while simultaneously inhaling deeply, using the middle scalene muscle (Fig. 71-2).

## Ribs Two to Ten: Pump Handle Motion

1. **Patient position:** supine.
2. **Physician position:** standing at the side of the table, facing the patient's head.
3. **Technique:**
   a. The patient places his hand, palm up, on his forehead.
   b. The physician reaches behind the patient with her near hand and grasps the posterosuperior part of the rib being treated.
   c. The physician places her other hand on top of the patient's hand.
   d. The patient is instructed to lift his hand and arm toward the ceiling while inhaling deeply. The physician provides isometric resistance (Fig. 71-3). This is maintained 3 to 5 seconds.
   e. Simultaneously, the physician pulls down on the posterior aspect of the rib.
4. In this technique, the patient uses the pectoralis and serratus anterior muscles to elevate the anterior part of the rib as the physician pulls down on the posterior rib to aid anterior elevation

## Ribs Two to Ten: Bucket Handle Motion

1. **Patient position:** supine.
2. **Physician position:** standing at the side of the table, facing the patient's head.

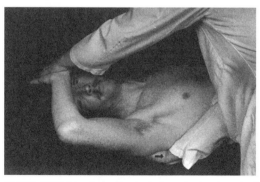

■ **FIG. 71-2** Muscle energy technique for treatment of inhalation restriction of first rib bucket handle motion.

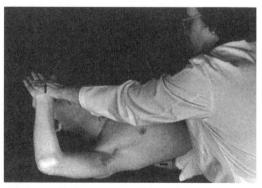

■ **FIG. 71-3** Muscle energy technique for treatment of inhalation restriction of the second through tenth ribs (pump and bucket handle motions).

3. **Technique:**
   a. The patient places his hand, palm up, on his forehead.
   b. The physician reaches behind the patient with her near hand and grasps the posterosuperior part of the rib being treated.
   c. The physician places her other hand on top of the patient's hand on the dysfunction side.
   d. The patient is instructed to lift his hand and arm up and laterally at a 45-degree angle from the vertical while simultaneously inhaling deeply. The physician provides isometric resistance (see Fig. 71-3). This is maintained for 3 to 5 seconds.
   e. As the patient inhales, the physician pulls down on the posterior aspect of the involved rib.
   f. These steps are repeated at least three times and the dysfunction is reassessed.
4. The lateral part of the serratus will then elevate the lateral part of the ribs to improve the bucket handle motion.

## Ribs Eleven and Twelve

1. **Patient position:** prone.
2. **Physician position:** standing at the side of the table, opposite the rib being treated.
3. **Technique:**
   a. The patient's legs are pulled toward the physician.
   b. The patient's arm on the involved side is placed above his head.
   c. With her near hand, the physician grasps the anterior inferior iliac spine on the side of the dysfunction and rotates the pelvis posteriorly.
   d. The palm of the physician's opposite hand is placed over the involved rib(s).
   e. The patient is asked to inhale deeply.
   f. As the patient inhales, the physician pushes laterally on the rib, separating it from its articulation to allow the breath to carry it into inhalation (see Fig. 71-6).
4. The patient's arm position uses the latissimus dorsi to facilitate the movement of the dysfunctional rib upward and outward while resisting the downward pull of the quadratus lumborum.

## ■ INHALATION DYSFUNCTIONS (EXHALATION RESTRICTIONS)

When a rib is restricted in its ability to move into exhalation and is held in an elevated, inhalation position, the following techniques are useful:

## Rib One: Pump Handle Motion

1. **Patient position:** supine.
2. **Physician position:** standing or seated at the head of the table.
3. **Technique:**
   a. The patient's neck is bent forward and supported by the physician's hand and arm.
   b. The physician places her thumb on the superior surface of the dysfunctional rib between the two heads of the sternocleidomastoid muscle.
   c. The patient is instructed to inhale deeply, and then exhale completely.
   d. The physician resists the anterior motion of the rib during inhalation and then presses down on the rib, following it into exhalation.
   e. The physician holds the rib down as the patient takes a shallow breath and exhales again.
   f. The technique is repeated three times and then the rib dysfunction is reassessed.

## Rib One: Bucket Handle Motion

1. **Patient position:** supine, with the head side-bent slightly toward the affected rib.
2. **Physician position:** standing or seated at the head of the table.
3. **Technique:**
   a. The patient's neck is bent forward, side bent to the dysfunctional side and supported by the physician's hand and arm.
   b. The physician places her thumb of the hand on the side of the dysfunction on the superior surface of the rib lateral to the clavicular attachment of the sternocleidomastoid muscle.
   c. The patient is instructed to inhale deeply, and then exhale completely.
   d. The physician resists the lateral upward motion of the rib during inhalation and

then presses down on the rib, following it into exhalation.

e. The physician holds the rib down as the patient takes a shallow breath and exhales again.

f. The technique is repeated three times.

g. The rib dysfunction is reassessed.

## Ribs Two to Five: Pump Handle Motion

1. **Patient position:** supine.

2. **Physician position:** standing or seated at the head of the table.

3. **Technique:**

   a. The physician places her fingers on the superior surface of the costal cartilage of the rib being treated and the on the one below it, lateral to the sternum.

   b. The patient's neck is bent forward fully. The physician places her knee on the table and supports the patient's head and neck on her thigh.

   c. The patient is instructed to exhale fully as the physician follows the inferior motion of the rib and encourages the rib to move further into a position of exhalation.

   d. The physician holds down the rib as the patient inhales, then moves it farther into exhalation as the patient exhales forcefully (Fig. 71-4).

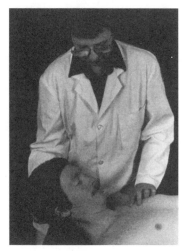

■ **FIG. 71-4** Muscle energy technique for treatment of exhalation restriction of the second through fifth ribs (pump handle motion).

e. The above steps are repeated three times and then the dysfunction is reassessed.

f. The intercostal muscles and the alteration of the thoracic cavity by descent of the diaphragm are thus used to pull down on the ribs as the physician presses them down with her finger.

## Ribs Two to Five: Bucket Handle Motion

1. **Patient position:** supine, with the shoulders and neck side-bent toward the affected side.

2. **Physician position:** standing or seated at the head of the table.

3. **Technique:**

   a. The patient's neck is bent forward, side bent to the side of the dysfunction and supported by the physician's hand and arm.

   b. The physician places her fingers on the lateral surface of the costal cartilage of the rib being treated in the mid-axillary line and on the one below it as well.

   c. The patient is instructed to inhale and then exhale fully as the physician follows the inferior motion of the rib and encourages the rib to move further into a position of exhalation.

   d. The physician holds the rib down as the patient inhales, then moves it farther into exhalation as the patient exhales forcefully an additional time.

   e. The above steps are repeated three times and then the rib dysfunction is reassessed.

   f. The intercostal muscles and the alteration of the thoracic cavity by descent of the diaphragm are thus used to pull down on the ribs as the physician presses them down with her fingers.

## Ribs Six to Ten: Pump Handle Motion

1. **Patient position:** supine, with the shoulders lifted up by the physician's hand placed between the scapulae or with the upper back resting on the physician's thigh. The upper trunk is thus bent forward.

2. **Physician position:** standing at the head of the table, supporting the patient.

3. **Technique:**
   a. The physician places her fingers on the lateral surface of the costal cartilage of the rib being treated lateral to the sternum and on the one below it as well.
   b. The patient is instructed to inhale and then exhale fully as the physician follows the inferior motion of the rib and encourages the rib to move further into a position of exhalation.
   c. The physician holds the rib down as the patient inhales and then moves it farther into exhalation an additional time.
   d. The above steps are repeated three times and then the rib dysfunction is reassessed.
   e. The intercostal muscles and the alteration of the thoracic cavity by descent of the diaphragm are thus used to pull down on the ribs as the physician presses them down with her finger. The rectus abdominus may also contribute.

## Ribs Six to Ten: Bucket Handle Motion

1. **Patient position:** same as for treating pump handle motion, except that the upper trunk is side-bent toward the affected rib as well as forward bent (Fig. 71-5).

2. **Physician position:** standing at the head of the table, supporting the patient.
3. **Technique:** same as for treating pump handle motion.

## Ribs Ten, Eleven, and Twelve

1. **Patient position:** prone.
2. **Physician position:** standing at the side of the table, opposite the involved rib.
3. **Technique:**
   a. The patient's legs are pulled toward the physician.
   b. The patient's arm remains at his side (the only position difference from the treatment of inhalation restrictions).
   c. Using her near hand the physician grasps the anterior inferior iliac spine and rotates the pelvis posteriorly.
   d. With the thenar eminence on the involved rib, the physician pushes it away from its articulation as the patient exhales forcefully (Fig. 71-6).
4. The patient's arm position reduces any tension on the patient's latissimus dorsi to facilitate the movement of the dysfunctional rib downwards. The tension on the quadratus lumborum can facilitate the caudad pull on the lowest rib.

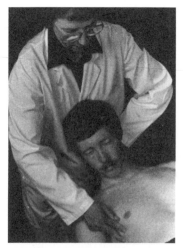

■ **FIG. 71-5** Muscle energy technique for treatment of exhalation restriction of the sixth through tenth ribs (bucket handle motion).

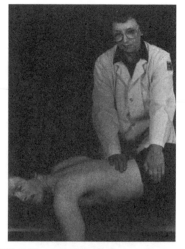

■ **FIG. 71-6** Muscle energy technique for treatment of exhalation restriction of ribs eleven and twelve. (Patient's arm at side for exhalation; arm above head for inhalation restrictions.)

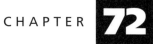

# Counterstrain Techniques for the Ribs

*Eileen L. DiGiovanna*

For the purposes of counterstrain treatment, rib somatic dysfunctions are generally classified as either depressed or elevated. *Depressed ribs* are held in exhalation and restricted in their movement into inhalation. *Elevated ribs* are held in inhalation and restricted in their movement into exhalation.

## ■ ANTERIOR TENDER POINTS

### Ribs One and Two (Depressed, Inhalation Restriction)

The locations of the tender points of the anterior rib cage are shown in Figure 72-1. The tender point for the first rib is lateral to the sternum, at the level of the angle of Louis, just below the sternoclavicular joint. The tender point for the second rib is in the mid-clavicular line at the level of the second rib interspace.

1. **Patient position:** supine.
2. **Physician position:** standing at the patient's side near the head of the table.
3. **Technique:**
   a. The tender point is continually monitored with the physician's finger.
   b. The patient's head is slightly flexed, rotated, and side-bent toward the tender point (Fig. 72-2).
   c. Slightly more flexion is required for the second rib than for the first.
   d. When the point is no longer tender, the position is held for 120 seconds. The pa-

tient is slowly returned to neutral and the tender point reassessed for tenderness.

### Ribs Three to Six (Depressed, Inhalation Restriction)

The anterior tender points for the third through sixth ribs lie along the anterior axillary line on the ribs, or more medially along the sternal border at the rib interspaces.

1. **Patient position:** seated on the table.
2. **Physician position:** standing behind the patient.
3. **Technique:**
   a. The physician places her foot on the table opposite the side of the tender point and drapes the patient's arm over her thigh.
   b. The physician moves her thigh laterally so that the patient, who is leaning on the thigh, side-bends to the side of the tender point.
   c. The patient is asked to curl his legs onto the table toward the side of the tender point (Fig. 72-3).
   d. The free arm is crossed over the patient's lap.
   e. When the point is no longer tender, the position is held for 120 seconds. The patient is then slowly returned to a neutral position and the tender point reassessed.

## ■ POSTERIOR TENDER POINTS

The posterior tender points lie along the angles of the ribs. Their locations are shown in Figure 72-4.

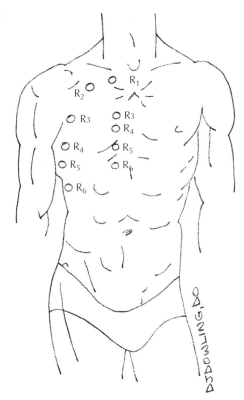

■ **FIG. 72-1** Tender point location, anterior rib cage.

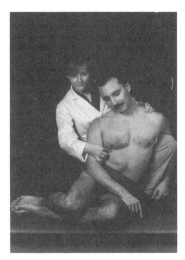

■ **FIG. 72-3** Counterstrain technique for depressed ribs three to six.

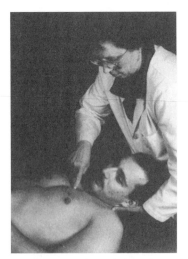

■ **FIG. 72-2** Counterstrain technique for a depressed first or second rib.

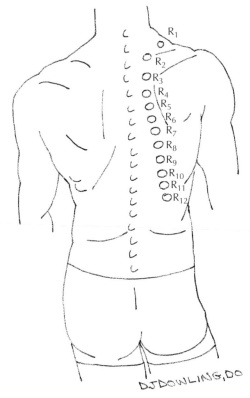

■ **FIG. 72-4** Tender point location, posterior rib cage.

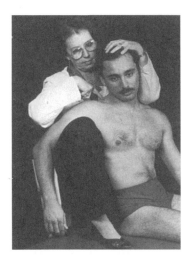

■ **FIG. 72-5** Counterstrain technique for an elevated first rib.

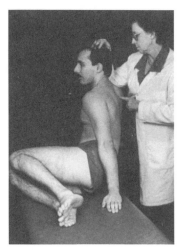

■ **FIG. 72-7** Lateral view of counterstrain technique for elevated ribs.

## Rib One (Elevated, Exhalation Restriction)

1. **Patient position:** seated on the table.
2. **Physician position:** standing behind the patient.
3. **Technique:**
   a. The physician places her foot on the table on the side of the tender point and drapes the patient's arm over her thigh.
   b. The patient leans on the physician's thigh, which is moved laterally, causing elevation of the first rib.
   c. The head is side-bent toward the tender point. It is then bent forward or backward,

whichever gives maximal softening of the tissues (Fig. 72-5).

## Ribs Two to Eight (Elevated, Exhalation Restriction)

1. **Patient position:** seated on the table.
2. **Physician position:** standing.
3. **Technique:**
   a. The physician places her foot on the table on the side of the tender point and drapes the patient's arm over her thigh.
   b. The thigh is moved laterally with the patient leaning on it, further elevating the ribs on that side.
   c. For upper ribs the head is side-bent and rotated away from the tender point.
   d. For lower ribs the patient is asked to curl his legs onto the table on the side opposite the tender point (Figs. 72-6 and 72-7).
   e. The free arm is placed behind the patient.
   f. When the point is no longer tender, the position is held for 120 seconds. The patient is then returned to a neutral position and the tender point is reassessed.

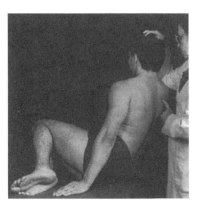

■ **FIG. 72-6** Counterstrain technique for elevation of second through eighth ribs.

### REFERENCES

DiGiovanna E, Schiowitz S. *An Osteopathic Approach to Diagnosis and Treatment, 2nd ed.* Philadelphia: Lippincott-Raven, 1997.

Jones LH, et al. *Jones Strain-Counterstrain.* Boise, ID: Jones Strain-Counterstrain Inc, 1995.

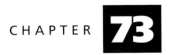

# Facilitated Positional Release

*Stanley Schiowitz*

This chapter contains the methods for treating rib somatic dysfunctions with facilitated positional release techniques.

## ■ FIRST RIB SOMATIC DYSFUNCTION

1. **Patient position:** supine.
2. **Physician position:** standing beside the table, on the side of the dysfunction, facing the head of the table.
3. **Technique:**
   a. The physician places his near hand over the patient's rib with the fingers on the posterior aspect of the first rib (right hand on right rib). The hand placement may be modified to treat soft tissue only, or at the costovertebral junction to obtain first rib articular release. His fingers should identify the area of greatest tension to treat the muscle.
   b. The physician bends the patient's elbow and places his far hand over the patient's flexed elbow, and then brings the humerus up to 90 degrees of flexion.
   c. The physician compresses down on the patient's elbow with the force directed toward his monitoring fingers (Fig. 73-1).
   d. Maintaining this compression, the physician adds internal rotation of the shoulder joint. This is accomplished by placing the patient's right forearm on the ventral aspect of the physician's near forearm and turning the patient's forearm outwards by a caudal motion of the physician's forearm. This should create tissue release or articular motion.

e. The position is held for 3 seconds.
f. Maintaining the compressive torsional force, the physician adducts the patient's arm toward the midline and then circumducts the arm down to the table top until the arm is along the patient's side (Fig. 73-2).
g. The position is released and the dysfunction reevaluated.

## ■ ANTERIOR RIB CAGE AND COSTOCHONDRAL DYSFUNCTIONS OR MUSCLE HYPERTONICITY

### Example: Fourth, Left, Costochondral Dysfunction

1. **Patient position:** seated.
2. **Physician position:** standing behind the patient.
3. **Technique:**
   a. The physician places his right arm around the front of the patient with the index finger of that hand on the tender tissue or on the rib somatic dysfunction.
   b. The physician's left hand is on the patient's cervicothoracic junction, with the left arm resting on the superior aspect of the patient's shoulder and his elbow over the acromion process.
   c. The patient is instructed to sit up straight until the thoracic kyphosis flattens slightly.
   d. The physician applies compression at the cervicothoracic junction and left shoulder,

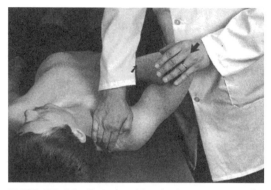

■ **FIG. 73-1** Facilitated positional release treatment for first rib dysfunction: application of compression with internal rotation of the shoulder.

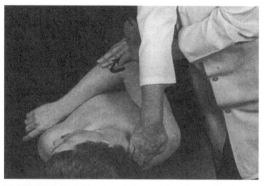

■ **FIG. 73-2** Adduction followed by circumduction to release the arm.

directly toward the floor (Fig. 73-3). (Do not allow forward bending.)

e. Maintaining the compressive force, the physician bends the patient's body forward to the monitoring finger. (The patient may be told to drop his head forward.)

f. The physician adds left side-bending until motion is felt at the monitoring finger. Rotation may have to be added (Fig. 73-4).

g. The position is held for 3 seconds and then released and the dysfunction is reevaluated.

## ■ POSTERIOR RIB DYSFUNCTIONS OR MYSCLE HYPERTONICITY

### Patient Prone Technique

1. **Patient position:** prone
2. **Physician position:** standing at the side of the table opposite the somatic dysfunction.
3. **Technique:**
   a. The physician reaches his caudad hand across to the patient's contralateral shoulder.
   b. He places the index finger of his cephalad hand on the costotransverse articulation to monitor motion.

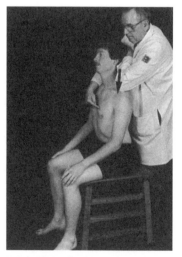

■ **FIG. 73-3** Facilitated positional release treatment for anterior rib cage somatic dysfunction: application of compression at the cervicothoracic junction.

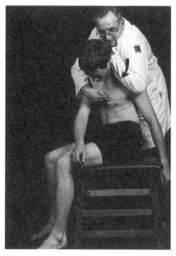

■ **FIG. 73-4** Facilitated positional release treatment for anterior rib cage somatic dysfunction with forward bending, side-bending, and rotation added.

c. With the hand on the shoulder, he introduces a compressive force toward the patient's feet, introducing side-bending of the contralateral thoracic spine until motion is felt at the somatic dysfunction.

d. A rotational or torsional force may be added until the tissue texture softens.

e. This position is held for 3 to 5 seconds.

f. The shoulder is returned to a neutral position and the somatic dysfunction is reassessed.

## Patient Seated Technique

1. **Patient position:** seated on the edge of the table or on a stool.
2. **Physician position:** standing behind the patient on the side of the somatic dysfunction at a 90 degree angle with the patient's back.
3. **Technique:**
   a. The physician monitors the somatic dysfunction with the hand farthest from the patient.
   b. The patient is asked to sit up straight and push his chest forward.
   c. The physician's flexed elbow of his near arm is placed anterior to the patient's shoulder with the forearm on top of the shoulder. With this arm he compresses the thoracic region downward and side-bends the region to the side of the dysfunction. With his elbow he adds a rotary force drawing the patient's shoulder posteriorly localizing to the site of the somatic dysfunction.
   d. This position is held for 3 to 5 seconds.
   e. The forces are released and the somatic dysfunction is reassessed.

Note: This technique is very similar to that performed for the posterior somatic dysfunctions of the thoracic spine performed in the seated position. The major difference is the point at which the monitoring finger detects the forces at the site of the dysfunction.

## ■ LATERAL RIB DYSFUNCTIONS OR MUSCLE HYPERTONICITY

### Example: Fifth Right Rib

1. **Patient position:** seated.
2. **Physician position:** standing on the patient's right side. Initially he is oriented approximately 90 degrees away from the patient (his back near the patient's right shoulder).
3. **Technique:**
   a. The physician places his left axilla over the patient's right shoulder as close to the cervicothoracic junction as possible.
   b. The physician uses his left hand to grasp the patient's right elbow. The patient's elbow is flexed and the shoulder is brought to approximately 45 degrees of flexion and abduction.
   c. The physician uses his right index finger to monitor the dysfunction.
   d. The patient is instructed to sit up straight.
   e. The physician adds a compressive force from his axilla down onto the patient's shoulder parallel to the spine.
   f. A slight force is also added from the patient's right elbow up toward the shoulder.
   g. By further adding pressure on the shoulder, side-bending is introduced down to the monitoring finger.
   h. Rotation toward the physician's monitoring finger is introduced. If tissue tension increases, rotation away may be attempted.
   i. The position is held for 3 seconds and then released and the dysfunction is reevaluated.

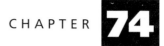

# Rib Still Techniques

*Dennis J. Dowling*

Still technique for treating rib somatic dysfunctions generally relates to the positional finding, anterior or posterior, of the involved rib. A simple relationship between an anterior rib and an inhalation dysfunction and a posterior rib and an exhalation dysfunction is drawn, which also contributes to the initial placement into the freedom of motion followed by engagement of the barriers. Some modification can also be included for pump or bucket handle components as well.

Rib one often has a component of elevation, possibly caused by the pull of the anterior and medial scalene muscles, as well as the medial upward pull of the sternocleidomastoid on the rib via the medial clavicle.

Compression is most commonly used, but some of the techniques involve an element of traction and/or torsion. Occasionally, the portion of the treatment involving movement toward the barriers may result in an articulatory "pop."

## ■ UPPER EXHALATION/POSTERIOR RIB (POSTERIOR SECOND RIB ON RIGHT)—SEATED

1. **Patient position:** seated.
2. **Physician position:** standing behind the patient on the dysfunctional side (right side in this example).
3. **Technique:**
   a. The physician places the pad of the thumb of his monitoring hand on the angle of the rib somatic dysfunction (the left finger contacts the patient's R2 right rib in this example). The palm of that hand can contour to the back and the fingers extend toward and over the shoulder on the side of the dysfunction.
   b. With the other hand, the physician grasps the patient's elbow on the side of the dysfunction (right hand holds right elbow).
   c. The physician uses the arm as a lever and extends the shoulder by bringing the elbow posteriorly and up to the level of the monitoring finger. Some amount of slight abduction may occur as the shoulder extends.
   d. Compression is introduced from the elbow along the humerus toward the rib (Fig. 74-1A).
   e. The physician introduces further abduction of the shoulder by moving the elbow laterally and then into adduction–flexion by bringing the elbow anteriorly through an arc (Fig. 74-1B).
   f. The upper arm will come to rest against the patient's chest.
   g. Compression is released.
   h. The arm is brought back to the patient's side and the rib somatic dysfunction is reassessed.

## ■ UPPER INHALATION/ANTERIOR RIB (ANTERIOR SECOND RIB ON RIGHT)—SEATED

1. **Patient position:** seated.
2. **Physician position:** standing behind the patient on the dysfunctional side (right side in this example).

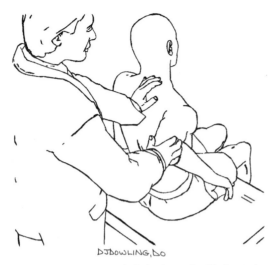

■ **FIG. 74-1A** Upper exhalation/posterior Rib (posterior second rib on right), seated.

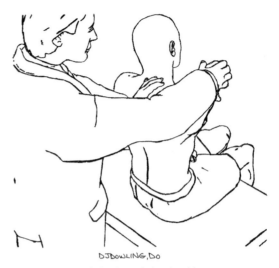

■ **FIG. 74-1B** Abduction of the shoulder.

3. **Technique:**
   a. The physician places the pad of the thumb of his monitoring hand on the angle of the rib somatic dysfunction (the left finger contacts the patient's R2 right rib in this example). The palm of that hand can contour to the back and the fingers extend toward and over the shoulder on the side of the dysfunction.
   b. With the other hand, the physician grasps the patient's elbow on the side of the dysfunction (right hand holds right elbow).

   c. The physician uses the arm as a lever and abducts the shoulder by bringing the elbow laterally and up to the level of the monitoring finger. Some small amount of extension is also introduced until localization is noted at the monitoring finger. (A variation can be used whereby the patient is directed to shrug the shoulder toward the ipsilateral ear, the physician maintains the position by holding and lifting the elbow, and the patient is then told to relax.) (Fig. 74-2A).

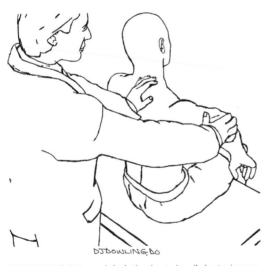

■ **FIG. 74-2A** Upper inhalation/anterior rib (anterior second rib on right), seated.

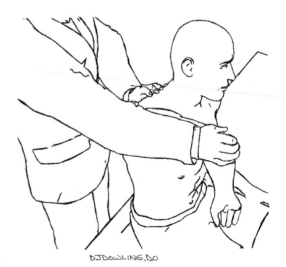

■ **FIG. 74-2B** Shoulder into further flexion.

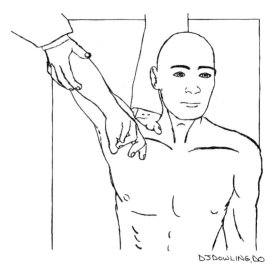

■ **FIG. 74-2C** Upper inhalation/anterior rib (anterior second rib on right), supine adaptation.

d. Compression is introduced from the elbow along the humerus toward the rib.

e. The physician introduces further abduction of the shoulder by moving the elbow laterally in the coronal plane. As the elbow is raised higher, a combined shoulder abduction-flexion-internal rotation occurs.

f. The elbow is brought anteriorly through an arc by bringing the shoulder into further flexion (Fig. 74-2B).

g. Compression is released.

h. The arm is brought back to the patient's side and the rib somatic dysfunction is reassessed.

Note: This technique can easily be adapted to the patient in the supine position and the physician seated or standing at the head of the table. The major difference is that a monitoring finger or thumb is more comfortably placed beneath the patient (Fig. 74-2C).

## ■ ANTERIOR/INHALATION RIB (ANTERIOR THIRD RIB ON THE RIGHT)—PATIENT SEATED

1. **Patient position:** seated.
2. **Physician position:** standing facing the patient.
3. **Technique:**
   a. Both of the physician's forearms are placed on the patient's shoulders as close to the patient's neck as is possible.

b. The physician places the pad of the index or middle finger of his monitoring hand on the angle of the involved rib on the side of the somatic dysfunction (the left finger contacts the patient's R3 right rib in this example).

c. The proximal part of the physician's forearm, which is anterior to the patient's shoulder opposite the dysfunction, pushes the shoulder on that side posteriorly (right forearm pushes the left shoulder posteriorly, which causes the right side and especially the rib somatic dysfunction to be rotated anteriorly).

d. The physician's forearm on the side of the dysfunction pushes downward on that shoulder to introduce side-bending to the level of the rib dysfunction.

e. The physician introduces a downward pressure through the patient's shoulders with slightly more pressure exerted on the side of the dysfunction toward the monitoring finger (Fig. 74-3).

f. While maintaining the compression, the patient's upper body is gently carried through the side-bending and rotation into the opposite directions (side-bending left and rotating right in this case).

g. The patient's body is brought back to the neutral position and the thoracic somatic dysfunction is reassessed.

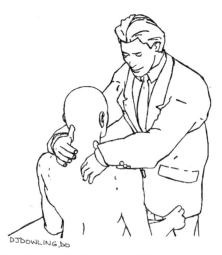
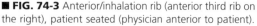

■ **FIG. 74-3** Anterior/inhalation rib (anterior third rib on the right), patient seated (physician anterior to patient).

## ■ POSTERIOR/EXHALATION RIB (POSTERIOR THIRD RIB ON THE RIGHT)—PATIENT SEATED

1. **Patient position:** seated.
2. **Physician position:** standing facing the patient.
3. **Technique:**
   a. Both of the physician's forearms are placed on the patient's shoulders as close to the patient's neck as is possible.
   b. The physician places the pad of the index or middle finger of his monitoring hand on the angle of the involved rib on the side of the somatic dysfunction (the left finger contacts the patient's R3 right rib in this example).
   c. The proximal part of the physician's forearm on the same side as the dysfunction, which is anterior to the patient's shoulder, pushes the shoulder on that side posteriorly (left forearm pushes the right shoulder posteriorly, which causes the right side and especially the rib somatic dysfunction to be rotated posteriorly).
   d. The physician's forearm on the side of the dysfunction pushes downward on that shoulder to introduce side-bending to the level of the rib dysfunction.
   e. The physician introduces a downward pressure through the patient's shoulders with slightly more pressure exerted on the side of the dysfunction toward the monitoring finger (Fig. 74-4).
   f. While maintaining the compression, the patient's upper body is gently carried through the side-bending and rotation into the opposite directions (side-bending left and rotating left in this case).
   g. The patient's body is brought back to the neutral position and the thoracic somatic dysfunction is reassessed.

## ■ POSTERIOR/EXHALATION RIB (POSTERIOR SIXTH RIB ON THE RIGHT) OR ANTERIOR/ INHALATION RIB (SIXTH RIB ON THE RIGHT)—PATIENT SEATED

1. **Patient position:** seated.
2. **Physician position:** standing behind the patient.

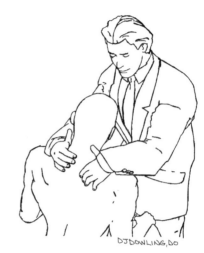

■ **FIG. 74-4** Posterior/exhalation rib (posterior third rib on the right), patient seated (physician anterior to patient).

3. **Technique:**
   a. The physician places the pad of the thumb of his monitoring hand on the angle of the rib somatic dysfunction (the right thumb contacts the patient's R6 right rib angle). The palm of that hand contours to and supports the patient's back.
   b. The patient is instructed to take his or her hand on the side of the somatic dysfunction and reach anteriorly and across to hold the opposite side shoulder (right hand on left shoulder).
   c. The physician places his axilla on the shoulder opposite to the rib somatic dysfunction and reaches the non-monitoring hand anterior and across to hold the shoulder on the side of the dysfunction (the physician's left axilla is on the patient's left shoulder and the physician's left hand is upon the patient's right shoulder).
   d. The physician side-bends the patient toward the side of the rib dysfunction
   e. If the rib dysfunction is posterior, the physician rotates the patient posterior on that side (rotates right side backwards) down to and toward the posterior rib angle (Fig. 74-5A). If the rib dysfunction is anterior, the physician rotates the patient anterior on that side (rotates right side forward) down to the posterior rib angle (Fig. 74-

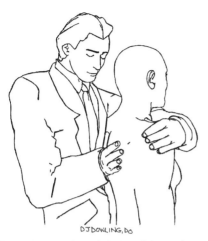

■ **FIG. 74-5A** Posterior/exhalation rib (posterior sixth rib on the right), patient seated (physician anterior to patient).

5B). The physician can further exaggerate this if necessary until softening of the underlying tissue is noted. Slight flexion or extension is added, depending on the reaction to the positioning.

f. The physician puts downward compression with the contacts of the palm of his (left) hand on the patient's right shoulder and through his (left) axilla on the patient's left shoulder until further softening of the tissue is noted at the monitoring finger.

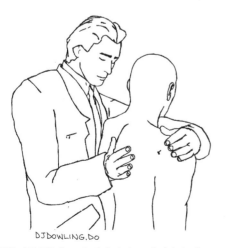

■ **FIG. 74-5B** Anterior/inhalation rib (sixth rib on the right), patient seated (physician anterior to patient).

g. While maintaining the compression, the patient's body is gently carried through neutral position and into the barrier directions (side-bending left and rotating left for a posterior right rib; side-bending left and rotating right for an anterior right rib in this case).

h. The patient's body brought back to the neutral position and the rib somatic dysfunction is reassessed.

## ■ POSTERIOR/EXHALATION RIB (POSTERIOR SIXTH RIB ON THE RIGHT) OR ANTERIOR/ INHALATION RIB (SIXTH RIB ON THE RIGHT) ANTERIOR—PATIENT SIDE-LYING

1. **Patient position:** lying on side with somatic dysfunction side up.
2. **Physician position:** standing facing the patient.
3. **Technique:**
   a. The patient's arm on the side of the rib somatic dysfunction is flexed and abducted and the hand is placed on his or her own neck.
   b. The physician places his cephalad arm through the opening created by the patient's bent arm and places the palm and fingers of that hand over the scapula on that side (physician's right hand on patient's right scapula).
   c. The physician places the pad of his index or middle finger of the other (caudad) monitoring hand on the rib angle at the level of the somatic dysfunction (the left finger contacts the patient's right sixth rib angle in this example). The palm and fingers of this hand contour to the patient's body and maintain position of the trunk throughout much of the treatment. The physician may rest his elbow or forearm on the patient's iliac crest on that side as well (left elbow on right hip).
   d. If the diagnosis is a posterior rib, the patient's (right) shoulder is pushed posterior by the physician's cephalad (left) hand, rotating the patient's upper body toward the direction of the freedom of motion of

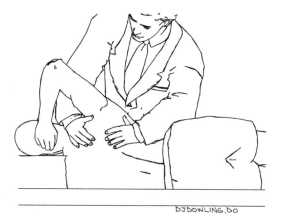

■ **FIG. 74-6A** Posterior/exhalation rib (posterior sixth rib on the right), patient side-lying.

the somatic dysfunction (Fig. 74-6A). If the diagnosis is an anterior rib, the patient's (right) shoulder is pulled anterior by the physician's cephalad (left) hand, rotating the patient's upper body forward and toward the direction of the freedom of motion of the somatic dysfunction (Fig. 74-6B).

e. Compression (approximately 5 pounds of pressure) and side-bending are introduced by the physician using his cephalad arm to push the patient's shoulder (right in this example) toward the hip on the same side until relaxation is noted in the soft tissue being monitored over the rib.

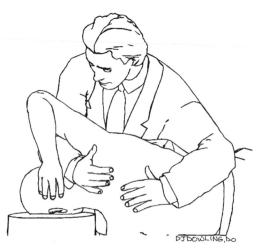

■ **FIG. 74-6B** Anterior/inhalation rib (sixth rib on the right) anterior, patient side-lying.

f. Compression is maintained.

g. If the diagnosis is of a posterior rib, the physician uses his caudad arm on the patient's hip and rolls the pelvis posterior. The cephalad hand and arm pull the patient's shoulder anteriorly and pulls the scapula up towards the patient's head (side-bending left and rotating left in this case into the barrier directions). If the diagnosis is of an anterior rib, the physician uses his caudad arm on the patient's hip and rolls the pelvis anterior. The cephalad hand and arm pull the patient's shoulder posteriorly and pulls the scapula up toward the patient's head (sidebending left and rotating right in this case into the barrier directions).

h. The patient's body is brought back to the neutral position and the rib somatic dysfunction level is reassessed.

## ■ POSTERIOR/EXHALATION RIB (POSTERIOR SIXTH RIB ON THE RIGHT)—PATIENT SUPINE

1. **Patient position:** supine with the shoulder on the involved side slightly off the edge of the table.

2. **Physician position:** standing facing the patient.

3. **Technique:**

   a. The physician places the pad of the index or middle finger of his caudad monitoring hand on the costal cartilage on the side and at the level of the rib somatic dysfunction (the right finger contacts the patient's sixth rib somatic dysfunction in this example).

   b. The physician takes hold of the patient's wrist on the side of the rib somatic dysfunction (the physician's left hand holds the patient's right wrist in this example).

   c. The physician introduces long axis traction by pulling the patient's (right) arm toward the patient's feet until relaxation is noted at the monitoring finger.

   d. The physician introduces shoulder extension, abduction, and external rotation while maintaining traction (Fig. 74-7A).

   e. While maintaining the traction, the pa-

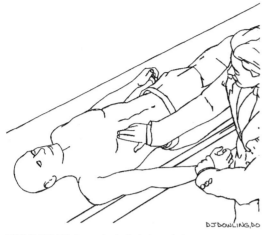

■ **FIG. 74-7A** Posterior/exhalation rib (posterior sixth rib on the right), patient supine.

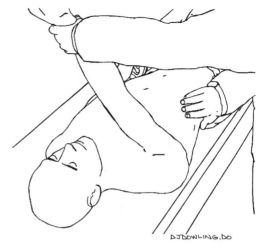

■ **FIG. 74-8A** Anterior/inhalation rib (anterior sixth rib on the right), patient supine.

tient's arm is flexed and adducted across the patient's body (Fig. 74-7B).

 f. Eventually the patient's arm is brought across to the opposite shoulder or higher.

 g. The patient's arm is brought back to the neutral position and the rib dysfunction is reassessed.

## ■ ANTERIOR/INHALATION RIB (ANTERIOR SIXTH RIB ON THE RIGHT)—PATIENT SUPINE

1. **Patient position:** supine with the shoulder on the involved side slightly off the edge of the table.

2. **Physician position:** standing facing the patient.

3. **Technique:**

 a. The physician places the pad of the index or middle finger of his caudad monitoring hand on the costal cartilage on the side and at the level of the rib somatic dysfunction (the right finger contacts the patient's sixth rib somatic dysfunction in this example).

 b. The physician holds the patient's wrist of the arm on the side of the rib somatic dys-

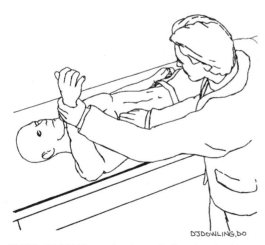

■ **FIG. 74-7B** The patient's arm is flexed and adducted across the patient's body.

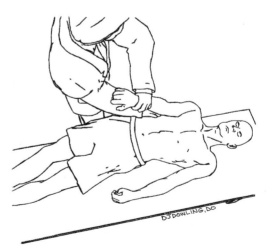

■ **FIG. 74-8B** The patient's arm is further flexed and abducted.

function (the physician's left hand holds the patient's right wrist in this example).

c. The physician introduces a long axis traction by pulling the patient's (right) arm toward the patient's feet until relaxation is noted at the monitoring finger.

d. The physician introduces shoulder flexion, adduction across the anterior side of the patient's body and internal rotation while maintaining traction (Fig. 74-8A).

e. While maintaining the traction, the patient's arm is further flexed and abducted anteriorly and laterally from the patient's body (Fig. 74-8B).

f. The patient's arm is brought back to the neutral position and the rib dysfunction is reassessed.

### REFERENCES

Van Buskirk RL. A manipulative technique of Andrew Taylor Still. *J Am Osteopath Assoc* 1996;96:597–602.

Van Buskirk RL. *The Still Technique Manual.* Indianapolis, IN: American Academy of Osteopathy, 1999.

Van Buskirk RL. Treatment of somatic dysfunction with an osteopathic manipulative method of Dr. Andrew Taylor Still. In Ward RC, ed. *Foundations for Osteopathic Medicine.* Philadelphia: Lippincott Williams & Wilkins, 2003: 1094–1114.

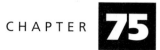

# PINS Techniques

*Dennis J. Dowling*

This chapter describes progressive inhibition of neuromusculoskeletal structures (PINS) techniques for treating somatic dysfunctions of the thoracic cage region. The examples provided are not the only ones that are possible (Fig. 75-1 *A* and *B*). The ones shown are fairly common. Occasionally, patterns in the thoracic cage region may continue into or from adjacent regions.

The patient is most commonly treated in the prone position but could be treated seated. In fact, treatment of rib dysfunction and intercostals is best performed with the patient seated because it allows easier continuous access to the patient's anterior and posterior chest. The physician should be positioned comfortably facing the region to be treated or alongside the table.

The principles and methods of PINS can be applied:

1. Locate a sensitive point in the region of the symptoms.
2. Analyze the structures that are deep to that point
3. Locate another sensitive point at the other end of a connecting structure (i.e., muscle, ligament, nerve, etc.). The more sensitive point is the primary point and the less sensitive point is the endpoint.
4. Apply inhibitory pressure to both points for 30 or more seconds. The soft tissue at the more sensitive point will typically lessen in tension.
5. Beginning at the more sensitive of the two points, locate another sensitive point approximately 2 to 3 centimeters toward the less sensitive point.
6. Repeat the procedure progressively toward the endpoint.

7. Reassess the status of the dysfunction. Determine if additional treatment or the application of other modalities is necessary.

## ■ PECTORALIS MINOR AND PECTORALIS MAJOR

1. **Technique:**
   a. The physician places the pad of his index or middle finger on the medial attachments of the muscles and lateral to the sternum. A finger of the physician's other hand locates a sensitive point laterally. The lateral point is located at the coracoid process for the *pectoralis minor* and at the medial border of the bicipital groove of the humerus for the *pectoralis major*.
   b. The pattern of intervening points is usually straight but the depth of pressure may indicate the muscles involved (deeper is the pectoralis minor and the pectoralis major is more shallow).
2. **Clinical Correlation:**
   a. Postmyocardial infarction
   b. Chest wall pain
      (1) Postmyocardial infarction
      (2) Costochondritis
   c. Shoulder pain
   d. Radiation of chest wall pain to shoulder and arm

## ■ RIB DYSFUNCTION AND INTERCOSTAL MUSCLES

1. **Technique:**
   a. The physician places the pad of his index or middle finger lateral to the transverse

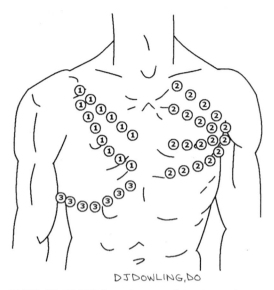

**■ FIG. 75-1A** PINS thoracic cage point patterns. 1, pectoralis minor; 2, pectoralis major; 3, rib dysfunction and intercostal muscles; 4, serratus anterior.

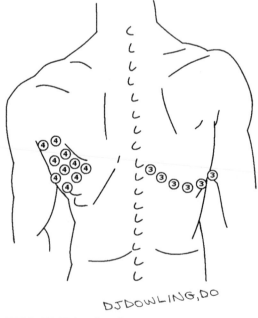

**■ FIG. 75.1B** (continued)

process that articulates with the involved rib posteriorly. A finger of the physician's other hand locates a sensitive point anteriorly. For the intercostal points, the posterior point may be located more laterally and slightly inferior to the bony rib. Another point is located anteriorly on the same rib. The intercostal pattern may actually be found between ribs.

b. The pattern of intervening points is generally slightly curved. The location of the points may correspond to the location of anterior and/or posterior counterstrain tender points. This should be especially kept in mind when counterstrain treatment appears to be ineffective.

2. **Clinical Correlation:**
   a. Back pain
   b. Flank pain
      (1) Nephrolithiasis (can mimic or be related to renal calculi)
      (2) Cholelithiasis/cholecystitis
   c. Respiratory difficulties
      (1) Asthma
      (2) Chronic obstructive pulmonary disease
      (3) Pneumonia
   d. Chest wall pain
      (1) Postmyocardial infarction
      (2) Costochondritis

### ■ SERRATUS ANTERIOR

1. **Technique:**
   a. The physician places the pad of his index or middle finger on a point in the lower thoracic cage region lateral to the lateral edge of the scapula. An anterior sensitive point may be found lateral to the costochondral junctions of the ribs.
   b. The pattern of intervening points is generally straight (muscle pattern) but may be slightly zigzag in following the course of the knife-like serratus muscles. Because of the overlapping nature of the muscle(s), there may be several patterns present.

2. **Clinical Correlation:**
   a. Back pain
   b. Rib pain
   c. Flank pain

## REFERENCES

Dowling DJ. Progressive inhibition of neuromuscular structures (PINS) technique. *J Am Osteopath Assoc* 2000;100: 285–286, 289–298.

Dowling DJ. Progressive inhibition of neuromuscular structures (PINS) technique. In Ward RC, ed. *Foundations for Osteopathic Medicine, 2nd ed.* Philadelphia: Lippincott Williams & Wilkins, 2003:1026–1033, Appendix II.

Dowling DJ. Progressive inhibition of neuromuscular structures (PINS) technique. In Chaitow L, ed. *Modern Neuromuscular Techniques.* Churchill Livingstone, 2003: 225–250.

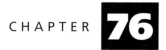

# CHAPTER 76

# Articulatory and Thrusting Techniques for the Ribs

*Eileen L. DiGiovanna, Barry Erner, and Dennis J. Dowling*

There are two direct methods used to move the rib articulations: *rib-raising techniques*, which are articulatory, and *thrusting* techniques, which are generally high-velocity, low-amplitude. Each has its own special applications as described here.

## ■ RIB-RAISING TECHNIQUES (ARTICULATORY)

Rib-raising techniques are techniques designed to articulate the rib heads by lifting and rotating them and, through the fascial attachments, to beneficially affect the sympathetic innervation at the chain ganglia.

In certain pulmonary diseases it is helpful to loosen tenacious mucus and to articulate the ribs to improve their motion. Rib-raising techniques achieve both these goals as the physician purposefully elevates groups of ribs.

### For the Bedridden Patient

This technique is especially useful for the patient who is unable to sit up, for a weakened and/or sick patient, or for a comatose patient.

1. **Patient position:** supine.
2. **Physician position:** standing or seated at the side of the table or bed.
3. **Technique:**
   a. The physician places her hands, palm up, on the bed, with her fingers under the patient's rib cage, at the costotransverse junctions.

   b. With the wrist as a fulcrum, the physician uses her fingers to raise and lower the ribs (Fig. 76-1), separating the articular surfaces. Generally, muscle tension in the region and restricted rib motion decrease during the treatment
   c. This process is repeated up and down the thorax.

### Rib Raising and Thoracic Pump in the Bedridden Patient

This technique serves the dual purpose of rib-raising and combining a *thoracic pump* for treating bedridden patients.

1. **Patient position:** supine.
2. **Physician position:** standing at the head of the table or bed.
3. **Technique:**
   a. The patient raises his arms above his head and clasps his hand behind the physician's thighs if able to do so, or the physician grasps the patient's upper arms.
   b. The physician grasps the patient's upper arms. The pads of the fingers can be placed in the axillae while the fingers curl around the pectoral muscles at the anterior axillary fold.
   c. As the physician rocks back and forth, performing the thoracic pump, the patient's chest is elevated through the pull on his arms.
   d. The technique can be coordinated with the patient's respiration by a pull on the

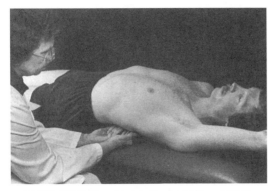

■ **FIG. 76-1** Rib raising in the bedridden patient.

muscle during inhalation and release during exhalation.

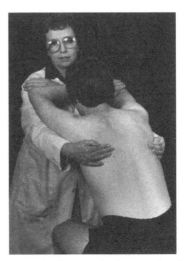

■ **FIG. 76-2** Rib raising in the seated patient.

## The Seated Patient

This technique is applicable to patients who are able to sit upright, and especially to patients who have difficulty breathing when supine and prefer to be upright.

1. **Patient position:** seated on the edge of the bed or on a chair.
2. **Physician position:** standing in front of the patient.
3. **Technique:**
   a. The patient crosses his arms in front of him with the elbows resting on the physician's upper arms near the shoulders.
   b. The physician reaches behind the patient's back, with the fingers of each hand grasping a group of ribs at the costotransverse junctions (Fig. 76-2).
   c. The physician rocks back while pressing down on the posterior ribs. At the same time, the patient falls forward onto his arms, which elevates the anterior rib cage.
   d. The physician repeats this maneuver rhythmically, moving her hands up and down the rib cage.
   e. The patient may assist in the treatment by inhaling deeply as the physician rocks back and exhaling fully as the physician moves forward. It can be performed for a few minutes or as long as the patient tolerates the treatment.

## Alternative Technique

1. **Patient position:** seated on a bed, chair, stool, or straddling table.
2. **Physician position:** standing behind the patient.
3. **Technique:**
   a. The physician places the thumbs of each hand pointing toward the spine and spreads her fingers over the ribs bilaterally near the costotransverse junctions.
   b. The patient places his hands on the table in front of him or on his knees.
   c. The physician pushes forward on the rib cage as the patient inhales and leans forward between his arms (Fig. 76-3).
   d. This maneuver is repeated rhythmically as the physician moves her hands up and down the thorax.
   e. The patient's inhalation elevates the ribs anteriorly as the physician assists motion posteriorly.

## ■ HIGH-VELOCITY, LOW-AMPLITUDE (HVLA) THRUSTING TECHNIQUES FOR THE RIBS

### Posterior Rib Head Somatic Dysfunction

1. **Patient position:** supine.
2. **Physician position:** Standing at the side of

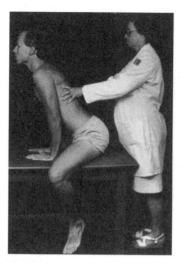

■ **FIG. 76-3** Alternate approach to rib raising in the seated patient.

the table on the side opposite the somatic dysfunction.

3. **Technique:**
   a. The patient crosses the arm closest to the physician over his chest and grasps his opposite shoulder. With his far arm, the patient reaches across and grasps the opposite iliac crest (Fig. 76-4)
   b. The physician places the thenar eminence of his localizing hand under the posterior rib being treated just lateral to the costotransverse joint.
   c. The physician rests his other hand over the patient's crossed arms and anterior chest wall, stabilizing the rib cage.

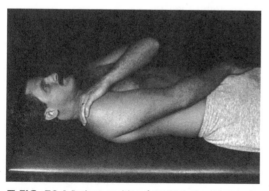

■ **FIG. 76-4** Patient position for HVLA thrusting technique for a posterior rib head somatic dysfunction.

   d. After the patient has exhaled completely, the physician exerts a rapid thrust through the patient's crossed arms toward his thenar eminence, which is resting on the posterior rib dysfunction (Fig. 76-5).

Note: As with high-velocity, low-amplitude thrusting techniques of the thoracic spine, flexion of the spine down to the segment of dysfunction may be necessary for rib dysfunctions lower in the thorax. Flexion is achieved by the physician grasping and cradling the patient behind the shoulders with his nonlocalizing hand and then flexing the patient to create localization down to the necessary point.

## Upper Rib Somatic Dysfunction (Ribs One to Four)

This technique is used for restricted motion at the costovertebral junction.

1. **Patient position:** prone.
2. **Physician position:** standing at the side of the table, opposite the dysfunction.
3. **Technique:**
   a. The patient cups his chin with the palm of his hand on the same side as the rib dysfunction, keeping the head in the midline.
   b. The physician places his thenar or hypothenar eminence on the rib dysfunction at

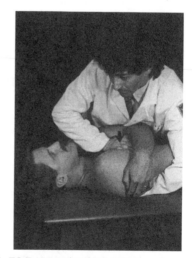

■ **FIG. 76-5** HVLA thrusting technique for a posterior rib head somatic dysfunction.

the costotransverse joint. Firm contact is maintained throughout.

c. The patient's elbow of the arm cupping the chin is moved cephalad as far as possible until motion is palpated at the dysfunction.

d. The physician's other hand is placed on the patient's head. The patient's head is rotated into the motion barrier while the chin remains firmly planted on his hand. This entails rotating the patient's head toward the rib dysfunction. The targeted rib may feel as if it is rising against the physician's hand. This should be resisted. A downward tension is exerted with the thrusting hand.

e. The physician maintains rotational and side-bending positioning of the patient's head, creating a locking at the cervico-thoracic spinal junction.

f. Additional rotation and lateral flexion are induced by the physician until spring is noted under the hand placed over the rib head somatic dysfunction.

g. The physician exerts a rapid thrust on the dysfunctional rib. The force vector exaggerates the lateral cephalic springing motion noted in Figure 76-6.

Note: No thrust should be applied to the patient's head or neck.

## First Rib Somatic Dysfunction (Exhalation Restriction)

1. **Patient position:** sitting on a stool or the treatment table, feet flat on floor.
2. **Physician position:** standing behind the patient with his knee and hip flexed and placed on the stool opposite the side of the rib dysfunction.
3. **Technique:**
   a. The patient drapes his arm on the side opposite the dysfunction over physician's flexed knee.
   b. The patient leans on the physician's knee, allowing his torso to become limp.
   c. The patient places his arm on the same side as the rib dysfunction between his legs.
   d. The physician flexes the cervical spine laterally toward the dysfunction until all the slack is removed from the cervicothoracic junction with the hand on the side opposite to the rib dysfunction.
   e. The physician places his thrusting hand with the metacarpophalangeal border (between the thumb and index finger) in the crease created by the patient's neck and the trapezius muscle on the posterior superior aspect of the first rib.
   f. The physician simultaneously applies a downward and medial thrust while rapidly exaggerating full cervical spine lateral flexion to the side of the rib dysfunction (Fig. 76-7).

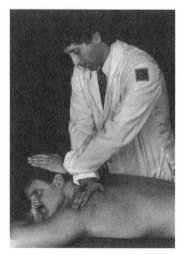

■ **FIG. 76-6** HVLA thrusting technique for upper rib somatic dysfunction, patient prone.

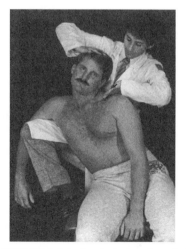

■ **FIG. 76-7** HVLA thrusting technique for a first rib somatic dysfunction.

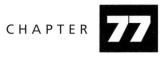

# Exercises for the Thoracic Cage

*Stanley Schiowtiz and Eileen DiGiovanna*

When evaluating a patient for an exercise program of the thoracic cage, it is important to consider including exercises for the thoracic spine (Chapter 44) and the shoulder girdle (Chapter 89).

## ■ PECTORAL MUSCLE STRETCH

1. **Patient position:** standing, facing a corner, with hands on adjacent walls and feet away from the wall.
2. **Instructions:**
   a. Drop your body forward, supported by your hands. This will bring the shoulder blades together and create pectoral muscle stretch (Fig. 77-1).
   b. Hold this position for 5 to 15 seconds.
   c. Return to starting position, relax, rest, and repeat.

## ■ INHALATION RIB STRETCH

1. **Patient position:** supine, both knees bent, feet on floor, entire spine flattened.
2. **Instructions:**
   a. Raise both fully extended arms off the floor while breathing in deeply (Fig. 77-2).
   b. Hold this position for 4 to 5 seconds.
   c. Lower both arms to floor as you slowly breathe out.
   d. Relax, rest, and repeat.

## ■ INHALATION RIB ISOMETRICS

1. **Patient position:** supine, both knees bent, feet on table, hands on sides of the rib cage.

2. **Instructions:**
   a. Inhale deeply while pressing firmly against your rib cage (Fig. 77-3). Try to prevent lateral chest expansion.
   b. Hold this position for 4 to 5 seconds.
   c. Exhale while you maintain your hand pressure.
   d. Relax, rest, and repeat.

## ■ EXHALATION ABDOMINAL STRETCH

1. **Patient position:** supine, hips and knees flexed to 90 degrees, feet supported by chair.
2. **Instructions:**
   a. Place both hands on your upper abdomen and breathe out slowly while contracting the abdominal muscles.
   b. Press both hands firmly down on abdomen to create forced exhalation (Fig. 77-4).
   c. Maintain firm hand pressure on abdomen as you slowly inhale, resisting abdominal stretch.
   d. Hold full inhalation 4 to 5 seconds.
   e. Relax, rest, and repeat.

## ■ ABDOMINOTHORACIC STRETCH

1. **Patient position:** supine, knees bent, feet on floor, both hands over head, elbows bent to 90 degrees.
2. **Instructions:**
   a. Inhale deeply. Try to use the abdomen only, with maximum abdominal muscle stretch (Fig. 77-5A).

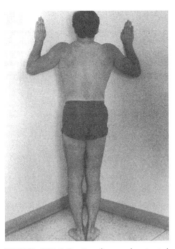

**■ FIG. 77-1** Pectoral muscle stretch

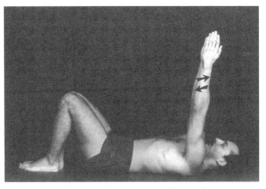

**■ FIG. 77-2** Inhalation rib stretch.

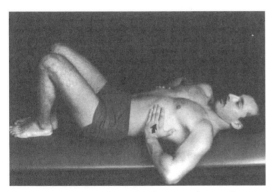

**■ FIG. 77-3** Inhalation rib isometric stretch.

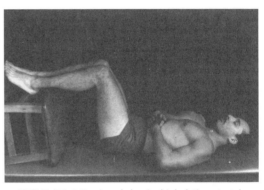

**■ FIG. 77-4** Passive abdominal inhalation stretch.

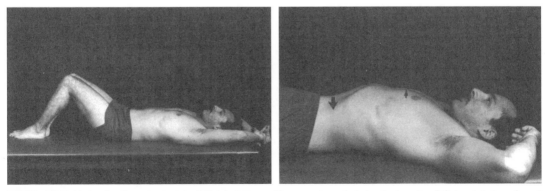

**■ FIG. 77-5** Abdominothoracic stretch. **(A)** Inhalation with expansion of abdominal cavity. **(B)** As air is transferred to the thoracic cage, the abdominal muscles are contracted and the chest is expanded.

b. Close your throat to prevent the escape of air.

c. Transfer the air to your upper chest by contracting your abdominal muscles. Your rib cage should rise (Fig. 77-5B).

d. Hold this position for 4 to 5 seconds. Release the air.

e. Relax, rest, and repeat.

## ■ STANDING INHALATION/ EXHALATION DIAPHRAGMATIC EXERCISE

1. **Patient position:** standing comfortably with feet separated approximately 6 inches.

2. **Instructions:**

a. Slowly raise your arms out from your side to a position straight over your head. As you raise your arms, inhale slowly so that you have achieved full inhalation by the time your arms are over your head.

b. Hold this position for 4 to 5 seconds.

c. Slowly lower your arms back to your side as you exhale so that you have achieved full exhalation by the time your arms are at your side.

d. Rest 4 to 5 seconds and then repeat this process. This should be performed eight to ten times, fully inhaling and exhaling as your arms are raised and lowered.

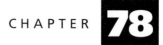

# Practical Applications and Case Histories of the Thoracic Cage

*Eileen L. DiGiovanna*

The thoracic cage plays a significant role in respiration, protection of major visceral organs of the chest, including the heart, lungs, blood vessels, and in pumping of the lymph into and out of the cysterna chyli. Freedom of motion is important for all of these functions. It is subject to a variety of traumas, infections, inflammatory processes, and somatic dysfunctions.

## ■ COSTOCHONDRITIS

Costochondritis is an inflammation of the costochondral junction. It is sometimes known as *anterior chest wall syndrome.* It is characterized by chest pain aggravated by coughing, sneezing, or deep inhalation. The patient often believes he is having cardiac pain, so this can be a frightening condition. Adding to the diagnostic problem is the fact that the pain can radiate to the shoulder.

Palpation of the costochondral junction elicits tenderness. There seldom is swelling. It must be differentiated from *Tietze syndrome*, which is similar in symptomatology. However, Tietze syndrome is generally more localized and swelling is usually present. Costochondritis must also be differentiated from somatic dysfunction, another cause of anterior chest wall pain. Evaluation of rib motion will usually allow a diagnosis; however, motion may be restricted in the presence of costochondritis as well.

It may be necessary to correct the rib motion restrictions to make an accurate diagnosis. The pain of somatic dysfunction should disappear or be markedly improved after treatment. If the pain and tenderness persist, it is likely costochondritis. In this case, anti-inflammatory medication and moist heat will usually give relief.

## ■ COSTOCHONDRAL SEPARATION

Blunt forces to the chest wall may separate the bony rib from its cartilaginous attachment. The patient will report pain in the anterior chest wall that must be differentiated from a fracture. The tenderness will be localized at the costochondral junction. This may occur iatrogenically during a thrusting technique used on the chest wall. It is almost universally the result of excessive force used during the thrust and represents a complication of a thrusting force passing through the chest wall.

This condition is self-limited and will heal in a few weeks without treatment other than reassurance and mild analgesia.

## ■ FRACTURES

Because of their size, the ribs may be fractured by less trauma than other larger bones. They are often involved in the early stages of osteoporosis and, thus, subject to fracture. A good history regarding trauma to the chest is essential in raising the suspicion of fracture of the ribs. X-rays may be helpful, but it is important to remember that hairline fractures may not show on x-ray until callus forms at the site of the fracture. Pinpoint tenderness of the shaft of the rib is the best indication in the presence of a history of trauma.

The application of force to the chest should be avoided when there is a suspicion of fracture or when there is a strong possibility of the presence of osteoporosis or osteopenia. Postmenopausal women, persons who have been using steroid medication for a period of time, and older men should not have a thrusting force applied to the chest unless the bone density has been evaluated.

Fractures of the sternum, scapulae, or clavicles are also possible, but generally they require a more forceful trauma for them to occur in adults. The clavicle is the most commonly fractured bone in children, however.

Once the fracture has healed, the area can be treated with gentle osteopathic manipulation to correct associated somatic dysfunctions.

## ■ DIAPHRAGM

The thoracic diaphragm is the major muscle of respiration. Disease processes in the thoracic cavity or in the abdominal cavity can affect its ability to function normally. When diaphragmatic tone increases, it tends to flatten. As it flattens, the motion of the lower ribs may be reversed and a decrease in the transverse diameter of the chest cavity may occur. This may be the result of acute or chronic obstructive lung disease. A flattened diaphragm will result in less efficient respiration and a decrease in the pressure gradients necessary for the movement of lymph.

*Doming the diaphragm* is an osteopathic technique used to decrease the hypertonicity of the muscle by stretching it. Along with the doming of the diaphragm, the ribs to which it attaches must be freed to allow for maximal motion during respiration.

## ■ SOMATIC DYSFUNCTION

Somatic dysfunction of the thorax may occur anteriorly, involving ribs, sternum, or clavicle, or posteriorly, involving costovertebral articulations or the scapulae. Muscle attachments connect the thoracic cage to the cervical spine, the thoracic spine, the lumbar spine, the innominate bones, and the upper extremities. These regions must be evaluated when problems occur in the thoracic cage.

The first rib is probably the rib most commonly involved in somatic dysfunction of all the ribs. It is affected by trauma, stress, and posture as well as by dysfunction of the C7–T1 complex. The patient may report "shoulder" pain, stiff neck, upper back or neck pain, and an inability to turn the head while driving. The first rib can impinge the neurovascular bundle as it passes between it and the clavicle through the costoclavicular space. The anterior and middle scalene muscles, which raise the first rib, may likewise compress the brachial plexus when they are in spasm and result in *thoracic outlet syndrome* symptoms. The patient's symptoms are then described as pain, numbness, or paresthesias of the arm or hand on the involved side. The physician needs to be aware that this may cause confusion should the patient demonstrate a herniated cervical disc on magnetic resonance imaging (MRI). The symptoms may be caused by the rib dysfunction rather than the herniated disc, so evaluation of the rib for normal motion and treatment of any dysfunction should be performed in these cases. Osteopathic manipulation may save the patient unnecessary surgery.

## Case 1

R.T. was a 48-year-old man who came to the clinic with a report of numbness and "pins and needles" in his right forearm and hand. This had been present for several months. He gave a history of an automobile accident approximately 1 year previously. He had undergone an MRI 1 month previously that demonstrated a herniation of the intervertebral disc between C6–C7, with apparent impingement on the foramen. He had a history of a mild elevation of his blood pressure, which was controlled with verapamil. He had been scheduled for surgery for the cervical disc for the following week and requested that a trial of manipulation be performed in an attempt to prevent surgery.

Examination showed R.T. to be overweight. His seated blood pressure was 130/84 in his left arm. His heart and lung sounds were normal. The range of motion of the cervical spine was decreased in right rotation and side-bending. The right first rib was depressed and had no motion on springing. The right trapezius, supraspinatus, and rhomboid muscles were hypertonic. Somatic dysfunctions were also present at C7–T1 and T3–4. Deep tendon reflexes were present in both upper extremities but slightly diminished on the right. Pulses were normal. The costoclavicular test was positive on the right and the Spurling maneuver was negative.

R.T. was treated with osteopathic manipulation. He received soft tissue myofascial techniques to the neck and upper back. The somatic dysfunctions were treated with facilitated positional release techniques, as was the first rib. The T3–4 somatic dysfunction was also treated with high-velocity, low-amplitude thrusting technique.

He was seen 1 week later and reported that beginning the day after the first treatment, he had had no further symptoms in his right arm and had cancelled the surgery. He was treated at that visit for some remaining hypertonicity of the muscle with soft tissue techniques. Although the first rib had better motion, it still was resistant to springing and so was treated a second time.

He was not seen again for almost 3 years, at which time he brought his daughter to the clinic to be examined for scoliosis. He reported that he had never experienced the numbness or paresthesias of the right arm again and had not had the surgery.

## ■ DISCUSSION

This case presents an example of the confusion sometimes caused by a first rib somatic dysfunction in the presence of an MRI-diagnosed cervical disc. Surgery had actually been scheduled for this man. Because the disc was obviously not the cause of his symptoms, it would have ended up being a "failed" surgery. First rib somatic dysfunction can cause symptoms severe enough to incapacitate some patients, with the inability to turn the head toward the dysfunctional rib, pain, or impingement of the neurovascular bundle to the upper extremity. Simply treating with osteopathic manipulation can relieve these symptoms quickly.

### REFERENCES

DiGiovanna EL. Schiowitz S. *An Osteopathic Approach to Diagnosis and Treatment, 2nd ed.* Philadelphia: Lippincott-Raven, 1997.

Schumacher HR. Klippel JH. Koopman WJ. *Primer on the Rheumatic Diseases, 10th ed.* Atlanta: Arthritis Foundation, 1993.

Ward RC. *Foundations for Osteopathic Medicine.* Philadelphia: Lippincott Williams & Wilkins, 2003.

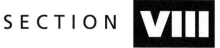

# Upper Extremities

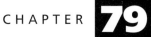

# CHAPTER 79

# Shoulder Anatomical Considerations

*Eileen L. DiGiovanna and Stanley Schiowitz*

The shoulder joint is the articulation between the head of the humerus and the glenoid fossa of the scapula. It is the most mobile joint in the body, as well as the most unstable. The *glenohumeral articulation* functions within the setting of the shoulder girdle. The *shoulder girdle* consists of three bones (the clavicle, humerus, and scapula), three true synovial joints (glenohumeral, sternoclavicular, and acromioclavicular), two functional joints (suprahumeral articulation and scapulothoracic), two accessory joints (costosternal and costovertebral), and the muscles that move the three bones.

## ■ BONES

The bones of the true shoulder joint are the head of the humerus and the scapula, specifically the glenoid fossa located on its lateral surface beneath the acromion. The clavicle plays a significant role in the motion of the shoulder and is, therefore, considered the third bone of the shoulder girdle.

The humerus is the long bone of the upper arm and at its proximal end is a neck with a smooth, round head that is covered with cartilage and forms one articulating surface of the true shoulder joint. The scapula is a flat, triangular bone overlying the ribs posteriorly. Easily palpable are its borders, spine posteriorly, coracoid process anteriorly, and the acromion process supero-laterally.

The clavicle lies on the upper thorax with articulations at either end. It is "crank-"shaped to allow for greater motion at its lateral end. It articulates with the sternum medially and with the acromion process laterally.

## ■ JOINTS

Five joints are primarily involved in shoulder girdle function. Three, the glenohumeral, acromioclavicular, and sternoclavicular, are true joints. The suprahumeral and scapulothoracic joints are pseudojoints (Fig. 79-1). These joints may be divided into two functional groups. Joints in the first group, the glenohumeral and suprahumeral joints, act in unison to produce the early motion of shoulder abduction. Joints in the second group, the scapulothoracic, sternoclavicular, and acromioclavicular joints, act in unison to produce the mid to late motions of shoulder abduction.

The *sternoclavicular* joint has a sellar or saddle-shaped articular surface, frequently with an interposed meniscus. This joint affords three planes of movement of the clavicle, in a frontal and horizontal plane, as well as rotation on its long axis.

The *acromioclavicular* joint is a planar joint. Occasionally there is an intra-articular plate between the surfaces that acts much as a disc. The acromioclavicular joint permits motion of the lateral end of the clavicle in an anteroposterior or cephalad–caudal direction, as well as rotation. More motion is possible at the lateral end of the clavicle because of the crank-like shape of the bone.

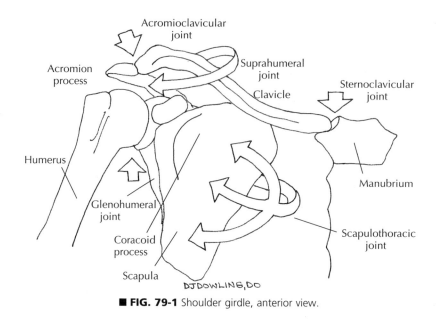

■ **FIG. 79-1** Shoulder girdle, anterior view.

The *glenohumeral* joint allows greater freedom of motion than any other joint in the body. The humeral head is convex and has a larger surface area than the concave glenoid fossa on which it moves. The humeral head slides along the surface of the fossa and rolls in various angular motions.

The capsule of the glenohumeral joint is loose and pleated. The ligaments, which are merely thickenings in the capsule, provide little support. The major support of the humerus into the fossa is provided by the rotator cuff muscles, which hold the head into the fossa. These muscles include the supraspinatus, infraspinatus, teres minor, and subscapularis. Abduction–adduction and axial and horizontal rotations are coupled in that angular motions are accompanied by translatory slides. The caudal slide of the humeral head with abduction confers increased freedom of motion on the supraspinatus tendon beneath the coracoacromial ligament.

The movements of the individual joints are as follows:

1. The glenohumeral joint has three degrees of cardinal motion: flexion and extension, abduction and adduction, and internal and external rotation.
2. The suprahumeral joint acts in concert with the glenohumeral joint as the humeral head articulates with the coracoacromial ligaments.
3. The scapulothoracic joint movements are related to scapular motions. The motions are medial and lateral movements of the scapula on the thorax (abduction–adduction), elevation of the scapula, and upward and downward rotation of the scapula (tilt), all relative to the glenoid fossa.
4. The sternoclavicular joint moves cephalad and caudad in the frontal plane, moves ventrad and dorsad in the horizontal plane, and rotates on its mechanical axis (Fig. 79-2). All cephalad–caudad and ventrad–dorsad movements are accompanied by translatory slides.
5. The primary motion of the acromioclavicular joint is axial rotation.

Total abduction of the shoulder joint can be divided into three phases. During the *first phase* (0 to 90 degrees), the supraspinatus and deltoid muscles are involved. At the beginning of the movement the supraspinatus is very efficient in abduction and in maintaining joint stability, whereas the deltoid is very inefficient and tends to produce superior dislocation. As abduction progresses, the deltoid's efficiency increases whereas that of the supraspinatus decreases.

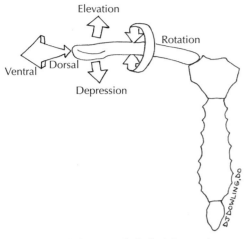

■ **FIG. 79-2** Sterno-clavicular joint motion.

These actions are a direct result of the changes in position of the muscles' origins and insertions that accompany the motion.

In the *second phase* (90 to 150 degrees), upward rotation of the scapula causes the glenoid fossa to tilt and face upwards as the humerus locks on the glenoid fossa. The trapezius and serratus anterior primarily contribute. The movement is restricted to some extent by the pectoralis major and latissimus dorsi but is facilitated by concomitant rotations of the sternoclavicular and acromioclavicular joints.

In the *third phase* (150 to 180 degrees) the spinal column is displaced laterally by the action of the contralateral spinal muscles. Bilateral abduction would require an exaggeration of the lumbar lordosis, because the spinal column would be otherwise synergistically balanced. These combined motions are known as the *scapulohumeral rhythm*.

Total flexion of the shoulder joint can also be divided into three phases. In the *first phase* (0 to 60 degrees), the muscles used are the anterior fibers of the deltoid, the coracobrachialis, and the clavicular fibers of the pectoralis major. Motion is limited by the tension of the coracohumeral ligament and by the resistance offered by the teres minor, teres major, and infraspinatus muscles.

In the *second phase* (60 to 120 degrees) the function is similar to the second phase of abduc-tion in that scapular rotation is added and the glenoid fossa is facing upward and anteriorly. In the *third phase* (120 to 180 degrees), unilateral and bilateral flexion require the same motion of the spinal column as for complete abduction.

## Functional Joints (Pseudojoints)

The two functional joints in the shoulder girdle are the *suprahumeral joint* and the *scapulothoracic* joint. As mentioned, both figure prominently in shoulder biomechanics and pathology. The suprahumeral joint is formed by the articulation of the head of the humerus with the coracoacromial arch, composed of the acromion, the coracoid process, and the ligament between them. Articulation occurs during abduction.

At rest, there is a space in the joint through which pass the tendon of the long head of the biceps, the supraspinatus muscle and supraspinatus tendon, the subacromial bursa, and the capsule—all important and sensitive structures. These soft tissues are normally compressed during abduction at approximately 90 degrees (Fig. 79-3). Internal rotation of the humerus causes impingement to occur at approximately 60 degrees. During external rotation, the head of the humerus glides posteriorly and inferiorly and impingement does not occur until 120 degrees of abduction. For this reason, persons with habitually slouched shoulders and internally rotated arms are more prone to degenerative processes such as tendinitis and bursitis.

The second functional joint is the scapulothoracic joint. This is formed by the scapula and the posterior thorax (ribs). Because muscle and fascia lie between the articulating surfaces, it is not a true joint with approximated articular surfaces and is also lacking a capsule.

## Accessory Joints

The accessory joints are the *costosternal joints* anteriorly, especially those of the first and second ribs, and the *costovertebral joints* posteriorly. The accessory joints are not anatomically involved in the shoulder joint or shoulder girdle, but dysfunction of these joints can interfere with free shoulder motion.

A minor degree of motion also occurs at *the Angle of Louis*, the point where the manubrium

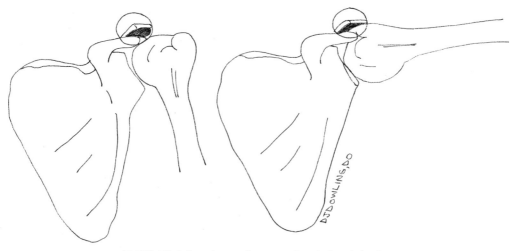

**■ FIG. 79-3** Suprahumeral compression during abduction.

joins the body of the sternum. There is some motion here during respiration and with abduction of the humerus. Restriction of motion here may affect normal glenohumeral motion.

## ■ MOTION OF THE SHOULDER BONES

### Humerus

The humerus moves in the following ways:

1. *Flexion* to 180 degrees in the sagittal plane.
2. *Extension* to 45 degrees in the sagittal plane.
3. *Abduction* to 180 degrees in the coronal plane, placing the arm in the same position as flexion to 180 degrees.
4. *Adduction* in the coronal plane, but only achieved with slight flexion or extension to clear the trunk.
5. *Horizontal flexion and extension* in the horizontal plane, after the arm has been abducted to 90 degrees.
6. *Internal and external rotation* around the long axis of the humerus in the horizontal plane, for a total of 180 degrees.
7. *Circumduction*, a combination of movements causing the arm to describe an irregular cone, with the humeral head moving in a small irregular circle and the hand moving in a wide sweeping circular motion.

### Scapula

Motion of the scapula is essential to normal functioning of the shoulder girdle. The motions of the scapula are the following:

1. *Elevation*, upward and parallel to the spine, and *depression*, a return from elevation (Fig. 79-4).
2. *Abduction* or *protraction* away from the spine, which is combined with a lateral tilt around the thorax (Fig. 79-5).
3. *Adduction* or *retraction*, moving closer to the spine (Fig. 79-6).
4. *Upward or forward tilt*, turning on a horizontal axis so that the posterior surface faces upward and the inferior angle protrudes. This motion is accompanied by a longitudinal axis rotation of the clavicle (Fig. 79-7).
5. *Upward and downward rotation* in relation to the glenoid fossa's elevation or depression: a frontal plane rotation (Fig. 79-8).

The glenoid fossa rotates upward during abduction, and this movement accomplishes several important functions:

1. The humerus impinges on the acromial arch at 90 degrees. To prevent impingement and permit abduction to 180 degrees, the scapula must rotate.
2. The fossa moves under the head of the humerus and increases the stability of the joint when the arm is elevated, preventing a downward dislocation.

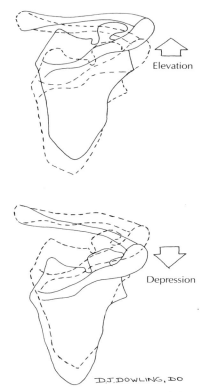

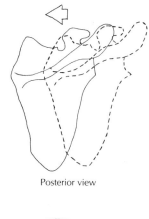

Posterior view

■ **FIG. 79-4** Elevation and depression of the scapula.

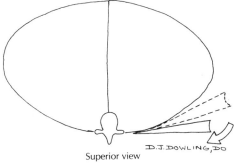

■ **FIG. 79-6** Scapular adduction (retraction).

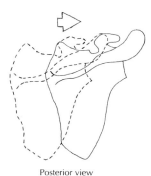

Posterior view

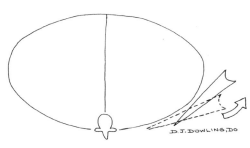

Superior view

■ **FIG. 79-5** Scapular abduction (protraction).

3. The fibers of the deltoid, attached from the scapula to the humerus, contract to abduct the arm to 90 degrees, at which point they are maximally contracted. As the fossa rotates upward, it maintains the deltoid in position for maximal contraction, allowing the humerus to continue to 180 degrees.

## ■ JOINT RHYTHMS AND MECHANISMS

The *scapulohumeral rhythm* is a free-flowing and synchronous movement of the scapula and humerus. During abduction, the scapula rotates as the humerus elevates. For every 15 degrees of abduction, humeral elevation accounts for 10 degrees and scapular rotation accounts for 5 degrees. Dysfunction of humeral elevation or of scapular rotation can disturb this rhythm and interfere with shoulder function. Dysfunction of clavicular motion can also interfere with this rhythm.

*Glenohumeral movement* requires a synchronous posterior downward glide of the humeral

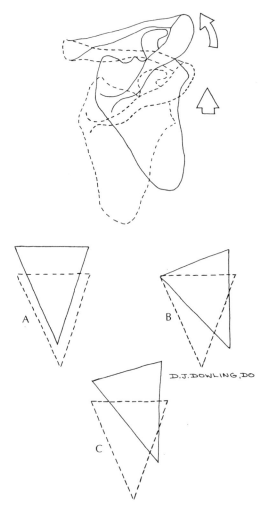

■ **FIG. 79-7** Scapular elevation with upward tilt. **(A)** Pure elevation. **(B)** Pure tilt. **(C)** Coupled motions.

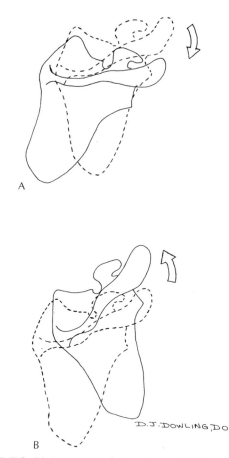

■ **FIG. 79-8** Rotation of the scapula. **(A)** Downward. **(B)** Upward.

head during abduction to prevent impingement on the coracoacromial arch. This necessitates an external rotation of the humerus to turn the greater tuberosity away from the arch.

Another mechanism indirectly involved in shoulder function is the *bicipital mechanism*. The tendon of the long head of the biceps passes through a groove between the greater and lesser tuberosities of the humerus and attaches to the rim of the glenoid. The tendon glides through the groove whenever the humerus is moved. Contraction of the muscle does not move the tendon. Biceps tendinitis, capsulitis, or adhesions may prevent free gliding of the tendon and interfere with normal motions.

The clavicle moves during most shoulder activity. Dysfunctions in clavicular motion can interfere with normal shoulder movement. The combined axial rotation of the sternoclavicular joint (30 degrees) and the acromioclavicular joint (30 degrees) allows the normal 60 degrees of rotation of the scapula on full abduction of the shoulder.

### REFERENCES

Bateman JE. The *Shoulder and Neck*, Philadelphia: WB Saunders, 1978.

DiGiovanna E. Shoulder kinetics. *Osteopath Ann* 1981;9: 75–79.

DiGiovanna E, Schiowitz S. *An Osteopathic Approach to Diagnosis and Treatment, 2nd ed.* Philadelphia: Lippincott-Raven, 1997.

Kapandji IA. *The Physiology of the Joints, vol. i.* Upper Limb. Edinburgh: Churchill Livingstone, 1972.

Quiring DP. *The Extemities.* Philadelphia: Lea & Febiger, 1960.

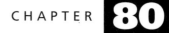

# Evaluation of the Shoulder

*Eileen DiGiovanna*

$A$s with any medical examination, the first step of the evaluation is a good history of the patient's symptom. The most common shoulder symptom will be pain, with limited motion a close second. The questioning must include a history of the pain and restriction as well as questions regarding trauma, either recent or distant, and whether sudden or gradual in onset. The patient's occupation, hobbies, sports activities, and posture may be involved in the condition and must be considered.

When evaluating the shoulder girdle during the physical examination, it is helpful to have an organized plan as with any evaluation. The following is a model that the student may follow to assure that parts of the examination are not overlooked.

## ■ OBSERVATION

Observation is the first step in evaluating the shoulder girdle. The physician should look for a smooth contour and symmetry between the two shoulders. Blemishes or signs of trauma, such as bruising, swelling, or lacerations, should be noted. Comparison should always be made to the normal shoulder.

The ability of the patient to move the shoulder during routine arm motions, such as removing an article of clothing or during gait, should be noted.

## ■ PALPATION

The shoulder should then be palpated. This is best begun with the physician standing behind the patient. Symmetry, smoothness of contour,

swelling, and tenderness should be noted. Quality of muscle tone should be evaluated. Abnormal temperature increases may be noted, especially around the joints. Bony changes of the clavicle, humerus, or scapula may be palpated.

It is helpful to identify significant bony landmarks during this part of the examination.

## ■ RANGE OF MOTION TESTING

The range of joint motion should be tested both passively and actively, with any restrictions noted. A general motion screening is performed by asking the patient to raise both arms slowly and touch the backs of his hands over the head. The physician observes scapular motion and symmetry of shoulder, elbow, and wrist angles. The inability to perform this test indicates motion restriction in the upper extremity. The areas of restriction must then be identified.

The Apley scratch test is a good method to test active range of motion. The patient is instructed to reach across his chest, over the shoulder, and touch the opposite scapula. Then he reaches behind his back and touches his opposite scapula. Finally, he reaches behind his head and touches the opposite scapula. These maneuvers actively test all the ranges of motion in the shoulder joint. If one of these maneuvers cannot be performed, it is then necessary to identify which shoulder motion is restricted and evaluate it more carefully.

The physician should then passively put the upper extremity through the ranges of motion. This assists in differentiating muscle from joint pain or restriction. Passive motion relieves the muscle of work so that if they are the source of the pain, the patient will not experience any pain they may have noted on active motion.

# ■ MUSCLE STRENGTH TESTING

Muscle strength should be tested. Each muscle group should be tested individually, e.g., the flexors, the extensors, etc. Individual muscles may be tested if one group of muscles is found to be weak. Muscle weakness may be neurologic in origin or from muscle injury, overuse, or lack of tone.

## Sensation Testing

There are no specific neurologic reflexes associated with the shoulder, but sensation testing may be helpful if a cervical problem is suspected. Testing of the dermatomal patterns of the skin over the shoulder and upper arm may be performed with a sharp object and wisp of cotton. This is not a common part of the shoulder evaluation.

## Special Tests for the Shoulder

Several specific tests may be used to detect a particular shoulder dysfunction. These are described.

### Arm Drop Test

The patient's arm is elevated to 90 degrees of abduction and released. If there is a tear in the rotator cuff muscles, the arm will drop. If the tear is partial, by tapping on the arm the physician will cause it to drop.

### Apprehension Test

This test is for a chronically dislocating shoulder. The shoulder is abducted, extended, and externally rotated. At the point where the shoulder is about to dislocate, the patient will appear apprehensive. Many patients are already aware that their shoulder dislocates spontaneously and will mention this in the history before the examination.

### Yergason Test

The Yergason test is performed to assess the stability of the biceps tendon in the bicipital groove. The physician applies traction to the elbow and externally rotates the arm. The patient attempts to internally rotate the arm against resistance. If

the tendon is unstable in the groove, it will pop out with a snap, and the patient will experience discomfort (Fig. 80-1).

All patients with a history of shoulder problems must be evaluated for dysfunctions of the cervical spine, upper thoracic spine, sternum and upper ribs.

# ■ EVALUATION FOR SOMATIC DYSFUNCTION

In diagnosing somatic dysfunctions involving shoulder girdle motion, the clinician must be aware that dysfunctions limiting motion reflect involvement of multiple joints, muscles, tendons, ligaments, the synovium, and the joint capsules. Functional anatomic knowledge and diagnostic ability should include knowledge of the following:

1. The functioning of accessory and coupled motions
2. The origins and insertions of the shoulder muscles
3. The influence of these muscles on the entire spinal column
4. The relationship of the thorax and rib cage to all scapular motion
5. How the first rib, at its sternal attachment, is directly influenced by clavicular and sternal motion

## Glenohumeral Joint

The glenohumeral joint can be evaluated during its range of motion testing. Somatic dysfunction is diagnosed if there is no pathology of the joint. Arthritis, tendonitis, or other pathology may be treated with appropriate osteopathic manipulation, but most responsive will be true somatic dysfunctions.

## Test for Clavicular Motion

In *abduction,* the distal end of the clavicle moves superiorly and the proximal end moves inferiorly. The physician tests motion in abduction by placing her index finger on the clavicular head next to the sternum while the patient is supine; the physician then asks the patient to shrug (Fig. 80-2). A caudad movement should be palpated with normal motion at the sternoclavicular joint.

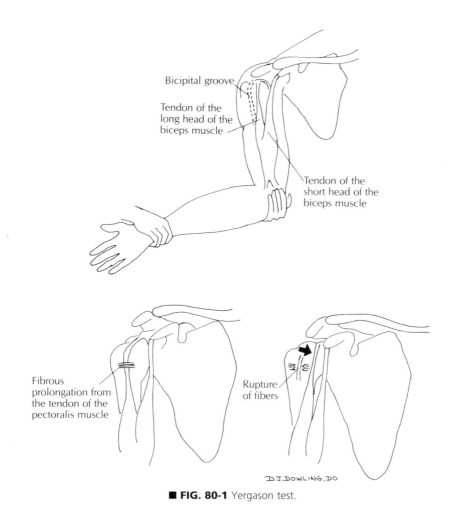

Bicipital groove

Tendon of the
long head of the
biceps muscle

Tendon of the
short head of the
biceps muscle

Fibrous
prolongation from
the tendon of the
pectoralis muscle

Rupture
of fibers

D.J.DOWLING,DO

■ **FIG. 80-1** Yergason test.

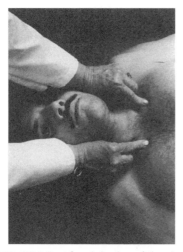

■ **FIG. 80-2** Test for abduction of the clavicle.

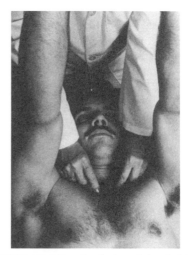

■ **FIG. 80-3** Test for flexion of the clavicle.

In *flexion*, the distal end of the clavicle moves anteriorly and the proximal end moves posteriorly on the sternum. The physician tests motion in flexion by placing her index finger on the clavicular head next to the sternum; the physician then asks the patient to flex his shoulder to 90 degrees and to reach up to the ceiling forcefully (Fig. 80-3). A posterior movement of the clavicle should be palpated with normal motion at the sternoclavicular joint.

The entire shoulder girdle, thorax, rib cage, and vertebral column must be evaluated for a comprehensive diagnosis of somatic involvement in shoulder girdle dysfunction. The plan for treatment should be similarly comprehensive.

## REFERENCES

Bateman JA. *The Shoulder and Neck.* Philadelphia: WB Saunders, 1982.

DiGiovanna E. Schiowitz S. *An Osteopathic Approach to Diagnosis and Treatment.* Philadelphia: Lippincott-Raven, 1997.

Hoppenfeld SA. *Physical Examination of the Spine and Extremities.* Norwalk, CT: Appleton-Century-Croft, 1995.

Polley HF, Hunder GA. *Physical Examination of the Joints.* Philadelphia: WB Saunders, 1987.

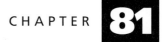

# Elbow Anatomic Considerations

*Eileen L. DiGiovanna, Stanley Schiowitz, and Dennis J. Dowling*

The elbow links the forearm with the upper arm and, in concert with the shoulder, allows motion of the hand through space. The elbow functions as a ginglymus or hinge joint. It is formed by the articulation of the proximal ends of the radius and ulna with the distal end of the humerus.

The distal end of the humerus articulates with the ulna and radius, forming two articulations: the *humeroulnar*, between the trochlea of the humerus and the trochlear notch of the ulna, and the *humeroradial*, between the capitellum of the humerus and the head of the radius (Fig. 81-1).

The motions observed in the elbow joint are flexion, extension, and rotation (supination and pronation). Flexion and extension are the only motions that involve the *true elbow joint*, the ulna with the humerus. The elbow joint has the composite motions of elbow flexion, with forearm supination, and elbow extension, with forearm pronation. Therefore, the superior radioulnar joint and its motions complicate, and are part of, elbow joint motion.

Flexion may be active or passive. Active flexion ends at approximately 145 degrees and is primarily limited by opposition of the contracting muscles of the arm and forearm. The range of passive flexion is slightly larger as the muscles relax and are flattened. There is some restriction as well that comes with the approximation of the raised coronoid process of the ulna into the shallow corollary depression in the humerus. Bony opposition and tension in the triceps and posterior capsular ligaments also limit flexion. The primary flexor muscle is the brachialis, which is assisted by the biceps brachii and the brachioradialis.

Extension of the elbow from the anatomic position is limited (5 to 10 degrees) by contact of the olecranon process with the fossa, tension in the anterior ligament, and resistance of anterior muscles. The triceps brachii is the only significant elbow muscle that functions in extension. There is some minor contribution by the anconeus. Because most elbow extension is accomplished by gravity, the triceps functions primarily against resistance.

Besides flexion and extension, the forearm can rotate around its longitudinal axis. Rotation involves the proximal radioulnar joint of the elbow and the distal radioulnar joint, which lies above the wrist. These motions are observed with the forearm flexed to 90 degrees.

Supination is the rotary motion that turns the palm of the hand toward the ceiling; pronation is the rotary motion that turns the palm toward the floor. In neutral rotation, the palm faces medially with the thumb up. The total range of rotation is approximately 180 degrees. Proximally, the olecranon process has minor coupled motions during pronation and supination. Supination is accompanied by a slight amount of adduction of the olecranon process while some slight amount of abduction occurs during pronation.

During supination, the interosseous membrane between the radius and ulna becomes taut. Supination is produced by contraction of the supinator and biceps muscles; pronation involves the pronator quadratus and pronator teres. The pronators are less powerful than the supinators.

During pronation and supination, the cupped radial head rotates about the knob of the capi-

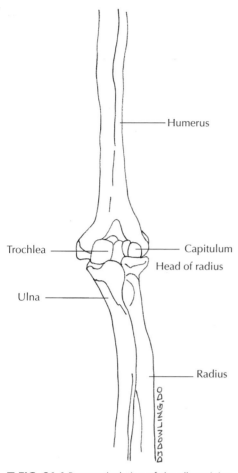

■ **FIG. 81-1** Bony articulation of the elbow joint.

tellum, a rounded portion of the humerus on its lateral aspect. It is held in place by the annular ligament, which attaches at both ends to the ulna and wraps about the neck of the radius. There are also secondary motions that accompany those of flexion, extension, supination, and pronation of the radiohumeral motion. Because of the concave–convex relationship, roll and slide most typically occur in the same direction when the elbow is flexed and extended. There is coupled motion of pronation with posterior slide and supination with anterior slide. These secondary, minor motions are the ones that become restricted in somatic dysfunction.

## ■ JOINTS

*Humeroradial articulation* consists of the concave head of the radius articulating with the convex-shaped capitellum of the humerus. Motion of this articulation must accompany humeroulnar flexion–extension. This angular motion is accompanied by ventral and dorsal translatory slide of the radius on the humerus: dorsal radial slide with extension and ventral radial slide with flexion (Fig. 81-2). Extension stress is the major cause of posterior radial head somatic dysfunction.

The proximal radioulnar articulation consists of the cylindrical rim of the head of the radius articulating with the radial notch of the ulna. The annular ligament encompasses the head of the radius and is attached to the anterior and

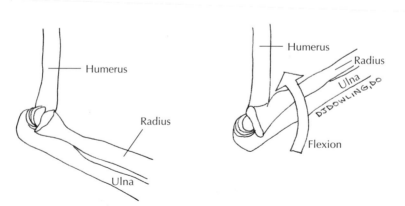

■ **FIG. 81-2** Translatory slide of the radius on the capitulum. Roll and slide occur in the same direction.

posterior margins of the radial notch. In conjunction with the distal radioulnar articulation, its main motions are supination and pronation. The axis of these motions is represented by a line drawn through the center of the head of the radius, with the distal end of the radius swinging around and in front of the ulna. The proximal end of the ulna moves backward and laterally during pronation and forward and medially with supination (Fig. 81-3). This means that the axis of rotation of the head of the radius does not remain constant. The accessory motions therefore consist of the previously mentioned dorsal–ventral radial slide on the capitulum, similar motion on the radial notch, and dorsal and ventral ulnar slide on the radius. All of these motions may contribute to somatic dysfunctions.

The joint capsule and several ligaments support the elbow joints. Maintaining the most support and resisting valgus and varus strains are the medial and lateral collateral ligaments, respectively. Other anatomical considerations include the relatively weaker contribution to flexion of the flexor muscles of the wrist and hand originating from the supracondylar ridge of the medial humerus. The wrist and hand extensor muscles originate from the lateral supracondylar ridge of the humerus. Several nerves pass from the proximal arm to the hand through the elbow region. Most notable are the ulnar nerve passing through a groove in the humerus and the median nerve that passes between the two heads of the pronator teres muscle in the antecubital fossa.

## ■ CARRYING ANGLE

When the arm is in the anatomic position, the upper arm and the forearm form an angle at the elbow, with the forearm directed away from the body in a valgus position. This is known as the *carrying angle* and is normally greater in women than in men (10 to 15 degrees in women, 5 degrees in men). If the carrying angle exceeds 15 degrees, it is called *cubitus valgus*. A decrease or

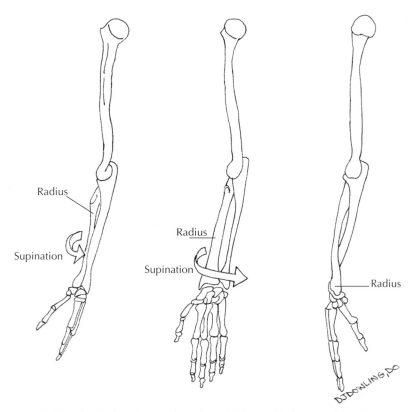

■ **FIG. 81-3** Supination to pronation. The radial head tilts downward and laterally.

reversal is known as *cubitus varus* or "gunstock" deformity.

# ■ SOMATIC DYSFUNCTION

Somatic dysfunctions can involve contraction of the related muscles, compression of the neural elements, strain of the ligamentous aspects, and restriction primarily of the secondary motions of the joint components. The radial head typically entails posterior or anterior dysfunctions and may involve the muscles, the annular ligament, and the lateral collateral ligament. The humero-olecranon dysfunctions can involve the muscles, the medial collateral ligament, and can be related to symptoms involving the ulnar nerve. Restriction of elbow extension (flexion dysfunction) and supination can involve the flexor muscles and compression of the median nerve. An extension dysfunction most likely will require treatment of the triceps component. Because of the overlapping of structures of the region, including the nerves, fascia, and especially the muscles that cross two joints, the search for the cause of dysfunction most frequently involves the adjacent regions of the shoulder and wrist/hand.

**REFERENCES**

DiGiovanna EL, Schiowitz S. *An Osteopathic Approach to Diagnosis and Treatment, 2nd ed.* Philadelphia: Lippincott-Raven, 1997.

Greenman PE. *Principles of Manual Medicine, 2nd ed.* Baltimore: Williams & Wilkins, 1996.

Kapandji IA. *The Physiology of the Joints,* Vol 1. Upper Limb. Edingburgh: Churchill-Livingston, 1972.

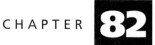

# Evaluation of the Elbow

*Eileen L. DiGiovanna*

$\mathbf{A}$ history of the elbow problem should be taken first. A pain history is essential if that is the chief symptom. The elbow is important in various arm movements and restriction of motion may be the primary symptom. A history of trauma, acute or chronic, should be noted. Occupation, hobbies, sports activities, and activities of daily living should be evaluated. This must be followed by a thorough examination of the elbow as well as the joints above and below it.

## ■ OBSERVATION

The elbow should be examined first by observation. The *carrying angle* of the elbow should be noted, as should any swelling, which may be diffuse or localized to the olecranon bursa posteriorly. Signs of old or new trauma should be noted, such as scars, abrasions, bruises, and the like.

## ■ PALPATION

The soft tissues and bony structures are then palpated to evaluate the integrity of the bones and the presence of any tenderness, masses, asymmetries, or crepitus. Any temperature changes should be noted, especially over the bursa and around the joints. Bony landmarks should be identified and compared between elbows. Swelling, especially over the olecranon bursa, should be noted. The olecranon bursa should not be palpable unless it is filled with fluid or thickened.

The ulnar nerve may be palpated in the groove between the medial epicondyle and the olecranon. The physician checks for scar tissue around the nerve that might compromise it.

## Range of Motion Testing

Range of motion should be checked actively and passively. Extension is minimal because of bony impingement. Flexion will be limited by the size of the biceps muscle. Besides the gross motions of flexion, extension, supination and pronation, the motion of the head of the radius must be evaluated as it glides on the lateral ulna. The motions of abduction and adduction of the ulna on the humerus should be evaluated.

## Muscle Strength Testing

The muscle strength of each muscle group should be tested and, if found to be weak, the individual muscle strength should be evaluated. Muscle groups to be tested are flexors, extensors, pronators, and supinators.

## Neurologic Examination

The skin around the elbow and in the forearm may be tested for sensation. This is especially important with complaints of paresthesias or numbness.

When examining the elbow, it may be appropriate to test the deep tendon reflexes at the elbow and forearm. This is most commonly performed to rule out the compression/impingement of the nerves exiting from the foramina of the cervical spine.

1. **Biceps reflex:** elicited by tapping the biceps tendon in the antecubital fossa: tests primarily C5.

2. **Brachioradialis reflex:** elicited by tapping the tendon on the lateral aspect of the lower forearm above the wrist: tests C6.
3. **Triceps reflex:** elicited by tapping the triceps tendon on the posterior arm just above the olecranon: tests C7.

## ■ SPECIAL TESTS

1. *Tinel test:* This is performed by tapping over the ulnar nerve as it passes between the olecranon and medial epicondyl. Marked sensitivity may be indicative of a neuroma or inflammation of the ulnar nerve.
2. *Tennis elbow test:* This test is performed by stabilizing the forearm. Instruct the patient to make a fist and extend his wrist. Press against the dorsum of the patient's hand as he resists. When tennis elbow (lateral epicondylitis) is present, the patient will experience pain at the lateral epicondyle.
3. *Ligamentous stability:* It may be necessary to test the elbow for ligamentous stability. This is performed by placing first a valgus stress and then a varus stress on the elbow, using one hand as a fulcrum and the other as an opposing force.

## ■ EVALUATION FOR SOMATIC DYSFUNCTION

## Adduction/Abduction of the Elbow

Adduction and abduction are accessory rocking motions of the upper part of the ulna on the trochlea of the humerus. Abduction is an accessory motion of pronation. Adduction is an accessory motion of supination.

The patient's elbow is semi-flexed approximately 45 degrees. The physician palpates the articulation by placing a finger on the dorsal aspect of the radial and ulnar sides of the olecranon, then tries to palpate into the trochlea. With his other hand, the physician grasps the patient's forearm and, starting from a neutral position, fully supinates the forearm, inducing a rocking, adduction motion of the ulna. Reversing the forearm motion into full pronation induces a rocking abduction motion. The elbow is tested for restriction of either motion.

## Radial Head Motion

The radial head is palpated by flexing and extending the elbow. The physician grasps the radial head and moves it in an anterior direction and in a posterior direction, noting any restriction to either motion. Posterior glide of the radius is coupled with pronation/extension and anterior glide is coupled with supination/flexion.

The most common dysfunction is a posterior radial head. This is diagnosed from the ability to move the radial head dorsally with restriction of motion ventrally. An anterior radial head is restricted in motion dorsally and free motion ventrally.

## REFERENCES

DiGiovanna EL. Schiowitz S. *An Osteopathic Approach to Diagnosis and Treatment, 2nd ed.* Philadelphia: Lippincott-Raven, 1997.

Hoppenfeld SA. *Physical Examination of the Spine and Extremities.* Norwalk, CT: Appleton-Century-Croft, 1995.

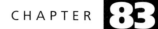

# Wrist and Hand Anatomic Considerations

*Eileen L. DiGiovanna, Stanley Schiowitz, and Dennis J. Dowling*

## ■ THE WRIST

### Bones

The wrist or carpus is the distal articulation of the radius and the articular disk with the proximal row of carpal bones. The disk joins the ulna and radius and lies between the ulna and the proximal row of carpal bones. Laterally to medially, these bones are the scaphoid (navicular), lunate, and the triquetrum. A small bone, the pisiform, lies slightly anterior to the triquetrum.

The wrist joint consists of fifteen bones, each with multiple articulations. A good example is the capitate bone, which articulates with the second, third, and fourth metacarpals and with the lunate, scaphoid, trapezoid, and hamate bones (Fig. 83-1). The wrist acts as a functional unit, exhibiting flexion, extension, adduction (ulnar deviation), abduction (radial deviation), and circumduction.

### Joints

The articular complex of the wrist can be divided into three functional units:

1. The radiocarpal joint, consisting of the distal end of the radius articulating with the scaphoid and lunate
2. The midcarpal joint, consisting of the combined articulations between the proximal and distal rows of the carpal bones (Fig. 83-2)
3. The ulnomeniscotriquetral pseudojoint, consisting of the distal end of the ulna, the triquetrium, and the meniscus between the two

The movements that occur at the radiocarpal and midcarpal joints can be considered together because these joints act as a combined mechanism. Flexion involves the combined motion of both units, with midcarpal motion somewhat greater than radiocarpal motion. The roles are reversed in extension: radiocarpal motion is greater (Fig. 83-3). In adduction, most of the motion occurs at the radiocarpal and the ulnomeniscotriquetral joints. Abduction involves primarily the midcarpal joint. There is a complex torsion movement of the carpal bones about their long axes during abduction and adduction. Circumduction of the hand is not axial rotation, but a series of movements: flexion followed by adduction, extension, and abduction, or the same movements in reverse order.

The wrist moves in two planes. In the *sagittal plane,* it flexes to approximately 85 degrees and extends to approximately 45 degrees. Flexion and extension appear to occur around more than one axis. In the *coronal plane,* the wrist moves into abduction (radial deviation) and adduction (ulnar deviation). Abduction is approximately 15 degrees and adduction 45 degrees. Pronation and supination occur at the radioulnar joint and, combined with flexion, extension, abduction, and adduction, permit circumduction so that the hand can lie in any plane.

Accessory movements are greatest at the radioscaphoid and radiolunate articulations. These movements are ventral–dorsal slide, axial rotation, slight side-to-side slide, and long-axis trac-

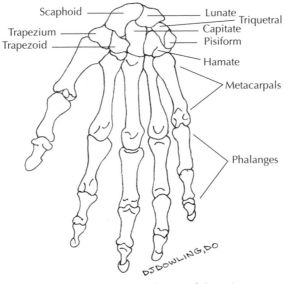

■ **FIG. 83-1** Bony articulations of the wrist.

tion. Similar accessory motions can be found at all carpal articulations, but in greatly diminished degrees.

The close-packed position of the wrist is full extension. Falling on the wrist in this position will readily cause fracture. In a relaxed, loosely packed position, the joints are relatively mobile. For the performance of any task involving wrist action, the articulations must enter into a combination of interdependent locked positions, creating a solid structure that can bear the strain of torsional motion. In turning a doorknob, for example, the wrist joint changes from a sack of loose bones into a solid functional unit for the transmission of force.

A nearly infinite number of partially close-packed positions of the wrist articulation can be created by muscle contraction and tightening of the ligaments. The close-packed articulation transmits force to the end of its total unit. Acting as a lever, it produces maximum force impact at one end, which would be the first "open pack" articulation. Somatic dysfunctions may easily develop in this manner, without sustaining direct trauma to the joint involved.

## Muscles

The wrist is moved by four groups of muscles:

1. **Flexor carpi ulnaris:** flexes the wrist and adducts the hand.
2. **Extensor carpi ulnaris:** extends the wrist and adducts the hand.
3. **Flexor carpi radialis and palmaris longus:** flex the wrist and abduct the hand.
4. **Extensor carpi radialis longus and brevis:** extend the wrist and abduct the hand.

The bodies of these muscles lie close to the elbow, and the corresponding tendons are long, passing down the forearm to attach to the wrist.

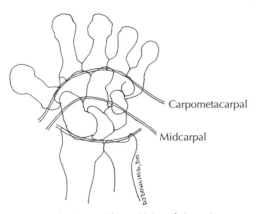

■ **FIG. 83-2** Midcarpal joint of the wrist.

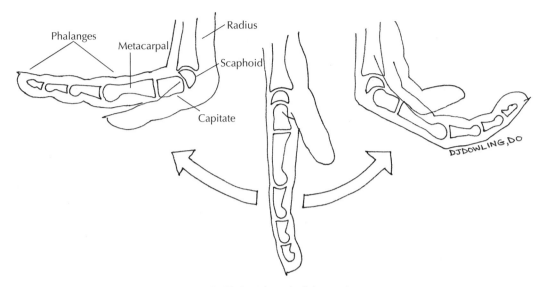

**■ FIG. 83-3** Major wrist joint motion.

## Tunnels

The carpal bones form an arch spanned by the *flexor retinaculum*. The concavity of the arch lies on the palmar surface between the bones and the transverse ligament (the flexor retinaculum) and is called the *carpal tunnel*. Through this tunnel pass the tendons of the wrist and finger flexors and the median nerve. It is the site of origin of the thenar and hypothenar muscles.

Another tunnel, the *tunnel of Guyon*, is formed by the ligament attaching the hook of the hamate and the pisiform. Through this tunnel pass the ulnar nerve and artery.

These two tunnels in particular are significant in that each contains a major nerve to the hand, which has a small diameter space through which the nerve passes. Tendons of the wrist and fingers occupy the greater part of that space. This makes impingement of the nerve a possibility when the diameter is narrowed by swelling, displacement of a bone, fibrous bands, or scar tissue.

## Anatomic Snuffbox

On the lateral aspect of the wrist is a small depression known as the anatomic snuffbox. The floor of the snuffbox is the scaphoid or navicular bone. It lies distal to the radial styloid and becomes prominent when the thumb is maximally extended. The abductor pollicis longus, the extensor pollicis brevis, and the extensor pollicis longus tendons bound it. This area will be tender to palpation if there is a fracture of the scaphoid.

## ■ THE HAND

The human hand is prehensile to a degree not attained in other species. Only in humans can the thumb be brought into opposition with each of the other fingers. This is a remarkable organ of sense, capable of measuring thickness and distance as well as perceiving light touch and temperature. The delicate movements of the hand allow grasping and fine movements.

## Bones and Joints

The hand consists of five metacarpal bones that articulate proximally with four carpal bones in the distal row. The second and third metacarpals remain relatively fixed while the first, fourth, and fifth move around this fixed segment. The five metacarpals articulate distally with the proximal phalanges of the fingers. These are usually considered ginglymus or hinge joints. They permit flexion–extension, abduction, adduction, and circumduction.

An extensor tendon lies along the dorsal aspect of each joint, and there are fibrocartilaginous plates over the palmar surface, known as palmar or volar plates. These plates lie between the joint and the flexor tendons.

Each finger, except the thumb, has a proximal and a distal interphalengeal joint. Because there are only two phalengeal bones in the thumb, there is only one joint. The interphalangeal joints are hinge joints, allowing flexion and extension with some axial rotation.

With the exception of the thumb, the movements of the carpometacarpal articulations consist almost exclusively of flexion–extension and abduction–adduction. The accessory motions are dorsal–ventral slide, axial rotation, and long-axis traction. These either occur when the structures conform to the shape of an object or are passively introduced. The thumb has a sellar articulation, permitting the motions of flexion–extension, abduction–adduction, rotation, and circumduction. The accessory motions are axial rotation and long-axis traction.

The intermetacarpal joints are limited to slight gliding of one on another. The accessory motion is axial rotation. The metacarpophalangeal articulations have the following movements: flexion–extension, adduction–abduction, limited rotation, and circumduction. The accessory motions are axial rotation, dorsal–ventral slide, and long-axis traction.

The interphalangeal joints are limited to flexion-extension motions. Flexion is usually accompanied by a conjunct rotation to assist in thumb–finger approximation. The accessory motions are dorsal–ventral slide, abduction–adduction, axial rotation, and long-axis traction. The early motion dysfunctions caused by arthritic involvement of the hands are manifested in loss of accessory motions.

## Muscles

The muscles of the fingers lie in the forearm. The tendons cross the wrist with the wrist muscle tendons. The flexor muscles cross the palm through numerous fibro-osseous tunnels. The extensor tendons pass along the dorsum of the hand through fewer tunnels. The flexor and extensor muscles are all extrinsic muscles.

Intrinsic muscles include the interosseous and lumbrical muscles. In addition to assisting with flexion and extension, they abduct and ad-

duct the fingers. At the base of the thumb on the palmar surface is the *thenar eminence*, which is made up of the intrinsic muscles of the thumb: the adductor pollicis, opponens pollicis, abductor pollicis brevis, and flexor pollicis brevis. These muscles are innervated by the median nerve. The thenar eminence atrophies when the median nerve is trapped, as in carpal tunnel syndrome. On the medial aspect of the palm, at the base of the fifth digit, is *the hypothenar eminence*, which contains three muscles: the flexor digiti minimi, abductor digiti minimi, and opponens digiti minimi.

## Prehensile Motions of the Hand

The skin over the palm of the hand is thicker than over the dorsum and is firmly attached to the fascia at the palmar creases. This permits the hand to grasp objects securely. Also important to know is the ability of the hand to change shape to conform to the object being grasped. It can flatten and spread out to conform to a flat surface or it can form a hollow cup-like depression.

According to Kapandji, there are six ways in which the hand can grasp objects: the thumb is involved in four kinds of prehensile motions.

1. **Prehension by terminal opposition** is the finest and most precise form of grasp. The tip of the finger pad or fingernail makes contact when the thumb and index finger grasp a thin object.
2. **Prehension by subterminal opposition** is the most common form of grasp. The object is held between the pads of the thumb and index fingers.
3. In **prehension by subterminolateral opposition,** the pad of the thumb holds an object, such as a coin, pressed against the radial surface of the first phalanx of the index finger.
4. **Palmar prehension** is used to grasp heavy, relatively large objects. The entire hand is wrapped around the object. The thumb opposes the force of the other four fingers.
5. **Prehension by digitopalmar opposition** entails grasp of a small-diameter object by the fingers pressing against the palm. The thumb is not involved.
6. **Prehension between lateral aspects of the fingers** is exemplified by holding a cigarette.

This grip is weak, and the object must be small. The thumb is not involved.

## Somatic Dysfunctions

As with many of the arthritic conditions, the primary dysfunction of the wrist and hand occur with the secondary motions more than the primary motions. Some dysfunctions of the carpal joints occur involving multiple joints. One of the most typical of the carpal dysfunctions involves restriction of glide of the lunate bone. It tends to have a preferential glide into the ventral direction and can contribute to the narrowing of the space of the carpal tunnel. The dysfunctions of the metacarpals can be addressed, but note should be taken of the immobile second and very nearly so third metacarpals as not being dysfunctions.

### REFERENCES

DiGiovanna EL, Schiowitz S. *An Osteopathic Approach to Diagnosis and Treatment, 2nd ed.* Philadelphia: Lippincott-Raven, 1997.

Kapandji IA. *Physiology of the Joints, Vol 1.* Upper Limb. Edinburgh: Churchill-Livingstone, 1972.

Sucher BM, Hinrichs RN. Manipulative treatment of carpal tunnel syndrome: biomechanical and osteopathic intervention to increase the length of the transverse carpal ligament. *J Am Osteopath Assoc* 1998;98:679–686.

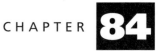

# Evaluation of the Wrist and Hand

*Eileen L. DiGiovanna*

The wrist and hand are an important part of a person's ability to function in activities of daily living. Any pain, dysfunction, or disability requires a careful and thorough evaluation of the area. This examination may include the forearm and even other joints of the upper extremity and neck. As with other joints of the upper extremity, a history of the symptom and related information is the first step in the evaluation process. Then the examination may proceed.

## ■ OBSERVATION

The hand should be observed while in use, such as while unbuttoning a shirt, and at rest. At rest, the hand should lie in slight flexion with mild extension at the wrist. The presence of all fingers should be noted.

Any joint or soft tissue swelling should be noted. Infection may spread rapidly through the soft tissues of the hand so signs of inflammation such as swelling should be evaluated. Fusiform swelling of the proximal interphalangeal joints is indicative of rheumatoid arthritis. Discrete bony nodules on the distal interphalangeal joints are called *Heberden's nodes* and are indicative of osteoarthritis. Rheumatoid arthritis of the hands may cause other notable deformities, including a *swan's neck deformity* or ulnar deviation

The nails should be inspected for clubbing, color (abnormal pallor or cyanosis), or infection around the edges (paronychia). Calluses of the finger pads should be noted. Any atrophy of the thenar or hypothenar areas should be noted.

## ■ PALPATION

The wrist and hand joints should be palpated for swelling, asymmetries, and tenderness. The skin of the wrist and hand should be evaluated for temperature and moisture changes. Tendons or joints may be tender. The anatomic snuffbox should be palpated. In case of trauma, any tenderness in this area should be noted, because the navicular is the most commonly fractured of the carpal bones.

The tunnels across the dorsum of the wrist should be palpated for swelling or tenderness. The volar tunnels should be similarly evaluated. Ganglia may occur in the tendon sheaths. These are firm, sometimes tender, nodules that are generally benign and of no significance but may be of concern to the patient.

### Range of Motion Testing

The wrist should be put through the ranges of flexion, extension, ulnar deviation, and radial deviation. Ulnar deviation should be greater than radial. These should be performed both passively and actively.

All joints should be put through their passive range of motion and the patient asked to demonstrate active range of motion. The digits are evaluated together and individually. The fingers and thumb should be flexed and extended, and finger abduction and adduction should be tested. When the patient touches the thumb to the tip of each of the other fingers, the wrist should flex, extend, abduct, and adduct.

## Muscle Strength Testing

A general screening of hand strength is to ask the patient to squeeze two or three of the examiner's fingers. If a weakness is found, each finger flexor is tested individually. The extensors are checked by trying to force the fingers into flexion against the patient's resistance.

To test the intrinsic muscles, the patient spreads his fingers while the examiner tries to close them. Then the patient tries to close his fingers against the examiner's resistance.

The pinch mechanism is tested by having the patient form an "O" with his thumb and index finger as the examiner hooks his fingers into the "O" and tries to pull it apart.

Wrist flexion and extension strength should be tested with the hand made into a fist.

## Sensation Testing

The peripheral nerves may be tested for sensation at the following sites:

1. **Radial nerve:** dorsum of web space between thumb and index finger
2. **Median nerve:** tip of index finger
3. **Ulnar nerve:** tip of fifth finger

The dermatome levels are the following:

1. C6: thumb and index finger and lateral palm
2. C7: middle finger
3. C8: fourth and fifth fingers and medial palm

## ■ SPECIAL TESTS

*Bunnel–Littler test* evaluates the tightness of the intrinsic muscles of the hand. The metacarpophalangeal joint is held in extension and the patient tries to move the proximal interphalangeal joint into flexion. If the proximal interphalangeal joint does not flex, then the intrinsic muscles are tight or the joint capsule is contractured. The metacarpophalangeal joint is rested briefly and then retested. If the proximal interphalangeal joint still cannot flex, the problem is in the joint capsule.

*Allen test* evaluates functioning of the medial and ulnar arteries. Occlude the two arteries and have the patient open and close his fist. The palm should be pale. Release one artery and the hand should flush. Repeat with the other artery.

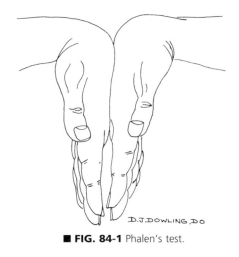

■ **FIG. 84-1** Phalen's test.

*Phalen's test* is for carpal tunnel syndrome. The patient flexes the wrists and presses the backs of his hands together. He holds this position for a minute. In carpal tunnel syndrome this will produce pain or paresthesias in the affected hand (Fig. 84-1).

*Tinel sign:* by tapping over the volar carpal ligament, pain or paresthesias may be produced over the distribution of the median nerve in a case of carpal tunnel syndrome (Fig. 84-2).

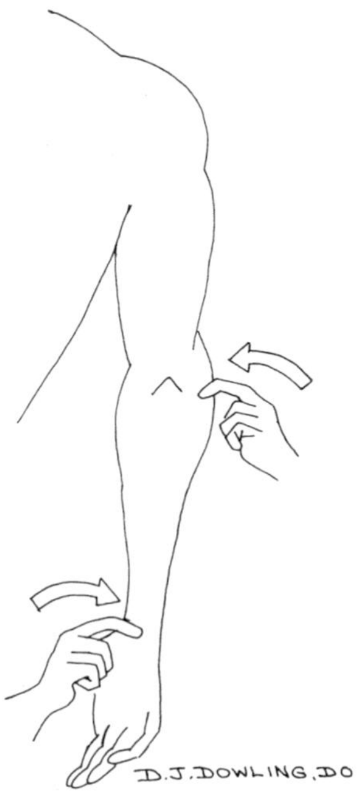

■ **FIG. 84-2** Tinel sign at the wrist and elbow.

*Finkelstein test* is used to rule out de Quervain's disease. The patient closes his fingers around his thumb and then ulnar deviates his wrist. Pain along the lateral wrist is a positive test.

## ■ EVALUATION FOR WRIST SOMATIC DYSFUNCTION

Gross motion is tested in flexion, extension, and radial and ulnar deviation. Both passive and active techniques may be used.

Somatic dysfunction of the wrist permits motion toward the dysfunction; motion away from the dysfunction will be restricted. The technique described may be used to test motion of the radionavicular joint and each of the intercarpal joints. It may also be used to test the carpometacarpal and metacarpophalangeal joints.

1. **Physician position:** seated facing the patient.
2. **Technique:**
   a. The physician grasps the bones adjacent to the joint to be tested between his thumb and forefinger.

b. The bones are moved through their range of motion and any restriction is noted.
c. The motions tested are gliding in all directions and long-axis traction.

Gross motion is tested in flexion, extension, and radial and ulnar deviation. Both passive and active techniques may be used.

## ■ TESTS FOR HAND SOMATIC DYSFUNCTION

1. **Physician position:** seated facing the patient.
2. **Technique:**
   a. The physician grasps the bones adjacent to the joint being tested between his thumb and index finger.
   b. The bones are moved through their range of motion as gentle traction is applied.

### REFERENCES

DiGiovanna EL, Schiowitz S. *An Osteopathic Approach to Diagnosis and Treatment, 2nd ed.* Philadelphia: Lippincott-Raven, 1997.

Hoppenfeld S. *Physical Examination of the Spine & Extremities.* Norwalk, CT: Appleton & Lange, 1976.

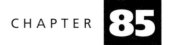

# Muscle Energy Treatment of the Upper Extremities

*Eileen L. DiGiovanna and Dennis J. Dowling*

Muscle energy may be applied efficiently and effectively to the upper extremity joints. It is useful as a primary treatment and as a preparatory technique for high-velocity low-amplitude techniques.

## ■ SHOULDER GIRDLE

### Glenohumeral Joint Restriction

Please see the isometric resistance modification of the Spencer techniques in Chapter 88.

### Restricted Abduction of the Sternoclavicular Joint (Adduction Dysfunction)

1. **Patient position:** supine.
2. **Physician position:** standing at the side of the table, next to the affected shoulder.
3. **Technique:**
   a. The physician places one hand on the proximal clavicular head. With her other hand, she grasps the patient's wrist and holds the arm extended and internally rotated (Fig. 85-1).
   b. The patient is instructed to raise his arm against the physician's hand, hold it in position for 3 to 5 seconds and then relax. The physician provides isometric resistance against each patient effort.
   c. The joint can be brought into the barrier direction after each effort.

d. The technique is repeated twice more and the joint motion is reassessed.

### Restricted Flexion of the Sternoclavicular Joint (Extension Dysfunction)

1. **Patient position:** supine.
2. **Physician position:** standing at the side of the table, next to the affected shoulder.
3. **Technique:**
   a. The physician places one hand on the restricted clavicle and with the other reaches behind the axilla to cover the scapula.
   b. The patient holds the physician's shoulder with the hand of the affected side (Fig. 85-2).
   c. The physician flexes the clavicle toward the manubrium until movement is palpated in the sternoclavicular joint. This is performed by straightening the body and pulling the scapula anteriorly.
   d. The patient is instructed to pull his shoulder down, hold this position for 3 to 5 seconds and then relax. The physician provides isometric resistance against each patient effort.
   e. The joint can be brought into the barrier direction after each effort.
   f. The maneuver is repeated twice more. The joint motion is reassessed.

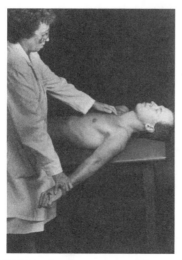

**■ FIG. 85-1** Muscle energy treatment for restricted abduction of the sternoclavicular joint.

## ■ ELBOW

### Abduction (Pronation) Dysfunction—Adduction (Supination) Restriction

1. **Patient position:** seated or supine.
2. **Physician position:** standing or seated at the side of the table.
3. **Technique:**
   a. The physician places the patient's flexed elbow into full supination.

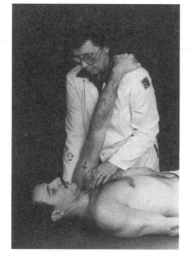

**■ FIG. 85-2** Muscle energy treatment for restricted flexion of the sternoclavicular joint.

   b. The patient gently tries to pronate his forearm against the physician's equal, restraining, isometric force.
   c. This position is held for 3 to 5 seconds and then the patient relaxes.
   d. The joint can be brought into the barrier direction after each effort.
   e. The technique is repeated twice more. The joint motion is reassessed.

### Adduction (Supination) Dysfunction—Abduction (Pronation) Restriction

1. **Patient position:** seated or supine
2. **Physician position:** standing or seated at the side of the table.
3. **Technique:**
   a. The physician places the patient's flexed elbow into full pronation.
   b. The patient gently tried to supinate his forearm against the physician's equal, restraining isometric force.
   c. The position is held for 3 to 6 seconds and then the patient relaxes.
   d. The joint can be brought into the barrier direction after each effort.
   e. This maneuver is repeated twice more. The joint motion is reassessed.

## ■ WRIST

### Wrist Dysfunction in Radial Deviation—Wrist Restriction in Ulnar Deviation

1. **Patient position:** seated or supine
2. **Physician position:** standing or seated at the side of the table.
3. **Technique:**
   a. The joint is moved into ulnar deviation to the barrier to motion.
   b. The patient is asked to push toward the radial aspect as the physician provides isometric resistance.
   c. This position is held for 3 to 5 seconds, then released.
   d. The joint is moved to its new barrier.
   e. The maneuver is repeated three or four times. The joint motion is reassessed.

## Wrist Dysfunction in Ulnar Deviation—Restriction in Radial Deviation

1. **Patient position:** seated or supine
2. **Physician position:** standing or seated at the side of the table.
3. **Technique:**
   a. The joint is moved into radial deviation to the barrier to motion.
   b. The patient is asked to push toward the ulnar aspect as the physician provides isometric resistance.
   c. This position is held for 3 to 5 seconds and then released.
   d. The joint is moved to its new barrier.
   e. The maneuver is repeated three or four times. The joint motion is reassessed.

Other restricted motions of the wrist or hand may be treated in a similar fashion by taking the joint to the barrier to motion, having the patient push against isometric resistance toward the freedom of motion, relax, and repeat the process three times. Any muscle energy technique may be followed by a passive stretch.

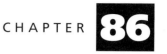

# Counterstrain of the Upper Extremities

*Eileen L. DiGiovanna*

## ■ SHOULDER

### Tender Point Locations

The common anterior tender points for the shoulder (Fig. 86-1) are the following:

1. Anterior acromioclavicular: anterior surface of distal clavicle
2. Long head of biceps: over the tendon
3. Short head of biceps: inferolateral to the coracoid process

The posterior tender points (Fig. 86-2) are the following:

1. Posterior acromioclavicular: behind the lateral end of the clavicle
2. Supraspinatus: in the supraspinatus fossa

The following lie in the axilla:

1. Subscapularis tender point: on the anterior surface of the scapula
2. Latissimus dorsi tender point: deep in the axilla on the medial surface of the humerus

### Anterior Acromioclavicular Tender Point

1. **Patient position:** supine.
2. **Physician position:** at the side of the table opposite the tender point.
3. **Technique:** The tender point is monitored as the arm is adducted across the chest 30 to 50 degrees and slightly internally rotated. The physician applies traction by pulling on the arm at the wrist (Fig. 86-3). The position is maintained for 90 seconds, then the arm is returned to a neutral position and the tender point is re-assessed.

### Long Head of Biceps Tender Point

1. **Patient position:** supine.
2. **Physician position:** at the side of the table, next to the tender point and facing the head of the table.
3. **Technique:** The patient's arm is supinated and flexed to 90 degrees at the elbow and shoulder. The physician applies downward pressure at the elbow along the humerus to the monitoring finger (Fig. 86-4). The position is held for 90 seconds, then the arm is returned to a neutral position and re-assessed.

### Short Head of Biceps Tender Point

The short head of biceps tender point is treated in the same manner as the long head, except that some fine-tuning into adduction is needed. Some internal rotation may be added for comfort.

### Posterior Acromioclavicular Tender Point

1. **Patient position:** prone.
2. **Physician position:** at the side of the table opposite the tender point.
3. **Technique:** The patient's arm is adducted across his back. The physician applies traction by pulling at the wrist (Fig. 86-5). The position is held for 90 seconds, then the arm is returned to a neutral position and the tender point re-assessed.

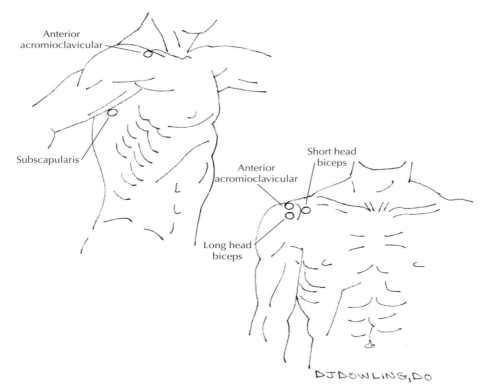

■ **FIG. 86-1** Location of the anterior tender points of the shoulder girdle.

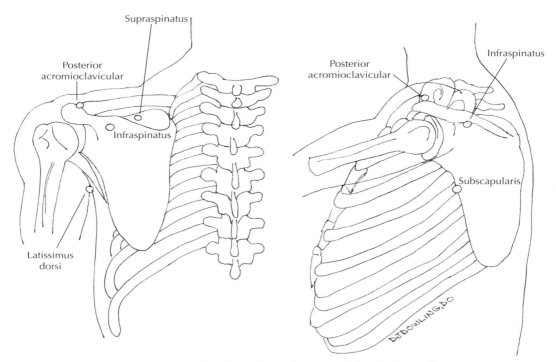

■ **FIG. 86-2** Location of posterior tender points of the shoulder girdle.

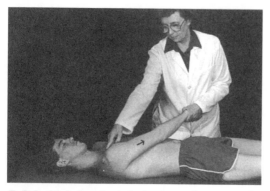

■ **FIG. 86-3** Counterstrain treatment for an anterior acromioclavicular tender point.

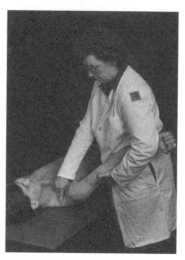

■ **FIG. 86-6** Counterstrain treatment for a supraspinatus tender point.

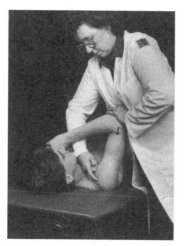

■ **FIG. 86-4** Counterstrain treatment for a tender point of the long head of the biceps.

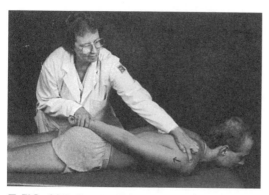

■ **FIG. 86-5** Counterstrain treatment for a posterior acromioclavicular tender point.

## Supraspinatus Tender Point

1. **Patient position:** supine.
2. **Physician position:** at the side of the table next to the tender point.
3. **Technique:** The patient's arm is flexed and abducted to 120 degrees. The humerus is markedly externally rotated. The muscle should become very soft in this position (Fig. 86-6). After the 90 seconds, the arm is returned to a neutral position and the tender point is reassessed.

## Subscapularis Tender Point

1. **Patient position:** supine.
2. **Physician position:** at the side of the table next to the tender point.
3. **Technique:** The patient's arm is held posteriorly over the side of the table and toward his feet. His arm is internally rotated. No traction is applied. The position is maintained for 90 seconds, then the arm is returned to a neutral position and the tender point is reassessed.

## Latissimus Dorsi Tender Point

The latissimus dorsi tender point is treated in the same manner as the subscapularis tender point except that traction is applied along the length of the arm. After 90 seconds, the arm is returned to a neutral position and the tender point is reassessed.

## ■ ELBOW

The tender points associated with the elbow are shown in Figure 86-7. Radial head or lateral epicondyle tender points may be treated in the same manner.

### Radial head/lateral epicondyle tender points

1. The elbow is held in full extension. This may be over a fulcrum of the table edge or the physician's hand or knee.
2. The arm is then supinated and abducted with varying amounts of force.
3. The position is maintained for 90 seconds, then the arm is returned slowly to a neutral position and the tender point reassessed. (Fig. 86-8).

### Coronoid Tender Points

1. The elbow is fully flexed.
2. The forearm is pronated and abducted gently.
3. The position is held for 90 seconds, then the arm is slowly returned to a neutral position. The tender point is re-assessed.

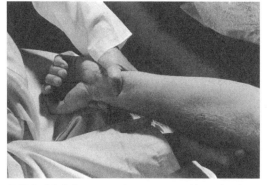

■ **FIG. 86-8** Counterstrain treatment of lateral epicondyle or radial head tender point.

### Olecranon

The elbow is hyper extended and the forearm is abducted slightly and supinated.

## ■ WRIST

The locations of the tender points associated with the wrist are shown in Figure 86-9 and Figure 86-10. All of these tender points respond to extending (posterior points) or flexing (ante-

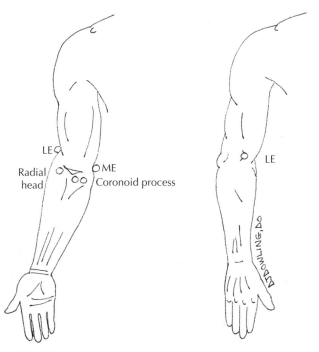

■ **FIG. 86-7** Tender points associated with the elbow. *LE*, lateral epicondyle, *ME*, medial epicondyle.

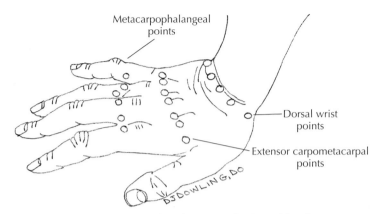

■ **FIG. 86-9** Dorsal tender points of wrist and hand.

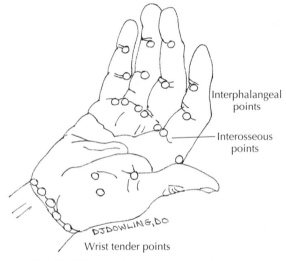

■ **FIG. 86-10** Ventral tender points of wrist and hand.

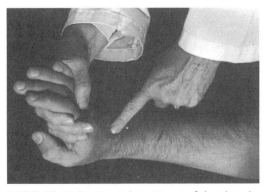

■ **FIG. 86-11** Counterstrain treatment of dorsal tender points of the wrist using extension of the wrist.

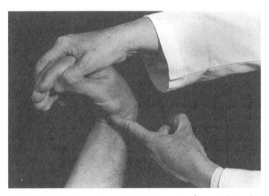

■ **FIG. 86-12** Counterstrain treatment of ventral tender points of the wrist using flexion of the wrist.

rior points) the wrist over the tender points (Figs. 86-11 and 86-12). It may be helpful to ulnar deviate and pronate the wrist for the more medial tender points and radial deviate and supinate the wrist for more lateral ones. Each position is held for 90 seconds, and then the hand is returned to a neutral position and the tender point is re-assessed.

## ■ HAND

The locations of the tender points associated with the hand are shown in Figures 86-9 and 86-10.

## Carpometacarpal Joint

A tender point of the first carpometacarpal joint that is associated with pain and weakness of the thumb is treated by markedly rotating the thumb toward the palm, with a slight amount of flexion.

## Interossei Tender Points

The tender points for the interossei muscles may be associated with either flexion or extension (anterior or posterior). The anterior or volar interossei tender points are treated by flexing the joint and applying some traction. The posterior or dorsal carpometacarpal tender point is treated by extending the joint and applying traction.

### REFERENCES

DiGiovanna EL, Schiowitz S. *An Osteopathic Approach to Diagnosis and Treatment, 2nd ed.* Philadelphia: Lippincott-Raven, 1997.

Jones L. *Strain and Counterstrain.* Colorado Springs: American Academy of Osteopathy, 1981

Yates HA, Glover JC. *Counterstrain Handbook of Osteopathic Technique.* Tulsa, OK: Y Knot Publishers, 1995.

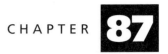

# Facilitated Positional Release of the Upper Extremities

*Stanley Schiowitz*

## ■ SHOULDER

### Muscle Hypertonicity (Point Tenderness) of the Shoulder Region (Right)

1. **Patient position**: Supine on the table, with arms at the side.
2. **Physician's position**: Standing on the right side of the table, facing the patient's head.
3. **Technique**:
   a. The physician places one finger of his right hand on the hypertonic muscle to monitor the motion and tissue changes.
   b. The physician uses his left hand to flex the patient's right shoulder to 90 degrees.
   c. The physician pushes the patient's right elbow down toward the table, causing a compressive force felt at the monitoring finger.
   d. The physician places the patient's shoulder into adduction and internal rotation until motion and tissue softening is felt at his monitoring finger. He should feel release of the hypertonicity (Fig. 87-1).
   e. Hold the position for 3 to 5 seconds, release, and reevaluate.

*Note:* If the hypertonic muscle is located above the mid-line of the shoulder joint, the flexion used is reduced accordingly. If the hypertonic muscle is located below the mid-line of the shoulder joint, the flexion is increased, accordingly, above the 90 degrees.

If the dysfunction is lateral to the middle of the shoulder joint, the final motions are abduction and external rotation.

## ■ ELBOW

### Muscle Hypertonicity (Tenderness) at the Radial Epicondyle (Right)

1. **Patient position**: Supine on the table with arms at the side.
2. **Physician's position**: Sitting at the right side of the table, facing towards the patient's head.
3. **Technique**:
   a. The physician places one finger of his left hand on the hypertonic muscle to monitor motion and tissue change.
   b. The physician uses his right hand to flex the patient's elbow to 90 degrees.
   c. The physician pushes the patient's right hand downward toward the table, causing a compressive force, felt at the monitoring finger.
   d. The physician places the elbow joint into abduction and external rotation to his monitoring finger. He should feel release of the hypertonicity (Fig. 87-2).
   e. Hold the position for 3 to 5 seconds, release, and re-evaluate.

*Note*: The amount of flexion and whether abduction–external rotation or adduction–internal rotation is applied will follow the same notes as for the shoulder joint.

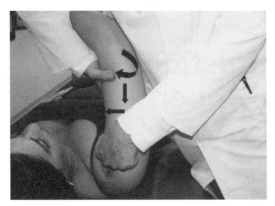

■ **FIG. 87-1** Facilitated positional release treatment for hypertonicity at the medial aspect of the right shoulder.

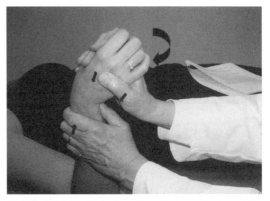

■ **FIG. 87-3** Facilitated positional release treatment for hypertonicity at the medial aspect of the right wrist joint.

## ■ WRIST

## Muscle Hypertonicity (Point Tenderness) of the Wrist Joint at the Mid-Radial Side of the Carpal Bones (Right)

1. **Patient position**: sitting on the table facing the physician.
2. **Physician position**: standing, facing the patient.

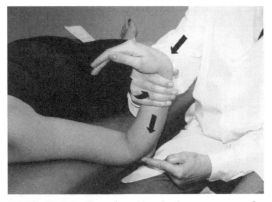

■ **FIG. 87-2** Facilitated positional release treatment for hypertonicity at the radial aspect of the right elbow.

3. **Technique**:
   a. The physician grasps the patient's right arm just below the wrist joint, with his right hand, and grasps the patient's hand firmly, above the wrist joint, with his other hand.
   b. The physician uses one finger of his left hand to monitor the motion and tissue changes at the dysfunction.
   c. The physician pushes his hands towards each other, causing a compression of the wrist joint.
   d. The physician places the patient's wrist into radial deviation and slightly pronated, up to his monitoring finger. He should feel release of the hypertonicity (Fig. 87-3).
   e. Hold the position for 3 to 5 seconds, release, and re-evaluate.

*Note*: The direction and deviation and pronation–supination of the wrist will change as the site of the hypertonicity changes. It is best to remember that the motions used to release the hypertonicity are toward and up to the monitoring finger.

Using a modification by adjusting the physician's hands, the compressive force applied can modify the procedure as shown, and each of the patient's finger joints can be similarly treated.

# CHAPTER 88

# Articulatory and Thrusting Techniques for the Upper Extremities

*Eileen L. DiGiovanna*

The two major goals of osteopathic manipulation of the upper extremity are to restore function and to prevent motion loss. The upper extremity is generally considered one unit when treating with articulatory or thrusting techniques. Each restricted joint must be returned to normal function.

## ■ SHOULDER GIRDLE

### Spencer Techniques

The Spencer techniques are seven gentle stretching/articulatory maneuvers used to treat/prevent shoulder restriction caused by hypertonic muscles, early adhesive capsulitis, healed fractures and dislocations, and any other traumatic or degenerative condition in which improved motion is required.

Although the Spencer techniques do allow the physician to assess the passive range of motion of the glenohumeral joint, they are primarily a treatment and not a diagnostic procedure. They are designed to articulate the humeral head throughout its ranges of motion in the fossa while stretching the periarticular soft tissues.

The general guidelines for performing all seven steps of the techniques are as follows:

1. **Patient position:** lateral recumbent position with the affected shoulder up. The patient's knees and hips are flexed, his back is straight and perpendicular to table, his lower arm is down and comfortable, and his head is supported by a pillow.
2. **Physician position:** standing at the side of the table, facing the patient.
3. **Technique:** The physician grasps the patient's forearm with one hand, flexing the patient's elbow. The physician's other hand is placed on top of the patient's shoulder to lock the shoulder girdle, limiting scapular movement.

Each technique is repeated six to eight times; one should stop when it becomes painful to the patient or motion is significantly restricted. With each movement, the physician tries to exceed the point reached in the previous excursion.

1. **To increase extension:** The physician moves the patient's arm in a horizontal plane, extending the shoulder and returning it to a neutral position, gently increasing the excursion. The patient's elbow is kept in flexion (Fig. 88-1).
2. **To increase flexion:** The physician flexes the patient's shoulder, straightening the elbow, until the arm is over the patient's ear (Fig. 88-2). This maneuver is gently repeated in rhythmic motion, with the shoulder returned close to neutral position each time. The physician may have to change the position of the hand locking the scapula to be comfortable during this maneuver.

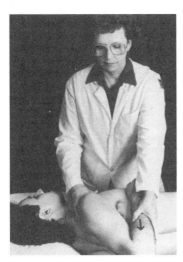

■ **FIG. 88-1** Spencer technique to increase shoulder extension.

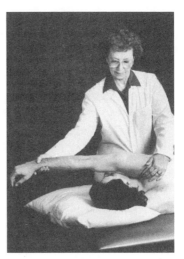

■ **FIG. 88-2** Spencer technique to increase shoulder flexion.

3.  **To increase circumduction:** The patient's elbow is flexed sharply and the shoulder is abducted to a 90-degree angle. The physician locks the patient's shoulder in this position and, using the patient's elbow as a pivot, gently rotates the shoulder in gradually increasing circles, clockwise and then counterclockwise (Fig. 88-3).

4.  **Circumduction with traction:** The physician extends the patient's elbow and abducts the arm to 90 degrees. The physician then locks the patient's scapula in this position and, using the patient's forearm as a pivot, gently rotates the humerus in gradually increasing circles, clockwise and then counterclockwise, maintaining a *traction* force at the patient's wrist (Fig. 88-4).

5a.  **To increase abduction:** The physician places her upper hand on the patient's shoulder. The patient's elbow is flexed and his hand rests on the physician's forearm below the elbow joint. The physician's lower

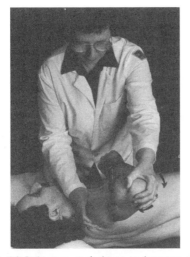

■ **FIG. 88-3** Spencer techniques to increase shoulder circumduction.

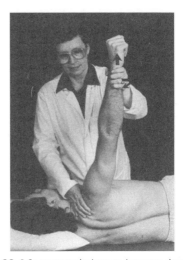

■ **FIG. 88-4** Spencer technique to increase shoulder circumduction, with traction.

arm gently exerts an upward pressure on the patient's flexed elbow, bringing the shoulder into abduction (Fig. 88-5).

5b. **To increase adduction:** Maintaining the above position, the physician's hand at the elbow gently exerts a downward pressure on the patient's flexed elbow bringing the patient's upper arm into adduction.

6. **To increase internal rotation:** The patient's hand, with the elbow flexed, is placed behind his lower ribs. The physician's upper hand locks the scapula; her lower hand gently draws the patient's elbow forward and down (Fig. 88-6). The patient's elbow is released and the maneuver is repeated. Care must be used in the motion because it may be the most painful to the patient. An external rotation force may also be used in this position.

7. **Traction stretch:** The patient's hand is placed on the physician's shoulder, with his elbow straight. The physician clasps her hands around the patient's upper arm. The physician may then provide a gentle pull, lifting the humeral head away from the fossa. By leaning back, the physician uses her body weight rather than muscular force (Fig. 88-7).

*Note:* Patriquin reports that the original techniques designed by Spencer had step five carry-

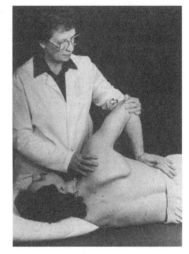

■ **FIG. 88-6** Spencer technique to increase internal rotation of the shoulder.

ing the shoulder into adduction by moving the elbow toward the table. Over time, the technique was changed to create an abduction force. Both abduction and adduction are now generally taught as part of step five.

## Isometric Variations of Spencer Techniques

The positions used in the Spencer techniques may also be used to treat the shoulder with isometric or muscle energy treatment. The physician moves the arm to a barrier. The patient ac-

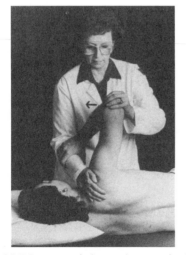

■ **FIG. 88-5** Spencer technique to increase shoulder abduction.

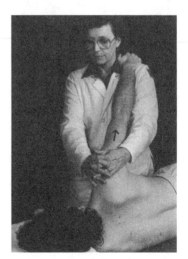

■ **FIG. 88-7** Spencer technique for traction stretch.

tively moves his arm away from the barrier against equal resistance in extension, flexion, abduction, adduction, and internal or external rotation.

For example, in the case of restricted motion in extension, the patient is first placed in a position of maximum comfortable extension. The patient then tries to move his arm into flexion while the physician applies a mild isometric resistive force. This position is held for 4 seconds, then the patient relaxes. The physician increases the patient's arm extension and the maneuver is repeated.

## ■ ARTICULATORY TECHNIQUES FOR CLAVICULAR RESTRICTIONS

The clavicle may be elevated or depressed at the sternal end. The techniques described are for an elevated clavicle.

### Technique 1

1. **Patient position:** supine.
2. **Physician position:** seated at the head of the table.
3. **Technique:** The patient's neck, fully flexed, rests against the physician's chest. This position locks out spinal motion. The physician places her thumb over the sternal end and exerts a downward and caudal pressure on the clavicle (Fig. 88-8). The patient is instructed to inhale and exhale fully. During

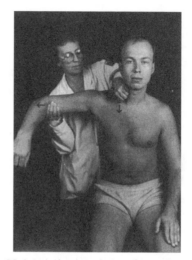

■ **FIG. 88-9** Articulatory technique for an elevated clavicle, patient seated.

exhalation the physician springs the clavicle to release the restriction.

### Technique 2

1. **Patient position:** seated.
2. **Physician position:** standing close behind the patient.
3. **Technique:** The physician reaches under the affected arm and grasps the abducted humerus. With her other hand, she reaches over the patient's shoulder and places the thumb or hypothenar eminence on the sternal end of the clavicle. The hand holding the humerus applies a lateral traction. The other hand provides a downward force on the clavicle (Fig. 88-9). This may be an articulatory or a high-velocity, low-amplitude force.

## ■ HIGH-VELOCITY, LOW-AMPLITUDE THRUSTING TECHNIQUES FOR THE SHOULDER GIRDLE

### Glenohumeral Thrusting Technique

1. **Patient position:** prone.
2. **Physician position:** standing at the side of the table, on the side of the dysfunction.
3. **Technique:**
   a. The physician grasps the patient's glenohumeral joint by encircling the joint with both hands.
   b. The physician's thumbs rest in a crossed

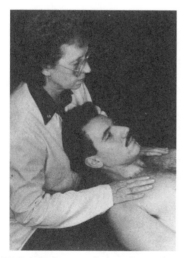

■ **FIG. 88-8** Articulatory technique for an elevated clavicle, patient supine.

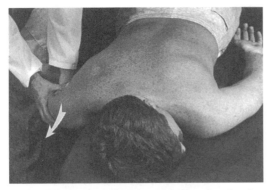

■ **FIG. 88-10** HVLA thrusting technique for glenohumeral joint somatic dysfunction.

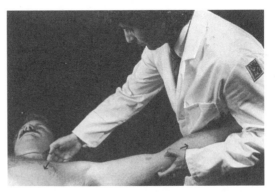

■ **FIG. 88-11** HVLA thrusting technique for superior clavicle.

pattern on the posterior aspect of the patient's glenohumoral joint.

  c. The physician exerts a rapid downward and slightly lateral force through the patient's glenohumoral joint (Fig. 88-10).

## Superior Clavicular Somatic Dysfunction

1. **Patient position:** supine.
2. **Physician position:** standing at the side of the table, on the same side as the dysfunction.
3. **Technique:**
  a. The physician grasps the superior surface of the restricted clavicle with the fingers of his monitoring hand.
  b. With his other hand, the physician flexes the patient's arm to 90 degrees (ipsilateral to the dysfunction).
  c. The physician exerts a simultaneous downward thrust on the clavicle and lateral traction on the patient's arm to produce the corrective force (Fig. 88-11).

## Sternoclavicular Somatic Dysfunction

1. **Patient position:** supine.
2. **Physician position:** standing at the head of the table.
3. **Technique:**
  a. The physician rests the thenar eminence of his monitoring hand over the sternoclavicular joint that is restricted.
  b. The physician grasps the patient's arm on

the side of the dysfunction and exerts a cephalad traction force on the arm.

  c. The physician achieves correction by exerting a downward thrust through the sternoclavicular joint while simultaneously inducing a rapid traction force through the patient's arm (Fig. 88-12).

## ■ ELBOW

## High-Velocity, Low-Amplitude Thrusting Technique for Elbow

Abduction/adduction restrictions:

1. **Patient position:** seated.

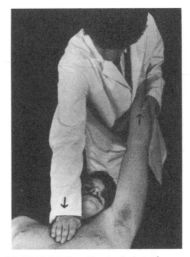

■ **FIG. 88-12** HVLA thrusting technique for somatic dysfunction of the sternoclavicular joint.

2. **Physician position:** standing facing the patient.
3. **Technique:**
   a. The physician grasps the patient's elbow. The fingers of his monitoring hand are on either side of the olecranon. The other hand is used to hold and stabilize the patient's forearm in supination/extension.
   b. The physician tests the motion of the radioulnar joint in adduction and abduction.
   c. If restriction of motion is noted in abduction, the physician places the patient's elbow into abduction and exerts a hyperabduction corrective thrust. This is performed with the elbow locked in extension.
   d. If restriction of motion is noted in adduction, the physician places the patient's elbow into adduction and exerts a hyperadduction corrective thrust. This is performed with the elbow locked in extension (Fig. 88-13).

### Anterior Radial Head Dysfunctions

1. **Patient position:** seated.
2. **Physician position:** standing facing the patient.
3. **Technique:**
   a. The physician grasps the patient's dysfunctional arm, flexing it at the elbow and pronating it at the wrist.
   b. The physician places the second and third digits of his other hand into the crease of the patient's elbow, directly over the radial head.
   c. The physician exerts a rapid hyperflexion force on the elbow while simultaneously thrusting the radial head dorsally with the fingers of the other hand (Fig. 88-14).

## Posterior Radial Head Dysfunctions

1. **Patient position:** seated.
2. **Physician position:** standing facing the patient.
3. **Technique:**
   a. The physician encircles the patient's dysfunctioned elbow with both hands and extends it.
   b. The physician places his thumbs over the head of the radius anteriorly and the phalanx of his index finger over the radial head posteriorly.
   c. The physician exerts a rapid hyperextension force on the patient's elbow while simultaneously inducing a ventral counterforce through the radial head (Fig. 88-15).

## ■ ARTICULATORY TECHNIQUE FOR THE HAND

### Intersegmental Articulations

1. **Physician position:** seated or standing, facing the patient.
2. **Technique:**
   a. The physician locks one metacarpal between the thumb and index finger of one hand.

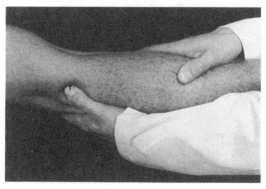

■ **FIG. 88-13** High-velocity, low amplitude thrusting technique for adduction restriction of the elbow.

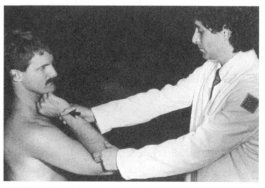

■ **FIG. 88-14** High-velocity, low-amplitude thrusting technique for anterior radial head.

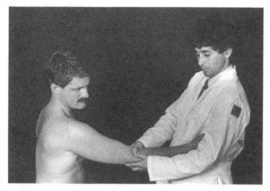

■ **FIG. 88-15** High-velocity, low-amplitude thrusting technique for posterior radial head.

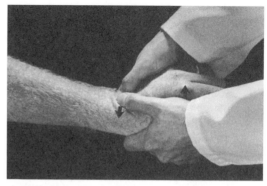

■ **FIG. 88-16** High-velocity, low amplitude thrusting technique for carpal dysfunction.

b. With the thumb and index finger of his other hand, the physician maneuvers the neighboring metacarpal into anterior or posterior glide or rotation, as desired.

## Fingers

1. **Physician position:** seated or standing, facing the patient.
2. **Technique:**
   a. The physician locks the metacarpal, in this instance the second, between the thumb and index finger of one hand.
   b. The physician places the thumb of his other hand on the dorsum of the first phalanx and the index finger on the volar surface of the first phalanx.
   c. The physician applies long-axis extension (straight-line traction) or rotation or anteroposterior glide.

## ■ HIGH-VELOCITY, LOW-AMPLITUDE THRUSTING TECHNIQUE

### Carpal Somatic Dysfunction

1. **Patient position:** seated on the table.
2. **Physician position:** standing facing the patient.
3. **Technique:**
   a. The physician grasps the patient's hand on the side of the dysfunction and localizes the dorsal radiocarpal joint with his thumbs.
   b. The physician exerts a whip-like thrust on the hand, moving it into rapid hyperflex-

ion while simultaneously exerting a downward counterforce through the carpal somatic dysfunction (Fig. 88-16).

## Phalangeal Somatic Dysfunction

1. **Patient position:** seated on the table.
2. **Physician position:** standing facing the patient.
3. **Technique:**
   a. With one hand, the physician holds and stabilizes the patient's wrist.
   b. The physician localizes the dysfunctional joint and exerts a simultaneous traction

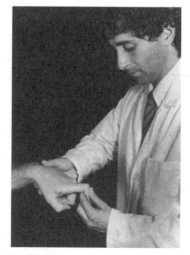

■ **FIG. 88-17** High-velocity, low-amplitude thrusting technique for phalangeal dysfunction.

and hyperflexion thrust through the somatic dysfunction (Fig. 88-17).
  c. To treat the second or third phalanges, the
     physician holds the phalanx above the ar-
     ticulation being treated and maneuvers
     the distal phalanx through the desired mo-
     tion.

## REFERENCES

DiGiovanna EL Schiowitz S. *An Osteopathic Approach to Diagnosis and Treatment, 2nd ed.* Philadelphia: Lippincott-
  Raven, 1997.
Patriquin D. Evolution of osteopathic manipulative techniques: the Spencer technique. *J Am Osteopath Assoc*
  1992;92:1134–1136, 1139–1146.

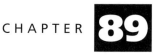
# Exercise Therapy for the Upper Extremity

*Stanley Schiowitz and Albert R. DeRubertis*

## ■ THE SHOULDER GIRDLE

The function and biomechanics of the shoulder girdle were reviewed in Chapter 79. The physician prescribing exercise therapy must take into account the three true articulations, the two pseudoarticulations, and the origins and insertions of all the muscles used in joint function.

## Glenohumeral Joint Exercises

A. **Pendulum exercise, acute phase—passive** (Fig. 89-1)
  1. **Patient position:** bent forward, body supported by the other arm holding on to a table or chair, the back comfortable.
  2. **Instructions:**
     a. Allow your painful arm to hang down away from your body.
     b. Move your body forward and backward, then side to side. This creates shoulder joint motion without active participation of the shoulder muscles.
     c. Gradually increase body motion. Do not create pain. Start with 5 to 10 seconds of exercise.
     d. Slowly bring your body back to an upright position. Passively move the painful arm back to your side, using your other arm to move it if necessary.
     e. Relax, rest, and repeat.
B. **Pendulum exercise, after acute phase—active** (Fig. 89-2)

1. **Patient position:** bent forward, body supported by the other arm holding on to a table or chair, the back comfortable.
2. **Instructions:**
   a. Allow your painful arm to hang down, away from your body.
   b. Swing your arm forward and backward, side to side, and in circles.
   c. Gradually increase the excursion of the arm motion. A weight may be held in your hand to increase the force used.
   d. Continue for 5 to 15 seconds, then slowly bring your body into the upright position.
   e. Relax, rest, and repeat.

  *Note:* Do not increase or create pain when performing this exercise.

C. **Flexion stretch** (Fig. 89-3)
  1. **Patient position:** standing facing a wall, an arm's length away.
  2. **Instructions:**
     a. Place the hand of the arm to be exercised against the wall with the elbow fully extended.
     b. Walk your fingers up the wall slowly, increasing flexion at the shoulder.
     c. After reaching the limit of painless flexion, hold your arm in this position for 10 to 15 seconds. Then slowly walk your fingers higher on the wall, 1 inch at a time, to increase flexion.

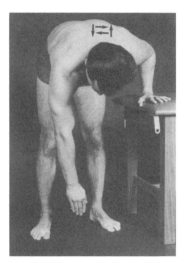

■ **FIG. 89-1** Pendulum exercise, acute phase—passive motion.

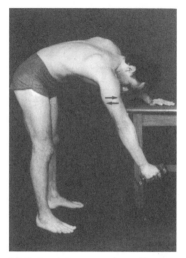

■ **FIG. 89-2** Pendulum exercise with active use of shoulder.

Hold your arm for 10 to 15 seconds at each new plateau of flexion, then walk the fingers higher.

d. At the end of 2 or 3 minutes, or if fatigued, slowly walk the arm down the wall.

e. Relax, rest, and repeat.

D. **Abduction stretch** (Fig. 89-4)

1. **Patient position:** standing with the side of the painful arm toward the wall.

2. **Instructions:** Repeat the technique de-

scribed for flexion stretch, walking the arm up into abduction.

*Note to physician:* If the cause of the dysfunction is supraspinatus impingement, do not prescribe this exercise.

E. **Abduction—external rotation stretch** (Fig. 89-5).

1. **Patient position:** standing or sitting with both hands clasped behind the head and the elbows brought together in front of the body.

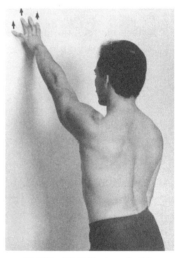

■ **FIG. 89-3** Flexion stretch.

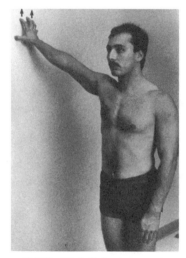

■ **FIG. 89-4** Abduction stretch.

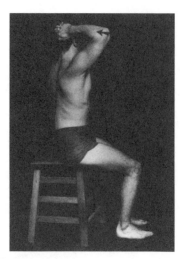

■ **FIG. 89-5** Abduction—external rotation stretch.

2. **Instructions:**
   a. Slowly separate your elbows as far back as they can be painlessly stretched.
   b. Hold this position for 5 to 15 seconds.
   c. Return to the starting position.
   d. Relax, rest, and repeat.
F. **Adduction—internal rotation stretch (passive)** (Fig. 89-6)
   1. **Patient position:** standing with the arms at the sides.
   2. **Instructions:**
      a. Turn the hand of the arm to be treated inward (internal rotation).
      b. Grasp that wrist with your other hand and pull it slowly across your chest to shoulder height.

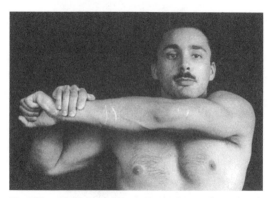

■ **FIG. 89-6** Adduction—internal rotation stretch (passive).

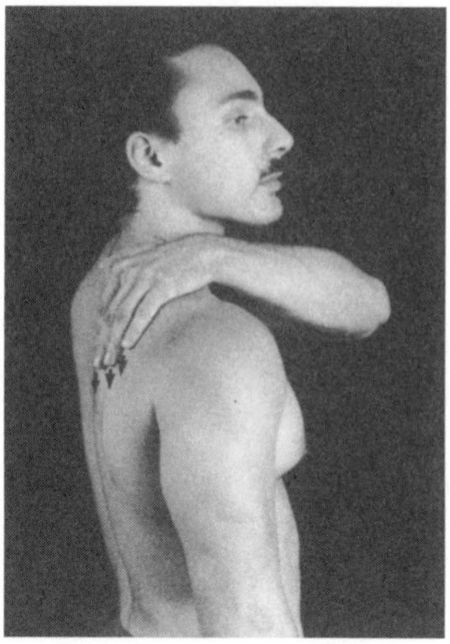

■**FIG. 89-7** Adduction—internal rotation stretch (active).

   c. Gradually increase your pull to maximum painless stretch. Hold for 5 to 15 seconds.
   d. Return arm to the starting position.
   e. Relax, rest, and repeat.
G. **Adduction—internal rotation stretch (active)** (Fig. 89-7)
   1. **Patient position:** standing with both arms at the sides.
   2. **Instructions:**
      a. Bring the arm that is to be treated across your body and up over the opposite shoulder. Keep your palm pointing down.
      b. Reach back over your shoulder and touch your scapula.
      c. Walk your fingers down the scapula to achieve maximum painless stretch. Hold for 5 to 15 seconds.
      d. Return your arm to the starting position.
      e. Relax, rest, and repeat.

## ■ FROZEN SHOULDER FORCED STRETCH EXERCISES

These exercises are not performed during the acute phase of injury. Moderate wet heat should be applied as an aid to muscle relaxation before the patient begins exercising. If analgesics or nonsteroidal anti-inflammatory drugs are prescribed, they should be taken 20 minutes before exercise. At the conclusion of these exercises, an ice pack should be applied for 20 minutes.

A. **Forced flexion stretch** (Fig. 89-8)
1. **Patient position:** seated facing a table, with the elbow on the side of the shoulder to be treated on the table on a towel.
2. **Instructions:**
   a. Place the back of the elbow joint on the table, making a 90-degree angle between the forearm and the elbow.
   b. Drop your body forward and downward, increasing shoulder flexion. Remain in this position for 15 seconds.
   c. Allow your entire weight to rest on your elbow joint. With the increased flexion (stretch), you may feel mild discomfort.
   d. Hold this position for 15 seconds. Raise your body up.
   e. Relax, rest, and repeat.
   f. Attempt to increase flexion motion with each repetition.
B. **Forced rotation stretch** (Fig. 89-9)
1. **Patient position:** seated facing a table, with the elbow on the side of the shoulder to be treated on the table on a towel. Hold a 3- to 5-pound weight in your hand.
2. **Instructions:**
   a. Allow your arm to pivot on the elbow inward, toward the table. The weight you are holding should slowly create forced internal rotation.
   b. Remain in this position for 10 sec-

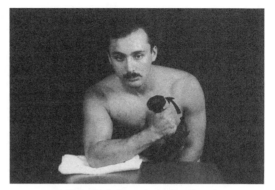

**■ FIG. 89-9** Forced rotation stretch.

onds, then pivot the arm outward, creating external rotation.
   c. Return your arm to the midline.
   d. Relax, rest, and repeat.
   e. Increase the weight held in your hand gradually, to force the rotation.
C. **Forced extension stretch** (Fig. 89-10)
   a. Gently perform a deep knee bend, resting your weight on your fist. This maneuver increases shoulder extension.
   b. Gradually increase the deep knee bend, resting all your weight on your fist.
   c. Hold this position of forced extension for 15 seconds.
   d. Return to the upright position.
   e. Relax, rest, and repeat.

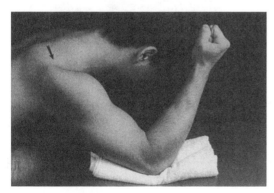

**■ FIG. 89-8** Forced flexion stretch.

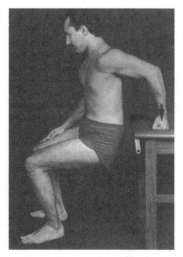

**■ FIG. 89-10** Forced extension stretch.

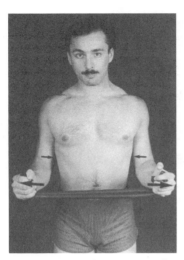

■ **FIG. 89-11** External rotator strengthening.

## ■ STRENGTHENING EXERCISES WITH MECHANICAL AIDS

A. **External rotators** (Fig. 89-11)
   1. **Patient position:** standing, both arms at the sides, elbows bent to 90 degrees, holding a length of rubber tubing in both hands.
   2. **Instructions:**
      a. Pull the tubing horizontally between your hands as far as possible. Keep your elbows and arms against your body.
      b. Hold this position for 5 to 15 seconds.
      c. Return to the starting position.
      d. Relax, rest, and repeat.
B. **Extensors** (Fig. 89-12)

   1. **Patient position:** standing, both arms at the sides, holding a length of rubber tubing in both hands.
   2. **Instructions:**
      a. Pull the rubber tubing horizontally as far as possible while simultaneously raising both arms to shoulder height. Try to stretch out the arms fully.
      b. Hold this outstretched position for 5 to 15 seconds.
      c. Return to starting position.
      d. Relax, rest, and repeat.
C. **Flexors** (Fig. 89-13)
   1. **Patient position:** standing, one hand holding a length of rubber tubing firmly below the waist at the mid-body line.
   2. **Instructions:**
      a. Grasp the other end of the rubber tubing with the arm to be treated.
      b. Pull on the tubing in a forward direction until your elbow is fully extended.
      c. Swing your fully extended arm over your head into full flexion.
      d. Hold this position for 15 seconds.
      e. Slowly return to the starting position.
      f. Relax, rest, and repeat.
D. **Abductors** (Fig. 89-14)
   1. **Patient position:** standing, one hand holding a length of rubber tubing firmly below the waist at the mid-body line.

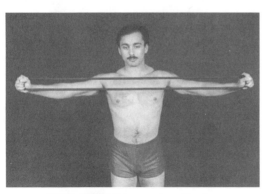

■ **FIG. 89-12** Extensor strengthening.

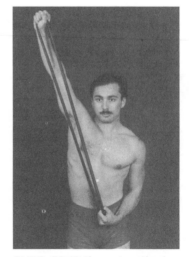

■ **FIG. 89-13** Flexor strengthening.

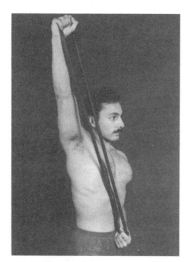

■ **FIG. 89-14** Abductor strengthening.

2. **Instructions:**
   a. Grasp the other end of the rubber tubing with the arm to be treated.
   b. Pull sideways, stretching the tubing, until your elbow is fully extended.
   c. Swing your fully extended arm over your head into full abduction.
   d. Hold this position for 15 seconds.
   e. Slowly return to the starting position.
   f. Relax, rest, and repeat.
E. **Internal rotators** (Fig. 89-15)
   1. **Patient position:** seated next to a table with the side to be treated beside a leg of the table.

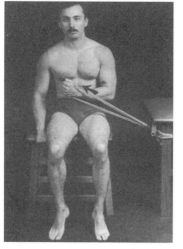

■ **FIG. 89-15** Internal rotator strengthening.

2. **Instructions:**
   a. Place a length of rubber tubing around the table leg and grasp it with the hand next to the table leg.
   b. Keep that elbow flexed to 90 degrees and held firmly against your body.
   c. Pull and stretch the tubing by rotating your hand toward the mid-body line. This creates internal rotation.
   d. Hold this position for 15 seconds.
   e. Slowly return to the starting position.
   f. Relax, rest, and repeat.

## ■ ELBOW JOINT

The exercises described in this section stretch the agonist muscles while strengthening the antagonist muscles. Each motion is performed slowly. The difficulty of the exercise is enhanced as the patient increases the weight used. To ensure maximum stretch, the patient uses his other arm to increase passively the motion after the extreme of voluntary stretch has been reached.

A. **Flexion–extension pronation stretch** (Fig. 89-16)
   1. **Patient position:** seated, with the side to be exercised next to a table. The elbow is placed near the edge of the table, with a towel or small pillow between it and the table.
   2. **Instructions:**
      a. Hold a 3- to 5-pound weight in your hand. Turn your hand so that the palm faces down (*pronation*).
      b. Allow the elbow to extend down to the table with the weight creating ex-

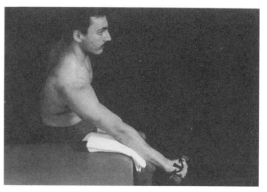

■ **FIG. 89-16** Flexion–extension pronation stretch.

tension off the table. The elbow acts as a fulcrum. Use your other hand to gently push the elbow into forced extension. Hold this position for 5 seconds.

c. Bring your arm up off the table into full elbow flexion. With your other hand, gently push the elbow into forced flexion. Hold for 5 seconds.

d. Repeat the entire motion. Remember to keep your palm down in full wrist pronation at all times.

B. **Flexion–extension supination stretch** (Fig. 89-17)

1. **Patient position:** seated, with the side to be exercised beside a table. The elbow is placed near the edge of the table, with a folded towel or small pillow between it and the table.

2. **Instructions:**

a. Hold a 3- to 5-pound weight in your hand. Turn your hand so that the palm faces up (*supination*).

b. Allow the elbow to extend down to the table with the weight creating extension off the table. The elbow acts as a fulcrum. With your other hand, gently push the elbow into forced extension. Hold this position for 5 seconds.

c. Bring your arm up off the table into full elbow flexion. With your other hand, gently push the elbow into forced flexion. Hold for 5 seconds.

d. Repeat the entire motion. Remember to keep your palm up in full wrist supination at all times.

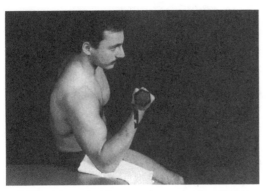

■ **FIG. 89-17** Flexion–extension supination stretch.

## ■ WRIST

### Wrist Stretch

A. **Extension—dorsiflexion stretch** (Fig. 89-18)

1. **Patient position:** standing, with the side to be treated next to a wall but far enough away to allow full elbow extension.

2. **Instructions:**

a. Place your palm, fingers pointing up, flat on the wall so that the elbow is fully extended.

b. Lean on to the wall, causing extension stretch of the wrist. Hold for 5 seconds.

c. Relax, rest, and repeat.

B. **Extension—palmar flexion stretch** (Fig. 89-19)

1. **Patient position:** standing, with the side to be treated next to a wall but far enough away to allow full elbow extension.

2. **Instructions:**

a. Place your palm, fingers pointing down, flat on wall so that the elbow is fully extended.

b. Lean on to the wall, causing extension stretch of the wrist. Hold for 5 seconds.

c. Relax, rest, and repeat.

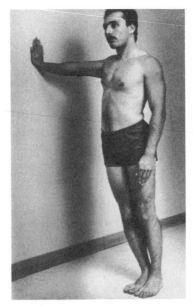

■ **FIG. 89-18** Wrist extension—dorsiflexion stretch.

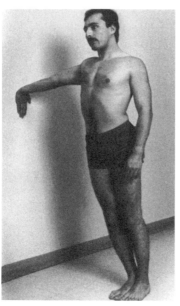

■ **FIG. 89-19** Wrist extension—palmar flexion stretch.

C. **Flexion–palmar flexion stretch** (Fig. 89-20)
  1. **Patient position:** standing, with the side to be treated next to a wall but far enough away to allow full elbow extension.

  2. **Instructions:**
    a. Place the back of your hand, fingers pointing up, flat on the wall so that the elbow is fully extended.
    b. Lean on to the wall, causing flexion stretch of the wrist.
    c. Hold for 5 seconds.
    d. Relax, rest, and repeat.

D. **Flexion–dorsiflexion stretch** (Fig. 89-21)
  1. **Patient position:** standing, with the side to be treated next to a wall but far enough away to allow full elbow extension.

  2. **Instructions:**
    a. Place the back of your hand, fingers pointing down, flat on the wall so that the elbow is fully extended.
    b. Lean on to the wall, causing flexion stretch of wrist.
    c. Hold for 5 seconds.
    d. Relax, rest, and repeat.

## Wrist Strengthening

A. **Wrist flexors** (Fig. 89-22)
  1. **Patient position:** seated, with the side to be treated beside a table. The forearm rests on the table on a towel with the elbow at approximately 90 degrees of flexion. The wrist is off the table.

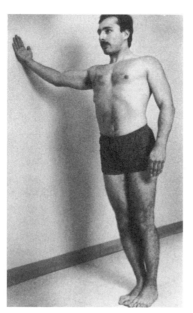

■ **FIG. 89-20** Wrist flexion—palmar flexion stretch.

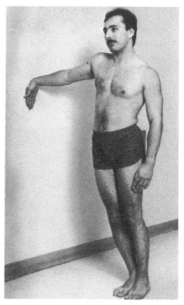

■ **FIG. 89-21** Wrist flexion—dorsiflexion stretch.

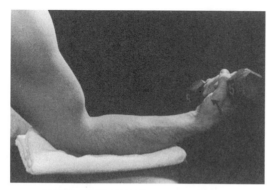

**■ FIG. 89-22** Wrist flexor strengthening.

2. **Instructions:**
   a. Hold a 3- to 5-pound weight in your hand. The palm faces up, putting the wrist in *supination*.
   b. Move the hand holding the weight up toward the ceiling (flex the wrist). Your forearm remains flat on the table.
   c. Hold for 5 to 15 seconds.
   d. Slowly lower the weight off the table, extending the wrist fully.
   e. Relax, rest, and repeat.

B. **Wrist extensors** (Fig. 89-23)
   1. **Patient position:** seated, with the side to be treated beside a table. The forearm rests on the table with the elbow at approximately 90 degrees of flexion. The wrist is off the table.
   2. **Instructions:**
      a. Hold a 3- to 5-pound weight in your hand. The palm faces down, placing the wrist in *pronation*.

b. Bring the hand holding the weight up toward the ceiling (extend the wrist). The forearm remains on the table.
c. Hold this position for 5 to 15 seconds.
d. Slowly lower the weight off the table, flexing the wrist fully.
e. Relax, rest, and repeat.

C. **Wrist rotators** (Fig. 89-24)
   1. **Patient position:** seated, with the side to be treated beside a table. The forearm rests on the table with the elbow at approximately 90 degrees of flexion. The wrist is off the table.
   2. **Instructions:**
      a. Hold a 3- to 5-pound weight in your hand. The palm faces down.
      b. Slowly rotate your forearm, keeping the wrist stiff, until the palm faces up.
      c. Hold this position for 5 seconds.
      d. Slowly rotate your wrist back to the starting position.
      e. Hold this position for 5 seconds.
      f. Repeat the technique.

D. **Ulnar–radial adduction**
   1. **Patient position:** seated, with the side to be treated beside a table. The forearm rests on the table with the elbow at approximately 90 degrees of flexion. The wrist is off the table.
   2. **Instructions:**
      a. Hold a 3- to 5-pound weight in your hand. The palm faces down. The wrist is held stiff.
      b. Bend your wrist to the side, trying to touch your thumb to your arm.
      c. Hold this position for 5 seconds.

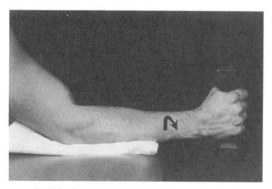

**■ FIG. 89-23** Wrist extensor strengthening.

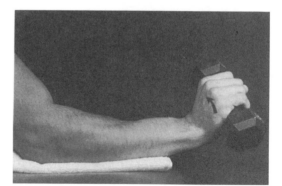

**■ FIG. 89-24** Wrist rotator strengthening.

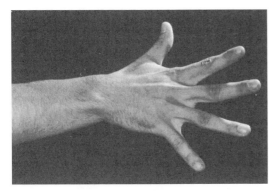

■ **FIG. 89-25** Finger stretch.

d. Bend your wrist to the side in the opposite direction, trying to touch your small finger to your arm.
e. Hold this position for 5 seconds.
f. Repeat the technique.

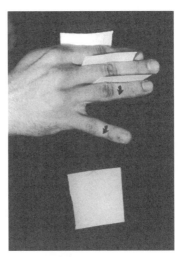

■ **FIG. 89-27** Finger coordination.

and fingertips. Let go suddenly, so that the card falls to the floor.
c. Repeat, using the thumb and different fingers.
d. Repeat the entire process.

C. **Finger coordination** (Fig. 89-27)
1. **Patient position:** sitting or standing.
2. **Instructions:**
a. Hold your hand with the palm down.
b. Place a card between each of the fingers (four cards).
c. Release one card at a time by separating the fingers.
d. Repeat the technique, releasing the cards in different order.

D. **Finger strengthening** (Fig. 89-28)
1. **Patient position:** sitting or standing.

## ■ THE HAND

A. **Finger stretch** (Fig. 89-25)
1. **Patient position:** sitting or standing.
2. **Instructions:**
a. Make a tight fist and hold it for 5 seconds.
b. Open your fist and stretch your fingers as far out as possible.
c. Hold this position for 5 seconds.
d. Repeat the procedure.

B. **Finger coordination** (Fig. 89-26)
1. **Patient position:** sitting or standing.
2. **Instructions:**
a. Hold your hand with the palm down.
b. Hold a card firmly between the thumb

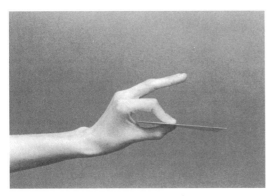

■ **FIG. 89-26** Finger coordination.

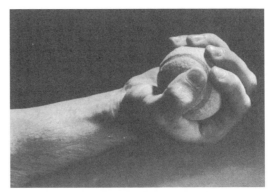

■ **FIG. 89-28** Finger–palm strengthening.

2. **Instructions:**
   a. Hold a rubber ball in the hand to be treated.
   b. Alternately squeeze the ball between your thumb and little finger, thumb and ring finger, thumb and middle finger, and thumb and index finger.
   c. Squeeze the ball with all your fingers.
   d. Hold each squeeze for 3 to 5 seconds.
   e. Repeat the sequence.

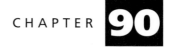

# Practical Applications and Case Histories of the Upper Extremities

*Eileen L. DiGiovanna*

The upper extremities are prone to acute problems such as infection and acute trauma. They are also affected by degenerative processes and overuse injuries. Because of the importance of the ability to use the hands, the physician must be alert for anything affecting the motion of any joint in the upper extremity and seek to prevent permanent disability when possible.

Although arm pain may be caused by some intrinsic joint or soft tissue problem, there are several extrinsic sources of arm pain that must be kept in mind, such as cervical pathology, a problem with the joint above or below the affected one, cardiac pathology, e.g., myocardial infarction or angina, pleurisy, or an irritation of the diaphragm by cholecystitis, peritonitis, or a gas bubble from laparoscopic surgery. The shoulder in particular is probably the most common site of referred pain in the body.

## ■ INFECTION

Infection of the skin or other soft tissues of the upper extremities will be apparent as an acute inflammatory event with the usual signs and symptoms of pain, heat, swelling, redness, and tenderness to palpation. Infections may be localized or may be more diffuse as in cellulitis.

Most significant in the upper extremity is an infection of the hand because this can spread rapidly through the open network of fascia and tunnels in the compartments of the hand. A localized infection of the tuft of the finger pad is known as a *felon*. Infections around the nails are

called *paronychia*. Infection may spread proximally and red streaks may appear along the forearm. In these cases, the lymph nodes of the axilla should be evaluated. All such infections should be treated aggressively.

## ■ ACUTE TRAUMA

Acute trauma will usually have an easily obtained history from the patient. Occupation, a variety of sports, vehicular accidents, falls onto the arm, twisting of the arm, and blows to the upper extremity account for most of the causes of acute trauma. Observation is most helpful in identifying cases not reported by the patient: bruises, abrasions, lacerations, and swelling are some of the items to be noted.

### Fractures

Fracture of the shoulder is most commonly seen at the surgical neck of the humerus in adults. Children are more likely to present with clavicular fractures. Falls onto the outstretched arm are probably the most common cause of fractures in the shoulder girdle. Motion must be restored to the shoulder girdle as quickly as is possible after healing of the fracture to assure a return of normal mobility.

Fracture of the elbow is least common in the upper extremity, but when it occurs it can have serious consequences if not properly diagnosed and treated.

The hand and wrist are commonly fractured in falls on the outstretched arm. The ulna, the radius, or both are prone to break as an individual attempts to catch oneself when falling. Blows to the forearm or hand may result in fractures. A fracture of the scaphoid at the base of the *anatomic snuff box* is one that is slow to heal or may result in non-union and must be watched carefully.

## Dislocations

Any joint in the upper extremity may dislocate if sufficient force is applied to it. The glenohumeral joint is especially prone to dislocating, usually in an anterior direction. A prominent end of the clavicle and loss of roundness of the shoulder may indicate a dislocation. Frequently there is an associated tear of the capsule. With any joint dislocation, radiographic imaging should be obtained to rule out an associated fracture.

Chronic dislocation may be a problem if there was a tear of the capsule at the time of original insult. The humeral head may dislocate through this tear when the arm moves into extension, abduction, and external rotation. The *apprehension test* is helpful in making the diagnosis if the patient is not aware of the cause of his pain.

## Soft Tissue Injuries

The shoulder girdle is most prone to two types of soft tissue injury. A separation at the *acromioclavicular joint* may occur from a blow to the acromion process causing a torquing of the scapula around the coracoid process. The acromioclavicular ligament is torn, causing an instability at the joint. There may be either a complete or a partial tear of the ligament. An x-ray with a weight in the ipsilateral hand may be required to make this diagnosis.

The second injury is a *tear of the rotator cuff muscles*. This is frequently a tendinous tear, although the muscle itself may be torn. A tear can be caused in young people by a significant force at the shoulder or in older people by a wearing away of the fibers of the tendon, which weakens it so that a lesser force may tear the tendon. Rotator cuff tears may vary in degree of severity. The supraspinatus is the most likely of the rotator cuff muscles to rupture caused by its passing

through the *suprahumeral* space between the humeral head and the acromioclavicular ligament and acromion and a generally inadequate blood supply.

Although not as common, the biceps muscle or tendon may also rupture. When this happens, the belly of the muscle is seen in a position more distal than is normal.

Occasionally, the biceps tendon is unstable in its groove, usually when the transverse ligament has been damaged by trauma or worn by repeated microtrauma. The tendon then will snap out of the groove on certain motions, such as the Yergason test.

## ■ DEGENERATIVE PROCESSES
### Tendinitis

Approximately 90% of nontraumatic shoulder pain is caused by tendonitis. The two tendons of the shoulder most commonly involved in an inflammatory process are those of the long head of the biceps and the supraspinatus tendon. Both pass through the suprahumeral space and are compressed during abduction of the shoulder.

The tendons, especially the supraspinatus, lack adequate circulation at the area where a gap occurs between vessels entering the tendon from the muscle and vessels entering from the bone. This area is known as the *critical zone*. The critical zone is also the most likely site of deposition of calcium in calcific tendonitis. Calcium deposits in the tendon, *calcific tendonitis*, may become chronic and delay recovery from the tendonitis.

Osteopathic treatment of all tender points around the shoulder girdle, especially those associated with the involved tendon, is helpful in diminishing the pain. All restrictions to motion and circulation should be removed.

### Capsulitis

Capsulitis of the shoulder seldom occurs in isolation. It is usually associated with other inflammatory processes of the shoulder. Adhesive capsulitis is the most common form (see Frozen Shoulder).

### Bursitis

Although bursitis is a common diagnosis in shoulder pain, only a small percentage of shoulder pain is actually caused by bursitis. The most commonly affected bursa is the *subacromial bursa*, because of its location in the suprahumeral space. Occasionally, a calcium deposit in a tendon will rupture through into the bursa, leading to *calcific bursitis*.

## Frozen Shoulder

Also known as *adhesive capsulitis*, frozen shoulder results from prolonged immobilization of the shoulder. Frozen shoulder may result from application of a splint or sling, or from failure to move the shoulder because of pain from trauma or an inflammatory process in the shoulder. Inflammatory and fibrous changes occur in all the periarticular soft tissues. The range of motion of the shoulder can be markedly restricted, with abduction and internal rotation usually the most affected. Patients should be instructed to exercise the shoulder. Complete immobilization should not be continued for more than 48 hours except under supervision of a physician; then, physical therapy should be begun as quickly as possible.

Prevention is the best treatment. Spencer techniques are especially helpful in preventing a loss of motion in a painful shoulder and in restoring motion to a shoulder involved in adhesive capsulitis.

## Epicondylitis

Epicondylitis is a common elbow problem, generally called *tennis elbow* if the lateral epicondyle is involved and *golfer's elbow* if the medial epicondyle is involved. This is an overuse syndrome that is associated with any activity that requires repetitive pronation and supination, such as gripping a tennis racquet, golf club, screwdriver, or doorknob. The wrist extensor muscles are involved in lateral epicondylitis.

Pain is located over the epicondyl and radiates down the arm. It is aggravated by dorsiflexion of the wrist while grasping an object or flexion of the wrist against resistance. Calcification within the tendon may be seen in the area of degeneration.

Somatic dysfunction of the radial head is often mistaken for lateral epicondylitis. When pain is in the lateral arm and there is weakness of grip, the radial head should be evaluated. Counterstrain treatment assists in diminishing the pain of a true inflammatory process. Correcting the cause of the problem is essential to prevent recurrences.

## Carpal Tunnel Syndrome

In carpal tunnel syndrome, the median nerve is compressed in the tunnel by fibrous bands, scar tissue from chronic inflammation or microtrauma, arthritis, or myxedema caused by hypothyroidism. The edema of pregnancy can create a carpal tunnel syndrome. Somatic dysfunction of the carpal bones can be a cause of carpal tunnel syndrome.

The syndrome is characterized by pain or paresthesias such as tingling in the hand, particularly along the distribution of the median nerve. Numbness may be the presenting symptom. Weakness of the hand frequently occurs. On examination, the thenar eminence may be atrophied. The flexor tendons might be slightly swollen. The Tinel sign and a positive Phalen test are valuable diagnostic clues.

Osteopathic treatment is aimed at stretching soft tissues, freeing restricted carpal bones, removing edema fluid, and improving circulation and nerve function.

## DeQuervain Syndrome

This condition is a *stenosing tenosynovitis* of the thumb. It is more common in women than in men and is related to repetitive movements of the thumb that cause inflammation within the tendon sheath. The main symptoms are pain and difficulty moving the thumb. Swelling around the anatomic snuffbox may be noted. There is pain on circumduction of the thumb. The specific test for this condition is the *Finkelstein test*. Injection with steroids may be necessary. Osteopathic treatment is directed to improving motion of the joint, decreasing swelling, and treating tender points with counterstrain.

## Dupuytren's Contracture

This condition is characterized by contracture of the palmar fascia and nodule formation in the palm. There appears to be a genetic predisposition to the disease. It is frequently found in alcoholics. It can be triggered or aggravated by trauma. The nodules are tender. The palmar fascia contracts, flexing the fingers, particularly on the ulnar side. Finger and hand function can be severely limited.

Osteopathic treatment is aimed toward keeping the palmar fascia as free as possible: the metacarpophalangeal and proximal interphalangeal joints should be mobilized to prevent secondary joint immobilization and tethering of the flexor tendons. Myofascial release techniques and stretching is useful. Surgical intervention may be required.

## Arthritis

Any type of arthritis may involve any of the shoulder girdle joints. The sternoclavicular joint is most commonly affected. Osteoarthritis of the glenohumeral joint is less common than in some of the other upper extremity joints.

Rheumatoid arthritis and osteoarthritis may involve the joints of the wrist and hand. Psoriatic arthritis and gouty arthritis may also affect this area. Many of the findings and specific deformities were mentioned previously. In the arthritides, the small accessory motions of the joint are lost first. The osteopathic physician must articulate all joints once the acute inflammation has subsided. Placing traction on the joint as it is articulated decreases the discomfort for the patient. The patient should be encouraged to exercise the joints gently to maintain mobility.

## ■ SOMATIC DYSFUNCTION

Most articular somatic dysfunctions of the shoulder girdle occur at the sternoclavicular or acromioclavicular joints. These dysfunctions are characterized by pain at the involved joint and restricted motion in one or more of the planes of joint motion.

The most common articular somatic dysfunction at the elbow involves the head of the radius. Restriction in anterior or posterior motion is tested by moving the radial head in an anteroposterior direction. This condition often mimics the pain of tennis elbow. The anterior slide of the radial head is coupled with supination–flexion, and the posterior slide with pronation–extension. Tender points are located on either epicondyle, over the radial head, in the antecubital fossa, or on the olecranon.

Somatic dysfunction can occur between any of the carpal or hand bones. Tender points lie over the dorsal and volar surfaces of the wrist. A common tender point of the hand is found in the thenar eminence.

## ■ CASE HISTORY—SHOULDER PAIN

A 24-year-old man is seen in the clinic with a symptom of pain in his right shoulder for the past 3 days. The pain had been unresponsive to over-the-counter medication. He stated that he had played pitch and catch with his nephew the day before the onset of the pain. He was sleeping poorly because of the pain, which was most severe on lifting objects, putting on his shirt, and reaching for objects overhead.

Examination of the shoulder revealed no bruising, swelling, or inflammation. Motion of the right shoulder was restricted in comparison to the left in flexion, abduction, extension, and external rotation, both passively and actively. He was unable to perform the Apley scratch test fully. Muscle strength was relatively normal, although it was difficult to test because of pain. The neck, elbow, and wrist were normal on examination. There was marked tenderness to palpation of the biceps tendon and some tenderness of the supinator tendon. There was no tenderness or swelling of the bursa of the shoulder.

A diagnosis of biceps and supraspinatus tendonitis was made. The patient was given a prescription for a non-steroidal anti-inflammatory medication, told to ice the shoulder two to three times per day, and to perform normal activities but to refrain from lifting objects or reaching. Tender points on the long and short head of the biceps tendons and the supraspinatus muscle were treated with counterstrain, and the trapezius, rhomboids, and pectoralis muscles were gently stretched.

At the next visit 1 week later, he was improved and was placed on a gradually increasing program of home exercise to restore motion, prevent adhesive capsulitis, and strengthen the shoulder muscles.

## Discussion

Tendonitis is a common finding in shoulder pain. Because the biceps tendon and the supraspinatus muscle and tendon pass through the suprahumeral space, it is common for them to be irritated during forceful use of the shoulder, especially when the shoulder has not been prepared for such activity. Strengthening of the rotator cuff muscles and warming up of all shoulder muscle groups should be done prior to strenuous use of the shoulder.

Because tendonitis is an inflammatory process, anti-inflammatory medication and ice are useful. Osteopathic treatment is directed to decreasing the associated pain and to improving the circulation in the area. Stretching of adjacent muscles assists in freeing the shoulder girdle to prevent further injuries. The home exercise program should include stretching and strengthening exercises.

When evaluating a patient for shoulder pain, it is imperative to remember that all shoulder pain does not indicate intrinsic shoulder problems but may be caused by some extrinsic source such as referral from some cervical spine pathology, myocardial infarction, pleurisy or irritation of the diaphragm by the gall bladder, an abscess, or a gas bubble after laparoscopic surgery.

## ■ CASE HISTORY—TENNIS ELBOW

R.F. is a 54-year-old man who played tennis two to three times per week. After a particularly rigorous game, pain developed in his right elbow. He iced it and took acetaminophen with little relief. He was unable to play tennis, and he found that his grip on doorknobs and when opening jar lids was weakened. He had never experienced trauma to his right upper extremity. He always stretched before activity

Examination showed a healthy middle-aged man who was trim and fit. He was in good health other than the pain in the elbow. The lateral epicondyle was tender to palpation, as were the muscles of the lateral forearm. His grip was weaker on the right than the left, and supination against resistance was painful.

He was given an anti-inflammatory medication, told to ice the elbow, and was treated with osteopathic manipulation. The tender point over the lateral epicondyle was treated with counterstrain technique. He was told to wear a tennis elbow brace on his arm until he was completely pain-free.

## Discussion

Tennis elbow is generally the result of overuse of the elbow joint in a supination motion. It occurs in tennis players who are using a backhand motion incorrectly. The tendonous attachment at the lateral epicondyl becomes inflamed, causing pain with supination. This is most commonly an inflammatory process and requires treatment with anti-inflammatory medication or sometimes injection with a steroid. Icing helps relieve the inflammation. A brace of the forearm is sometimes helpful. If tennis is the cause of the problem, having a professional evaluate the backhand swing will prevent aggravation of the condition from an incorrect use of the racquet. Osteopathic treatment is directed to treatment of the tender point at the epicondyle. This provides some but not complete relief.

It is important to evaluate the radial head as a somatic dysfunction of the radial head frequently mimics tennis elbow and responds well to osteopathic manipulative treatment.

The physician must also consider "tennis elbow" in persons who do not play tennis. It can occur whenever there is a strong grip while supinating and pronating the arm, as in the use of a screwdriver or turning a resistant object such as a doorknob or jar lid.

## ■ CASE HISTORY—IMPINGEMENT SYNDROMES

A.M., a 50-year-old mail carrier was seen and reported pain and tingling in his right arm and hand that had been evident for approximately 8 months. He gave a history of a fall onto his outstretched right arm. After the fall, he experienced pain in his wrist and shoulder. He was previously cared for by the Veteran's Hospital with a diagnosis of carpal tunnel syndrome.

Examination of the upper extremity revealed several areas of dysfunction. Most of the muscle groups of the arm were weaker than those of the left arm. Range of motion was normal except in the wrist, which was restricted in abduction/

adduction. Sensation in the hand was decreased. The cervical range of motion was decreased. The first rib on the right was elevated and restricted. Reflexes were normal. The thenar eminence was atrophied and thumb grasp was weak. There was a tender point in the pronator teres and pronation was weak and painful.

He was treated with a variety of osteopathic techniques. The cervical spine was treated with muscle energy and normal motion was restored. The first rib was treated with facilitated positional release. The pronator teres and the wrist were treated with counterstrain. The wrist was treated with articulatory techniques.

At the time of the second visit, he was much improved with less pain. He still had numbness and tingling in his fingers and the musculature was still weak.

## Discussion

This case is a good example of multiple impingement syndromes. Besides the obvious carpal tunnel, A.M. had some additional impingement of the median nerve as it passes by the pronator teres. The tension in the soft tissues at the thoracic inlet impinged the nerves of the brachial plexus as they passed through the costoclavicular space. It is important to remember that when there is a fall on the rigid arm, the force is transmitted all the way to the neck. In A.M.'s case, this resulted in dysfunctions of bone and soft tissue that resulted in multiple nerve impingements: "thoracic outlet syndrome," "pronator teres syndrome," and "carpal tunnel syndrome."

## REFERENCES

Arminio JA. DeQuervain's disease: The forgotten syndrome. *Resident Staff Physician* 1982;28:84–88.

Cailliet R. *Shoulder Pain*. Philadelphia: F.A. Davis, 1966.

DiGiovanna E, Schiowitz S. *An Osteopathic Approach to Diagnosis and Treatment, 2nd ed.* Philadelphia: Lippincott-Raven, 1997.

Hoppenfeld S. *Physical Examination of the Spine and Extremities*. Norwalk, CT: Appleton-Century-Crofts, 1995.

Janecki CJ, Field JH. Washerwoman's sprain, working woman's pain. *Aches Pains* 1984;14:20.

Leddy JP, Hamilton JJ. Tennis elbow: Not just a case for the courts. *Aches Pains* 1984;14:21.

Lipscomb PR. Carpal tunnel syndrome: Guide to office diagnosis. *J Musculoskel Med* 1984;35:41.

Nirschl RP. The prevention and management of tennis elbow. *Pain Analg* 1984;6:10.

Paletta FX. Dupuytren's contracture. *Am Fam Physician* 1981; 23:85–90.

Roland AC, Cawley PW. Common elbow injuries. *Family Practice Recertifications*. MRA Publications, Inc., September 1984.

Salter RB. *Textbook of Disorders and Injuries of the Musculoskeletal System, 3rd ed.* Baltimore: Williams & Wilkins, 1999.

Sucher BM, Hinrichs RN. Manipulative treatment of carpal tunnel syndrome, Biomechanical and osteopathic intervention to increase the length of the transverse carpal ligament. *J Am Osteopath Assoc* 1998;98:679–686.

Weiss TE. Painful hands: Differential diagnosis by physical examination only. *Consultant* 1984;24:51–65.

# Lower Extremities

# CHAPTER 91

# Anatomical Considerations of the Hip

*Stanley Schiowitz*

## ■ ARTICULATION

The hip joint joins the pelvis to the lower extremity. It is a ball-and-socket articulation that allows motion in three planes and circumduction. Its bony components are the acetabulum, which is at the junction of the ilium, ischium, and pubic bones; and the head of the femur. The convex femoral head fits into the concave acetabulum. The articular surfaces are reciprocally curved but are not coextensive, nor are they fully congruent. The close-packed position of the hip joint is full extension, abduction, and medial rotation.

The anatomic relationships of the hip joint are similar to those of the glenohumeral joint. It is a ball and socket articulation, allowing 3 degrees of motion plus circumduction (Fig. 91-1). The entire weight of the body is transmitted through the hip joints, which, therefore, must have a greater degree of stability than the glenohumeral joints. A deeper acetabulum, the acetabular labrum, and the strong supportive ligaments afford increased stability. The acetabulum is in the innominate bone and relates to spinal, sacral, and ilial movements.

## ■ LIGAMENTS

The hip joint is strongly maintained by its capsule and its ligaments—the iliofemoral ligament, the pubofemoral ligament, the ischiofemoral ligament, and the ligament of the head of the femur. The ligaments slacken or tauten with mo-

tion, thereby stabilizing and limiting hip movement.

## ■ OSTEOLOGY

In an upright human, the femoral head and neck face medially, anteriorly, and cephalad. Any change in direction will influence pelvic tilt and gait.

The shaft of the femur descends medially, creating a mechanical genu valgus. The femoral shaft also undergoes torsional osseous changes so that the femoral condyles can articulate with the tibial condyles in a frontal plane. The genu valgus is exaggerated with increased pelvic width and contributes to the unstable gait patterns in elderly women.

A major bony landmark is the greater trochanter, easily palpated on the lateral superior aspect of the shaft. The lesser trochanter is on the medial aspect of the inferior end of the femoral neck. This trochanter, although not palpable, is very important, because it is the site of attachment of the iliopsoas tendon. At its distal end, the femoral condyles and epicondyles are easily palpable at the knee joint.

## ■ GROSS MOTION

Movements of the hip joint, which should be measured, include flexion–extension, internal and external rotation, and abduction–adduction. The range of flexion depends on the action of the knee joint. Hip flexion is greater with

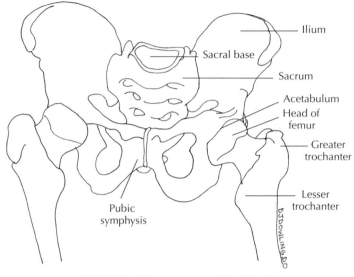

■ **FIG. 91-1** Bony anatomy of the hip joint.

the knee flexed (Fig. 91-2). Greater hip flexion can be achieved passively than actively. Both hips undergo full passive flexion when both knees are approximated to the chest and this is accompanied by a posterior pelvic tilt and lumbar flattening. Hip extension is greater when the knee is in extension (Fig. 91-3). Passive extension is greater than active extension.

All hip joint motions should be measured with one hand stabilizing the pelvis. Average normal measurements are as follows:

1. Abduction–adduction, hip and knee flexed: 70 to 75 degrees.
2. Abduction, hip and knee extended: 40 to 45 degrees.
3. Adduction, crossing the anterior aspect of the opposite extended leg: 20 to 30 degrees.
4. Rotation, hip and knee extended or flexed similarly: external rotation approximately: 45 degrees and internal rotation approximately 35 degrees.
5. Flexion, knee flexed: 120 to 130 degrees.
6. Flexion, knee extended: usually less than 90 degrees, because it is limited by extensor muscle action.
7. Extension, subject prone: 20 to 30 degrees. If the opposite leg is placed in 90 degrees of flexion, hip extension is 90 to 120 degrees.

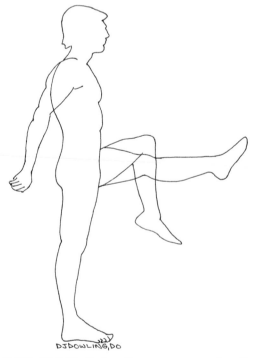

■ **FIG. 91-2** Hip flexion. Shown are ranges of motion with the knee in different positions.

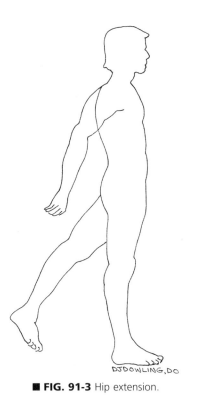

DJDOWLING,DO

■ **FIG. 91-3** Hip extension.

The accessory hip motions consist of slide with abduction–adduction and internal–external rotation as well as long axis traction.

## ■ MAJOR MUSCLES

1. **Iliopsoas** The *iliopsoas* muscle is a major flexor of the hip on the trunk. Its origins are very extensive, involving the vertebrae and their disks from the twelfth thoracic vertebra to the sacrum, and the anterior ilium and sacrum. The iliopsoas muscle is affected by a wide variety of dysfunctions. Except in cases of nerve damage, it is always slightly hypertonic. The clinician should be aware of this when prescribing an exercise program and should avoid iliopsoas contracting and strengthening programs, especially for patients with low back pain. Athletes involved in major hip flexion sports, such as skating, soccer, and running, have overly developed iliopsoas muscles, creating an exaggerated lumbar–thoracic lordosis.

2. **Tensor fascia lata.** The tensor fascia lata originates in the anterior part of the external lip of the iliac crest and deep fascia lata and inserts on to the iliotibial tract of the fascia lata. This

muscle flexes, medially rotates, and abducts the hip joint. Chronic dysfunction may manifest with a number of seemingly unrelated symptoms, including knee pain (especially at the fibular head), buttock pain, and a burning feeling in the lateral upper thigh.

3. **Gluteus medius.** The gluteus medius originates on the external surface of the ilium, below and between the iliac crest and the posterior gluteal line, and inserts on to the lateral surface of the greater trochanter. It is a major abductor of the hip joint and assists slightly in medial rotation and flexion. Hypotonic dysfunctions will affect stance and gait; hypertonic dysfunctions will usually be point-sensitive and mimic sciatic nerve symptoms.

4. **Gluteus maximus.** The gluteus maximus originates at the posterior gluteal line of the ilium, the posterior lower sacrum and coccyx, the aponeurosis of the erector spinae, the sacrotuberous ligament, and the gluteal aponeurosis. The major actions of this muscle are to extend and laterally rotate the hip. Hypotonic dysfunctions will affect stance and gait. Hypertonic dysfunctions are usually greater in scope than those of the gluteus medius, involving sacral motion and ilial motion as well as hip joint motion.

   The gluteus maximus follows the *law of muscle detorsion*. Therefore, to increase hip extension, as in ballet movement, the ilium must be rotated. Somatic dysfunction of the lumbar spine will limit lumbar regional motion, pelvic rotation, and hip extension

5. **Hamstrings.** The hamstrings are three muscles, the semimembranosus, semitendinosus, and biceps femoris. All originate at the tuberosity of the ischium and insert on to various areas of the fibula and tibia. They are two-joint muscles that extend the hip and flex the knee. Both motions are interdependent and will affect each other's function. Dysfunctions are commonly found at the ischium, at the lateral aspect of the knee, and at the pes anserinus bursa.

6. **Piriformis.** The piriformis muscle originates on the pelvic surface of the sacrum, at the margin of the greater sciatic foramen, and at the sacrotuberous ligament. It inserts on to

the superior border of the greater trochanter. The piriformis muscle is a lateral hip rotator, and its proximity to the sciatic nerve makes it a common site for dysfunction. When hypertonic, it is readily palpable in the lateral rectal mucosa. The piriformis symptom complex follows a sciatic neuritic pain distribution. Specific point tenderness can usually be evoked at a point in the buttocks halfway between the posterosuperior iliac spine and the superolateral aspect of the greater trochanter.

Of major importance in evaluating hip joint function and dysfunction is the fact that many of the large hip joint muscles involve the function of both the knee and hip joints. Contraction of these muscles always involves an attempt at motion of both joints. Limiting the motion of one joint requires stabilization of the other joint by other muscles.

Somatic dysfunctions related to hip joint dysfunction may involve the lower spine, sacrum, ilium, acetabulofemoral joint, femoral shaft, and the knee joint.

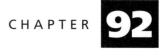

# Evaluation of the Hip

*Dennis J. Dowling and Eileen L. DiGiovanna*

$A$s a fairly competent ball and socket joint, the major concerns for examination of the hip are to determine any neurological conditions, screen for orthopedic dysfunction, evaluate muscular asymmetries, locate counterstrain tenderpoints, and integrate the localized findings with those noted from other regions.

## ■ OBSERVATION

Observation of the hip should take place with the patient standing and during gait. With the patient standing, the physician should inspect for swelling, muscle asymmetry, and evidence of trauma. It should be noted if the hip is held in flexion, a common position suggesting pain or dysfunction of the joint. External rotation of the lower extremity may indicate spasm of the iliopsoas. During gait, the patient should be watched for any abnormality of the gait, including a limp or stiffness of the hip with motion. A painful hip may cause the patient to tilt his body toward that hip.

## ■ PALPATION

The physician should palpate the soft tissues of the hip, looking for muscle changes, fascial strains, tenderness, particularly counterstrain tender points, and temperature changes of the skin, possibly indicating an inflammatory process. The tensor fascia lata and iliotibial band should be palpated. Tenderness of the inguinal ligament should be noted. The bony landmarks should be palpated, including the greater trochanter and pelvic structures where ligaments of many hip muscles attach.

Two bursas in particular should be palpated for tenderness and swelling:

1. Trochanteric—over the greater trochanter of the hip
2. Ischial—over the ischial tuberosity, known as "weaver's bottom" when enlarged

## ■ RANGE OF MOTION TESTING

The gross motions of the hip joint are flexion–extension, abduction–adduction, internal and external rotation, and circumduction. Passive motion should generally exceed active motion. In both cases, the effect of the position of the knee is also important. Several of the muscles are two joint muscles and knee flexion or extension will affect the findings (i.e., hip flexion is greater with knee flexion than with knee extension).

Many hip joint motions should be measured with one hand stabilizing the pelvis. Both sides should be tested and asymmetry may be a more important finding than absolute amount of motion. Average normal measurements are as follows:

## ■ PARAMETERS:

1. Abduction–adduction, hip and knee flexed: 70 to 75 degrees.
2. Abduction, hip and knee extended: 40 to 45 degrees.
3. Adduction, crossing the anterior aspect of the opposite extended leg: 20 to 30 degrees.
4. External rotation: 45 degrees; internal rotation approximately 35 degrees.

5. Flexion, knee flexed: 120 to 130 degrees.
6. Flexion, knee extended: usually less than 90 degrees, because it is limited by extensor muscle action.
7. Extension, subject prone: 20 to 30 degrees. If the opposite leg is placed in 90 degrees of flexion, hip extension is 90 to 120 degrees.

## Seated–Active Motion Testing

1. **External rotation**
   a. Procedure:
      (1) The patient is instructed to place the lateral malleolis of the ankle on the knee of the opposite leg.
      (2) The procedure is repeated for the opposite leg and the extent of rotation is compared.
   b. Interpretation
      (1) The patient can indicate which side is more comfortable when crossing the ankle over the knee.
      (2) The leg with the more horizontal position has the greater range of motion.
2. **Adduction**
   a. Procedure:
      (1) The patient is instructed to cross his legs by placing the popliteal portion of one knee on the anterior knee of the opposite leg.
      (2) The procedure is repeated for the opposite leg and the extent of rotation is compared.
   b. Interpretation
      (1) The patient can indicate which side is more comfortable when crossing one knee over the other
      (2) The leg with the greater ease of crossing has the greater range of motion

## Supine–Passive Motion Testing

1. **Flexion**
   a. The patient's leg is raised with:
      (1) Knee extended
      (2) Knee flexed
2. **Abduction**
   a. The nontested leg is held at midline
   b. The patient's leg is moved laterally

3. **Adduction**
   a. The nontested leg is held at midline
   b. The patient's hip is slightly flexed to bring it anterior to the other leg
   c. The leg is moved medially and across the other leg
4. **Internal Rotation**
   a. The patient's hip and knee are flexed to 90 degrees each
   b. The physician's cephalad hand stabilizes the patient's bent knee
   c. The physician's other hand pulls the patient's foot and lower leg laterally, creating internal rotation
5. **External Rotation**
   a. The patient's hip and knee are flexed to 90 degrees each
   b. The physician's cephalad hand stabilizes the patient's bent knee
   c. The physician's other hand pushes the patient's foot and lower leg medially creating external rotation

## Prone–Passive Motion Testing

1. **Extension**
   a. The patient's leg is raised with the knee extended, and then with
   b. Knee flexed
2. **Abduction**
   a. The nontested leg is held at midline
   b. The patient's leg is moved laterally
3. **Adduction**
   a. The nontested leg is held at midline
   b. The patient's leg is slightly extended to bring it posterior to the other leg
   c. The leg is moved medially and across the other leg
4. **Internal Rotation**
   a. The patient's knee is flexed to 90 degrees
   b. The physician's cephalad hand stabilizes the patient's pelvis by holding the sacrum
   c. The physician's other hand pulls the patient's foot and lower leg laterally creating internal rotation
5. **External Rotation**
   a. The patient's knee is flexed to 90 degrees
   b. The physician's cephalad hand stabilizes the patient's pelvis by holding the sacrum
   c. The physician's other hand pushes the patient's foot and lower leg medially creating external rotation

## ■ MUSCLE STRENGTH TESTING

Each muscle group should be tested for strength. Strength testing is accomplished by placing the hip into the direction opposite to that being tested (i.e., to test flexion strength, place the hip into extension and have the patient push into flexion).

The primary *flexors* are the psoas and iliacus. This may be tested in a seated position with the patient lifting the knee while the examiner stabilized the pelvis and evaluates strength with the application of graded resistance at the knee. It may also be evaluated with the patient supine and the knees extended.

The gluteus maximus, biceps femoris semitendinosus, and semimembranosus muscles create *extension*. This is best evaluated with the patient prone and the knees extended.

The prime mover of the hip into *abduction* is the gluteus medius muscle with some contribution by the tensor fascia lata and gluteus minimus. *Adduction* is provided by the adductor magnus, adductor brevis, adductor longus, the gracilis, and the pectineus. Both abduction and adduction can be tested with the patient lying on the side opposite the hip being tested. In all these tests, the physician applies a graded resistance to the motion.

*Internal* and *external rotation* can be tested with the patient seated and the resistance applied to the ankle of the leg being tested. External rotation occurs with contraction of the obturator externus and internus, piriformis, gluteus maximus, and gemelli muscles. Internal rotation is provided by the gluteus minimus and tensor fascia lata muscles.

## ■ STRENGTH TESTING—PATIENT SUPINE

1. **Extension**
   a. The patient's leg is raised with the knee extended
   b. The patient pushes downward against physician's resistance
2. **Adduction**
   a. The nontested leg is held at midline
   b. The patient's leg is moved laterally
   c. The patient pushes the leg medially against physician's resistance

3. **Abduction**
   a. The nontested leg is held at midline
   b. The patient's leg is slightly flexed to bring it anterior to the other leg
   c. The leg is moved medially
   d. The patient pushes the leg laterally against physician's resistance
4. **External Rotation**
   a. The patient's hip and knee are flexed to 90 degrees each
   b. The physician's cephalad hand stabilizes the patient's bent knee
   c. The physician's other hand pulls the patient's foot and lower leg laterally, creating internal rotation
   d. The patient pushes the foot medially against physician's resistance
5. **Internal Rotation**
   a. The patient's hip and knee are flexed to 90 degrees each
   b. The physician's cephalad hand stabilizes the patient's bent knee
   c. The physician's other hand pushes the patient's foot and lower leg medially, creating external rotation
   d. The patient pushes the foot laterally against physician's resistance

## ■ PRONE

1. **Flexion**
   a. The patient's leg is raised with knee extended
   b. The patient pushes downward against the physician's resistance
2. **Adduction**
   a. The nontested leg is held at midline
   b. The patient's leg is moved laterally
   c. The patient pushes the leg medially against the physician's resistance
3. **Abduction**
   a. The nontested leg is held at midline
   b. The leg is held in its medial position
   c. The patient pushes the leg laterally against the physician's resistance
4. **External Rotation**
   a. The patient's knee is flexed to 90 degrees
   b. The physician's cephalad hand stabilizes the patient's pelvis by holding the sacrum

c. The physician's other hand pulls the patient's foot and lower leg laterally, creating internal rotation

d. The patient pushes the foot medially against the physician's resistance

5. **Internal Rotation**

a. The patient's knee is flexed to 90 degrees

b. The physician's cephalad hand stabilizes the patient's pelvis by holding the sacrum

c. The physician's other hand pushes the patient's foot and lower leg medially creating external rotation

d. The patient pushes the foot laterally against the physician's resistance

(4) Extension—the physician puts tension into the position by pushing the knee toward the table (Fig. 92-1)

d. The procedure is repeated for the other side.

4. **Interpretation:**

a. The physician should note the quantity, quality, and symmetry of motion

b. Some reduction in motion may be caused by sacroiliac dysfunctions

c. The range of motion may be reduced and there may be a solid, grinding restriction indicating a bony impedance to movement

d. Reduction in motion that appears to be "softer" in restriction indicates muscular

## ■ SPECIAL TESTING

There are several tests that can be used to evaluate specific problems with the hip joint and its surrounding soft tissues.

### Patrick or Fabere Test

The *Patrick test* is also known as the *Fabere test*, which indicates the motions engaged during testing: *f*lexion, *ab*duction, *e*xternal *r*otation, and *e*xtension.

1. **Patient position**: supine
2. **Physician position**: Standing on the side to be treated facing the patient at the level of the patient's knee
3. **Procedure**:
   a. The physician's cephalad hand is placed on the patient's knee.
   b. The physician's other hand grasps the patient's ankle
   c. The patient's leg is brought progressively into:
      (1) Flexion—hip and knee flexion to the anatomic limit
      (2) Abduction—the patient's knee is abducted while the foot remains in line.
      (3) External Rotation—by bringing the knee to the furthest extent of abduction some external rotation is added to bring the leg to the extent of anatomic barrier

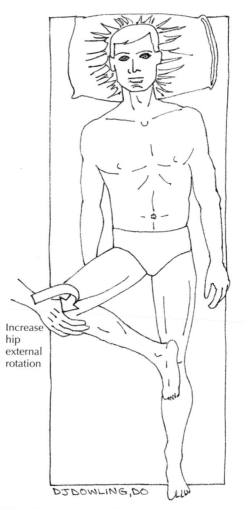

Increase hip external rotation

■ **FIG. 92-1** Patrick's (FABERE) test for hip joint motion restriction.

contractions, especially the adductors and iliopsoas muscles

   e. This maneuver should be painless. Any dysfunction of the hip will cause pain or inability to complete the test.

   f. Since the test may also be affected by dysfunction of the sacroiliac joint, localization of the pain is necessary to differentiate the cause of the problem.

## Ober Test

1. **Patient position**: side-lying with the side to be evaluated up and away from the table.
2. **Physician position:** standing behind patient.
3. **Procedure:**
   a. The uppermost leg, with the knee bent, is lifted.
   b. The leg is then released.
4. **Interpretation**:
   a. The leg should drop quickly
   b. A delay or slow drop of the leg indicates contracture of the tensor fascia lata or iliotibial band.

## Ortolani's Sign

Also known as the *Ortolani click*, this test evaluates for congenital dysplasia or dislocation of the hip. It is performed on newborns in the following manner:

1. **Patient position**: supine
2. **Physician position**: standing over patient
3. **Procedure**:
   a. The physician grasps the patient's thighs on each side close to the hips.
   b. The pads of the index fingers are placed on the hip joint over the greater trochanter
   c. The fingers are sunk into the buttocks
   d. The patient's hips and knees are flexed
   e. The thighs are gently externally rotated and abducted
   f. The physician notes any clicking and/or telescoping of the hip joints
4. **Interpretation**:

A click can indicate hip dysplasia and/or congenital dislocation of the hip

## Telescoping Sign

The *telescoping sign* is used to test for congenital dislocations as well. The femur is pulled and pushed in relation to the pelvis and appears to "telescope" into the fossa, shortening the leg.

## Thomas Test

The *Thomas test* is positive when there is a contraction or contracture of the psoas muscle present.

1. **Patient position**: supine. One version has the patient completely on the table. Another version has the patient with head, neck, trunk, and pelvis on the table but either the legs are able to hang off table or the legs are put into this position by a drop leaf on the table
2. **Physician position**: standing on the side to be evaluated
3. **Procedure**:
   a. The patient is instructed to flex both hips and knees and use his arms to hug them toward his chest
   b. The patient is instructed to release one leg and allow the hip and knee to extend while continuing to hug the other leg close to the chest.
   c. The physician can exaggerate the position of the flexed hip and knee by pushing them into further flexion.
   d. The physician can test if the extended leg is as far as is possible by pushing that leg toward the table/floor.
   e. The physician places one hand beneath the patient's lumbar spine to determine any change in lordosis.
   f. The physician then places a hand beneath the patient's knee of the outstretched leg. The distance between the popliteal line and the table can be measured in fingerbreadths or by a ruler.
   g. The procedure is repeated for the other side (Fig. 92-2).
4. **Interpretation**:
   a. An increase in lordosis can indicate psoas spasm on that side.
   b. The patient's outstretched leg should normally contact the table. Space between the popliteal line of the knee and the table indicates iliopsoas spasm
   c. The amount of space beneath each knee is compared. Asymmetry of height indicates

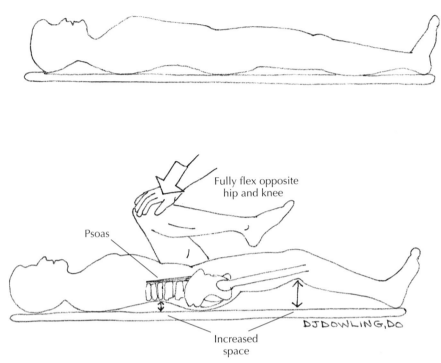

Fully flex opposite
hip and knee

Psoas

Increased
space

DJ DOWLING, DO

■ **FIG. 92-2** Thomas test for hip flexion contracture.

asymmetry in spasm. The higher the knee, the greater the relative tightness of the muscle.

## Trendelenberg Test

The *Trendelenberg test* is an evaluation for gluteus medius weakness, a dislocation of the hip, or a nonunion of the neck of the femur.

1. **Patient position**: standing
2. **Physician position**: kneeling or squatting behind patient with eyes at level of the patient's pelvis
3. **Procedure**:
   a. The physician's hands can be placed lightly alongside the patient's hips to help the patient balance.
   b. The physician notes the position of the patient's iliac crests.
   c. The patient is instructed to stand on one leg while lifting the opposite foot from the floor and bending the hip and knee on the nonstance leg.

   d. The position of the iliac crest on the non-stance side is noted (Fig. 92-3).
   e. The procedure is repeated with the opposite leg.
4. **Interpretation**:
   a. As the weight is shifted onto the dysfunctional leg, the pelvis on the opposite side will drop. Normally, that side should rise slightly.
   b. An iliac crest of a bent leg that drops below the level of the other side indicates a weakness of the opposite stance leg.
   c. The weakness is in the stance leg gluteus medius.
   d. Intact gluteus medius function of the stance leg should maintain the opposite iliac crest at either the same level or higher than the stance side.

## Squatting Test

1. **Patient position**: standing
2. **Physician position**: standing facing the patient

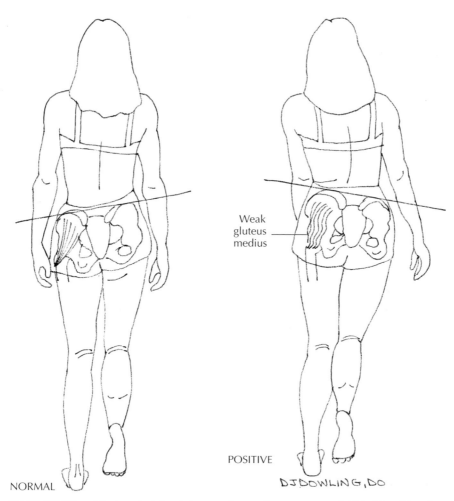

Weak
gluteus
medius

NORMAL

POSITIVE

DJDOWLING,DO

■ **FIG. 92-3** Trendelenberg test for gluteus medius weakness or congenital hip joint dislocation.

3. **Procedure**:
   a. The physician holds the patient's hands to steady him.
   b. The patient is instructed to squat with feet remaining in place and then to rise upward again to a standing position (Fig. 92-4).
4. **Interpretation**:
   a. Squatting involves intact neurological function of the lumbar plexus, but L4 specifically.
   b. Limitation of the hip joint may be noted in asymmetric or inability to perform maneuver.
   c. The weakness is in the stance leg gluteus medius.
   d. Inability to rise may indicate weakness of the quadriceps muscles.

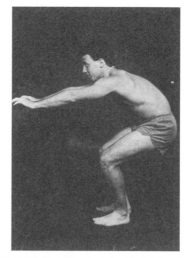

■ **FIG. 92-4** Squatting test for hip joint restriction.

## Erichsen's Test

1. **Patient position:** supine
2. **Physician position:** standing alongside the patient's pelvis looking toward the patient's head
3. **Procedure:**
   a. The physician places both hands on either side of the patient's pelvis in the iliac region.
   b. The physician places bilateral medial pressure towards the sacroiliac joints bilaterally (Fig. 92-5).
   c. The patient is requested to give feedback as to whether there is pain.
4. **Interpretation:**
   a. Pain on one side indicates a sacroiliitis on that side.
   b. Inflammatory changes of the sacroiliac joint may be noted on radiological studies.

## Straight Leg Raising—Seated

1. **Patient position:** seated.
2. **Physician position:** kneeling, squatting, or standing facing patient.

3. **Procedure:**
   a. The patient is instructed to sit straight upward.
   b. The patient is instructed to grasp the edge of the table.
   c. The physician takes the patient's foot on one leg and brings that knee into extension.
   d. The procedure is repeated for the other leg.
4. **Interpretation:**
   a. Pain that radiates indicates possible radiculopathy.
   b. If the patient is unable to maintain the straightened seated position or unable to fully extend knee, this indicates contraction of the hamstring muscles.

## Straight Leg Raising—Supine

1. **Patient position:** supine
2. **Physician position:** standing next to the patient on the side to be treated
3. **Procedure:**
   a. The physician's cephalad hand contacts and holds the ASIS on the same side to be tested.
   b. The physician's other hand grasps the patient's ankle on the same side.
   c. The physician raises the patient's leg and maintains knee extension and creates hip flexion (Fig. 92-6).

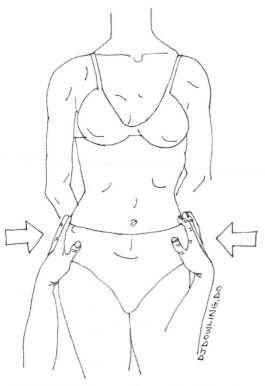

■ **FIG. 92-5** Erichsen test for sacroiliac dysfunction.

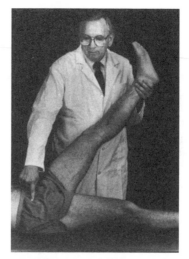

■ **FIG. 92-6** Straight leg raising test.

4. **Interpretation:**
   a. Pain radiating down the posterior leg indicates a possible radiculopathy.
   b. If the knee bends (positive "bow sign"), then there is contraction of the hamstring muscles.

## Ludloff Sign

1. **Patient position:** supine
2. **Physician position:** standing or sitting alongside patient
3. **Procedure:**
   a. The physician observes the femoral triangle from above the patient.
   b. Both sides are evaluated.
4. **Interpretation**
   a. Observation of an ecchymosis within the triangle indicates possible hip fracture.
   b. The test is more specific for an avulsion fracture of the lesser trochanter. The leg on the involved side may be:
      (1) Apparently shorter
      (2) Internally rotated
      (3) Weakness of hip flexion

## Tinel Test

1. **Patient position:** supine
2. **Physician position:** standing or seated next to the patient at the level of the thigh on the side to be evaluated

3. **Procedure:**
   a. The physician locates a line connecting the ASIS and the greater trochanter
   b. The physician taps the tip of a finger or reflex hammer onto positioned fingers approximately two-thirds of the way from the ASIS on the line.
   c. The patient is requested to give feedback as to what is felt after the procedure is finished.
4. **Interpretation:**
   a. Reproduction of pain or paresthesia indicates meralgia parasthetica

### REFERENCES

DiGiovanna EL. Schiowitz S. *An Osteopathic Approach to Diagnosis and Treatment 2nd ed.* Philadelphia: Lippincott-Raven, 1997.

Hoppenfeld S. *Physical Examination of the Spine and Extremities.* Norwalk, CT: Appleton-Century-Crofts, 1986.

Kapandji KA. *The Physiology of the Joints,* Vol. II. Edinburgh: Churchill-Livingstone, 1970.

Polley HF. Hunder GG. *Rheumatologic Interviewing and Physical Examination of the Joints, 2nd ed.* Philadelphia: WB Saunders Co., 1978.

Schiowitz S. The lower extremity: The hip joint. In: *An Osteopathic Approach to Diagnosis and Treatment 2nd ed.* DiGiovanna EL, Schiowitz S, eds. Philadelphia: Lippincott-Raven, 1997:319–324.

Schiowitz S. Diagnosis and treatment of the lower extremity: The hip. In: *An Osteopathic Approach to Diagnosis and Treatment, 2nd ed.* DiGiovanna EL, Schiowitz S, eds. Philadelphia: Lippincott-Raven, 1997:339–340.

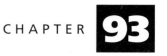

# Knee Anatomic Considerations

*Stanley Schiowitz*

The knee joint is the largest and most complicated articulation in the body. It is a compound joint comprising medial and lateral femoral–tibial articulations and a patella–femoral articulation, all within one joint capsule. Positioned midway in each supporting limb of the body, the knee is subjected to severe stresses as it performs its functions of weight-bearing and locomotion. The anatomic description of this articulation is simplified by considering it as two separate joints. The larger one, the femorotibial joint, consists of two condylar joints between corresponding femoral and tibial condyles. The second one, the femoropatellar joint, is between the patella and the femur.

## ■ THE FEMOROTIBIAL JOINT

The femoral condyles are convex in both planes and, viewed laterally, are spiral-shaped. The lateral condyle flattens more rapidly in the anteroposterior dimension than does the medial condyle, producing inequality in articular lengths. This is evident when the knee is placed in full extension. An automatic coupled rotation occurs to accommodate this inequality. Hoppenfeld describes a "screw home" motion in which the medial aspect of the tibia rotates laterally around the lateral femoral condyle, allowing the medial femoral condyle to complete its extension. This approximates a close-packed position, allowing prolonged periods of standing without relying to any great degree on muscle function.

The tibial condyles are concave and end toward the mid-tibial line in intercondylar eminences. The condyles are separated by the intercondylar area.

The femorotibial joint is one of the few articulations with menisci. The medial meniscus is semicircular. Its anterior end is attached to the anterior intercondylar area in front of the anterior cruciate ligament. The lateral meniscus is almost a complete ring. Its anterior end is attached in front of the intercondylar eminence of the tibia, blending partially with the anterior cruciate ligament.

The femoral condyles roll and slide on the tibial condyles during flexion and extension, accompanied by similar motions of the menisci. During extension, the menisci are pulled anteriorly; with flexion, they are moved posteriorly.

The femorotibial joint is stabilized by the capsule and its related ligaments and muscular attachments. Laterally, these attachments comprise the fibular collateral ligament, biceps tendon, popliteus tendon, and the iliotibial band; medially, they comprise the *pes anserinus*, the medial head of the gastrocnemius, the tibial lateral ligament, and a portion of the quadriceps tendon. Posteriorly the joint is stabilized by both heads of the gastrocnemius, the semitendinous muscle, the biceps tendon, the oblique popliteal ligament, and the arcuate ligament. The anterior aspect is stabilized by the quadriceps muscles, the quadriceps tendon, the patella, the patellar tendon, and the medial and lateral retinacula.

The cruciate ligaments are intra-articular but extra-synovial. They stabilize the knee in the anteroposterior direction and allow the joint to function as a hinge while keeping the articular surfaces together. The *anterior cruciate ligament* arises from the tibia and runs backward, upward, and laterally to insert on to the lateral femoral condyle. During flexion, the anterior cruciate ligament slides the femoral condyle forward. The *posterior cruciate ligament* arises from the posterior aspect of the tibia and runs forward and upward obliquely to insert onto the lateral aspect of the medial femoral condyle. During extension the posterior cruciate ligament slides the femoral condyle posteriorly.

## ■ THE FEMOROPATELLAR JOINT

The femoropatellar joint is a sellar joint; the articulating surface of the patella is adapted to the patellar surface of the femur. This femoral articulation involves the anterior surface of both condyles. An oblique groove divides it into a large lateral and smaller medial area. The quadriceps muscles, the quadriceps tendon, and the patellar tendon maintain the joint's stability. Its major motions are vertical up-and-down movement on the femur, and movement in a sagittal plane with respect to the tibia. This allows a pulley function during flexion and extension of the knee.

## Major Muscles

The quadriceps femoris is the extensor muscle of the knee. It consists of four muscles that have a common tendon of insertion on to the anterior tuberosity of the tibia. The rectus femoris arises from two tendinous heads, one from the anterior iliac spine and the second from a groove above the acetabulum and the hip joint capsule. It is directed downward along the anterior aspect of the thigh and ends in the common tendon. It functions as a two-joint muscle, producing both hip flexion and knee extension. The vastus lateralis is the largest part of the quadriceps. It arises from the upper intertrochanteric line and the anterior and inferior borders of the greater trochanter. The vastus medialis arises from the lower part of the intertrochanteric line, the spiral line, the medial lip of the linea aspera, the medial supracondylar line, and the tendons of the adductor longus and magnus. The vastus intermedius arises from the front and lateral surface of the upper shaft of the femur.

The flexor muscles of the knee are located in the posterior compartment of the thigh. They are the hamstrings, the gracilis, the sartorius, the popliteus, and the gastrocnemius muscles. All of these muscles are biarticular, with the exception of the popliteus and the short head of the biceps. Their action on knee flexion is related to the position of the hip. Rotation of the knee is also a function of these knee flexors.

## Knee Movements

The active motions of the knee are classified as flexion–extension and medial–lateral rotation. Normally the knee flexes to 135 degrees; extension is a return from flexion to zero degrees. Medial–lateral rotation, with the knee in flexion, is 10 degrees in each direction. With the foot on the ground, the last 30 degrees of extension is accompanied by a conjunct medial femoral rotation. With the foot off the ground, extension is accompanied by a conjunct lateral rotation of the tibia.

Accessory motions with the knee semi-flexed are: anteroposterior glide, abduction–adduction, and long-axis extension.

With the foot on the ground, the final 30 degrees of femoral extension is accompanied by a conjunct medial femoral rotation (Fig. 93-1). This conjunct rotation results from the geometry of the articulating surfaces and the action of the ligaments. In full extension, the knee is in close-packed position, which confers greater stability and strength on the joint. As in all close-packed joints, trauma can more easily cause fracture. However, the more common ligamentous tears occur in mid- or loose-packed positions. With the foot off the ground, extension is associated with conjunct lateral rotation of the tibia.

The voluntary movements of axial internal and external rotation also occur in the knee. These motions are best observed with the knee in a flexed position. Passive internal and external rotation are each approximately 10 degrees.

The accessory motions of the femorotibial joint consist of passive internal and external rotation, conjunct rotation, dorsal and ventral tibial slide, abduction, adduction, and long-axis traction.

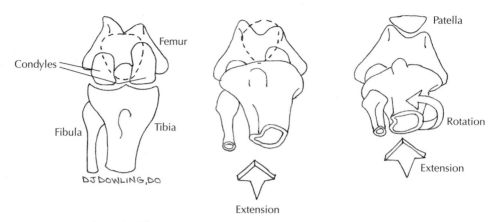

■ **FIG. 93-1** Tibial-femoral extension accompanied by conjunct rotation of the tibia.

Besides the possibility of multiple soft tissue dysfunctions, the major somatic dysfunctions of joint motion affect abduction and adduction, or dorsal and ventral slide.

The patella, with the knee semi-flexed, can be passively moved in the dorsal–ventral, cephalad, caudad, and side-to-side directions.

## ■ TIBIOFIBULAR JOINTS

The superior tibiofibular joint is a plane oval articulation. The tibial facet lies on the postero-lateral aspect of the rim of the lateral tibial condyle. It faces obliquely posteriorly, inferiorly, and laterally. The inferior tibiofibular joint is a syndesmosis. The tibial facet is a rough concave notch into which the convex fibular facet fits. The fibula has a distal articulation with the tibia and the talus at the ankle.

Dorsiflexion and plantar flexion of the ankle automatically create motion in both tibiofibular joints. Dorsiflexion causes the lateral malleolus to move laterally, to move vertically in a cephalad direction, and to rotate medially. This causes the superior tibiofibular joint to move in an upward posterior direction while rotating medially. The reverse occurs in plantar flexion.

The most common somatic dysfunction found in this area is a posterior fibula at the superior tibiofibular joint. This may be secondary to ankle dysfunction and marked inversion and plantarflexion of the ankle. To resolve the superior tibiofibular dysfunction, it is important to evaluate the ankle joint and treat any dysfunctions found in that region.

### REFERENCES

Basmajian JV. *Muscles Alive*. Baltimore: Williams & Wilkins, 1978.

Cailliet R. *Foot and Ankle Pain*. Philadelphia: F.A. Davis, 1968.

D'Ambrosia RD. *Musculoskeletal Disorders*. Philadelphia: J.B. Lippincott, 1977.

Hoppenfeld S. *Physical Examination of the Spine and Extremities*. Norwalk, CT: Appleton-Century-Crofts, 1986.

Jones L. *The Postural Complex*. St. Louis: Charles C Thomas, 1955.

Kapandji IA. *The Physiology of the Joints*. Vol II. Edinburgh: Churchill Livingstone, 1970.

MacConaill MA. The Movement of Bones and Joints. *J. Bone Joint Surgery* (AM) 1949;1:100–104.

MacConaill MA, Basmajian JV. *Muscles and Movements*. New York: Robert E. Krieger, 1977.

O'Donoghue DH. *Treatment of Injuries to Athletes*. Philadelphia: W.B. Saunders, 1970.

Rasch PJ, Burke RK. *Kinesiology and Applied Anatomy*. Baltimore: Lea & Febiger, 1978.

Warwick RB, Williams PL. *Gray's Anatomy*, 35th British ed. Philadelphia: W.B. Saunders, 1973.

Wells KF, Luttgens K. *Kinesiology*. Philadelphia: W.B. Saunders, 1976.

Wilson FC. *The Musculoskeletal System*, 2nd ed. Philadelphia: J.B. Lippincott, 1983.

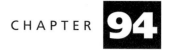

# Evaluation of the Knee

*Stanley Schiowitz and Eileen L. DiGiovanna*

The most common symptom relevant to the knee is pain. The knee is subject to a variety of injuries and is a common joint for the development of arthritis. It can also be involved in somatic dysfunction and is commonly influenced by problems originating in the hip or the foot and ankle.

## ■ OBSERVATION

The physical examination should begin with observation. Any evidence of trauma, such as bruises, abrasions, or scars, should be noted. Swelling is generally readily observable around the knee. With an inflammatory or infectious process, the knee may be erythematous.

With the patient standing, the physician should view the knees from the front, back, and side. Any abnormal posture should be noted. *Genu valgus* is a posture in which the knees are close together and the feet separated. This is often referred to as *knock-kneed*. It can be a normal variant and is more common in females. With *genu varus* the legs will appear bowed, with the knees not touching even when the feet are close together. This is colloquially referred to as *bow-legged*. Clincally, this can sometimes be correlated with rickets. From the lateral view it is possible to see a backward curvature of the knee joint known as *genu recurvatum*. These positions of the knee joints place abnormal stresses on the joint surfaces. Flexion deformities may be seen in the presence of osteoarthritis, as may some bony changes in the normal landmarks.

The knee should be observed during gait as well as statically. The range of motion during the swing phase and the length of the stride should be noted. A limp or antalgic gait may be observed.

## ■ PALPATION

The knee should be palpated and landmarks identified. Swelling may be palpated medial, inferior, or lateral to the patella or in the popliteal fossa. Tenderness detected during palpation may indicate the location of the source of pain, such as over the tibial tuberosity in the case of Osgood-Schlatter disease.

Landmarks to identify include:

1. Patella and patellar tendon
2. Head of the fibula
3. Tibial plateau
4. Medial joint line and medial collateral ligament
5. Lateral joint line and lateral collateral ligament
6. Tibial tuberosity

The tone and quality of the muscles and fascia of the knee joint should be identified during palpation.

1. The quadriceps femoris consists of four muscles of the anterior thigh. These knee extensor muscles are, perhaps, the most significant. Weakened quadriceps muscles decrease the stability of the knee and make it more prone to injury.
2. The hamstring muscles lie in the posterior compartment of the thigh. These are the flexors of the knee and are more likely to be hypertonic but may be weak as well. Tender-

**487**

ness of the hamstring tendons may be identified.

3. The attachment of the semitendinosus, sartorius, and gracilis, also knee flexors, below and medial to the knee joint may be tender in the presence of *pes anserine bursitis.*

4. The gastrocnemeus, a bi-articular calf muscle, may be palpated behind the knee joint.

5. The popliteus and the short head of the biceps are the only two knee flexors that are one joint muscles. All the others are two joint muscles.

6. The iliotibial band along the lateral thigh is often tender, which may indicate undue tension of the tissues between the hip and knee.

## ■ RANGE OF MOTION TESTING

The range of motion of the knee joint should be tested actively and passively. The patient should be instructed to flex and extend the knee while seated and, from the standing position, to squat and arise. The latter tests muscle strength as well as active range of motion. The physician should hold the hands of older patients to prevent them from falling.

Passively, the physician should put the knee through a full range of motion of flexion, extension, and medial and lateral rotation. Normally, the knee flexes to 135 degrees and extension is a return to zero degrees. Full extension is typically modified by the amount of hip flexion caused by the two-joint expanse of the hamstring muscles. Medial–lateral rotation with the knee flexed should be approximately 10 degrees in each direction. While moving the knee, the physician should monitor the patient's knee joint to sense any *crepitus.*

The patella should be articulated and any pain or crepitus noted. The accessory motions with the knee semi-flexed are *anteroposterior glide, abduction, adduction,* and *long-axis extension.* These are the motions most likely involved in somatic dysfunction of the tibia/femur articulation.

The fibular head, lateral to the knee joint, should be articulated in an anterior/posterior glide. Because of the combined mechanics with the ankle mortise, a posterior glide somatic dysfunction is the most common knee somatic dysfunction with anterior glide the next.

## ■ SPECIAL TESTS

There are a number of special tests that can be performed to evaluate dysfunctions of the knee joint. They may be used to differentiate the type of problem involved, whether of the ligaments, menisci, or other source. Some of them are described.

### Varus–Valgus Stress Test

This test evaluates the medial and lateral collateral structures. With the patient supine, the ankle joint is held between the examiner's side and arm, thus freeing both hands. The knee is tested in full extension by applying a valgus and then a varus force to the proximal tibia (abduction–adduction motion of leg) (Fig. 94-1). The examiner notes any instability or increased motion on application of force in either direction. Then the test is repeated with the knee slightly flexed. If the cruciate ligaments are intact, motion can be stable with the knee in full extension, even with collateral ligament rupture.

### Rotary Instability Testing

#### Anterior Draw Test

The anterior draw test evaluates anterior cruciate ligament dysfunction. The patient is supine, with his knee flexed 90 degrees and his foot on the table. The examiner sits on the patient's foot or otherwise holds it firmly to stabilize it. The examiner then grasps the back of the proximal tibia with one or both hands and pulls it forward (Fig. 94-2). The patient's leg and foot are internally rotated 30 degrees, then externally rotated 15 degrees, and in a neutral position. On internal rotation, anterior shift of the lateral tibial plateau in conjunction with medial rotation implies injury to the anterior cruciate and lateral ligament. On external rotation, anterior shift of the medial tibial plateau in conjunction with lateral rotation implies injury to the anterior cruciate and medial collateral ligaments. With the foot in neutral position (anterior draw sign), an anterior tibial shift indicates anterior cruciate ligament dysfunction, probably accompanied by medial and lateral ligamentous injury.

#### Lachman Maneuver

The Lachman maneuver is performed in a similar fashion to the anterior draw test, but the knee

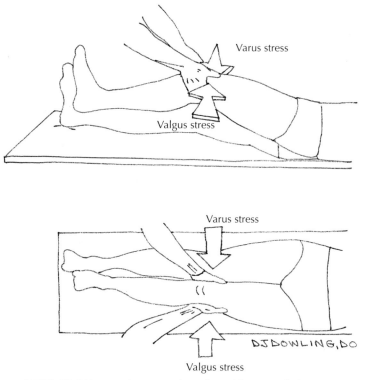

■ **FIG. 94-1** Varus–valgus stress for collateral ligament dysfunction.

is at approximately 10 degrees of flexion. It is considered more sensitive than the anterior draw test for anterior cruciate ligament tears. Both tests lose sensitivity if performed when there is mass effect of swelling that occurs with ligament disruption. They should be performed immediately upon injury or after the edema has subsided.

### Posterior Draw Test

The posterior draw test evaluates posterior cruciate ligament dysfunction. The patient's foot is placed in neutral position, as performed for the anterior draw test. The examiner applies force on the anterior tibia in a posterior direction (Fig. 94-3). The femoral condyles become prominent

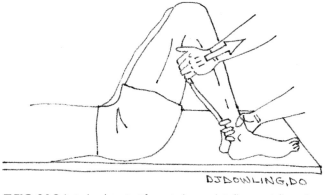

■ **FIG. 94-2** Anterior draw test for anterior cruciate ligament disruption.

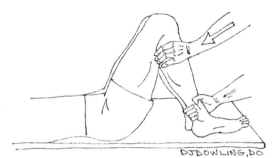

■ **FIG. 94-3** Posterior draw test for posterior cruciate ligament disruption.

anteriorly as the tibia subluxates posteriorly, indicating posterior cruciate ligament dysfunction.

### External Rotation—Recurvatum Test

With the patient supine, the examiner grasps one lower extremity under the heel. With his other hand he supports the calf. The knee is allowed to move from 10 degrees of flexion to full extension (Fig. 94-4). If the knee becomes hyperextended with external rotation of the tibia and tibial varus, the test is positive. This indicates injury to the arcuate ligament, popliteus, and fibular collateral ligament.

### McMurray Test

The McMurray test evaluates for meniscal tears. With the patient supine, the examiner grasps the foot with one hand and palpates the knee joint line with the other hand. The examiner acutely flexes the knee and rotates the tibia into medial and lateral rotation. With the tibia held in lateral rotation, the examiner applies a valgus stress and

extends the knee (Fig. 94-5). The maneuver is repeated with the knee held in medial rotation and a varus stress applied while extending the knee. A palpable or audible click, especially with pain, within the joint is considered a sign of a meniscal tear.

### Apley's Compression Test

With the patient prone, the knee is flexed to 90 degrees. The examiner stabilizes the patient's thigh and leans on the heel, compressing the menisci between the femur and tibia, then rotates the tibia medially while maintaining this compression (Fig. 94-6). Medial joint pain produced by this maneuver suggests a medial meniscal tear, whereas lateral joint pain suggests a lateral meniscal tear.

### Apley's Distraction Test

With the patient prone, the knee is flexed to 90 degrees. The examiner stabilizes the thigh by kneeling on it, then applies traction to the leg while rotating it medially and laterally (traction reduces meniscal pressure but increases ligamentous strain) (Fig. 94-7). Any pain elicited by

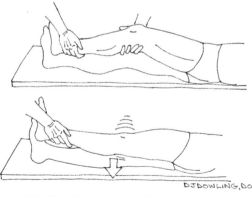

■ **FIG. 94-4** Recurvatum or "bounce home" test.

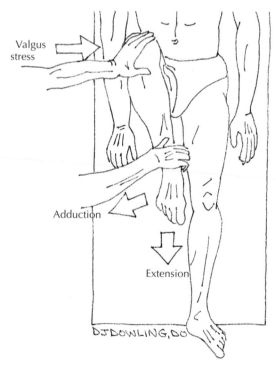

Valgus stress

Adduction

Extension

■ **FIG. 94-5** McMurray test for meniscal tears.

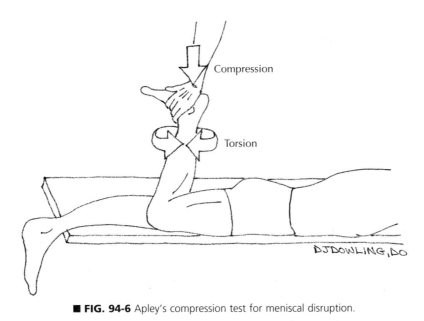

■ **FIG. 94-6** Apley's compression test for meniscal disruption.

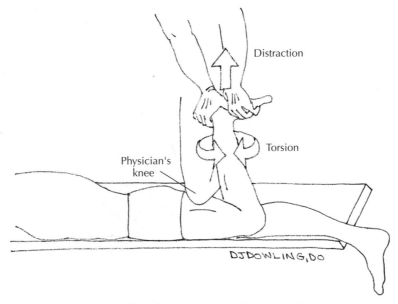

■ **FIG. 94-7** Apley's distraction test for ligamentous disruption.

this maneuver indicates medial or lateral ligamentous dysfunction.

## Knee Joint Effusion Test (Bounce–Home Test)

The knee joint effusion test is performed by supporting the patient's heel in one hand and the calf in the other. The knee is semi-flexed. The hand under the calf is removed carefully and the knee allowed to extend in the same manner as the recurvatum tests. Failure of the knee to extend fully indicates increased joint fluid. Normally the knee should extend fully and end, with a slight "bounce back" at the end point.

## Patella Femoral Grinding Test

The patient is supine with the knee extended and relaxed. The examiner pushes the patella caudad in the trochlear groove and then holds it in this position. The patient is instructed to tighten the quadriceps muscle against the examiner's resistance. Palpable crepitation or pain on patellar motion is an indication of roughness of the articulating surfaces, potentially caused by chondromalacia of the patella.

## ■ DIAGNOSIS OF SOMATIC DYSFUNCTIONS OF THE KNEE JOINT

### Abduction of Tibia on Femur

This is a condition of varus stress of the tibia on the femur. It can be created by a blow to the medial knee joint or by a twisting motion that produces lateral ligamentous sprain. The lateral joint structures are lax, the medial knee joint approximates, and tibial motion on the femur is restricted in medial translatory slide.

1. **Patient position:** supine, with the knee fully extended.
2. **Physician position:** standing on the side of the somatic dysfunction, facing the table.
3. **Technique:**
   a. The physician's cephalad hand grasps the patient's distal femur, holding it firmly and restricting its movement.
   b. With his other hand, the physician grasps the patient's lower ankle and creates val-

gus–varus stress of the tibia on the femur. The varus motion should be greater than the valgus motion.
   c. The physician moves his hand up to the proximal tibia, then induces a straight medial–lateral translatory slide of the tibia upon the femur (Fig. 94-8). The lateral translatory motion should be greater than the medial translatory motion.

### Adduction—Tibia on Femur

This is a condition of valgus stress of the tibia on the femur. It can be created by a blow to the lateral knee joint or by a twisting motion that produces medial ligamentous sprain. The medial joint structures are lax, the lateral knee joint approximates, and tibial motion on the femur is restricted in lateral translatory slide.

1. **Patient position:** supine, with the knee fully extended.
2. **Physician position:** standing on the side of the dysfunction, facing the patient.
3. **Technique:**
   All positions are as described for abduction; however, the findings are reversed: valgus motion is greater than varus, and medial translatory motion is greater than lateral.

### Internal and External Rotation—Tibia on Femur

1. **Patient position:** supine. A pillow is placed under the knee to be examined to maintain slight flexion.

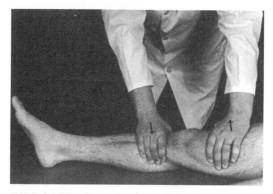

■ **FIG. 94-8** Motion testing for medial–lateral translatory slide dysfunctions.

2. **Physician position:** standing on the side of the dysfunction, facing the table.
3. **Technique:**
   a. The physician's cephalad (with respect to the patient) hand grasps the patient's distal femur, holding it firmly and restricting its movement.
   b. With his other hand the physician grasps the patient's lower ankle and induces internal and external rotary motion of the tibia on the femur (Fig. 94-9).
4. **Interpretation:**
   Increased internal rotation with restricted external rotation signifies internal rotation dysfunction; increased external rotation with restricted internal rotation signifies external rotation dysfunction.

## Anteroposterior Slide Dysfunction—Tibia on Femur

In this condition, the tibia is restricted in anterior or posterior slide. This motion is coupled to knee flexion–extension. Movement of the tibia on the femur into extension is coupled with anterior slide. Movement of the tibia on the femur into flexion is coupled with posterior slide. The initial symptoms or findings are restrictions of flexion or extension movements. The physician must look for these dysfunctions.

1. **Patient position:** supine, with the dysfunctional knee flexed and the foot flat on the table.

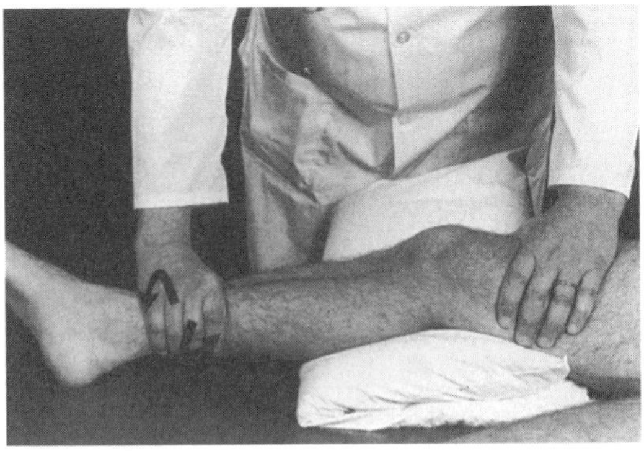

2. **Physician position:** sitting on the patient's foot, anchoring it to the table.
3. **Technique:**
   a. The physician wraps both hands around the proximal tibia with his thumbs in front of the medial and lateral condyles and pressing on them. The physician's hand encircles the leg and grasps it firmly below the popliteal space.
   b. The physician creates a direct anteroposterior translatory slide of the tibia on the femur by first pulling the tibia forward with both hands and then pushing it backward with both thumbs (Fig. 94-10).

*Note:* In performing this test, the physician is not evaluating for cruciate ligamentous tears. The anteroposterior force used must be greatly reduced.

4. **Interpretation:**
   Increased anterior slide with decreased posterior slide signifies anterior slide dysfunction; increased posterior slide with decreased anterior slide signifies posterior slide dysfunction.

## Proximal Fibular Head Dysfunction—Fibula on Tibia

The fibula is not anatomically part of the knee joint. However, the proximity of the fibular head to the knee joint and the overlapping symptom

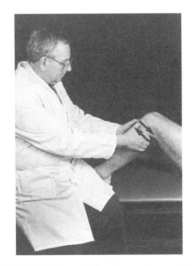

■ **FIG. 94-9** Motion testing for internal and external rotation of the tibia on the femur.

■ **FIG. 94-10** Motion testing for anteroposterior slide dysfunctions of the tibia on the femur.

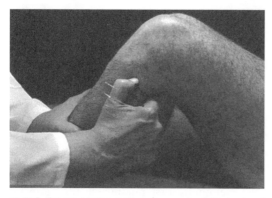

**■ FIG. 94-11** Motion testing for proximal fibular head dysfunctions.

complexes warrant inclusion of these somatic dysfunctions here. When evaluating or treating a fibular head dysfunction, the physician should completely examine the distal articulation as well as the ankle joint.

1. **Patient position:** supine, with the dysfunctional knee flexed and the foot flat on the table.

2. **Physician position:** sitting on the patient's foot.

3. **Technique:**
   a. The initial steps are as in the modified drawer test (see anteroposterior slide dysfunction).
   b. The physician grasps the head of the fibula with his thumb and index finger (Fig. 94-11).
   c. A firm anteroposterior slide motion of the fibular head on the tibia is created.

4. **Interpretation:**
   Increased anterior slide with decreased posterior slide signifies anterior fibular head dysfunction; increased posterior slide with decreased anterior slide signifies posterior fibular head dysfunction.

### REFERENCES

DiGiovanna EL, Schiowitz S. *An Osteopathic Approach to Diagnosis and Treatment, 2nd ed.* Philadelphia: Lippincott-Raven, 1997.

Hoppenfeld S. *Physical Examination of the Spine and Extremities.* Norwalk, CT: Appleton-Century-Crofts, 1986.

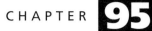
# Foot and Ankle Anatomic Considerations

*Stanley Schiowitz*

The foot and ankle make up a complex unit of twenty-eight bones. The unit must perform the functions of weight-bearing and adapting to terrain during walking or running, yet still remain sufficiently compliant to accommodate additional stress. Approximately 40% of the entire population has foot abnormalities, which makes knowledge of this region extremely important.

## ■ THE ANKLE

The ankle articulation consists of the distal end of the tibia and the medial and lateral malleoli, which together form a concave surface, the crural arch, into which is fitted the body of the talus. These bones are connected by the joint capsule and by the deltoid, anterior and posterior talofibular, and calcaneofibular ligaments. The tibial malleolus extends approximately one-third of the way down the medial surface of the talus and is anterior to the lateral malleolus. The fibular malleolus extends down the entire lateral aspect of the talus. When viewed from above, the entire articulation is laterally angled, thus creating a toeing-out of 15 degrees (Fig. 95-1).

The body of the talus is wedge-shaped and wider in its anterior portion. Dorsiflexion creates a close-packed position of the talus in the crural arch. Further dorsiflexion induces separation of the tibiofibular articulation, with lateral and caudal displacement of the distal fibula and medial rotation around the tibia. This motion of the fibula can be a major source of fibular head dysfunction.

The major joint motions of the ankle are plantar flexion (to 50 degrees) and dorsiflexion (to 20 degrees) (Fig. 95-2). Accessory motions of side-to-side glide, rotation, abduction, and adduction are present if the joint is in plantar flexion.

The triangular deltoid ligament is located medially and is attached above to the medial malleolus and below to the tuberosity of the navicular, the sustentaculum tali of the calcaneus, and the medial tubercle of the talus. The deltoid ligament is so strong that trauma often causes fractures of its bony attachments rather than rupture of the ligament itself.

The anterior talofibular ligament goes from the anterior margin of the lateral malleolus forward and medially to attach to the lateral aspect of the neck and the lateral articular facet of the talus. The posterior talofibular ligament runs from the lower part of the lateral malleolus to the lateral tubercle of the posterior process of the talus. The calcaneofibular ligament runs from the apex of the lateral malleolus downward and backward to the tubercle on the lateral surface of the calcaneus (Fig. 95-3).

The shape of the crural concavity, the extent of the lateral malleolus on the talus, and the strong ligamentous attachments deter joint dislocations unless accompanied by fracture of the malleoli.

The most common sprain represents an inversion and is usually caused by a combination of plantar flexion, internal rotation, and inver-

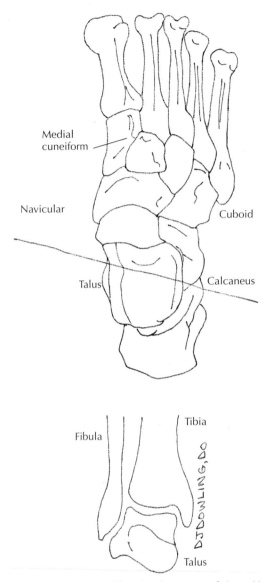

■ **FIG. 95-1** Regional functional anatomy of the ankle joint.

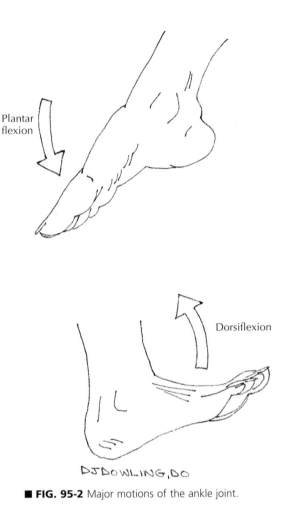

■ **FIG. 95-2** Major motions of the ankle joint.

sion. The lateral ankle ligaments sustain the initial impact. The type of ligamentous tear or fracture–dislocation will depend on the severity of the force. (Fig. 95-4)

The major muscle of ankle dorsiflexion is the tibialis anterior, assisted by the extensor digitorum longus, the extensor hallucis longus, and the peroneus tertius. The major muscles of ankle plantar flexion are the gastrocnemius and soleus, assisted by the plantaris, tibialis posterior, flexor hallucis longus, and flexor digitorum longus.

The subtalar articulation consists of the talus on the calcaneus. These bones have two separate concave–convex articulations. The major motions are calcaneal abduction (valgus) and calcaneal adduction (varus), in relationship to the fixed talus. The talus articulates with the navicular and the calcaneus articulates with the cuboid.

## ■ THE FOOT

The posterior portion of the foot consists of the talocalcaneal, talonavicular, and calcaneocuboid articulations. The calcaneus can move into abduction (valgus) or adduction (varus) in relation

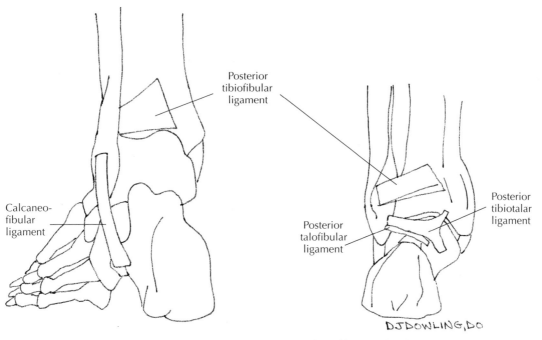

■ **FIG. 95-3** Ligamentous attachments at the ankle, posterior view.

to the talus (Fig. 95-5). The other motions are best described as combined talocalcaneal–navicularcuboid efforts. *Inversion* in relation to a stable talus can be described as a medial rotation of the calcaneus and navicular bone, increasing the height of the medial arch, accompanied by the cuboid rotating downward on the calcaneus

(Fig. 95-6). Motion of the anterior tarsus and plantar flexion will increase this movement. *Eversion* is the reverse of this.

The combined motions of the talonavicular and calcaneocuboid joints create foot *inversion* and *eversion* (see Fig. 95-4). Inversion is created by calcaneal adduction, navicular rotation, and

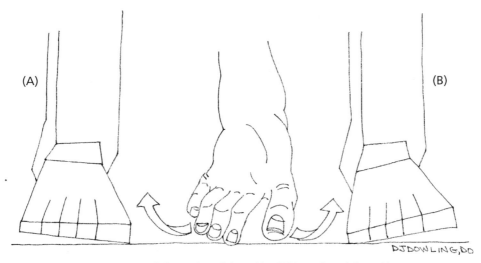

■ **FIG. 95-4 (A)** Eversion of the ankle. **(B)** Inversion of the ankle.

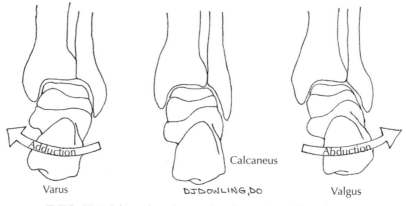

■ **FIG. 95-5** Calcaneal motion on the talus as viewed from the rear.

glide on the talus. These motions raise the navicular and the medial border and depress the lateral border of the foot. Eversion is produced by an opposite series of motions. The muscles involved in the motion of inversion are the tibialis anterior and posterior. The muscles involved in the motion of eversion are the peroneus longus and brevis. The cuboid motions on the calcaneus are glide with conjunct rotation. This usually accompanies the inversion–eversion motions of the combined articulations.

With weight-bearing, the distal tarsus and metatarsals become involved, creating the combined motions of pronation and suppination. *Pronation* of the foot consists of a combination of calcaneal abduction (valgus), eversion, foot ab-

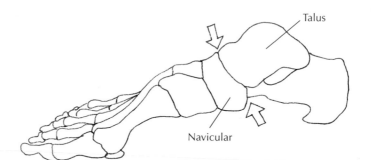

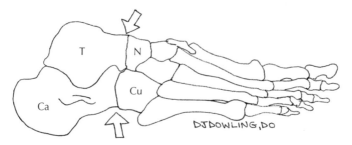

■ **FIG. 95-6** Forefoot inversion creating medial rotation of the cuboid **(Cu)** on the calcaneus **(Ca)** and the navicular **(N)** on the talus **(T)**.

duction, and dorsiflexion. The opposite motions, calcaneal abduction (varus), inversion, foot adduction, and plantar flexion produce supination.

The accessory motions of these articulations are slide and conjunct rotations.

The *forefoot* consists of the metatarsals and phalanges. These bones have a combined motion of forefoot abduction and adduction (Fig. 95-7). The primary motions of the tarsometatarsal joints are flexion and extension. The axis of flexion and extension of the fourth and fifth metatarsals is oblique. This raises and lowers the transverse metatarsal arch with flexion and extension movements of these metatarsals. The intermetatarsal joint movement is primarily that of slide. Accessory motions of the tarsometatarsal and intermetatarsal joints consist in exaggeration of all sliding motions, especially when accompanied by long-axis traction. The metatarsophalangeal articulations allow active motions of extension–flexion and adduction–abduction. Accessory motions are sliding, axial rotation, and long-axis traction.

The active interphalangeal motions are flexion and extension. The accessory motions are abduction and adduction, axial rotation, and long-axis extension.

## Arches of the Foot

The longitudinal curve of the foot can be divided into *medial* and *lateral longitudinal arches*.

To perform its weight-bearing and elastic mobile activities, the longitudinal arch is constructed in two different anatomical forms. The *lateral longitudinal arch* is a firm osseous structure consisting of the calcaneus, cuboid, and the fourth and fifth metatarsals. It resembles the classical architectural definition of an arch, having a keystone (the cuboid) with a flank stone (calcaneus and metatarsal) on each side. It is low, of limited mobility, and built to transmit weight and thrust to and from the ground (Fig.95-8). Its major articulation is the calcaneocuboid, which has a limited range of motion. Stress through this arch can create a typical cuboid somatic dysfunction. Torsion through the anterior aspect of this arch will readily cause fracture of the fifth metatarsal.

The *medial longitudinal arch* is composed of the calcaneus, the talus, the navicular, the cuneiforms, and the first three metatarsal bones. This arch is considerably higher and more mobile than its lateral counterpart. The plantar ligaments, plantar fascia, and the tibialis posterior, flexor digitorum longus, flexor hallucis longus, and intrinsic muscles of the foot assist in controlling the medial arch. The *medial arch* is without firm osseous support and can be increased or reduced to meet the needs of motion or terrain. MacConaill describes the subtalar area as functioning as a twisted plate. It is flattened transversely along the line of the

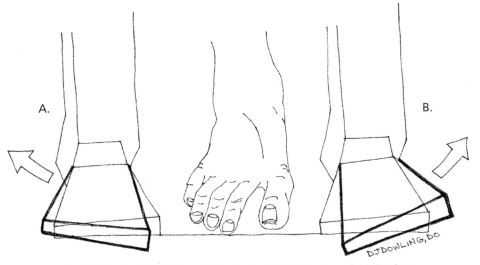

■ **FIG. 95-7 (A)** Abduction of the forefoot. **(B)** Adduction of the forefoot.

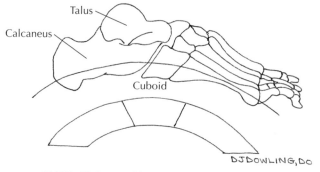

■ **FIG. 95-8** Lateral longitudinal arch of the foot.

metatarsal heads and vertically at the calcaneus. It can be elongated or untwisted in pronation, dropping the medial "arch," or, with supination, can become more twisted, raising the medial arch (Fig.95-9).

The medial arch is controlled by the rotation of the calcaneus on a longitudinal axis (calcaneal valgus–varus). Extreme adduction of the standing feet (crossing one foot over the other) causes posterior rotation of the calcaneus (varus) and a high medial arch. Extreme abduction of the standing foot with dorsiflexion of the ankle causes anterior rotation of the calcaneus (valgus) with a dropping of the medial arch. Therefore, the structure and motions of this area of the foot can be said to twist and untwist the foot in various positions.

Evidently, muscles contribute little to the maintenance of the arch, which instead is supported passively by the skeletal structure and ligaments. Muscles do play an active role in balance and gait.

Many authors describe a number of *transverse arches* (Fig. 95-10). With the exception of the metatarsal heads, these arches do not transmit forces to the ground. The anterior metatarsal transverse arch consists of the five metatarsal heads, with the second metatarsal as its highest point. With weight-bearing, this arch is flattened. Depression of the anterior metatarsal transverse arch increases the weight-bearing burden of the metatarsal heads, creating dysfunction. A second, posterior metatarsal arch consists of the bases of the five metatarsals. A third, tarsal arch has been described, consisting of the navicular, cuneiform, and cuboid bones. This arch assists in flexibility and the rotation motions of the foot. Diminution or absence of the tarsal arch is evident in *pes planus* (flat feet).

If on examination the foot arch changes in conformity with these principles, the feet are not structurally flat. Calcaneal valgus can have far-reaching structural and mechanical effects. It can

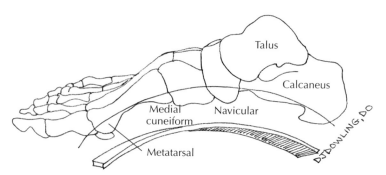

■ **FIG. 95-9** Medial longitudinal arch of the foot and its associated torsion.

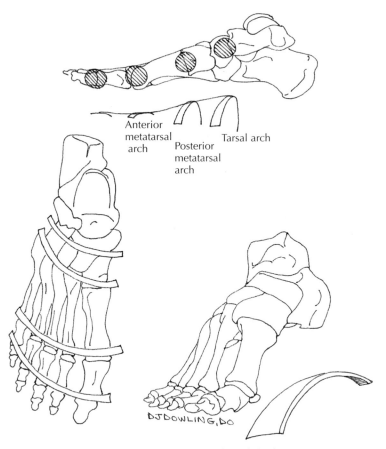

Anterior metatarsal arch    Posterior metatarsal arch    Tarsal arch

DJ DOWLING, DO

■ **FIG. 95-10** Transverse arches of the foot.

reduce the medial arch, exaggerating foot pronation and increasing toe abduction and the tendency for eversion. This is very evident when observing gait. Calcaneal valgus also increases genu valgus, anterior pelvic tilt, and lumbar lordosis. The evaluation and treatment of foot imbalance is an integral part of the osteopathic examination.

Somatic dysfunction restricting joint motion will affect the motions of slide and conjunct rotation. An example is the conjunct rotation of the cuboid on the calcaneus with eversion and inversion of the foot.

## REFERENCES

Basmajian JV. *Muscles Alive.* Baltimore: Williams & Wilkins, 1978.

Cailliet R. *Foot and Ankle Pain.* Philadelphia: F.A. Davis, 1968.

D'Ambrosia RD. *Musculoskeletal Disorders.* Philadelphia: J.B. Lippincott, 1977.

DiGiovanna EL, Schiowitz S. *An Osteopathic Approach to Diagnosis and Treatment, 2nd ed.* Philadelphia: Lippincott-Raven, 1997.

Hoppenfeld S. *Physical Examination of the Spine and Extremities.* Norwalk, CT: Appleton-Century-Crofts, 1986.

Jones L. *The Postural Complex.* St. Louis: Charles C Thomas, 1955.

Kapandji IA. *The Physiology of the Joints. Vol II.* Edinburgh: Churchill Livingstone, 1970.

MacConaill MA, Basmajian JV. *Muscles and Movements.* New York: Robert E. Krieger, 1977.

O'Donoghue DH. *Treatment of Injuries to Athletes.* Philadelphia: W.B. Saunders, 1970.

Rasch PJ, Burke RK. *Kinesiology and Applied Anatomy.* Baltimore: Lea & Febiger, 1978.

Warwick RB, Williams PL. *Gray's Anatomy, 35th British ed.* Philadelphia: W.B. Saunders, 1973.

Wells KF, Luttgens K. *Kinesiology.* Philadelphia: W.B. Saunders, 1976.

Wilson FC. *The Musculoskeletal System, 2nd ed.* Philadelphia: J.B. Lippincott, 1983.

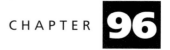

# Evaluation of Foot and Ankle Dysfunctions

*Stanley Schiowitz and Eileen L. DiGiovanna*

The walking foot is constantly adapting to terrain. Beyond the calcaneus, the tarsals, metatarsals, and phalanges act as stabilizers, rising, falling, twisting, and turning to accommodate to every change in the road or style of movement. These motions in turn are transmitted through the calcaneus, talus, and ankle mortice. The last articulation acts as a secondary balancing mechanism, allowing dorsiflexion and plantar flexion, rotation, abduction, and adduction at the ankle.

Unexpected or uncompensated stresses or strains of the foot will create dysfunctions. These can occur at the articulations of the foot or at the ankle joint. A diagnosis is based on loss of joint mobility and tissue changes. Because the foot and ankle are attached to the body, the physician must always search out secondary dysfunctions.

A thorough history, physical examination, and ancillary studies should be performed before treatment is instituted. The ankle joint is commonly involved in eversion and inversion strains or sprains, as well as in malleolar fractures. Dysfunction often follows immobilization treatment procedures. People with healed fractures may still have unresolved somatic dysfunctions.

## ■ OBSERVATION

The skin of the foot should be examined for evidence of infection, fungal infection, and signs of trauma. The ankle should be observed for any swelling or inflammation. The nails should be inspected for paronychia (infections of the cuticle of the nail) or for fungal infection of the nails. Calluses and corns may be present on the sole of the foot or any of the toes.

It is important to observe the foot and ankle in the standing and seated positions and during gait. With the patient standing, weight equally distributed on each extremity, the foot and ankle should be observed for toeing in or out and the height of the medial arch of the foot. If the arch is flattened, it is necessary to determine whether this is structural or caused by pronation of the foot. If the flattening remains with the patient seated, then it is a structural problem. If the arch returns to the foot when seated, then the problem is functional. If the foot pronates, it will be noted that the Achilles tendon is bowed when the foot is weight-bearing. Occasionally the arch is too high and this should be noted because of the foot problems that may occur.

The foot and ankle are observed during gait. The foot should first strike the ground on the heel, roll to the lateral edge of the foot, the weight should then roll back across the ball of the foot (the transverse arch), and the great toe should push the foot off the ground. The flexibility of the ankle should be noted during this process. Any abnormal turning in our out of the foot (inversion or eversion) or pronation should be noted.

Bone and joint asymmetries should be noted. *Hammer toes* have a flexion deformity of the middle phalangeal joint and an extension deformity of the distal phalangeal joint. A claw toe has flexion deformity of both joints. Frequently a callus forms over the top of the flexed middle phalangeal joint. A *bunion* is seen as a lateral deviation of the first metatarsal bone with a medial deviation of the proximal phalanx of the great toe. The proximal metatarsal–phalangeal joint is often enlarged, swollen, and tender.

## ■ PALPATION

The foot and ankle may be palpated with the patient seated or supine. Soft tissues are palpated for tenderness and swelling. Tissue texture changes should be noted. Bony landmarks are palpated for any asymmetry or arthritic changes.

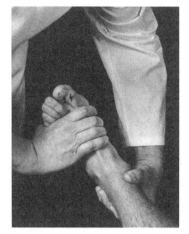

■ **FIG. 96-1** Motion testing for dorsiflexion and plantar flexion.

## ■ MOTION TESTING

The clinician should first examine a healthy extremity and test its motions. The findings in a healthy extremity provide a standard for comparison with a dysfunctional extremity. Restricted motion in a joint of the foot or ankle is often indicative of somatic dysfunction, especially when no arthritic changes have been palpated in that joint.

### Dorsiflexion and Plantar Flexion

1. **Patient position:** supine, with the knee slightly flexed and supported by a pillow.
2. **Physician position:** standing at the foot of the table, facing the patient.
3. **Technique:**
   a. With one hand, the physician grasps the anterior ankle, locking both malleoli.
   b. With the other hand, he grasps the forefoot close to but not on the talus.
   c. The physician inverts the forefoot and, while maintaining this position, places the foot into dorsi-flexion and then plantar–flexion (Fig. 96-1).
   d. Note degrees and freedom of motions as compared with the other foot.

### Abduction–Adduction (Subtalar)

1. **Patient position:** supine, with the knee slightly flexed and supported by a pillow.
2. **Physician position:** standing at the foot of the table, facing the patient.

3. **Technique:**
   a. The physician grasps the forefoot and places it into abduction and adduction (Fig. 96-2).
   b. Note degrees and freedom of motions as compared to the other foot.

### Calcaneal Inversion–Eversion

1. **Patient position:** supine, with the knee slightly flexed and supported by a pillow.
2. **Physician position:** standing at the foot of the table, facing the patient.

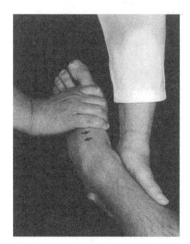

■ **FIG. 96-2** Motion testing for subtalar abduction–adduction.

3. **Technique:**
   a. The physician grasps the calcaneus in one hand. His other hand is on the forefoot, locking the talus.
   b. The physician inverts and everts the calcaneus on the talus (Fig. 96-3).
   c. Note degrees and freedom of motions as compared to the other foot.

## Cuboid Dysfunction

1. **Patient position:** prone.
2. **Physician position:** standing beside the table, with one knee on the table.
3. **Technique:**
   a. The patient's knee is flexed, with the foot resting on the physician's knee.
   b. The physician grasps the calcaneus with one hand, locking it.
   c. With the thumb and index finger of the other hand, the physician grasps the cuboid and moves it dorsally and ventrally (Fig. 96-4).
   d. Note degrees and freedom of motion as compared to the other foot.

## Fifth Metatarsal Dysfunction

1. **Patient position:** prone.
2. **Physician position:** standing beside the table, with one knee on the table.

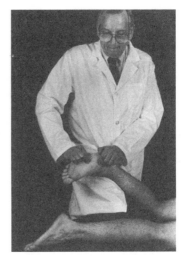

■ **FIG. 96-4** Motion testing for cuboid dysfunction.

3. **Technique:**
   a. The physician grasps the cuboid with one hand, locking it.
   b. With his other hand, he grasps the fifth metatarsal and moves it dorsally and ventrally (Fig. 96-5).
   c. To examine rotary motion of the metatarsal, the physician locks the fourth metatarsal and examines motion of the fifth. To examine motion of the fourth metatarsal, he locks the third metatarsal.
   d. Note degrees and freedom of motions as compared to the other foot.

## Navicular Dysfunction

1. **Patient position:** supine.
2. **Physician position:** seated at the foot of the

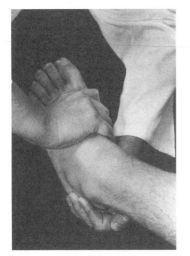

■ **FIG. 96-3** Motion testing for calcaneal inversion–eversion.

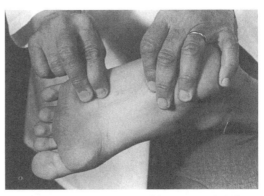

■ **FIG. 96-5** Motion testing for fifth metatarsal dysfunction.

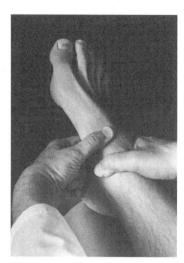

■ **FIG. 96-6** Motion testing for navicular dysfunction.

table with his back to the patient. The foot to be examined lies on a pillow on his lap.
3. **Technique:**
   a. The physician grasps the foot, including and locking the talus with one hand.
   b. With his other hand, he grasps the navicular and moves it dorsally and ventrally (Fig. 96-6).
   c. Note degrees and freedom of motions as compared to the other foot.

## Cuneiform Dysfunction

1. **Patient position:** supine.
2. **Physician position:** seated at the foot of the table with his back to the patient. The foot to be examined lies on a pillow on his lap.
3. **Technique:**
   a. The physician grasps and locks the navicular.
   b. The physician moves the cuneiform on the navicular

## First Metatarsal Dysfunction

1. **Patient position:** supine.
2. **Physician position:** seated at the foot of the table with his back to the patient. The foot to be examined lies on a pillow on his lap.

3. **Technique:**
   a. The physician grasps and locks the first cuneiform.
   b. He grasps the first metatarsal and moves it dorsally and ventrally.
   c. To examine for rotary motion of the metatarsals, the physician locks the second metatarsal to evaluate the first, and locks the third to evaluate the second.
   d. Note degrees and freedom of motions as compared to the other foot.

## Phalangeal Dysfunction

1. **Patient position:** supine.
2. **Physician position:** seated at the foot of the table with his back to the patient. The foot to be examined lies on a pillow on his lap.
3. **Technique:**
   a. The physician grasps the metatarsal and locks it with one hand.
   b. With his other hand, he grasps the first phalanx articulating with that metatarsal.
   c. After applying slight traction, the physician evaluates dorsal, ventral, abduction, adduction, and rotary motions (Fig. 96-7).
   d. Note degrees and freedom of motions as compared to the other foot.

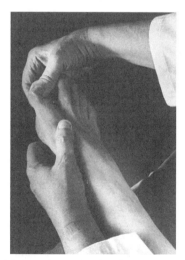

■ **FIG. 96-7** Motion testing for phalangeal dysfunction.

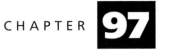

# Muscle Energy of the Lower Extremity

*Dennis J. Dowling*

**M**uscle energy treatment of the lower extremity is most easily performed with the patient in the supine or prone positions. However, by applying the principles of the modality, other positions are easily possible. Isolating the joint or muscle, placing it into its barrier, instructing the patient to push the extremity toward the freedom, and progressively challenging the altering barrier remain the steps for successful application. By convention, the description is the somatic dysfunction relative freedom (i.e., "flexion" indicates flexion freedom and extension barrier). The diagnoses listed in this chapter are according to joint and direction of motion. More specific adaptations can be performed for specific muscles.

## ■ HIP

1. **Flexion—Prone**
   a. **Patient position**: prone
   b. **Physician position**: physician stands on side opposite to the dysfunction at level of patient's legs facing the patient.
   c. **Technique**:
      (1) The physician's cephalad hand is placed on the patient's sacrum with his index finger at the posterior superior iliac spine of the side to be treated.
      (2) The physician's other hand reaches across the patient's legs and is placed anterior to the thigh above the knee.
      (3) The leg is extended at the hip until motion occurs at the ilium as moni-

tored by the physician's cephalad hand.
      (4) The patient is instructed to push his leg downward toward the table. The physician provides isometric resistance for 3 to 5 seconds.
      (5) The patient is instructed to relax for 3 to 5 seconds and then the physician repositions the patient into the new barrier.
      (6) The procedure is repeated until normal range of motion is accomplished or approximated.

2. **Flexion—Supine**
   a. **Patient position**: supine with lower legs off the end of the table and knees even with end of table.
   b. **Physician position**: physician stands on side to be treated at the end of the table.
   c. **Technique**:
      (1) The patient is instructed to flex both hips and knees and to use his arms to hug them toward his chest.
      (2) The patient is instructed to release the leg to be treated and allow the hip to extend and lower leg to hang off the end of the table while continuing to hug the other leg close to the chest.
      (3) The physician pushes the leg to be treated towards the table/floor.
      (4) The patient is instructed to push his leg upwards toward the ceiling. The physician provides isometric resistance for 3 to 5 seconds.

(5) The patient is instructed to relax for 3 to 5 seconds, and then the physician repositions the patient into the new barrier by pushing the leg further downward.

(6) The procedure is repeated until normal range of motion is accomplished or approximated.

3. **Extension**
   a. **Patient position**: supine
   b. **Physician position**: physician stands on the side of the dysfunction at level of patient's legs facing the patient.
   c. **Technique**:
   (1) The physician's cephalad hand is placed on the patient's anterior superior iliac spine of the side to be treated.
   (2) The physician's other hand holds the patient's leg above the ankle.
   (3) The leg is flexed at the hip until motion is limited. Occasionally, the patient's knee will bend. The barrier is just before this occurrs. The physician can support the patient's leg on his arm or shoulder.
   (4) The patient is instructed to push his leg downward toward the table. The physician provides isometric resistance for 3 to 5 seconds.
   (5) The patient is instructed to relax for 3 to 5 seconds, and then the physician repositions the patient into the new barrier.
   (6) The procedure is repeated until normal range of motion is accomplished or approximated.

4. **Adduction**
   a. **Patient position**: supine, closer to the opposite side of the table
   b. **Physician position**: physician stands at the foot of the table closer to the side to be treated.
   c. **Technique**:
   (1) The physician's hand is placed on the patient's knee or ankle on the non-treated side.
   (2) The physician's other hand holds the patient's leg to be treated above the ankle

(3) The leg to be treated is abducted until the limit of motion is limited palpated. The physician can stand in a position between the patient's legs as a means of resisting adduction of the side to be treated.

(4) The patient is instructed to push his leg medially towards the other leg. The physician provides isometric resistance for 3 to 5 seconds.

(5) The patient is instructed to relax for 3 to 5 seconds and then the physician repositions the patient into the new barrier.

(6) The procedure is repeated until normal range of motion is accomplished or approximated.

5. **Abduction**
   a. **Patient position**: supine, closer to the side of the table on the side to be treated
   b. **Physician position**: physician stands at the foot of the table closer to the side opposite to the side to be treated.
   c. **Technique**:
   (1) The physician's hand is placed on the patient's knee or ankle on the non-treated side.
   (2) The physician's other hand holds the patient's leg being treated above the ankle.
   (3) The leg to be treated is flexed enough to clear the other leg and then adducted until the limit of motion is palpated.
   (4) The patient is instructed to push his leg laterally. The physician provides isometric resistance for 3 to 5 seconds.
   (5) The patient is instructed to relax for 3 to 5 seconds, and then the physician repositions the patient into the new barrier.
   (6) The procedure is repeated until normal range of motion is accomplished or approximated.

6. **External Rotation—Supine**
   a. **Patient position**: supine
   b. **Physician position**: physician stands on the side of the dysfunction at level of patient's legs facing the patient.

c. **Technique**:
  (1) The patient's hip and knee are flexed to 90 degrees each.
  (2) The physician's cephalad hand stabilizes the patient's bent knee.
  (3) The physician's other hand pulls the patient's foot and leg laterally creating internal rotation.
  (4) The patient is instructed to push his foot medially. The physician provides isometric resistance for 3 to 5 seconds.
  (5) The patient is instructed to relax for 3 to 5 seconds and then the physician repositions the patient into the new barrier.
  (6) The procedure is repeated until normal range of motion is accomplished or approximated.

7. **External Rotation—Prone**
  a. **Patient position**: prone
  b. **Physician position**: physician stands on the side of the dysfunction at level of patient's legs facing the patient.
  c. **Technique**:
    (1) The patient's knee is flexed to 90 degrees.
    (2) The physician's cephalad hand stabilizes the patient's bent knee.
    (3) The physician's other hand pulls the patient's foot and leg laterally creating internal rotation.
    (4) The patient is instructed to push his foot medially. The physician provides isometric resistance for 3 to 5 seconds.
    (5) The patient is instructed to relax for 3 to 5 seconds, and then the physician repositions the patient into the new barrier.
    (6) The procedure is repeated until normal range of motion is accomplished or approximated.

8. **Internal Rotation—Supine**
  a. **Patient position**: supine
  b. **Physician position**: physician stands on the side of the dysfunction at level of patient's legs facing the patient.
  c. **Technique**:
    (1) The patient's hip and knee are flexed to 90 degrees each.

    (2) The physician's cephalad hand stabilizes the patient's bent knee.
    (3) The physician's other hand pushes the patient's foot and leg medially creating external rotation.
    (4) The patient is instructed to push his foot laterally. The physician provides isometric resistance for 3 to 5 seconds.
    (5) The patient is instructed to relax for 3 to 5 seconds and then the physician repositions the patient into the new barrier.
    (6) The procedure is repeated until normal range of motion is accomplished or approximated.

9. **Internal Rotation—Prone**
  a. **Patient position**: prone
  b. **Physician position**: physician stands on the side of the dysfunction at level of patient's legs facing the patient.
  c. **Technique**:
    (1) The patient's knee is flexed to 90 degrees.
    (2) The physician's cephalad hand stabilizes the patient's bent knee.
    (3) The physician's other hand pushes the patient's foot and leg medially and over the other leg creating external rotation.
    (4) The patient is instructed to push his foot laterally. The physician provides isometric resistance for 3 to 5 seconds.
    (5) The patient is instructed to relax for 3 to 5 seconds and then the physician repositions the patient into the new barrier.
    (6) The procedure is repeated until normal range of motion is accomplished or approximated.

## ■ KNEE

1. **Flexion**
  a. **Patient position**: supine
  b. **Physician position**: physician stands on the side of the dysfunction at level of patient's legs facing the patient.
  c. **Technique**:
    (1) The patient's knee is extended to the extent possible.

(2) The physician's cephalad hand stabilizes the patient's bent knee.

(3) The physician's other hand holds the patients leg above the ankle.

(4) The patient is instructed to bend his knee. The physician provides isometric resistance for 3 to 5 seconds.

(5) The patient is instructed to relax for 3 to 5 seconds, and then the physician repositions the patient into the new barrier.

(6) The procedure is repeated until normal range of motion is accomplished or approximated.

2. **Extension**
   a. **Patient position**: prone
   b. **Physician position**: physician stands on the side of the dysfunction at level of patient's legs facing the patient.
   c. **Technique**:
   (1) The patient's knee is flexed to the extent possible.
   (2) The physician's cephalad hand stabilizes the patient's bent knee.
   (3) The physician's other hand holds the patients leg above the ankle.
   (4) The patient is instructed to straighten his knee. The physician provides isometric resistance for 3 to 5 seconds.
   (5) The patient is instructed to relax for 3 to 5 seconds, and then the physician repositions the patient into the new barrier.
   (6) The procedure is repeated until normal range of motion is accomplished or approximated.

3. **Posterior Fibular Head**
   A posterior fibular head somatic dysfunction is accompanied by foot inversion, forefoot adduction, and lower leg internal rotation.

   a. **Patient position**: supine
   b. **Physician position**: physician stands on the side of the dysfunction at level of patient's legs facing the patient.
   c. **Technique**:
   (1) The patient's hip and knee are flexed to 90 degrees each.
   (2) The physician's cephalad hand stabilizes the patient's bent knee and holds the posterior fibular head between thumb and index finger (Figure 97-1).
   (3) The physician's other hand holds the patient's foot.
   (4) The physician everts and dorsiflexes the patient's foot and also creates external rotation of the lower leg.
   (5) The patient is instructed to push his foot medially. The physician provides isometric resistance for 3 to 5 seconds.
   (6) The patient is instructed to relax for 3 to 5 seconds, and then the physician repositions the patient into the new barriers.
   (7) The procedure is repeated until normal range of motion is accomplished or approximated.

4. **Anterior Fibular Head**
   An anterior fibular head is accompanied by foot eversion, forefoot abduction, and lower leg external rotation.

   a. **Patient position**: supine
   b. **Physician position**: physician stands on the side of the dysfunction at level of patient's legs facing the patient.
   c. **Technique**:
   (1) The patient's hip and knee are flexed to 90 degrees each.
   (2) The physician's cephalad hand stabilizes the patient's bent knee and holds the anterior fibular head with his thenar eminence.

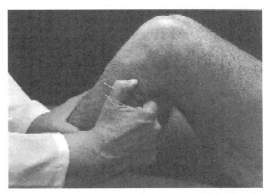

■ **FIG. 97-1** Muscle energy for posterior fibular head.

(3) The physician inverts the patient's foot and also creates internal rotation of the lower leg.

(4) The patient is instructed to push his foot laterally. The physician provides isometric resistance for 3 to 5 seconds.

(5) The patient is instructed to relax for 3 to 5 seconds and then the physician repositions the patient into the new barriers.

(6) The procedure is repeated until normal range of motion is accomplished or approximated.

## ■ ANKLE

1. **Dorsiflexion**
   a. **Patient position**: supine, seated, or prone
   b. **Physician position**: at level with foot to be treated
   c. **Technique**:
      (1) The physician grasps the patient's ankle with one hand at the level of the malleoli.
      (2) The physician's other hand is placed over the dorsum of the patient's foot (Fig. 97-2).
      (3) The patient's foot is brought into plantar flexion to the barrier.
      (4) The patient is instructed to push his foot into dorsiflexion. The physician provides isometric resistance for 3 to 5 seconds.

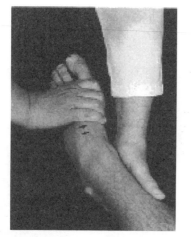

■ **FIG. 97-2** Muscle energy for ankle dorsiflexion dysfunction.

(5) The patient is instructed to relax for 3 to 5 seconds and then the physician repositions the patient into the new barriers.

(6) The procedure is repeated until normal range of motion is accomplished or approximated.

2. **Plantar Flexion**
   a. **Patient position**: supine, seated, or prone
   b. **Physician position**: at level with foot to be treated
   c. **Technique**:
      (1) The physician grasps the patient's ankle with one hand at the level of the malleoli.
      (2) The physician's other hand is placed under the plantar surface of the patient's foot.
      (3) The patient's foot is brought into dorsiflexion to the barrier.
      (4) The patient is instructed to push his foot into plantar flexion. The physician provides isometric resistance for 3 to 5 seconds.
      (5) The patient is instructed to relax for 3 to 5 seconds, and then the physician repositions the patient into the new barriers.
      (6) The procedure is repeated until normal range of motion is accomplished or approximated.

3. **Subtalar Adduction**
   a. **Patient position**: supine, seated, or prone
   b. **Physician position**: at level with foot to be treated
   c. **Technique**:
      (1) The physician grasps the patient's leg at the ankle with one hand.
      (2) The physician's other hand is placed the patient's heel.
      (3) The patient's calcaneus is deviated laterally to the barrier.
      (4) The patient is instructed to push his foot medially. The physician provides isometric resistance for 3 to 5 seconds.
      (5) The patient is instructed to relax for 3 to 5 seconds, and then the physician repositions the patient into the new barriers.

(6) The procedure is repeated until normal range of motion is accomplished or approximated.

4. **Subtalar Abduction**
   a. **Patient position**: supine, seated, or prone.
   b. **Physician position**: at level with foot to be treated.
   c. **Technique**:
      (1) The physician grasps the patient's leg at the ankle with one hand.
      (2) The physician's other hand is placed the patient's heel.
      (3) The patient's calcaneus is deviated medially to the barrier.
      (4) The patient is instructed to push his foot laterally. The physician provides isometric resistance for 3 to 5 seconds.
      (5) The patient is instructed to relax for 3 to 5 seconds, and then the physician repositions the patient into the new barriers.
      (6) The procedure is repeated until normal range of motion is accomplished or approximated.

5. **Calcaneal Eversion**
   a. **Patient position**: supine, seated, or prone.
   b. **Physician position**: at level with foot to be treated.
   c. **Technique**:
      (1) The physician grasps the patient's heel with one hand.
      (2) The physician's other hand is grasps the patient's forefoot.
      (3) The patient's calcaneus is deviated medially to the barrier (Fig. 97-3).
      (4) The patient is instructed to push his heel laterally. The physician provides isometric resistance for 3 to 5 seconds.
      (5) The patient is instructed to relax for 3 to 5 seconds, and then the physician repositions the patient into the new barriers.
      (6) The procedure is repeated until normal range of motion is accomplished or approximated.

6. **Calcaneal Inversion**
   a. **Patient position**: supine, seated, or prone
   b. **Physician position**: at level with foot to be treated.

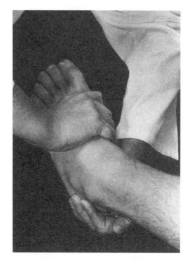

■ **FIG. 97-3** Muscle energy for calcaneal eversion.

   c. **Technique**:
      (1) The physician grasps the patient's heel with one hand.
      (2) The physician's other hand is grasps the patient's forefoot.
      (3) The patient's calcaneus is deviated laterally to the barrier.
      (4) The patient is instructed to push his heel medially. The physician provides isometric resistance for 3 to 5 seconds.
      (5) The patient is instructed to relax for 3 to 5 seconds, and then the physician repositions the patient into the new barriers.
      (6) The procedure is repeated until normal range of motion is accomplished or approximated.

## ■ FOOT

1. **Forefoot Dorsiflexion**
   a. **Patient position**: supine, seated, or prone.
   b. **Physician position**: at level with foot to be treated.
   c. **Technique**:
      (1) The physician grasps the patient's heel with one hand.
      (2) The physician's other hand is placed over the dorsum of the patient's foot.
      (3) The patient's foot is brought into plantar flexion to the barrier.

(4) The patient is instructed to push his foot into dorsiflexion. The physician provides isometric resistance for 3 to 5 seconds.

(5) The patient is instructed to relax for 3 to 5 seconds, and then the physician repositions the patient into the new barriers.

(6) The procedure is repeated until normal range of motion is accomplished or approximated.

2. **Forefoot Plantar Flexion**
   a. **Patient position**: supine, seated, or prone.
   b. **Physician position**: at level with foot to be treated.
   c. **Technique**:
      (1) The physician grasps the patient's heel with one hand.
      (2) The physician's other hand is placed under the plantar surface of the patient's foot.
      (3) The patient's foot is brought into dorsiflexion to the barrier.
      (4) The patient is instructed to push his foot into plantar flexion. The physician provides isometric resistance for 3 to 5 seconds.
      (5) The patient is instructed to relax for 3 to 5 seconds, and then the physician repositions the patient into the new barriers.
      (6) The procedure is repeated until normal range of motion is accomplished or approximated.

3. **Phalangeal Plantar Flexion**
   a. **Patient position**: supine, seated, or prone
   b. **Physician position**: at level with foot to be treated.
   c. **Technique**:
      (1) The physician grasps the patient's foot at the metatarsal head with the thumb and fingers of one hand just proximal to the phalanx to be treated.
      (2) The physician's other hand holds the phalanx to be treated.
      (3) The patient's toe is brought into dorsiflexion to the barrier.
      (4) The patient is instructed to push his toe into plantar flexion. The physician

provides isometric resistance for 3 to 5 seconds.

(5) The patient is instructed to relax for 3 to 5 seconds, and then the physician repositions the patient into the new barriers.

(6) The procedure is repeated until normal range of motion is accomplished or approximated.

4. **Phalangeal Dorsiflexion**
   a. **Patient position**: supine, seated, or prone.
   b. **Physician position**: at level with foot to be treated.
   c. **Technique**:
      (1) The physician grasps the patient's foot at the metatarsal head with the thumb and fingers of one hand just proximal to the phalanx to be treated.
      (2) The physician's other hand holds the phalanx to be treated.
      (3) The patient's toe is brought into to the plantar flexion barrier (Figure 97-4).
      (4) The patient is instructed to push his toe into dorsiflexion. The physician provides isometric resistance for 3 to 5 seconds.
      (5) The patient is instructed to relax for 3 to 5 seconds, and then the physician repositions the patient into the new barriers.

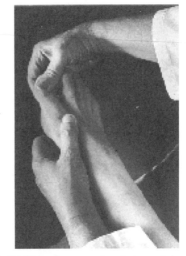

■ **FIG. 97-4** Muscle energy for phalangeal dorsiflexion.

(6) The procedure is repeated until normal range of motion is accomplished or approximated.

5. **Phalangeal Adduction or Abduction**
   a. **Patient position**: supine, seated, or prone.
   b. **Physician position**: at level with foot to be treated.
   c. **Technique**:
      (1) The physician grasps the patient's foot at the metatarsal head with the thumb and fingers of one hand just proximal to the phalanx to be treated.
      (2) The physician's other hand holds the phalanx to be treated.
      (3) The patient's toe is brought into to the adduction or abduction barrier.
      (4) The patient is instructed to push his toe into direction opposite the barrier, the freedom direction. The physician provides isometric resistance for 3 to 5 seconds.
      (5) The patient is instructed to relax for 3 to 5 seconds, and then the physician repositions the patient into the new barriers.
      (6) The procedure is repeated until normal range of motion is accomplished or approximated.

## REFERENCES

DiGiovanna EL, Schiowitz S. *An Osteopathic Approach to Diagnosis and Treatment, 2nd ed.* Philadelphia: Lippincott-Raven, 1997:339-360

Graham K. *Outline of Muscle Energy Techniques.* Tulsa, OK: Oklahoma College of Osteopathic Medicine, 1985.

Mitchell FL Jr, Moran PS, Pruzzo NA. *An Evaluation and Treatment Manual of Osteopathic Muscle Energy Procedures.* Valley Park, MO: Mitchell, Moran, and Pruzzo Associates, 1979.

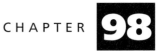

# Counterstrain Treatment for Lower Extremities

*Eileen L. DiGiovanna*

## ■ HIP

Three significant tender points are associated with the hip joint (Fig. 98-1). One might also consider the piriformis tender point when treating hip pain. The piriformis tender point is most closely associated with sacral dysfunctions and was discussed in Chapter 62, but because of its attachment to the posterior lateral trochanter, it is often interpreted as hip pain. Often it is necessary to treat the body of the piriformis tender point to relieve the trochanteric point.

### Posterolateral Trochanteric Tender Point

This point needs to be looked for whenever there is a piriformis syndrome or with a tender point in the belly of the piriformis muscle.

1. **Tender point:** on the posterolateral surface of the greater trochanter.
2. **Patient position:** prone.
3. **Physician position:** standing or seated beside the table.
4. **Technique:**
   a. The physician monitors the tender point with the finger of one hand.
   b. The patient's hip is extended and abducted (Fig. 98-2) until softening of the tissues of the tender point occurs and the point is no longer tender.
   c. External rotation may be needed.
   d. The position is held for 90 seconds and then the leg is returned to a neutral position and the tender point is reassessed.

### Lateral Trochanteric Tender Point

1. **Tender point:** 5 to 6 inches below the trochanter on the lateral thigh.
2. **Patient position:** prone.
3. **Physician position:** standing or seated beside the table.
4. **Technique:**
   a. The physician monitors the tender point with one hand.
   b. The patient's leg is abducted until the tissues of the tender point soften and the tender point is no longer tender (Fig. 98-3).
   c. Some flexion may be introduced as needed.
   d. The position is held of 90 seconds and then the leg is returned to a neutral position and the tender point reassessed.

### Posteromedial Trochanteric Tender Point

1. **Tender point:** 2 to 3 inches below the trochanter along posterior shaft of femur over to the ischial tuberosity.
2. **Patient position:** prone.
3. **Physician position:** standing beside the table, opposite the tender point.
4. **Technique:**
   a. The physician monitors the tender point with the finger of one hand.
   b. The patient's thigh is extended, adducted, and externally rotated (Fig. 98-4) until the

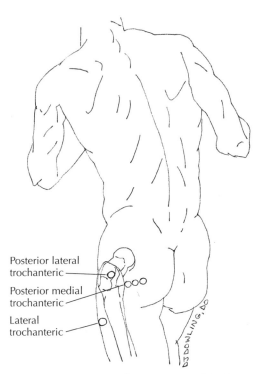

■ **FIG. 98-1** Location of tender points of the hips.

Posterior lateral trochanteric

Posterior medial trochanteric

Lateral trochanteric

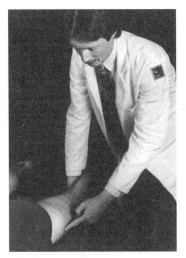

■ **FIG. 98-3** Counterstrain treatment for the lateral trochanteric tender point.

tissues of the tender point soften and the point is no longer tender.

c. The position is held for 90 seconds and then the leg is returned to a neutral position and the tender point is reassessed.

## ■ KNEE

The locations of the tender points around the knee are shown in Figure 98-5.

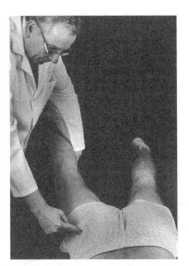

■ **FIG. 98-2** Counterstrain treatment for the posterolateral trochanteric tender point.

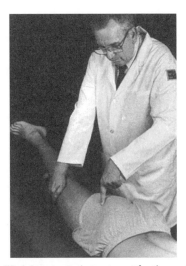

■ **FIG. 98-4** Counterstrain treatment for the posteromedial trochanteric tender point.

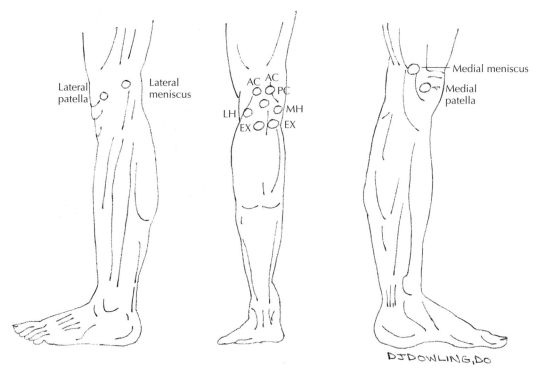

■ **FIG. 98-5** Location of the tender points around the knee. *PAT*, patellar; *LM*, lateral meniscus; *LH*, lateral hamstring; *MM*, medial meniscus; *MH*, medial hamstring; *EX*, gastrocnemius; *AC*, anterior cruciate; *PC*, posterior cruciate.

## Anterior Tender Points

### Medial or lateral patellar tender point

1. **Tender point:** on the patellar tendon just below the patella.
2. **Patient position:** supine.
3. **Physician position:** standing beside the table.
4. **Technique:**
   a. A rolled pillow is placed beneath the patient's calf near the ankle.
   b. The physician monitors the tender point with the finger of one hand.
   c. The knee is hyperextended by the physician pressing down on the anterior thigh just above the patella with a fair amount of force until the tissues have softened and the point is no longer tender (Fig. 98-6).
   d. The foot is internally rotated as needed.
   e. The position is held for 90 seconds and then the pressure is released and the tender point is reassessed.

## Medial and Lateral Patellar Tender Points

1. **Tender points:** on the medial or lateral surface of the patella.
2. **Patient position:** supine.
3. **Physician position:** standing at the side of the table.

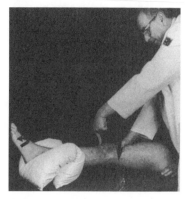

■ **FIG. 98-6** Counterstrain treatment of patellar tender point.

4. **Technique:**
   a. The physician monitors the tender point with the finger of one hand.
   b. The patient's patella is pushed laterally for a lateral tender point or medially for a medial tender point. Softening of the tender point should be felt and the tender point should no longer be tender.
   c. This position is held for 90 seconds and then the pressure is released and the tender point is reassessed.

## Posterior Tender Points

### Anterior Cruciate Tender Point

1. **Tender point:** on either the medial or lateral hamstring in the upper popliteal area.
2. **Patient position:** prone.
3. **Physician position:** standing beside the table.
4. **Technique:**
   a. The physician monitors the tender point with the finger of one hand.
   b. A rolled pillow is placed under the thigh of the involved leg.
   c. The physician presses down on the lower leg just below the joint with a large amount of force (Fig. 98-7). This technique shortens the anterior cruciate ligaments. Softening of the tender point should be felt and the tender point should no longer be tender.
   d. The position is held for 90 seconds and then the pressure is released and the tender point is reassessed.

### Posterior Cruciate Tender Point

1. **Tender point:** in the center of the popliteal fossa.
2. **Patient position:** supine.
3. **Physician position:** standing beside the table.
4. **Technique:**
   a. A rolled pillow is placed under the calf behind below the knee joint.
   b. The physician monitors the tender point with the finger of one hand.
   c. The physician presses down on the dorsum of the ankle with a large amount of force.
   d. The foot is internally rotated as needed (Fig. 98-8). This maneuver shortens the posterior cruciate ligament. Softening of the tissues should be felt and the tender point should no longer be tender.
   e. The position is held for 90 seconds and then the pressure is released and the tender point is reassessed.

### Gastrocnemius Tender Point

1. **Tender point:** lateral and medial attachments of the gastrocnemius muscle in the lower popliteal fossa.
2. **Patient position:** prone.
3. **Physician position:** standing beside the table with his foot on the table.

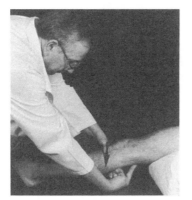

■ **FIG. 98-7** Counterstrain treatment for the anterior cruciate ligament tender point.

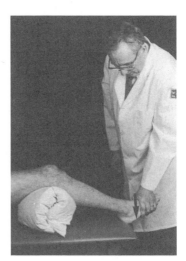

■ **FIG. 98-8** Counterstrain treatment for the posterior cruciate ligament tender point.

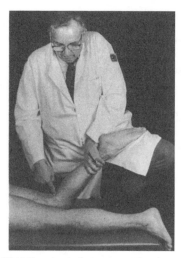

■ **FIG. 98-9** Counterstrain treatment for the gastrocnemius tender point.

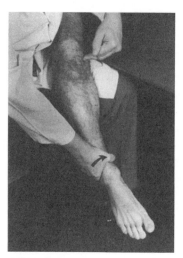

■ **FIG. 98-10** Counterstrain treatment for the medial meniscus tender point.

4. **Technique:**
   a. The physician monitors the tender point with the finger of one hand.
   b. The physician flexes the patient's knee and the foot is hyperextended over the physician's knee by a downward force on the posterior ankle (Fig. 98-9). This maneuver shortens the gastrocnemius muscle. Softening of the tissues should be felt and the tender point should no longer be tender.
   c. The position is held for 90 seconds and then the pressure is released. The leg is returned to a neutral position and then the tender point is reassessed.

## Medial Tender Points

### Medial meniscus tender point

1. **Tender point:** along the medial joint line, posterior to the medial patella.
2. **Patient position:** supine, involved leg off the table.
3. **Physician position:** seated beside the table.
4. **Technique:**
   a. The physician monitors the tender point with the finger of one hand.
   b. The physician grasps the patient's foot and internally rotates the lower leg, keeping the knee flexed to approximately 40 degrees.
   c. The knee is adducted slightly against the edge of the table (Fig. 98-10). Softening

of the tissues should be felt and the tender point should no longer be tender.
   d. The position is held for 90 seconds and then the leg is returned to a neutral position and the tender point is reassessed.

### Medial Hamstring Tender Point

1. **Tender point:** on the medial hamstring muscle near its distal attachment.
2. **Patient position:** supine.
3. **Physician position:** standing beside the table.
4. **Technique:**
   a. The physician monitors the tender point with the finger of one hand.
   b. The knee is flexed to approximately 60 degrees.
   c. The leg is externally rotated with a slight amount of adduction. This may be accomplished by grasping the patient's foot or ankle to use it as a lever. Softening of the tissue should be felt and the tender point should no longer be tender.
   d. This position is held for 90 seconds and then the leg is returned to a neutral position and the tender point is reassessed.

## Lateral Tender Points

### Lateral meniscus tender point

1. **Tender point:** along the lateral joint line, posterior to the lateral patella.

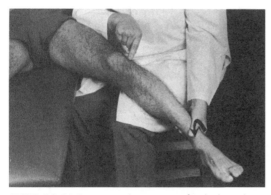

**■ FIG. 98-11** Counterstrain treatment for the lateral meniscus tender point.

2. **Patient position:** supine, with the leg off the table.
3. **Physician position:** seated beside the table.
4. **Technique:**
   a. The physician monitors the tender point with the finger of one hand.
   b. The leg is off the table with the knee slightly flexed.
   c. The physician grasps the patient's foot and internally rotates it (Fig. 98-11).
   d. The lower leg is slightly abducted. A softening of the tissues should be felt and the tender point should no longer be tender.
   e. Occasionally external rotation may be needed.
   f. The position is held for 90 seconds and then the leg is returned to a neutral position and the tender point is reassessed.

### Lateral Hamstring Tender Point

1. **Tender point:** on the lateral hamstring muscle at its attachment near the fibular head.
2. **Patient position:** supine, with the leg off the table.
3. **Physician position:** seated next to the table.
4. **Technique:**
   a. The physician monitors the tender point with the finger of one hand.
   b. The physician grasps the patient's foot and externally rotates it.
   c. The knee is flexed approximately 30 degrees and an abduction force is applied to the leg (Fig. 98-12).
   d. The position is held for 90 seconds and

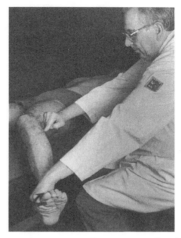

**■ FIG. 98-12** Counterstrain treatment for the lateral hamstring tender point.

then the leg is returned to a neutral position and the tender point is reassessed.

### ■ FOOT AND ANKLE

The locations of the tender points on the lateral and medial aspects of the ankle and the dorsum of the foot are shown in Figure 98-13. There is also a tender point on the sole of the foot at the distal end of the calcaneus (calcaveal tubercle).

### Calcaneal Tender Point

1. **Tender point:** distal end of the calcaneus on the sole of the foot.
2. **Patient position:** prone.
3. **Physician position:** standing at the side of the table with one knee resting on the table.
4. **Technique:**
   a. The patient's foot rests on the physician's knee.
   b. The physician monitors the tender point with the finger of one hand.
   c. The foot is plantar flexed against the physician's knee by downward pressure against the calcaneus while at the same time pushing it toward the toes until the tissues soften and the tender point is no longer tender (Fig. 98-14).
   d. The position is held for 90 seconds and then the pressure is released and the foot returned to a neutral position.
   e. The tender point is reassessed.

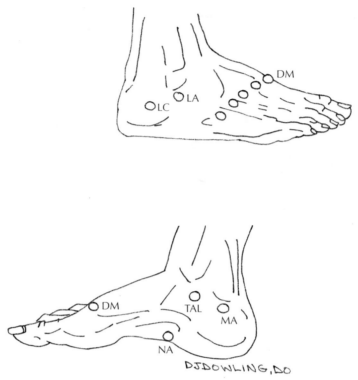

■ **FIG. 98-13** Locations of foot and ankle tender points. *DM,* dorsal metatarsal; *MA,* medial ankle; *LA,* lateral ankle; *TAL,* talus; *DC,* dorsal cuboid; *NA,* navicular; *LC,* lateral calcaneal.

## Dorsal Metatarsal Tender Points

1. **Tender points:** at the proximal ends of the metatarsals across the dorsum of the foot.
2. **Patient position:** prone, with knee flexed to 90 degrees.

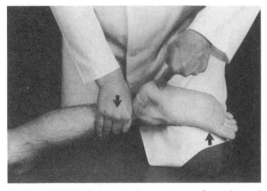

■ **FIG. 98-14** Counterstrain treatment for calcaneal tender point.

3. **Physician position:** standing beside the table.
4. **Technique:**
   a. The physician monitors the tender point with the finger of one hand.
   b. The physician strongly dorsiflexes the foot by putting a downward pressure on it (Fig. 98-15) until the tissues soften and the tender point is no longer tender.
   c. The position is held for 90 seconds and then the foot and leg are returned to a neutral position and the tender point is reassessed.

## Medial Ankle Tender Point

1. **Tender point:** below medial malleolus and slightly posterior on the medial calcaneus.
2. **Patient position:** lying on his side with the involved leg up.
3. **Physician position:** seated beside the table.

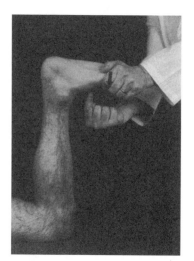

**FIG. 98-15** Counterstrain treatment for dorsal metatarsal tender points

## Lateral Ankle Tender Point

1. **Tender point:** below the lateral malleolus.
2. **Patient position:** lying on his side with the involved leg up.
3. **Physician position:** seated beside the table.
4. **Technique:**
   a. The physician monitors the tender point with the finger of one hand.
   b. The patient's foot is brought off the table.
   c. A rolled towel is placed under the anterior ankle.
   d. The physician everts the foot forcefully until the tissues soften and the tender point is no longer tender (Fig. 98-17).
   e. The position is held for 90 seconds and then the pressure is released. The foot and leg are then returned to a neutral position and the tender point is reassessed.

## Talar Tender Point

1. **Tender point:** on the anteromedial ankle deep to the talus.
2. **Patient position:** supine with the toes pointing upward.
3. **Physician position:** seated at the foot of the table.
4. **Technique:**
   a. The physician monitors the tender point with the finger of one hand.
   b. The foot is dorsiflexed, inverted, and internally rotated until the tissue softens and the tender point is no longer tender (Fig. 98-18).
   c. The position is held for 90 seconds and then the foot and leg are returned to a

4. **Technique:**
   a. The physician monitors the tender point with the finger of one hand.
   b. The patient's foot is brought off the table
   c. A rolled towel is placed under the anterior ankle.
   d. The physician inverts the foot by pressing forcefully on the lateral side of the foot until the tissue softens and the tender point is no longer tender (Fig. 98-16).
   e. The position is held for 90 seconds and then the pressure is released and the foot and leg are returned to a neutral position and the tender point is reassessed.

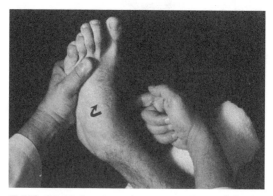

**FIG. 98-16** Counterstrain treatment for medial ankle tender point.

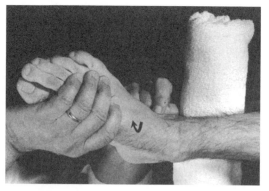

**FIG. 98-17** Counterstrain treatment for lateral ankle tender point.

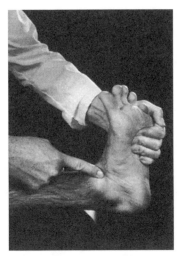

■ **FIG. 98-18** Counterstrain treatment for talus tender point.

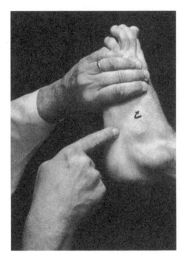

■ **FIG. 98-19** Counterstrain treatment for dorsal cuboid tender point.

neutral position and the tender point is reassessed.

## Dorsal Cuboid Tender Point

1. **Tender point:** on the lateral dorsum of the foot over the superior surface of the cuboid.
2. **Patient position:** supine.
3. **Physician position:** standing beside the table.
4. **Technique:**
   a. The physician monitors the tender point with the finger of one hand.
   b. The physician grasps the patient's foot and inverts it by applying pressure on the lateral side until the tissues soften and the tender point is no longer tender (Fig. 98-19).
   c. The position is held for 90 seconds and then the foot is returned to a neutral position and the tender point is reassessed.

## Navicular Tender Point

1. **Tender point:** on the medial arch of the foot over the navicular bone.
2. **Patient position:** supine.
3. **Physician position:** seated or standing beside the table.

4. **Technique:**
   a. The physician monitors the tender point with the finger of one hand.
   b. The physician places his thumb or two fingers over the navicular bone to cause an inversion of the navicular.
   c. A slight amount of flexion is used until the tissues soften and the tender point is no longer tender (Fig. 98-20).
   d. The position is held for 90 seconds and then the pressure is released and the foot returned to a neutral position and the tender point is reassessed.

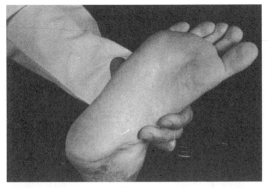

■ **FIG. 98-20** Counterstrain treatment for navicular tender point.

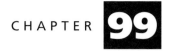

# Facilitated Positional Release of the Lower Extremities

*Stanley Schiowitz*

## ■ HIP

### Muscle Hypertonicity (Tenderness) of the Right Hip

1. **Patient position**: supine on the table with both legs fully extended.
2. **Physician's position**: standing at the right side of the table and facing towards the patient's head.
3. **Technique**:
   a. The physician places a finger of his left hand on the hypertonic muscle to monitor the motion and tissue changes.
   b. The physician uses his right hand to flex the patient's right hip joint to 90 degrees.
   c. The physician pushes the patient's right leg downward toward the table causing a compressive force, felt at the monitoring finger. In some instances, it might be easier for the physician to lean his weight on the patient's right knee to create the compressive force.
   d. The physician places the patient's leg into abduction and external rotation, up to his monitoring finger. He should feel a release of the hypertonicity (Fig. 99-1).
   e. Hold the position for 3 to 5 seconds, release, and re-evaluate.

*Note:* If the hypertonic muscle is located above the midline of the hip joint, the flexion used is reduced accordingly. If the hypertonic muscle is below the mid-line of the hip joint, the hip flexion is increased accordingly. If the hypertonicity is located medial to the mid-line of the hip joint, the final motions are adduction and internal rotation.

## ■ KNEE

### Muscle Hypertonicity (Point Tenderness) of the Knee at the Level of and Medial to the Midpoint of the Knee Joint (Left)

1. **Patient position**: prone on the table, with both legs in full extension.
2. **Physician's position**: standing besides the table, alongside the patient's left leg, and facing toward the patient's head.
3. **Technique**:
   a. The physician places one finger of his left hand on the hypertonic muscle to monitor the motion and tissue changes.
   b. The physician uses his right hand to flex the patient's left knee to 90 degrees.
   c. The physician pushes the patient's left leg downward toward the table causing a compressive force, felt at the monitoring finger.
   d. The physician adducts and internally rotates the patient's left leg up to the monitoring finger. He should feel a release of the hypertonicity (Fig. 99-2).
   e. Hold the position for 3 to 5 second, release, and re-evaluate.

*Note*: The amount of flexion and whether abduction–external rotation or adduction–inter-

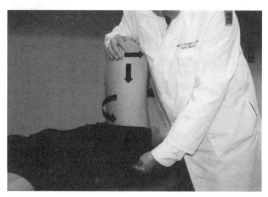

■ **FIG. 99-1** Facilitated positional release treatment for hypertonicity at the lateral aspect of the right hip.

nal rotation is applied will be the same as for the hip joint.

## ■ ANKLE AND FOOT

### Muscle Hypertonicity (Tenderness) of the Ankle Joint at the Midpoint and on Its Medial Aspect (Left)

1. **Patient position**: prone on the table with both legs fully extended.
2. **Physician's position**: standing at the left side of the table and facing toward the patient's head.
3. **Technique**:
   a. The physician has the patient flex the left knee up to 90 degrees.
   b. The physician places one finger of his left hand on the hypertonic muscle to monitor motion and tissue changes.

c. The physician uses his right hand to push the foot directly downward to create a compressive force of the ankle joint, felt at the monitoring finger.
   d. The physician places the ankle joint into internal rotation and side bending in a medial direction, up to the monitoring finger. He should feel release of the hypertonicity (Fig. 99-3).
   e. Hold the position for 3 to 5 seconds, release, and re-evaluate.

*Note*: As noted, the motions should be modified toward the monitoring finger, either side bending medially with internal rotation or laterally with external rotation.

### Hypertonicity (Point Tenderness) of the Foot (Left)

1. **Patient position**: prone on the table with both legs in full extension.
2. **Physician's position**: standing at the left side of the table and facing toward the table.
3. **Technique**:
   a. The physician places a finger of his right hand on the hypertonic muscle to monitor motion and tissue changes.
   b. The physician places the rest of his right hand around the forefoot and his left hand grasps the patient's heel.
   c. The physician brings both of his hands towards each other creating a compressive force up to the monitoring finger.
   d. The physician uses both of his hands to create a side-bending of the foot laterally

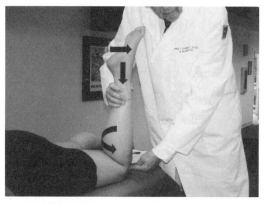

■ **FIG. 99-2** Facilitated positional release treatment for hypertonicity at the lateral aspect of the left knee.

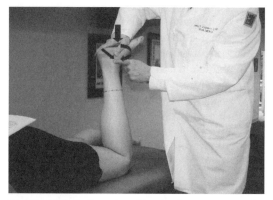

■ **FIG. 99-3** Facilitated positional release treatment for hypertonicity at the lateral aspect of the left ankle joint.

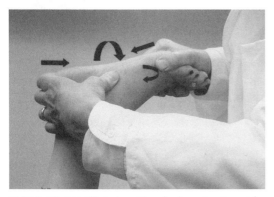

■ **FIG. 99-4** Facilitated positional release treatment for hypertonicity at the lateral aspect of the left foot.

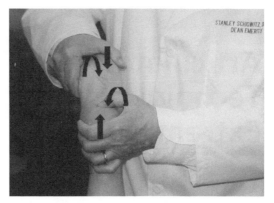

■ **FIG. 99-5** Facilitated positional release treatment for hypertonicity of the plantar fascia of the left foot.

to the monitoring finger and then adds external rotation of the forefoot until a release of the hypertonicity is felt (Fig. 99-4).

e. Hold the position for 3 to 5 seconds, release and reevaluate.

*Note:* If the hypertonicity is on the *plantar fascia*, the monitoring finger is placed at the site on the plantar aspect of the foot, the compression is applied as mentioned and followed by both hands creating a flexion of the plantar aspect of the foot up to the monitoring finger, and then side-bending the foot medially or laterally, depending on whether the hypertonicity is medial or lateral to the mid-point of the plantar aspect of the foot (Fig. 99-5).

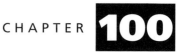

# Articulatory and Thrusting Techniques for the Lower Extremities

*Eileen L. DiGiovanna and Barry Erner*

Thrusting techniques are more useful for some extremity joints than for others. Thrusting of the hip joint, for example, is not commonly performed. The more common techniques are included in this chapter.

## ■ KNEE

Fibular head somatic dysfunctions are the commonly seen somatic dysfunctions of the knee. They are often the cause of lateral knee pain.

### Anterior Fibular Head Somatic Dysfunction

1. **Patient position:** supine.
2. **Physician position:** standing beside the table, on the same side as the dysfunction.
3. **Technique:**
   a. The physician grasps the patient's foot on the side of the somatic dysfunction with his non-thrusting hand. The foot is inverted, internally rotated, and slightly plantar flexed.
   b. The physician places the thenar eminence of his thrusting hand over the anterolateral aspect of the fibular head.
   c. The patient's knee is placed in the close-packed position and then slightly flexed.
   d. The physician exerts a rapid knee extension while simultaneously. introducing a downward and medial thrust through the fibular head (Fig. 100-1).

   e. Slight internal rotation of the tibia facilitates the motion.

### Posterior Fibular Head Somatic Dysfunction

1. **Patient position:** supine.
2. **Physician position:** standing beside the table, opposite the dysfunction.
3. **Technique:**
   a. The physician grasps the patient's foot and ankle on the side of the dysfunction with his non-thrusting hand.
   b. The physician flexes the patient's hip and knee to 90 degrees.
   c. The physician places the index finger of his thrusting hand into the patient's popliteal crease, monitoring the dysfunctional fibular head with his metacarpalphalangeal joint.
   d. The physician locks the patient's foot on the side of the dysfunction into eversion, dorsiflexion, and external rotation. This may be held by the physician's hand or in his axilla.
   e. The physician exerts a rapid knee flexion by a downward thrust on the distal tibia and fibula while simultaneously pulling the fibular head anteriorly with his index finger (Fig. 100-2).
   f. Slight external rotation of the tibia facilitates the motion.

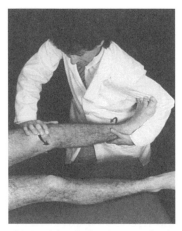

■ **FIG. 100-1** High-velocity, low-amplitude thrusting technique for an anterior fibular head dysfunction.

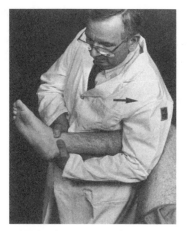

■ **FIG. 100-3** Combination articulatory treatment of the knee and ankle using long-axis traction.

## ■ COMBINED KNEE AND ANKLE—LONG-AXIS EXTENSION

This technique is a combination of myofascial ligamentous release and articulation of both the knee and ankle joints. It is especially useful when both the knee and ankle joints of the same leg are involved. It is designed to improve motion without a thrust.

1. **Patient position:** supine with the hip and knee on the side of the dysfunction in 90 degrees of flexion.
2. **Physician position:** standing beside the table on the side of the dysfunction, facing the foot of the table.
3. **Technique:**
   a. The physician places his flexed elbow (closer to the table) in the patient's popli-

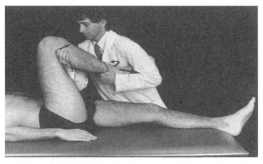

■ **FIG. 100-2** High-velocity, low-amplitude thrusting technique for a posterior fibular head somatic dysfunction. (Physician is on opposite side to allow viewing of hand positions.)

teal space and grasps the calcaneus with that hand.
   b. With his other hand, the physician grasps the anterior aspect of the patient's ankle at the talus. A small towel or pillow can be inserted between the physician's elbow and patient's thigh for comfort or if the patient's leg is longer than the physician's arm.
   c. As the physician rocks backward, his elbow should separate the femur from the tibia, while his hand on the calcaneus and talus should separate the talus from the crural arch (Fig. 100-3).
   d. This position can be held for 3 seconds, then the physician rocks forward to relax the traction force.
   e. Rest and repeat the maneuver.

## ■ ANKLE

### Eversion–Inversion Somatic Dysfunction of the Ankle

1. **Patient position:** supine.
2. **Physician position:** standing at the foot of the table.
3. **Technique:**
   a. The physician grasps the patient's foot on the side of the dysfunction, placing one hand on the dorsal mid-tarsal region and using the other to grasp the calcaneus.
   b. The physician applies traction to the patient's leg (Fig. 100-4).

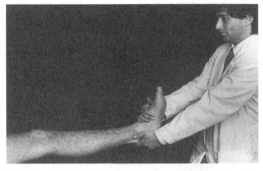

■ **FIG. 100-4** High-velocity, low-amplitude thrusting technique for an eversion–inversion ankle somatic dysfunction.

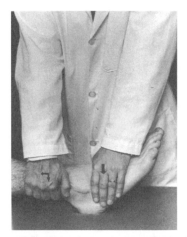

■ **FIG. 100-5** High-velocity, low-amplitude thrusting technique for tibiocalcaneal somatic dysfunction.

c. If an inversion somatic dysfunction (i.e., eversion restriction) is present, the physician exerts rapid long axis traction through the calcaneus with simultaneous hypereversion of the ankle.

d. If an eversion somatic dysfunction (i.e., inversion restriction) is present, the physician exerts traction through the calcaneus while simultaneously hyperinverting the ankle.

## Tibiocalcaneal Somatic Dysfunction

1. **Patient position:** supine.
2. **Physician position:** standing beside the table on the side of the somatic dysfunction.
3. **Technique:**
   a. The physician cups the patient's tibia and fibula with one hand and places the thenar eminence of the other hand over the dorsum of the patient's forefoot.
   b. The physician applies traction cephalad on the patient's leg, through the tibia/fibula.
   c. The physician exerts traction and a rapid posterior thrust through the hand on the patient's forefoot. The physician's other hand stabilizes the ankle joint (Fig. 100-5).

## ■ FOOT

## Metatarsal Somatic Dysfunction

1. **Patient position:** supine.
2. **Physician position:** standing beside the table on the side of the somatic dysfunction.
3. **Technique:**
   a. The physician grasps the patient's involved foot and places the pads of his thumbs, fac-

ing one another, over the junction of the metatarsal somatic dysfunction.

b. The physician exerts a downward thrust through the thumbs, separating the joint articulation (Fig. 100-6).

## Transtarsal Somatic Dysfunction

1. **Patient position:** supine.
2. **Physician position:** standing beside the table on the side of the somatic dysfunction.
3. **Technique:**
   a. The physician places the patient's knee in flexion, abduction, and external rotation.
   b. The physician places the thenar eminence of one hand over the calcaneus; the other hand is placed over the first metatarsal and talus.
   c. The physician exerts a clockwise or counterclockwise rotary thrust with the hand

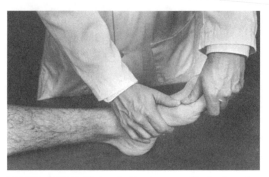

■ **FIG. 100-6** High-velocity, low-amplitude thrusting technique for metatarsal somatic dysfunction.

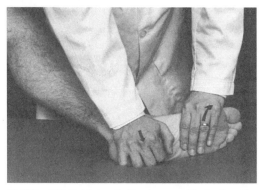

■ **FIG. 100-7** High-velocity, low-amplitude thrusting technique for transtarsal somatic dysfunction.

holding the talus while simultaneously exerting a downward thrust through the calcaneus with the other hand (Fig. 100-7).

## Modified Technique for Transtarsal Somatic Dysfunction

1. **Patient position:** supine with hip flexed, abducted, and externally rotated.
2. **Physician position:** standing beside the table.
3. **Technique:**
   a. The physician exerts a simultaneous downward, lateral, and rotary thrust with the hand over the calcaneus. His other hand stabilizes the foot (Fig. 100-8).

## Cuboid–Navicular Somatic Dysfunction

This technique is sometimes called the *Hiss whip technique* for J. M. Hiss, DO, who introduced it

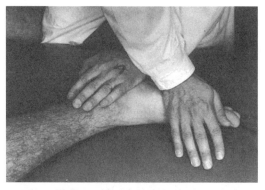

■ **FIG. 100-8** Modified high-velocity, low-amplitude thrusting technique for transtarsal somatic dysfunction.

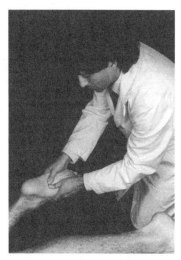

■ **FIG. 100-9** High-velocity, low-amplitude thrusting technique for a cuboid–navicular somatic dysfunction. (Hiss whip technique).

and for its whip-like thrust. It can be used for the navicular or the cuneiform bones.

1. **Patient position:** prone.
2. **Physician position:** standing beside the table on the side of the dysfunction.
3. **Technique:**
   a. The physician flexes the patient's hip and knee on the dysfunctional side and then drops the leg off the side of the table.
   b. The physician grasps the patient's foot with both hands and places his thumbs in a "V" shape over the plantar surface of the cuboid or navicular, whichever it is that is in a dropped position relative to the other metatarsals.
   c. The physician exerts a downward thrust through his thumbs while simultaneously inducing a whip-like action at the patient's ankle and knee (Fig. 100-9).
   d. A more medial thrust can be introduced for the medial tarsals and a lateral thrust is used for the lateral tarsals.

**REFERENCES**

DiGiovanna EL, Schiowitz S. *An Osteopathic Approach to Diagnosis and Treatment.* Philadelphia: Lippincott-Raven, 1997.

DiGiovanna EL. *An Encyclopedia of Osteopathy.* Indianapolis, IN: American Academy of Osteopathy, 2001.

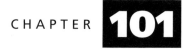

# Exercise Therapy for the Lower Extremity

*Stanley Schiowitz and Albert R. DeRubertis*

## ■ THE HIP

Related exercises are described in Chapter 67 ("Exercise Therapy for the Sacrum and Pelvis"). These exercises should be reviewed when prescribing exercise therapy for the hip.

### Muscle Stretch

A. **Groin muscle stretch** (Fig.101-1)
1. **Patient position:** standing, facing a firm support such as a table.
2. **Instructions:**
   a. Place the sole of the foot of the leg to be treated on the edge of the table (the left foot is used as an example). The other foot remains on the floor, with the knee fully extended.
   b. Flex your left hip and knee as you lean your body toward the table. Continue leaning until you have achieved maximum painless stretch of the left groin muscles.
   c. Hold this position for 5 to 15 seconds.
   d. Straighten out the left leg. Relax, rest, and repeat.
   e. The stretch should affect the muscles of the medial, anterior, and posterior groin. To stretch the right groin, repeat the exercise with your right foot on the table.

B. **Groin muscle stretch** (Fig. 101-2)
1. **Patient position:** standing, facing a firm support such as a table.

2. **Instructions:**
   a. Place the sole of the foot of the non-dysfunctional leg on the edge of the table (the left leg is used as an example). The right leg is fully extended with the foot on the floor and parallel to the table.
   b. Flex your left hip and knee as you lean your body toward the table. Continue leaning until you have achieved maximum painless stretch of the right medial groin muscles.
   c. Hold this position for 5 to 15 seconds.
   d. Straighten out the left leg. Relax, rest, and repeat.
   e. To stretch the left groin, repeat the exercise with your right foot on the table.

C. **Bilateral groin muscle stretch** (Fig. 101-3)
1. **Patient position:** seated on the floor, with the hips and knees flexed and the soles of the feet resting against each other. The hands hold the toes or ankles.
2. **Instructions:**
   a. Pull your body forward, bending from the hips, while keeping your back flat to avoid strain. Create a groin stretch.
   b. Place your elbows forward and resting on your legs. Lean on your elbows to push your thighs toward the floor.
   c. Hold a position of maximum painless stretch for 5 to 15 seconds.
   d. Relax, rest, and repeat.

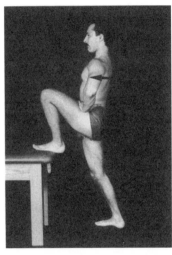

■ **FIG. 101-1** Groin muscle stretch.

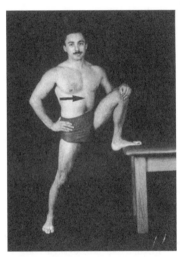

■ **FIG. 101-2** Groin muscle stretch.

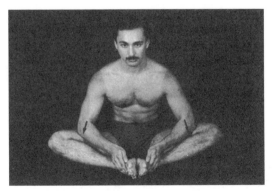

■ **FIG. 101-3** Bilateral groin muscle stretch.

## Muscle Strengthening

A. **Hip flexors** (Fig. 101-4)
1. **Patient position:** standing, holding on to a firm support that is behind the patient; or seated with the legs dangling off a high table. A 3- to 5-pound weight is attached to the ankle of the leg to be exercised.
2. **Instructions:**
   a. Slowly flex your knee and hip to 90 degrees.
   b. Hold this position for 5 to 15 seconds.
   c. Lower foot slowly to the floor.
   d. Relax, rest, and repeat.
B. **Hip extensors** (Fig. 101–5)
1. **Patient position:** standing, holding on to a firm support with the hand opposite the leg to be exercised, or prone. A 3- to 5-pound weight is attached to the ankle.
2. **Instructions:**
   a. Move your fully extended leg backward, keeping your low back flat.
   b. Hold this position for 5 to 15 seconds.
   c. Slowly return to the starting position.
   d. Relax, rest, and repeat.
C. **Hip abductors** (Fig. 101-6)
1. **Patient position:** standing, holding on to a firm support with hand opposite the leg to be exercised; or lying on the side. A 3- to 5-pound weight is attached to the ankle.

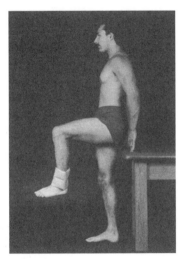

■ **FIG. 101-4** Hip flexor strengthening.

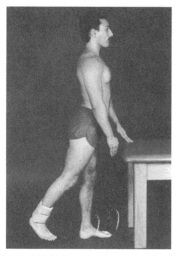

■ **FIG. 101-5** Hip extensor strengthening.

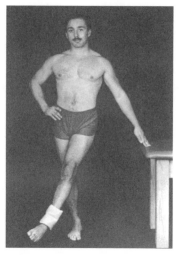

■ **FIG. 101-7** Hip adductor strengthening.

2. **Instructions:**
   a. Move the leg to be exercised directly sideways, fully extended, away from the midline of the body.
   b. Hold this position for 5 to 15 seconds.
   c. Slowly return to the starting position.
   d. Relax, rest, and repeat.
D. **Hip adductors** (Fig. 101-7)
   1. **Patient position:** standing, holding on to a firm support with the hand on the same side as the leg to be exercised. A 3- to 5-pound weight is attached to the ankle.

2. **Instructions:**
   a. Extend the leg to be exercised and move it in front of the other leg and across the midline of the body.
   b. Hold this position for 5 to 15 seconds.
   c. Slowly return to the starting position.
   d. Relax, rest, and repeat.
E. **Hip adductors** (Fig. 101-8)
   1. **Patient position:** lying on the side to be exercised. The upper leg rests on a box or a chair, 8 to 10 inches above the floor. A 3- to 5-pound weight is attached to the ankle.
   2. **Instructions:**
   a. Raise the leg to be exercised off the floor toward the other leg. Keep the leg fully extended.

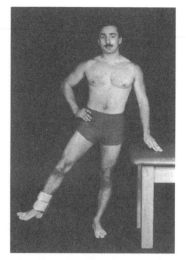

■ **FIG. 101-6** Hip abductor strengthening.

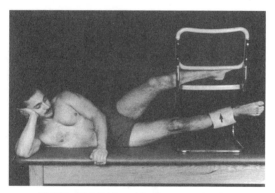

■ **FIG. 101-8** Hip adductor strengthening.

b. Hold for 5 to 15 seconds.

c. Slowly return to the starting position.

d. Relax, rest, and repeat.

## ■ THE KNEE

### Muscle Stretch

A. **Quadriceps** (Fig. 101-9)

1. **Patient position:** seated on a table with the hips and knees bent. The knee with contracted quadriceps will not fully flex to 90 degrees.

2. **Instructions:**

   a. Place increasingly heavier weights on the ankle, forcing the knee into flexion and quadriceps stretch. Or,

   b. Have someone push down on your leg slowly, creating quadriceps stretch.

   c. Hold for 5 to 15 seconds. Return to the starting position.

   d. Relax, rest, and repeat.

### Muscle Strengthening

A. **Knee flexors** (Fig. 101-10)

1. **Patient position:** standing, holding on to a support in front of the body. A 3- to 5-pound weight is attached to the ankle.

2. **Instructions:**

   a. Flex your knee as far as it will go. Keep your back straight.

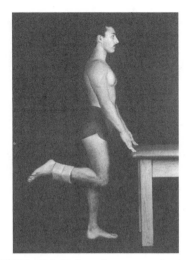

■ **FIG. 101-10** Knee flexor strengthening.

b. Lower your foot, slowly straightening out your knee. Count slowly to ten as you lower the foot to the floor.

c. Relax, rest and repeat.

B. **Knee flexors—prone position** (Fig. 101-11)

1. **Patient position:** prone, with a 3- to 5-pound weight attached to the ankle.

2. **Instructions:**

   a. Bend your knee to 90 degrees.

   b. Very slowly lower that leg down into full extension.

   c. Relax, rest and repeat.

C. **Terminal position of full knee extension** (Fig. 101-12)

1. **Patient position:** seated on the floor or a table. A rolled towel or pillow is placed under the knee to be exercised (about 6

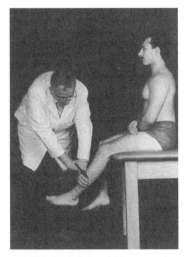

■ **FIG. 101-9** Quadriceps stretch.

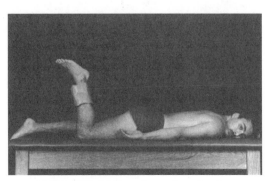

■ **FIG. 101-11** Knee flexor strengthening.

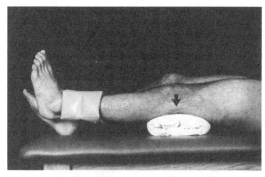

**■ FIG. 101-12** Terminal position of full knee extension.

inches high). A 3- to 5-pound weight is attached to the ankle.

2. **Instructions:**
   a. Push your knee down against the pillow, toward the floor, so that the weighted ankle comes off the table as the knee straightens out. Concentrate on pushing the knee down; do not try to extend the knee.
   b. Hold this position for 5 to 15 seconds.
   c. Slowly lower the weight to the table.
   d. Relax, rest, and repeat.

D. **Isometric quadriceps contraction** (Fig. 101-13)
   1. **Patient position:** seated, with one hand on the quadriceps muscle on the side to be treated.
   2. **Instructions:**
      a. Without moving your leg, try to contract the muscle you are touching so that the kneecap moves upward toward your hand.

b. If the exercise is performed correctly, you will see the kneecap move and feel the muscle tighten.

# ■ THE FOOT AND ANKLE

## Stretch

A. **Passive foot and ankle stretch** (Fig. 101-14)
   1. **Patient position:** sitting, holding the foot to be stretched with one hand above the ankle and the other hand on the forefoot.
   2. **Instructions:**
      a. Push your forefoot down. Hold for 3 seconds. Relax.
      b. Push your forefoot up. Hold for 3 seconds. Relax.
      c. Push your forefoot in. Hold for 3 seconds. Relax.
      d. Push your forefoot out. Hold for 3 seconds. Relax.
      e. Rotate your forefoot in a clockwise and then counterclockwise direction, four times each way. Relax.
      f. Rest and repeat the entire exercise.

## Stretch-Strengthening

A. **Heel-raising** (Fig. 101-15)
   1. **Patient position:** standing with both feet flat on floor, 6 to 8 inches apart.

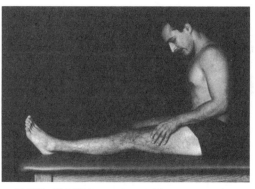

**■ FIG. 101-13** Isometric quadriceps contraction.

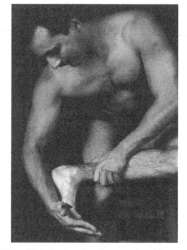

**■ FIG. 101-14** Passive foot and ankle stretch.

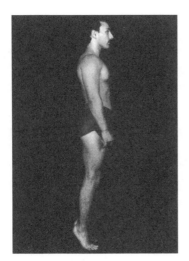

■ **FIG. 101-15** Heel raising to strengthen the gastrocnemius and stretch dorsiflexors.

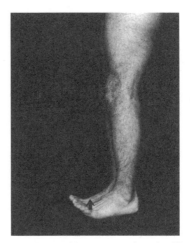

■ **FIG. 101-16** Toe raising to strengthen dorsiflexors and stretch the gastocnemius.

2. **Instructions:**
   a. Rise up on your toes. Hold on to something for balance, if necessary.
   b. Maintain this position for 5 to 15 seconds.
   c. Return to the starting position.
   d. Relax, rest, and repeat.
B. **Toe walking**
   1. Toe walking is performed in the same position as the heel-raising exercise. Walk forward on the toes for ten steps.
C. **Toe-raising** (Fig. 101-16)
   1. **Patient position:** standing, with both feet flat on floor and 6 to 8 inches apart.
   2. **Instructions:**
      a. Lean back on your heels.
      b. Maintain this position for 5 to 15 seconds.
      c. Return to the starting position.
      d. Relax, rest, and repeat.
D. **Heel walking**
   1. With the weight on the heels and the toes off the ground, walk backward on your heels for ten steps.
E. **Picking up marbles** (Fig. 101-17)
   1. **Patient position:** standing near support. Marbles are placed on the floor within reach of the foot to be exercised.
   2. **Instructions:**
      a. Pick up one marble with your toes.
      b. Lift this foot off the floor, cross it in front of the other leg, and release the

marble into a container placed 6 to 8 inches off the floor to the side of your stationary leg.
      c. In this manner pick up all the marbles on the floor, one at a time.
F. **Toe stretch** (Fig. 101-18)
   1. **Patient position:** seated, with both feet resting flat on a book resting firmly on the floor.
   2. **Instructions:**
      a. Lift up your toes only. Hold for 3 seconds. Relax.
      b. Put your toes over the edge of the

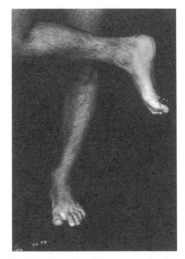

■ **FIG. 101-17** Toe stretch to stretch the arch and strengthen the peroneus longus.

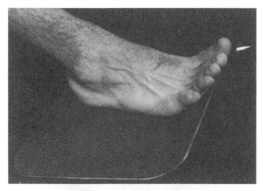

**■ FIG. 101-18** Toe stretch.

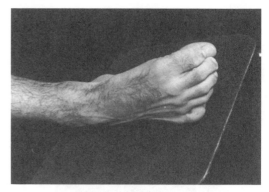

**■ FIG. 101-19** Toe curl.

book and push them down. Hold for 3 seconds. Relax.

c. Spread the toes far apart. Hold for 3 seconds. Bring them firmly together.

d. Curl your toes down as you bring your foot facing inward. Place your weight on the outer surface of your feet (Fig.101-19). Hold for 3 seconds. Relax.

e. Place one foot forward and resting on its heel, with the foot and toes pointing up. Press down on that heel as you turn your foot in clockwise and counterclockwise circles. Your big toe should make complete circles. Repeat three times.

f. Relax, rest, and repeat the entire exercise.

# CHAPTER 102

# Practical Applications and Case Histories of the Lower Extremities

*Stanley Schiowitz*

## ■ HIP

There are numerous musculoskeletal conditions that are found to be present in relation to the hip joint. In the following discussion, the pediatric patient is considered, and then common musculoskeletal conditions found in the adult are reviewed. This is not meant to be an all-inclusive review. Fractures, dislocations, and sprains, caused by trauma, can occur at any age. These are not discussed. The physician should be aware that recurrent fractures and other injuries seen in the pediatric patient must be investigated fully to rule out abuse. In many states, suspicion of child abuse must be reported to the proper authorities.

## Pediatric Considerations

### 1. Congenital dislocation of the hip in the newborn

This is a condition that is extremely important to diagnose before the onset of weight-bearing. The time of diagnosis can be the difference between simple conservative therapy and surgical intervention.

The only historical information that may be available is the presence of the condition in a sibling. This occurs approximately 5% of the time. In addition, the condition is found six times more frequently in females. The predominant signs will be asymmetry of the gluteal skin folds, with an apparent shorter leg. There will be a limitation of abduction of that hip present.

The use of the *Ortolani "click" test* and the telescoping of the hip will supply positive evidence of the presence of the hip dislocation. An x-ray of the pelvis should confirm the diagnosis.

The Ortolani "click" test is performed in the following manner. The baby is in the supine position. The physician brings both the baby's hips into 90-degrees of flexion and then abducts both hips fully, one hip at a time. There will be a distinct audible click sound heard as the dislocated hip(s) relocates into the socket.

Telescoping of the hip is tested with the baby in the supine position. The physician should create traction of that hip joint with one hand while stabilizing the hip with the other hand, extending one finger onto the greater trochanter. If he feels the greater trochanter move distally as traction is applied and then return to its previous position on the release of traction, it is a sign of dislocation of that hip.

### 2. Transient synovitis

This is a condition found four times as often in males as in females. It occurs between the ages of 3 and 12. There is a chief symptom of the child walking with a limp. There is generally no history of trauma elicited. On examination, a limitation of hip motions is found with the child maintaining the hip in flexion, abduction, and external rotation. There will be tenderness of the hip joint present. A low-grade temperature is usually found. A complete blood count will show a mild elevation of leukocytes. An x-ray of the hip will reveal a swelling of the joint capsule and widening of the joint space. This condition is self-limiting with the use of bed rest for approximately 3 weeks. Primarily assuring the parents of the nature of the condition is required.

### 3. Osteochondritis deformans juvenilis (Legg-Calve-Perthes disease)

This condition is usually found in the male child between the ages of 4 and 12. It is usually unilateral, with the chief symptoms being pain in the hip and a marked limp. The pain may radiate into the groin and to the knee joint. There will be a limitation of abduction, extension, and internal rotation present of that hip. Disuse atrophy may be present in the upper thigh.

The Thomas test (reviewed in chapter 92) will be positive because of contracture of the psoas and adductor muscles. The blood sedimentation rate test may be elevated. An x-ray of the hip joint will confirm the diagnosis.

There are four stages in the development of this condition, starting with joint swelling and no femoral head deformity, to severe deformity of the femoral head being present. The treatment will depend on the stage found when making the diagnosis. Discontinuing all weight-bearing on that hip joint is advised in milder cases; hip joint replacement will be necessary once the femoral head has been destroyed.

### 4. Slipped capital femoral epiphysis

This condition is found in males approximately four times as often as in females, usually from the ages of 4 to 12. It may be found at earlier ages in females. The male will have typical findings of female fat distribution and sexual underdevelopment. It is present bilaterally in 40% of patients. The patient will report a limp and mild pain of the involved joint, around the groin, thigh, and knee. There will be tenderness over the joint region.

The foot is turned outwards because of an external rotation of the hip. Motion of the hip is limited. In severe cases, with marked displacement of the epiphysis, the gait may be a waddling type of gait. A Trendelenburg test will be positive. An x-ray of the hip will confirm the diagnosis as well as the severity of the condition. The treatment provided, similar to that for osteo-

chondrits deformans, will depend on the stage of development of the condition.

## Considerations in the Adult

### 1. Ischiogluteal bursitis

Ischiogluteal bursitis is commonly found in patients who have a sedentary occupation. It was once called *tailor's bottom,* because tailors tended to sit all day on hard chair seats. The patient reports pain when they sit on a hard surface. The pain is usually unilateral. Point tenderness is present over the ischial tuberosity and will be relieved when the patient stands up. There will be no x-ray evidence found. An MRI or CAT scan may reveal a thickening of the bursa. The pain can be relieved by an injection of a local anesthetic into the area. The prescription of a non-steroidal anti-inflammatory medication (NSAID), the use of a cushion on the chair, as well as instructing the patient to stand up for 1 minute every hour while working will relieve the condition.

### 2. Trochanteric bursitis

Trochanteric bursitis is caused by a non-infectious inflammation of the bursa that is lateral to the greater trochanter of the involved hip. The patient reports pain overlying the lateral trochanter and radiating down the lateral aspect of the leg. The pain is present with weight bearing, walking, or lying on the involved side. There is no history of trauma.

The major physical finding is point tenderness right over the bursa. There is usually no x-ray evidence found, but as mentioned, an MRI or CAT scan may show evidence of bursal thickening.

The question that must be answered when this diagnosis is made is, what was the underlying condition that caused this condition? The function of the bursa is in relationship to muscle function. The muscle(s) involved include those used for hip motion as well as knee motion. Pelvic function and balance is involved as well. Somatic dysfunctions are a common finding and must be addressed. The finding of an anatomical short leg should be sought. Simply treating the local symptoms will not "cure" the condition.

### 3. Meralgia paresthetica

Meralgia paresthetica is an inflammation of the lateral cutaneous nerve of the femur. The nerve appears at the lateral border of the psoas muscle and then crosses the iliacus muscle deep to its fascia in a direction toward the anterior superior iliac spine. It divides into two branches, an anterior and a posterior branch. The anterior branch, the larger of the two, passes beneath the inguinal ligament and supplies the skin on the lateral aspect of the thigh to the knee. The posterior branch supplies the skin of the lateral buttock distal to the greater trochanter. This condition is caused by trauma to the area causing inflammation of the nerve. The difficulty arises when there is no history of an immediate direct trauma to the area followed by symptoms. The trauma can be chronic, such as a belt rubbing or tight clothing that is rubbing over the nerve. Clinically it is also correlated with obesity or pregnancy. The patient will report persistent paresthesia, anesthesia, or hypoesthesia at the lateral buttock, down the thigh to the knee. There seems to be no apparent reason. There is no point tenderness present and no limp or gait changes. There may be a positive Tinel sign present over the nerve. X-rays and MRI or CAT scan will be of no assistance in the confirming of the diagnosis.

A very careful history has to be taken with suspicion that this condition may be present. Whatever has caused the trauma is to be removed. There will be multiple somatic dysfunctions present, with the lumbar region being involved significantly. These must be treated as well.

### 4. Psoas muscle dysfunction

There are a number of causes for the creation of psoas dysfunction. Among these are trauma to the lumbar spine, lesser trochanter or pubes, myosistis or psoatic bursitis, or visceral dysfunction in relationship to the psoas muscle, such as an acute appendicitis, renal or urethral dysfunctions, fallopian tube inflammation, and iliac or femoral artery phlebitis. Any musculoskeletal condition that causes a low back imbalance and lumbar and pelvic somatic dysfunctions must be evaluated. It is important that any and all of the findings be actively treated.

The patient will report pain in the groin and down the leg. There will be a typical psoatic gait present with the patient limping with the foot and hip in abduction and the body flexed toward that side. On standing, the patient will have a pelvic tilt to the involved side and hold the knee and hip in a flexed posture. In the supine position, there will be an exaggerated lumbar lordosis. The Thomas test will be positive.

### 5. Osteoarthritis of the hip

Osteoarthritis of the hip is a common condition found in the geriatric patient. However, it can be found at any age, usually secondary to trauma of the joint. The predominant symptom is one of progressive pain, worse with movement of the hip and relieved with rest. Typically, the patient will state that after rest, the joint is stiff but loosens up with motion, such as walking, but soon after the pain returns. There is tenderness found on palpation of the groin area. There is limitation of all hip motions, both active and passive. *Crepitus*, a grinding sensation that may be heard as well, may be felt and/or heard with motion. There is an antalgic gait present. This condition can cause muscle atrophy when present for a long period of time.

An x-ray may show evidence of joint space narrowing and changes in the subchondral bone. In early conditions, there will be no evidence noted, but usually an MRI or CAT scan will show evidence of cartilage changes. Etiological causes can include chronic trauma such as is caused by a short leg syndrome or chronic pelvic imbalance. Dysfunctions of the knee, foot, and ankle, which create any change in posture, weight-bearing, or gait, can be the cause of hip dysfunction. It is important, regardless of the age at onset, that a complete postural evaluation is completed and all changes, including somatic findings be corrected.

In all conditions that affect the lower extremities, the physician should prescribe exercises as indicated. Even in bed rest, atrophy of muscles caused by lack of use should be prevented. In other conditions, exercises to increase motion or strength are needed.

## ■ KNEE

## Osteochondritis of the Tibial Tubercle (Osgood-Schlatter Disease)

Osgood-Schlatter disease is a condition that is usually found in adolescent boys in which the tibial tubercle fractures or enthesopathy of the tendon occurs. It is frequently bilateral. It has a gradual asymptomatic onset. The patient eventually becomes aware of pain, tenderness, and swelling at the tibial tubercle. There is generally no history of trauma. It may occur during growth spurts, with increased tension on the patellar ligament. The symptoms are worsened with direct pressure applied to the area, such as in kneeling. Early in the disease there may be no evidence seen, although an MRI will usually show evidence of the condition, even at an early stage. Later it can be identified on x-ray examination. This disease is self-limiting with the fusion of the tubercle to the tibia.

The treatment is usually conservative in nature with avoidance of excessive activity that will create the symptoms. An explanation of the condition assists the child and the parents in understanding the cause of the pain and the necessity of resting the knee during the healing process. Occasionally, the tubercle may be pinned to the tibia to create early fusion.

## Prepatellar Bursitis

This is a condition of inflammation of the bursa overlying the patella. The patient reports swelling and tenderness at that site. The pain is worsened with flexion of the knee because of the swelling present. The inflammation is usually created by an acute trauma, but there is also the possibility of chronic trauma (i.e., kneeling) as the cause. This is a condition of inflammation of the bursa overlying the patella and is often called "housemaid's knee." It is usually treated conservatively. Occasionally, the bursa requires drainage to relieve the pressure. Non-steroidal anti-inflammatory medication (NSAIDs) may be prescribed to relieve the inflammation and pain.

## Baker's Cyst

Baker's cyst is usually asymptomatic and the patient's primary symptom is of a large mass or swelling in the posterior aspect of the knee. This bursal swelling may communicate with the knee joint space. It may be associated with osteoarthritis of the involved knee. It usually requires no treatment. Occasionally, it may require aspiration because of its size interfering with joint function. The injection of a steroid has on occasion been effective.

## Chondromalacia Patella

Chondromalacia patella is a softening of the articular cartilage on the underside of the patella accompanied by some degree of fibrosis, fissuring, and erosion. In severe cases, the entire articular surface of the patella may be destroyed. The etiological factors may be diverse, from acute or chronic traumas, to any instability of the structural integrity of the knee, i.e., genu–varus, valgus, tibial torsion, or osteoarthritis with meniscal deformity.

The patient will report pain with sitting down, climbing stairs, and prolonged walking or running. He may say that he hears a grating or grinding noise when he bends his knee, exaggerated with squatting, or he will note swelling of the front of the knee. The patella femoral grinding test is positive. An x-ray may show positive changes, as will an MRI or CAT scan.

The treatment rendered will depend on the condition of the articulation. It is important to diagnose this condition at the onset and remove all etiological factors, especially those that are creating the instability of the knee. As in the hip region, the influence of problems in other areas of the body on knee joint stability, especially those found below the knee at the foot or ankle joint, must be considered.

## Tears of the Menisci

Tears of the medial or lateral meniscus are the most common cause of internal derangement found in the knee joint. Most lesions involve the medial meniscus because of the nature of its attachment about its periphery, which makes it less mobile than the lateral meniscus and more subject to injuries. A "bucket handle" lesion is usually found in young people, whereas a horizontal, posterior lesion is more apt to be found in the middle aged and the elderly patient. There usually is a history of acute trauma, which resulted in swelling, pain, and disability of the knee.

Once the swelling has been reduced, an MRI will easily determine the nature of the tear, if one is present. Examination at the onset may reveal swelling, inflammation, and point tenderness. A McMurray test will be positive. Arthroscopy for diagnosis and for surgical correction is used most commonly.

There are two additional, interesting dysfunctions often seen in the knee region, which really are not part of the knee joint function. These are the *pes anserine bursitis* and the *fibular head somatic dysfunction*.

## Pes Anserine Bursitis

This bursa is located at the medial aspect and immediately below the knee joint. It is in relationship to the insertion of the semitendinosus muscle. This muscle has as its origin the ischial tuberosity and its insertion is at the medial aspect of the tibia, just below the knee joint. The other muscles attaching in this area are the sartorius and gracilis muscles.

The bursitis has as its cause trauma to the area, acute or chronic, as well as any dysfunction affecting the ischium or the structural integrity of the knee joint. The patient reports pain at the medial aspect of the knee, but careful palpation will elicit point tenderness below the knee joint that is very specific and localized in its nature. The pain will be made worse with contraction of the semitendinous, sartorius, and gracilis muscles. An evaluation for somatic dysfunctions of the pelvis, sacrum, and lumbar region, as well as the postural balance of the lower extremity, must be performed. Treatment can be a local injection of a steroid, a prescription for a NSAID, ice, exercises, and osteopathic manipulative treatment (OMT) of all somatic dysfunctions, including knee, hip, and pelvic region.

## Posterior Fibular Head Somatic Dysfunction

This dysfunction, including its diagnosis and treatment, has been discussed in previous chapters of this section. This diagnosis must be considered when the patient reports pain at the lateral aspect of and immediately below the knee joint. In addition, it should be recognized that there is a relationship between the development of this type of dysfunction and acute sprain of the ankle joint that creates dorsiflexion of the ankle. Always examine the ankle to insure that it is not creating a chronic dysfunction above it.

## ■ FOOT AND ANKLE

## Ankle Sprain

The most common injury to the ankle is an acute sprain. Its intensity may vary from a mild strain of the ligaments to tearing of the ligaments with avulsion of the bone at its attachments. In addition, severe trauma may cause fractures and dislocations. The most common strain is caused by inversion stress. This is when the foot is slightly plantar flexed and inversion of the foot causes stretch of the lateral collateral ligaments. The patient will give a history of an acute onset and report pain, swelling, and ecchymosis of the lateral aspect of the ankle joint. The patient will limp and the symptoms worsen with weight-bearing and walking. If the patient says that he heard a snap at the time of the inversion, you must be aware of a possible fracture or ligamentous tear. Treatment will depend on the severity of the condition; however, at the onset, ice packs for the swelling with the patient forbidden to bear weight on that ankle is mandated.

A marked dorsi-flexion dysfunction of the ankle joint will create a close-packed joint and create a posterior fibula somatic dysfunction. This posterior fibula somatic dysfunction is easily diagnosed and treated. If the condition chronically reoccurs, the physician must evaluate the postural integrity of the foot. Calcaneal valgus is a common cause for chronic sprain of the ankle.

## ■ FOOT

## Pediatric Patient

### Pes planus

Pes planus is the flattening of the longitudinal arches. This may be a normal finding in the infant that will eventually improve as the child starts walking. To test for a normal flattening, try to mold the dorsum of the foot to create a longitudinal arch. The normal foot can be molded. The abnormal foot will have dropping of the bones that can not be molded into place. An attempt should be made to create motion of these bones and to mold them into an arch. Train the parents in these maneuvers and have them perform them daily at home.

## Talipes equinovarus (club foot)

In Tapipes equinovarus, or club foot, the foot is in a position of inversion, adduction of the forefoot, calcaneal varus, and equines. The calf muscles are contracted. In the infant, these muscles can be manually stretched. Again, train the parents to perform this function at home. In addition, the child can be measured for a Dennis Brown splint, which is applied to maintain the correction after treatment and can be removed and reapplied by the parents. Gentle osteopathic manipulation of the bones of the feet and legs will assist in a return to normal more quickly.

## Metatarsus varus

This is a condition characterized by calcaneal valgus. The forefoot is adducted and there is a convex lateral border of the foot present. Early treatment by manual stretching of the muscles daily should be instituted. A Dennis Brown splint can be applied.

## Tibial torsion

Tibial torsion is a condition in which the tibia is twisted on its longitudinal axis, usually internally, and the relationship between the patella and the foot is abnormal. It can be secondary to a femoral torsion. The torsion creates a toeing-in of both feet. In the infant, the parents can stretch the muscles of the feet and legs daily. Osteopathic manipulation, especially fascial release, is useful in this condition.

# ■ ADULTS

## Morton's Neuroma

Morton's neuroma is a fibro-tendinous reaction occurring between the heads of the third and fourth metatarsals. A small, inflamed neuroma forms. The pain is neuritic in type and radiates to the toes. The patient reports that taking off the shoe brings immediate relief. There is a finding of severe point tenderness at that spot. Treatment by injecting steroid into the neuroma is often effective. The patient's feet should be evaluated to determine if he needs a change in the type of shoes worn. The shoes may be too tight, have an improper last, or require the raising of the metatarsal heads.

# March Fracture

A March fracture is a stress fracture usually found at the shaft of the second or third metatarsal bones. It was originally named a *March fracture* because it was frequently found in soldiers immediately after long marches while wearing high boots. It is difficult to diagnose by x-ray, because it is a hairline fracture. It may show up on an MRI or a bone scan. It becomes easier to diagnose in a few weeks as callus, which is easily seen by x-ray, develops. A history of direct trauma is almost never obtained. There will be point tenderness at mid-shaft of the involved metatarsal, which is worsened with flexion or extension of the toes. Resting the foot for 3 to 4 weeks is usually all that is needed. The prevention of further reoccurrences is important. Check the shoes for fit and the structure of the foot for abnormalities. Using osteopathic manipulation to free the motion of all foot bones is helpful.

# Hallux Valgus

Hallux valgus is a lateral deviation of the proximal phalanx on the first metatarsal, sometimes referred to as a *bunion*. It is an extremely painful deformity. The protrusion of the proximal end of the phalanx laterally causes pressure on that part of the foot and eventually bunion formation. The first toe may be shorter and have a predisposition to valgus formation. The physician has to be aware of the effect on the great toe caused by women wearing high-heel shoes or pointed-toe shoes. It is important to educate them about the proper shoes to be worn and why. The treatment is usually conservative in nature, consisting of foot exercises, NSAIDs, moist heat, and, as noted, proper shoes. Osteopathic manipulation is a good adjunctive treatment if instituted before severe deformity occurs. If the deformity is advanced, surgical removal may be necessary.

# Plantar Fascitis

Plantar fascitis is an inflammation of the plantar fascia of the foot, usually at its insertion on the calcaneus. When chronic in nature, a calcification may develop at the site of insertion of the tendon and a diagnosis of a *heel spur* is made.

The fascia may be painful in any of its parts and it is common to have patients report pain of the plantar surface of their foot whenever they walk or perform specific tasks, such as going up on their toes or heels. A patient may use a heel cushion with or without a hole in the center for relief of the pain. Localized steroid injection into the region will relieve the pain. Properly fitting shoes are a necessity as is the use of osteopathic manipulative treatment directed to freeing motion of the bones of the foot and stretching hypertonic muscles of the calf as well as the fascia itself. Exercises to increase foot flexibility and stretching of the calf muscles and Achilles tendon are important.

## Pes Planus (Flat Feet)

Pes planus, commonly known as *flat feet,* is a very frequent diagnosis made by patients and physicians. It is a condition in which there is a dropping of the medial longitudinal arch. The patients will state that their feet are tired after standing or walking, and eventually pain will develop. They may have looked at their feet, noticed the dropping of the arch, and decided that this was their problem. Many will arrive with variously prescribed or over-the-counter arch supports that they have been using with limited results.

It first must be determined if there is a true dropping of this arch. While in the upright position, the patient is instructed to cross his right leg in front of his left and to place his foot alongside the lateral aspect of the left foot, with both feet placed on the ground. The height of the medial arch will normally change and be raised up if the arch is not truly dropped (flat), but is capable of being influenced by the function of the muscles. With this finding, arch supports are not the recommended treatment.

First, the position of the calcaneus must be evaluated. If it is in a valgus position, it must be corrected by the use of a medial heel wedge. In addition, exercises to strengthen the muscles involved must be prescribed. Correction of calcaneal valgus by the use of medial heel wedges will show an immediate change in gait. The foot will no longer be abducted as the patient walks. It is important that, in prescribing the wedge,

the size and shape of the shoes worn are evaluated. The shoes should have a straight last and be the correct size. Shoes with heels that are wider than needed will not hold a medial wedge properly.

## ■ CASE 1

A 64-year-old man was seen in the clinic with a chief symptom of pain in his right hip. The pain had started approximately 6 months before this visit, mild, gradually worsening, until it was present constantly and he felt that he was disabled. He noted that the pain was referred into the right groin, but not down his leg. In addition, he noted that in recent months he had seen a marked restriction in the movements of that hip. He could no longer walk for distances and had to give up playing tennis. He was a retired school teacher but had always been active, as noted, playing tennis at least three times weekly.

He had seen a number of physicians previously for this condition and had a number of different NSAIDs prescribed. These medications all gave him relief of pain, but all created severe gastrointestinal symptoms that made him stop using them.

All other histories were noncontributory.

Physical examination revealed, that the patient seemed to have a right pelvic tilt with a compensatory right convex lumbar scoliosis in the upright position. His standing flexion test was positive on the right. He was able to bend in all directions without difficulty. His gait showed a decided limp on the right leg, with marked restriction of normal hip movements.

Examination of his back and lower extremities revealed that the patient had restriction of his right sacrum, somatic dysfunctions at the level of his first and fifth lumbar segments, and severe restriction of passive motion of his right hip in all directions.

He brought with him previously taken x-rays as well as an MRI, which showed that he had osteoarthritis of the right hip joint, with early flattening of the head of the femur.

Further investigation for a possible short leg syndrome was postponed at this time, because it was felt that much of the pelvic tilt seen could have been secondary to the hip dysfunction. It was to be evaluated further when the hip and sacral motions were improved.

The patient was treated with osteopathic manipulation to resolve the somatic dysfunctions as well as to increase motion of his right hip in all directions. He was prescribed a series of hip exercises to perform for the purpose of increasing hip motion as well as muscle strength.

## Discussion

This is a typical history of unilateral osteoarthritis of the hip joint. The question of why the one joint was involved has not been answered. Because the patient had been an active tennis player, he could have had previous falls injuring the hip and had not recalled them. There could be an anatomical short leg syndrome present, which over the years could have created undue stress on the one hip joint with the resulting osteoarthritic changes. The original treatment and prescribed exercises should slow down the progression of the disease and reduce the symptom complex. As soon as the region's motion is improved, it was planned that a standing x-ray should be taken to evaluate the possibility of a short leg syndrome.

## ■ CASE 2

A 25-year-old woman was seen in the clinic with a chief symptom of pain in her left knee. The pain was sudden in onset and she believed that it was created when she twisted her ankle as she was jogging 2 weeks previously. The pain was relieved when sitting or lying down. She had not noticed any swelling of the knee joint. The pain caused her to limp after walking or standing for an hour. She jogged almost daily but had to stop because of the pain that developed. She denied any previous history of knee pain or injury. All other history was noncontributory.

An examination of the knee was performed. There was no obvious swelling, redness, or scars present. There was point tenderness elicited at the medial aspect of the joint. Multiple testing was performed, including full passive and active motion testing and those usually used to evaluate for ligamentous and menisci dysfunctions. When the valgus–varus stress test was applied, the pain was exaggerated when valgus stress was

applied. This test had created a stretching of the medial collateral ligaments and pain. There was limitation noted in the transverse sliding of the femur on the tibia in both directions. Muscle strength was good.

A diagnosis was made of medial collateral knee ligament sprain, with somatic dysfunction of the knee joint. The patient was treated with osteopathic manipulation to increase the knee motion and rest, NSAIDs, and exercises to maintain the strength of the muscles as well as to maintain joint motion.

## Discussion

This patient's problem developed as a result of a mild strain with twisting of the knee joint. Should the pain continue, an MRI should be performed to rule out ligamentous or meniscal tear. The patient should recover fully in a few weeks and be able to gradually return to full activity. When evaluating this type of report, the physician must be aware that the ankle joint and the fibular head could be involved.

## ■ CASE 3

A 32-year-old man was seen in the clinic with a symptom of pain and swelling of his right ankle. He had been running and twisted his ankle that morning. He denied any previous history of ankle injuries. His other history was noncontributory.

An examination of his ankle joint revealed swelling of the entire ankle joint with some redness and increased skin temperature present. There was no sign of ecchymosis present. The swelling was greater at the lateral aspect of the joint. There was severe point tenderness present at the lateral ankle joint. Motion was restricted in all directions. There was no point tenderness of the shaft of the tibia or fibula.

An x-ray was taken and reported as negative for fracture or dislocation. The prescribing of an MRI was postponed until the swelling had an opportunity to be reduced. There was no evidence of somatic dysfunctions at the knee joint or head of the fibula.

A diagnosis of an acute inversion sprain–strain of the right ankle was made. The degree of the strain was not identified until the swelling reduced, motion had improved, and further testing could be performed to evaluate for tear of the ligaments.

The patient was told to be off his feet for the next 3 days, apply ice packs to the area for the next 24 hours, and use prescribed NSAIDs. He was to be seen again in 3 days and re-evaluated for further diagnostic procedures or treatment as deemed necessary.

## Discussion

Ankle sprain is a very common diagnosis and almost everyone during his or her lifetime experiences it. The majority of times, the condition resolves itself after a few days of rest and ice. The greater problem is that a number of these sprains become chronic in nature and it takes less and less twisting force for an acute flare-up to occur. This is because many times a physician is not consulted or the follow-up visit is ignored. However, if there is a follow-up visit, the physician must be aware that a chronic condition can develop. He must evaluate for a minor tear and see that the patient performs specific exercises to maintain joint motion and muscle strength. In addition, the physician should evaluate the patient's extremities for underlying structural changes that might create the tendency for twisting of the ankle joint. The primary, undiagnosed condition found is usually a calcaneal valgus. This can be treated as can any somatic dysfunction that is found.

## ■ CASE 4

A 46-year-old woman was seen in the clinic with a chief symptom of pain in her left foot on the plantar aspect. The pain had been present for at least 6 months. The patient was not certain of the duration, because she stated that the pain had developed gradually over a period of months or up to a year. The pain was worse when she was walking or jogging, but it was relieved when she rested. The patient denied any previous history of foot disorders or any accidents to the area. Her other history was non-contributory.

Examination of her feet revealed that there was a mild calcaneal valgus of both heels as well

as early hallux valgus present. However, there was severe point tenderness present on the plantar surface of her left foot approximately 2 inches distal to the calcaneal tubercle. The area around the tubercle itself was not tender to touch. The fascia around that area seemed to be firmer and tighter than that of the right foot. There was mild tenderness of the gastrocnemius muscles on the left. Motion of the foot and ankle joint was good in all directions. There was no evidence of somatic dysfunctions of the extremity present. There were somatic dysfunctions of the sacrum and lumbar segments. An x-ray was reported as negative. Her gait was evaluated and it was noted that she was hesitant about putting weight on the left foot. Her shoes were examined and discussed with her. It was felt that the shoes she wore during the day were usually inflared and contributed to the development of her hallux valgus.

A diagnosis was made of plantar fascial strain and multiple somatic dysfunctions of the sacrum and lumbar area. The patient received osteopathic manipulation, which included specific treatment to the fascia of the foot involved, as well as the prescription for exercises to increase motion of her foot and ankle, strengthening of the muscles, and NSAIDs. She was educated about the proper fitting of her shoes to prevent further changes of her toes. The calcaneal valgus was to receive further treatment at the next visit.

## Discussion

This patient had early dysfunction of the fascia of one foot. She did not have flat feet or other foot deformities. She was a candidate for the development of these deformities because of the shoes she wore at work all day. In addition, she was a jogger and the sneakers she wore should have had built-in medial calcaneal supports. This type of sneaker is commercially available. The condition was resolved in a few weeks with one or two treatments, the wearing of the proper shoes/sneakers, and her performing the exercises as prescribed. It is anticipated that the performance of this regime as prescribed should avoid the development of chronic dysfunction in the future.

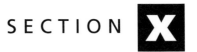

# Cranial Osteopathy

# CHAPTER 103

# Cranial Anatomic Considerations

*Hugh Ettlinger and Bonnie Gintis*

The ability to diagnose and treat dysfunctions related to cranial osteopathy and the primary respiratory mechanism (PRM) requires a solid knowledge of the anatomy of the cranium and the central nervous system, cerebral and spinal.

## ■ THE FLUCTUATION OF THE CEREBROSPINAL FLUID AND THE POTENCY OF THE TIDE

Fluctuation of the cerebrospinal fluid (CSF) is considered the first principle of the PRM. Movement of CSF involves both circulation and fluctuation. Circulation of the CSF occuring via hydrostatic forces at choroid plexuses and arachnoid granulations have been well documented. Seventy percent of CSF is formed at the choroid plexus in the ventricles. These plexi are formed by the pia and intracranial capillary beds and are part of the blood–brain barrier. The other 30% is formed as central nervous system (CNS) extracellular fluid moves into the subarachnoid space, providing a pathway for the brain (Fig. 103-1). The intraventricular and subarachnoid distribution of CSF is connected by two small foramina in the fourth ventricle, the foramen of Magendie and the foramen of Luschka. CSF is drained via arachnoid granulations, formed by arachnoid and the inner layer of the dura. Arachnoid granulations are found in the superior sagittal sinus and near the dorsal root ganglia in the spinal cord.

Forces generated by hydrostatic gradients of the choroid plexus and arachnoid granulations are not sufficient to account for the movement of CSF. Fluctuation, a back-and-forth movement of the fluid, contributes to this process.

Fluctuation of CSF has been documented recently by MRI studies. These studies demonstrate fluctuant movement of CSF in response to arterial pulse and respiration. The PRM also causes the CSF to fluctuate. This fluctuation provides a continuous mixing, which combined with the small circulatory forces allows for adequate movement of CSF, and exchange of the CSF with the circulation of the body. Circulatory forces alone are inadequate to account for this process.

Dr. Sutherland likened the fluctuation of the CSF to the tide in the ocean. In her book, *The Sea Around Us*, Rachel Carson describes the difference between waves, currents, and the tide. Her analogy illustrates concepts that also apply to circulation and fluctuation in the human body.

> There is no drop of water in the ocean, not even the deepest parts of the abyss that does not know and respond to the mysterious forces that create the Tide. No other force that affects the sea is so strong. Compared with the tide, the wind- created waves are surface movements. So despite their impressive sweep, are the planetary currents, which seldom involve more than the upper several hundred fathoms.
> —The Sea Around Us, Rachel Carson, 149

Currents are similar to circulation, carrying fluid from one place to another at relatively rapid speed. The tide is a fluctuation, which creates a mixing by to-and-fro movement of the fluid. Dr. Carson continues:

> The influence of the tide over the affairs of sea creatures as well as men may be seen all over the world. The billions upon billions of sessile animals like oysters, mussels, and barnacles owe their very existence to the sweep of the tides, which bring them the food, which they are unable to go in search of.

The sessile cells of the central nervous system also depend on a constant mix of their fluid sur-

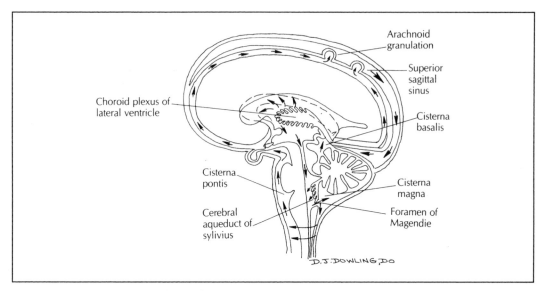

**■ FIG. 103-1** Circulation of cerebrospinal fluid. (Adapted from Netter, Ciba collection.)

roundings to maintain concentration gradients adequate for nutrition and waste disposal. The fluctuation of CSF helps maintain these gradients.

Dr. Sutherland referred to the effect of the fluctuation of the CSF on the physiologic centers in the body: "Through the functions of the PRM, the medulla relates to the secondary physiology of the living human body." The discovery of the circumventricular organs in the walls of the third and fourth ventricles 30 to 40 years after Dr. Sutherland's statement sheds light on a possible mechanism for this relationship. These organs are sensory apparatuses designed to monitor the CSF for the operation of various feedback mechanisms of the CNS. The circumventricular organs have been shown to be involved in the regulation of temperature, electrolyte balance, hypothalamic–pituitary function, and cardiovascular and respiratory function. Adequate exchange of the CSF is necessary for these organs to receive accurate information and appropriately regulate body function. The ability of osteopathic treatment to influence the function of the body's homeostatic feedback mechanisms expands the scope of clinical practice far beyond the biomechanics of the musculoskeletal system.

## ■ THE INTRACRANIAL AND INTRASPINAL MEMBRANES AND THE RECIPROCAL TENSION MEMBRANE

Membranous structures in the body are all composed of connective tissue derived from embryonic mesenchyme. All membranes are continuous with all other mesenchymally derived connective tissues of the body. The intracranial membranes are intimately related to the fascias of the rest of the body through foramina in the cranial base and throughout the entire spine, the foramen magnum, and all fascial attachments to the undersurface of the cranial base.

The newborn skull has no interlocking sutures. The only fully formed joint in the cranium is that between the condyles of the occiput and the atlas. A newborn's cranial bones develop within dura, and the shape of the skull is maintained by dura, by fluid, and by the central nervous system's motion within. Developmentally before bone formation, membranes provide shape and protection and also guide and limit motion.

The pia mater is a thin membrane, one cell in thickness, that is adherent to the brain and spinal cord. It is highly vascular. A cranial portion sheaths nerve roots, extending down into fissures and sulci. Its vessels for the choroid plexus of the ventricles. The spinal portion sheathes spinal nerves. Lateral extensions form the denticulate ligaments and blend with the filum terminale internally.

The arachnoid is a gauzy membrane, adherent to the internal dura that contains CSF in the space between itself and the pia and the subarachnoid space. Subarachnoid cisternae are enlargements of the arachnoid space containing CSF. Cisterns function as "waterbeds," cushioning the brain. Arachnoid granulations, also called Pacchionian bodies, lie along the longitudinal fissure and function to resorb CSF. There are also spinal arachnoid granulations along the arachnoid layer in the spinal canal.

The dura is described as having cranial and spinal portions. In actuality there is one continuous membrane. These two parts are named only for anatomical convenience (Fig. 103-2).

There are two layers of cranial dura. This membrane is tough and inelastic. In the adult, the layers are tightly adherent to each other, except where they form the venous sinuses.

The external layer of dura is the internal periosteum of cranial bones, the pericranium. Pericranium is continuous with periosteum of sutures and foramina, and with the external periosteum of the cranial bones. Compressive and tensile forces generated on the dura by the growing brain stimulate the membranous connective tissue to form bone between these layers of the dura. Therefore, the bones of the cranium develop within layers of dural membrane.

The periosteum of all cranial bones is continuous with all the dura. All adjacent membranous and fascial structures are continuous with each other. The dura and bone of the skull are examples of the continuity of connective tissues of differing densities.

## ■ CRANIAL STRUCTURES FORMED BY DURA

The internal layer of dura is called the *meningeal layer*. This layer surrounds the brain and comes together in two layers in replication to form the falx cerebri, the tentorium cerebelli and the falx cerebelli.

The falx cerebri is a sickle-shaped arc between the two hemispheres of the brain that has three poles of attachment (Fig. 103-3). The anterior inferior pole attaches to the crista galli of the ethmoid. The superior pole attaches to the surface of the skull along the metopic and sagittal sutures. The posterior pole attaches to the occiput and blends into the superior surface of the tentorium in the area of the straight sinus and the internal occipital protuberance.

The tentorium cerebelli is a double sickle-shaped membrane in the posterior fossa. It is formed by transversely oriented and concave anteriorly. The two layers of dura from which it is formed are derived from the coming together of the mesenchymal tissue that covers the occipital lobes superiorly and the cerebellum inferiorly. It is classically described as having poles of attachment that relate to the free and attached borders; however, current anatomical research is investigating the poles of attachment based on the borders of the upper and lower layers of dura.

The free or inner concave border forms the tentorial notch, which surround the midbrain and is classically described as attaching to the anterior clinoid processes of the sphenoid. The attached or outer convex border is classically described as attaching to five areas: the transverse ridge of the sulcus of the transverse sinus of the occiput, the posteroinferior angle of the parietal bone at the asterion, the mastoid portion of the temporal bone, the petrous ridge of the temporal bone, and the posterior clinoid process of the sphenoid.

The falx cerebelli is a small sickle of dura that extends between the two hemispheres of the cer-

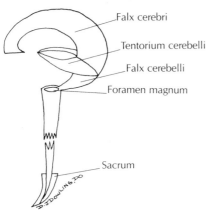

Falx cerebri

Tentorium cerebelli

Falx cerebelli

Foramen magnum

Sacrum

■ **FIG. 103-2** Dural membranes, lateral view.

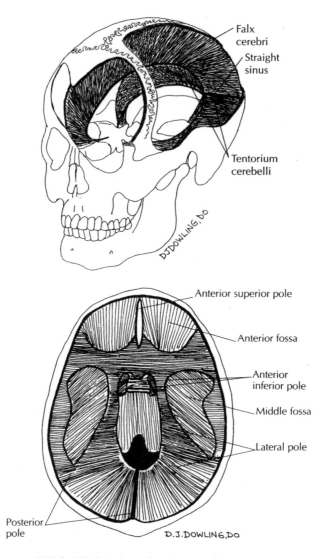

Falx
cerebri

Straight
sinus

Tentorium
cerebelli

DJDOWLING, DO

Anterior superior pole

Anterior fossa

Anterior
inferior pole

Middle fossa

Lateral pole

Posterior
pole

D.J.DOWLING, DO

■ **FIG. 103-3** Reciprocal tension membrane system.

ebellum. Its superior attachment blends into the inferior surface of the tentorium cerebelli in the area of the straight sinus. Its inferior attachment is to the vertical crest on the inner surface of the occiput. The inferior aspect of the attachment extends posteriorly, where it has a strong attachment to the foramen magnum. It is continuous with the dura of the spinal canal.

Dural membranes fold or form a sac to form three important structures. The diaphragma sellae is a small fold of dura that covers the hypophyseal fossa of the sella turcica of the sphenoid, encasing the pituitary. Dura completely encases the pituitary and blends with its capsule. This arrangement will alternately change the shape of the pituitary with the phases of the PRM and assist its portal circulation. Meckel's cave is formed from a fold of dura and sits on the anterior surface of the petrous portion of the temporal bone. It encases the semilunar ganglion, which is composed of three sensory branches of the fifth cranial nerve, the trigeminal nerve. At the anterior end of the ganglion, the dura blends with the capsule of the ganglion. Strain in the dura in this area can produce or contribute to trigeminal neuralgia. The endolymphatic sac is part of the membranous labyrinth system of the inner ear. It is composed of dura and is suspended from the inferior aspect of the petrous portion of the temporal bone.

The spinal portion of the dura is continuous with the inner layer of the cranial dura. Only one layer extends into the spinal canal. The other layer is continuous with the periosteum of the outside of the cranium. The spinal dura surrounds the spinal cord within the spinal canal. There are many attachments within the spinal canal. Firm attachments of spinal dura include the foramen magnum, the posterior aspect of the dens, the posterior aspect of the body of C3, the posterior aspect of the body of S2, the posterior aspect of the coccyx via the filum terminale, and minor fibrous slips to the posterior longitudinal ligament along the entire spine, most predominant in the lunar area.

The arterial supply to the dura is derived from terminal branches of the external and internal carotid arteries. Arteries passing through the dura are not just supplying the brain. The dura has its own rich blood supply.

The nerve supply to the dura is derived from all three branches of the trigeminal nerve, from sympathetic nerves from the carotid plexus and the superior cervical ganglion, and from cervical sensory nerves from C1 and C2.

## ■ DURAL VENOUS SINUSES

The venous sinuses are spaces within dural layers that convey venous blood from veins within the cranium to the systemic venous circulation (Fig. 103-4). Venous sinuses are devoid of the elastic and muscle tissue found in all other veins and therefore have no elasticity and muscular contraction to enhance drainage. Circulation is dependent on motion. During the inhalation phase, the sinuses change from "V"-shaped to ovoid, with a resultant increase in capacity. During this phase, the tributary veins increase drainage into the sinuses.

Venous sinuses drain 95% of blood from the cranium via the internal jugular vein. It is of crucial importance that there is proper relation and motion between the occipital and temporal bones, which comprise the jugular foramen, to have unimpeded venous drainage. The remaining 5% of venous blood drains via facial veins and the external jugular vein.

The superior sagittal sinus lies in the attached margin of the falx cerebri and drains primarily to the right transverse sinus, the sigmoid sinus, and then to the internal jugular vein. The inferior sagittal sinus lies in the posterior two-thirds of the free margin of the falx cerebri. It joins the great vein of Galen to form the straight sinus, which drains into the left transverse sinus, the

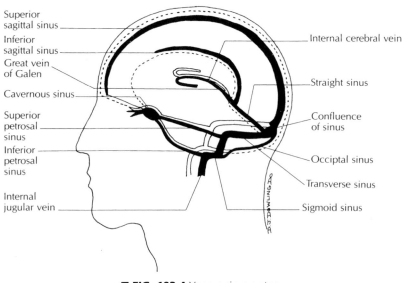

Superior sagittal sinus

Inferior sagittal sinus

Great vein of Galen

Cavernous sinus

Superior petrosal sinus

Inferior petrosal sinus

Internal jugular vein

Internal cerebral vein

Straight sinus

Confluence of sinus

Occipital sinus

Transverse sinus

Sigmoid sinus

■ **FIG. 103-4** Venous sinus system.

sigmoid sinus, and then to the internal jugular vein. The straight sinus is at the junction of the falx cerebri and the tentorium cerebelli. It is also the point of union of the great vein of Galen and the inferior sagittal sinus. These sinuses drain primarily to the left transverse sinus, the sigmoid sinus, and then to the internal jugular. The occipital sinus lies in the attached margin of the falx cerebelli, extending from the foramen magnum to the internal occipital protuberance. It drains primarily to the left transverse sinus, the sigmoid sinus, and then to the internal jugular vein.

The bilaterally paired cavernous sinuses are found lateral to the sella turcica and extend from the sphenoidal fissure to the apex of the petrous portion of the temporal bone. Cranial nerves III, IV, VI, the ophthalmic division of V, and the internal carotid artery are all found in relation to the cavernous sinuses. The sinuses are fed by ophthalmic veins, and drain to the superior and inferior petrosal sinuses, the sigmoid sinus, and then to the internal jugular vein. Dysfunction at the tip of the petrous portion of the temporal can interfere with the outflow of the cavernous sinus into the narrow petrosals.

The circular sinus or intercavernous sinus surrounds the pituitary and connects the cavernous sinus via two transverse vessels. The circular sinus drains to the superior and inferior petrosal sinuses, the sigmoid sinus, and then to the internal jugular vein. The circular sinus carries the outflow from the pituitary gland, including all of its hormones.

The superior petrosal sinuses lie in the attached margin of the tentorium cerebelli along the superior border of the petrous portion of the temporal bone. They drain into the sigmoid sinus, and then to the internal jugular vein. The inferior petrosal sinuses lie at the junction of the posterior border of the petrous portion of temporal bone with the basilar process of the occiput. They drain into the internal jugular vein.

The transverse sinuses lie in the attached margin of the tentorium cerebelli and extend from the area of the confluence of sinuses (internal occipital protuberance) to the jugular fossae. They lie in grooves in the occipital squama and mastoid angles of the parietals. The transverse sinuses become the sigmoid sinuses along the mastoid portion of the temporal bones and the jugular process of the occiput and drain into the internal jugular vein.

The basilar sinus or basilar plexus overlies the basisphenoid and basiocciput connection the inferior petrosal sinuses. This plexus consists of several interfacing vein between layers of the dura, connecting the circular sinus with the internal vertebral venous plexus.

## ■ RECIPROCAL TENSION MEMBRANE (RTM)

The RTM is a single unit of structure and function. All membranes change shape during the phases of the primary respiratory mechanism. Membranes balance and maintain a constant level of tension during the rhythmic, simultaneous alternating shape change of the phases of the PRM. Just as ligaments allow joints to move through a range of motion, the intracranial and intraspinal membranes allow a range of motion of the cranial bones. This reciprocal action functions around a fulcrum in a dynamic relationship, guiding and limiting motion in the cranium and responding to motion throughout the body.

The RTM functions in the phases of inhalation and exhalation around a suspended automatically shifting fulcrum. Dr. Magoun named this fulcrum the *Sutherland fulcrum* in honor of its discoverer. This fulcrum shifts and adjusts to maintain balanced tension in response to normal motion or trauma. The Sutherland fulcrum normally functions somewhere along the junction of the falx and the tentorium, along the straight sinus. It is not a fixed anatomical point. It is automatically shifting and suspended to be able to adapt to changing forces.

Dr. Sutherland stressed the importance of learning to observe the functioning of the fulcrum. If the membranes can be brought to a state of balanced membranous tension, the inherent forces within the body have an opportunity to influence dysfunctions.

## ■ THE INHERENT MOTILITY OF THE CENTRAL NERVOUS SYSTEM

The central nervous system (CNS) exhibits a rhythmic expansion and contraction of the brain and spinal cord during the phases of the PRM, which occurs simultaneously with movement of membrane, bone, and fluid. This is a coiling and uncoiling of the nervous system occurring about a fulcrum located at the lamina terminalis.

## Cranial Bones and Sutures

Study of the embryological development of cranial bone provides important information regarding their form and function. Compressive forces early in development create a cartilaginous matrix in the area that becomes the cranial base. Tensile forces create membrane in the area that develops into the cranial vault. Dr. Sutherland considered the motion in the cranial base primary, the motion in the vault being accommodative to the base.

The PRM is palpable in the newborn, whose cranium is predominantly cartilage and membrane and lacks sutures between the bones. As the skull ossifies, sutures form to accommodate this motion, which is already present. The shape of the suture therefore reflects the motion it accommodates. The basic suture types and their respective motions are shown in Figure 103-5 and are listed here:

1. **Serrate:** saw-toothed (e.g., the sagittal suture). It allows a rocking motion.
2. **Squamous:** scale-like or overlapping, such as the temporoparietal (squamoparietal) suture. Allows a gliding motion, determined by the bevel and groove direction of the two surfaces.
3. **Harmonic:** edge to edge (e.g., the lacrimo–ethmoidal suture). It allows shearing.
4. **Squamoserrate:** a combination, found in the lambdoidal and coronal sutures.

The motion of a bone may be deduced from the shape of its sutures, because the sutures were formed to accommodate motion that was present before the bone ossifies (Fig. 103-6). An axis of motion crossing a suture line causes the suture to change shape and develop a bevel, because motions on opposite sides of an axis are different. These points are called pivots (Fig. 103-7).

## The Sphenoid

The sphenoid articulates with 12 bones (Fig. 103-8). It is influential in the motion of the frontal and facial bones. It is important to note that the bones are not prime movers. They have mobility and the ability to change shape, and will

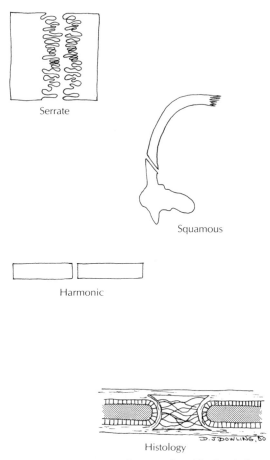

Serrate

Squamous

Harmonic

Histology

■ **FIG. 103-5** Types of sutures found in the skull.

therefore influence, not actually move, the other structures with which they are in contact.

Structurally, the sphenoid consists of the body, the greater and lesser wings laterally and the pterygoid plates inferiorly.

### Articulations

1. **Occiput:** The sphenoid articulates with the basilar portion of the occiput (the sphenobasilar joint), a synchrondrosis that is cartilaginous until age 20 to 25 years, and then converts to cancellous bone. It exhibits flexibility, not articular mobility.
2. **Temporals:** The sphenoid articulates with the temporal in three areas. The articulation of the squamosal border of the greater wing of the sphenoid with the inferior border of the temporal squama is important. Within this articulation is a change in bevel called

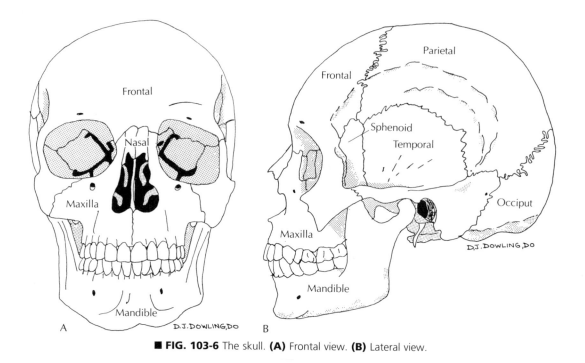

■ **FIG. 103-6** The skull. **(A)** Frontal view. **(B)** Lateral view.

the sphenosquamous pivot (SS pivot, Fig. 103-9). A line connecting the SS pivot on either side of the bone reflects the axis of motion of the sphenoid. It is found directly behind the zygomatic arch. Above the sphenosquamous pivot, the articulation is mostly squamous and the sphenoid is beveled on the external surface. The temporal bone is beveled on the internal surface. More simply, the temporal bone overlaps the sphenoid here and a primarily gliding motion exists.

Below the sphenosquamous pivot, the articulation is more serrate, less vertical, and more evenly beveled. The motion is more of a rocking motion.

3. **Parietals:** A small articulation exists at the pterion between the posterosuperior surface of the greater wing of the anterior inferior angle of the parietal bone. It is a squamous suture, allowing gliding motion. The sphenoid overlaps the parietal bone.

4. **Frontal bone:**

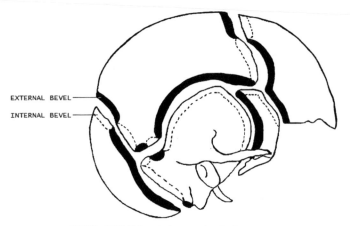

■ **FIG. 103-7** Bevel changes in skull sutures.

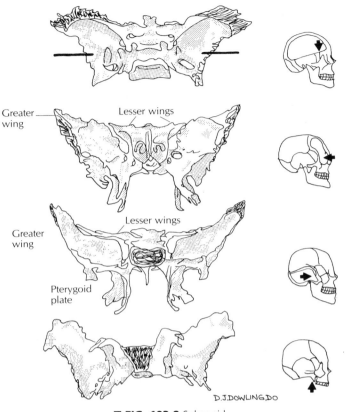

■ **FIG. 103-8** Sphenoid.

a. An "L"-shaped articulation exists between the anterosuperior surface of the greater wings of the lateral inferior surfaces of frontal bone. It is a serrate suture.

b. Two other articulations, also serrate, exist between the anterior border of the lesser wings laterally and the orbital surface of the frontal bone, and between the anterosuperior surface of the body medially and the

orbital surface of the frontal bone. Together, these two articulations allow the sphenoid to influence the lateral surfaces of the frontal bone laterally, anteriorly, and slightly superiorly as the sphenoid flexes.

5. **Ethmoid:**

a. The anterior body of the sphenoid (ethmoid spine) articulates with the posterior border of the cribriform plate. This articu-

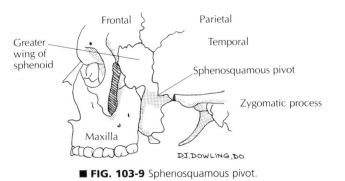

■ **FIG. 103-9** Sphenosquamous pivot.

lation is a gomphosis or peg-in-socket joint.

  b. Two other articulations, both harmonic, allow flexibility of motion in these areas of contact (laterally in the horizontal plane and midline in a vertical plane).

6. **Palatines (two)**
7. **Vomer**
8. **Zygoma (two)**

The palatines, vomer, and sygomae are intermediaries between the sphenoid and maxillae.

### Motion

In this text, the motion of each bone is simplified for beginner study. Although the descriptions are good presentations of the general motion present, it is important to consider that in the living body, other variables may be actively influencing the ability of a bone to move.

## The Occiput

The occiput is influential in the motion of the posterior part of the cranium.

### Parts

The structures of the occiput are shown in Figures 103-10 and 103-11.

1. **Basilar occiput (basiocciput):** anterior to and forming the anterior border of the foramen magnum.
2. **Condyles:** adjacent to and forming the lateral borders of the foramen magnum.

3. **Squama:** body of the occiput, forming the posterior border of the foramen magnum.

Ossification of all parts is not complete until approximately 5 years. This has important clinical significance in the timing of the treatment of certain problems in children.

### Articulations

Articulating with six bones, the occiput is influential in the movement of the temporal and parietals (Fig. 103-12).

1. **Sphenoid:** The articulation of the occiput with the sphenoid was discussed under the sphenoid bone.
2. **Parietals (two):** The lambdoidal suture between the superior surface of the occiput and the posteroinferior surface of the parietal bone is the site of articulation. The change in bevel along this articulation can be found by extending the superior temporal line from the parietal bone posteriorly to this suture (Fig. 103-13). The change in bevel occurs at the point at which the orientation of both bones changes from primarily the coronal plane (superior) to primarily the horizontal plane (inferior). From the midline to this point, the occiput is internally beveled, overlapping the parietal, and the suture is more serrate, although squamoserrate. Lateral to this point, the occiput is externally beveled, overlapped by the parietal bone, and the suture is less serrate, although still squamoserrate (see Fig. 103-13). The motion is primar-

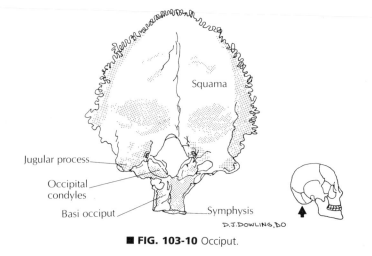

Jugular process

Occipital condyles

Basi occiput

Squama

Symphysis

D.J.DOWLING, DO

■ **FIG. 103-10** Occiput.

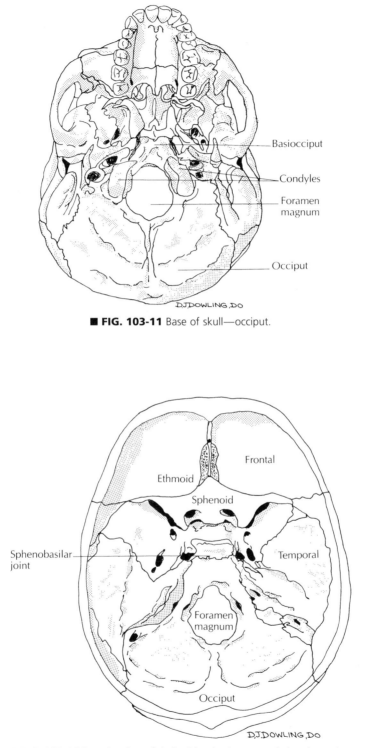

■ **FIG. 103-11** Base of skull—occiput.

■ **FIG. 103-12** Superior view of skull with calvaria removed, showing articulations of the occiput.

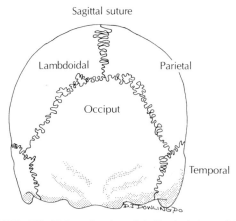

■ **FIG. 103-13** Posterior view of skull articulations of the occiput.

ily rocking, but there is some slide as the occiput slides anteriorly into flexion. The parietal motion is almost entirely lateral.

3. **Temporals (two):** There are three distinct areas of contact of the occiput and the temporal bones (Fig. 103-14).

   a. The lateral posterior surface of the occiput articulates with the mastoid portion of the temporal bone. The joint is convex on the temporal bone and concave on the occiput, almost describing an "L" shape. The point at which the legs meet is a point of bevel change, called *condylosquamomastoid pivot.* Superior and posterior to this point, the occiput is externally beveled, anterior to this point it is internally beveled or flat. The joint is serrate, accommodating a rocking motion.

   b. The jugular notch of the occiput articulates with the jugular surface of the temporal bone. There are two parts to this articulation.

      (1) The jugular notch of the occiput articulates with the jugular fossa of the temporal bone, forming a smooth, quadrangular articulation in the coronal plane.

      (2) An irregular, flat, rough surface posterior to the notch articulates with a surface on the temporal bone. It is in the horizontal plane. This is an extremely important articulation because it is the fulcrum around which the occiput and temporal bones move in relation to each other. The temporal bone moves anteriorly and superiorly posterior to this point, anteriorly and inferiorly anterior to this point, laterally above the point, and medially below it.

      (3) The upper edge of the lateral border of the basiocciput articulates with the petrous portion of the temporal bone (inferior border). This is a tongue-and-groove articulation, allowing a hinge and glide motion.

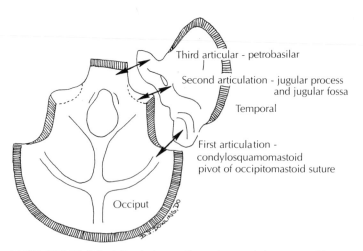

■ **FIG. 103-14** Articulation between the occiput and the temporal bone, superior aspect.

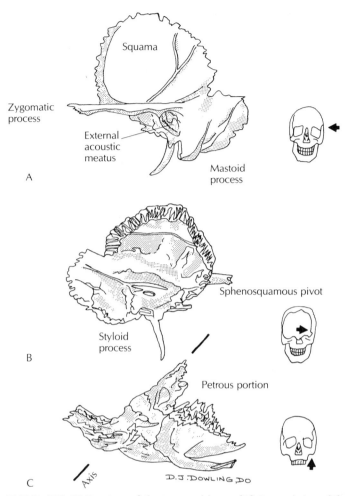

■ **FIG. 103-15** Structure of the temporal bone. **(A)** External view. **(B)** Internal view. **(C)** Inferior view.

5. **Atlas:** The occipitoatlantal articulation is a synovial joint. The articular surfaces converge anteriorly and inferiorly, predisposing the articulation to compression when hyperextended, such as in whiplash or the birth process. It is the only fully formed articulation in the cranium at birth. Birth trauma involving the craniocervical junction can have serious clinical consequences, because the condylar parts of the occiput are still separate and can be forced medially, changing the size and shape of the foramen magnum. The atlas is less often affected by birth trauma because the transverse ligament of the atlas prevents widening of the atlas facets.

## Motions

The primary motion of the occiput on the atlas is flexion-extension, with the occipital condyles convex and the superior articular facets of the atlas concave.

## The Temporal Bone

### Parts

The structure of the temporal bone is shown in Figure 103-15.

1. **Squama:** smooth body of the temporal bone.
2. **Mastoid portion:** posterior, including the mastoid process.
3. **Zygomatic arch:** anterior and lateral.

4. **Petrous portions:** medial, containing the auditory and vestibular apparatus. It is the surface for the attachment of the tentorium cerebelli.

### Articulation

The temporal bone articulates with seven other bones.

1. **Sphenoid:** The articulation of the temporal bone with the sphenoid was discussed under the sphenoid bone.
2. **Occiput:** The articulation of the temporal bone with the occiput was discussed under the occiput. This is the major influence on temporal motion.
3. **Zygoma (two):** The temporozygoma articulation forms the zygomatic arch, a serrate suture that allows rocking.
4. **Parietal (two):** The temporoparietal articulation can be considered as two separate articulations, or as one articulation with a change in bevel where the mastoid and squamous portions of the temporal bone meet. For present purposes it is considered as two separate articulations.
   a. The superior surface of the temporal bone, broadly beveled internally, articulates with the inferior anterior surface of the parietal bone, broadly beveled externally. This suture is squamous, allowing medial and lateral glide of both bones as they rotate internally and externally.
   b. The superior surface of the mastoid portion of the temporal bone articulates with the posteroinferior surface of the parietal bone, forming an irregular, cobblestone articulation. There is a change in bevel at the center. This suture accommodates the rotary motion of the petrous portion of the temporal bone.
1. **Mandible:** The temporomandibular articulation is a synovial joint found beneath the most posterior portion of the zygomatic arch.

## The Parietal Bones

### Parts

The parietal bone has only one part (Fig. 103-16).

### Articulations

The parietal bones articulate with five bones (Fig. 103-17).

1. **Parietal:** The interparietal (sagittal) suture is serrate, allowing a rocking motion as the parietal bones rotate internally and externally. It has fewer but wider serrations posteriorly to accommodate greater motion there.
2. **Frontal:** The coronal suture is squamoserrate with an external bevel medially and an internal bevel laterally on the parietal.
3. **Sphenoid**
4. **Occiput**
5. **Temporal**

## Frontal Bone

### Parts

1. **Nasal part:** inferior and midline, articulates with the ethmoid.
2. **Orbital parts:** lateral and inferior, forming the roof of the orbit.
3. **Squama:** forehead area, with frontal eminences laterally. A metopic suture exists in the midline in 10% of adults.

### Articulations

The frontal bone articulates with 12 bones (Fig. 103-17).

1. **Parietal bones (two)**
2. **Sphenoid**
3. **Ethmoid:** three sutures, two lateral, one in the midline anteriorly, all harmonic to accommodate gliding.
4. **Lacrimals (two)**
5. **Maxillae (two)**
6. **Nasal bones (two)**
7. **Zygomae (two)**

## Ethmoid

### Parts

1. **Horizontal cribriform plate:** where the falx cerebri attaches (Fig. 103-19).
2. **Lacrimal masses (two)**
3. **Perpendicular plate**

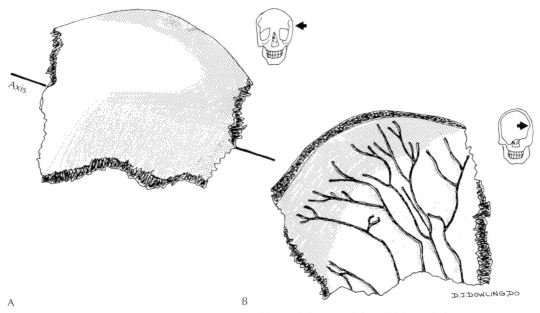

■ **FIG. 103-16** Structure of the parietal bone. **(A)** External view. **(B)** Internal view.

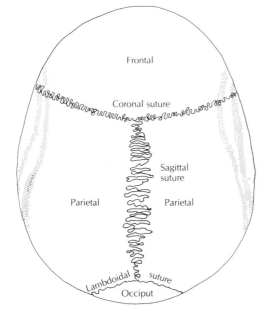

■ **FIG. 103-17** Sutures and articulations of the parietal bones of the skull, superior view.

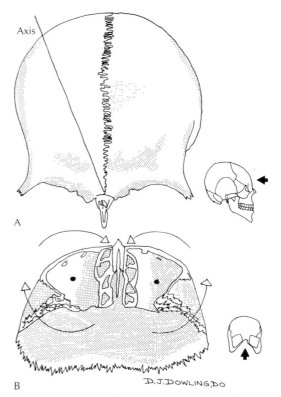

■ **FIG. 103-18** Frontal bone. **(A)** Anterior view. **(B)** Inferior view.

## Articulations

The ethmoid articulates with thirteen bones.

1. **Frontal bone**
2. **Sphenoid**
3. **Palatines (two)**
4. **Nasals (two)**
5. **Vomer**
6. **Inferior conchae (two)**
7. **Maxillae (two)**
8. **Lacrimals (two)**

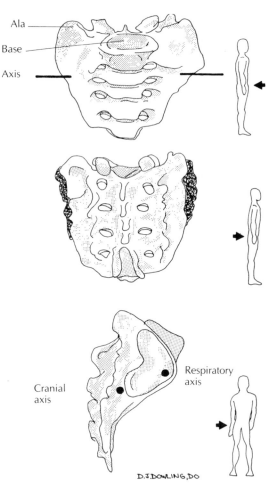

■ **FIG. 103-20** Axes of sacral motion.

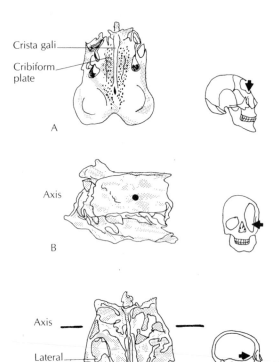

■ **FIG. 103-19** Structure and articulations of the ethmoid. **(A)** Superior view. **(B)** Lateral view. **(C)** Inferior view.

## Involuntary Motion of Sacrum Between Ilia

The sacrum rocks on a transverse axis through the articular pillar of the second sacral segment. The motion occurs in conjunction with the rocking of the basiocciput through the connection of the dura (Fig. 103-20).

# CHAPTER 104

# Cranial Motions and Dysfunction

*Hugh Ettlinger and Bonnie Gintis*

## ■ PATTERNS OF MOTION IN THE CRANIUM

No cranial bone moves independently. Restriction originating in any part of the cranium will cause changes in the motion of the entire cranium. The patterns of both functional and dysfunctional motions presented in this section should be considered in the context of variability that may influence the overall motion that presents itself. This approach provides an excellent basis for deepening understanding of the varieties of patterns that may present clinically.

Magoun has identified three factors essential for cranial articular motion.

1. **Plastic resiliency:** Every bone must be sufficiently resilient in itself and mobile in the sutures to move through its normal range without strain.
2. **Resiliency of contiguous bones:** The contiguous bones must be similarly resilient and mobile to accompany movement or compensate for it without strain.
3. **Unrestricted movement of dural membranes:** The dural membranes must be unrestricted in their areas of reciprocal tension to allow such movement to occur within normal limits.

To this list one may add the influence of cervical fascia and muscles attaching to the cranial base, as well as sacral articular mobility, and the effects of fluid fluctuation patterns.

Magoun emphasizes one further point referring to palpation of the cranium, "Do not look for movement as in other joints of the body. This is merely a resiliency—a combination of slight yielding or suppleness in the articulation plus the flexibility of live and pliant bone."

The sphenobasilar junction is the reference point around which diagnostic motion patterns are described. This does not imply that the dysfunction originated or is generated from the point. These general patterns represent the adaptation of the cranium to strain. The strain may be the result of dysfunction anywhere in the body. Cranial treatment is most effective when it is part of a complete osteopathic treatment plan.

The sphenobasilar junction is the reference point for the discussion of physiologic and nonphysiologic cranial motion patterns.

## Flexion and Extension

Flexion of the sphenobasilar junction results in a slight relative elevation of that articulation. The midline bones all rotate about a transverse axis into flexion (Fig. 104-1). Paired lateral bones move into external rotation. During extension, opposite motions occur (Fig. 104-2). All motions are subtle and may be sensed by hand contact. This motion is not generally perceptible by visual examination.

### Occiput

In flexion, the occiput rotates about a transverse axis directly superior to the foramen magnum at the level of the confluence of sinuses. As it rotates, the basilar part and the condyles move anteriorly and superiorly, directly influencing the temporal bones, and the squama moves posteriorly and slightly laterally. The greatest lateral deviation occurs at the lateral angles.

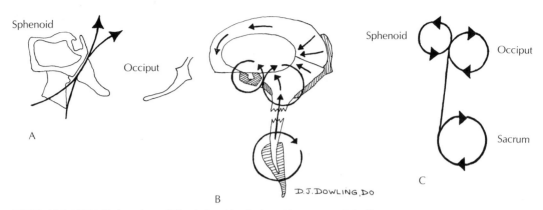

■ **FIG. 104-1** PRM, flexion phase. **(A)** Relationship of sphenoid to occiput. **(B)** Effects on reciprocal tension membrane system. **(C)** Direction of force in flexion.

## Sphenoid

The sphenoid rotates on a transverse axis through the center of the body at the level of the floor of the sella turcica. The greater wings move forward, slightly laterally, and inferiorly, influencing the lateral edges of the frontal bone anteriorly and laterally. The pterygoid processes move posteriorly and slightly internally.

## Temporal bone

The temporal bone externally rotates around an axis running from the jugular surface to the petrous apex. This approximates a line running through the petrous portion along its long axis. The squamous portion and zygomatic arch move anteriorly, laterally, and inferiorly, the mastoid

moves medially, superiorly, and slightly posteriorly, and the top of the petrous portion rotates laterally and slightly superiorly. The motion of the temporals has been likened to a "wobbly wheel."

## Parietal bones

The inferior surface of the parietal bone moves laterally around an axis connecting the anterior and posterior bevel changes. The posterior surface moves more laterally than the anterior surface.

## Ethmoid

Influenced by the sphenoid and falx cerebri, the ethmoid rotates about a transverse axis through

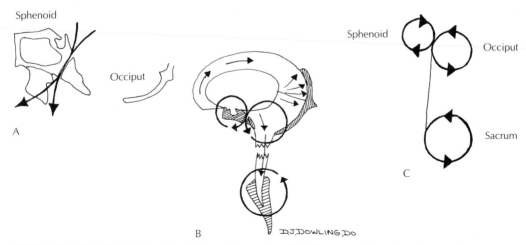

■ **FIG. 104-2** PRM. **(A)** Relationship of sphenoid to occiput. **(B)** Effects on reciprocal tension membrane system. **(C)** Directions of force in extension.

**TABLE 104-1 FINDINGS IN A FLEXION OR EXTENSION DYSFUNCTION OF THE SPHENOBASILAR SYMPHYSIS**

| PARAMETER EVALUATED | FLEXION DYSFUNCTION | EXTENSION DYSFUNCTION |
| --- | --- | --- |
| Restricted motion | Extension | Flexion |
| Head diameter | Increased in transverse dimension | Increased in longitudinal dimension |
| Forehead | Wide and sloping | Vertical |
| Eyes | Prominent | Receded |
| Paired bones | Externally rotated | Internally rotated |
| Ears | Protruding | Close to head |

the middle of the bone, in the same direction as the occiput. The lateral masses move as paired bones into external rotation.

### Frontal bone

The frontal bone acts as paired bones do, rotating externally under the influence of the sphenoid. The axis of motion runs from the frontal eminence through the center of the orbital plate. The inferior lateral angles move laterally and anteriorly. The glabella recedes slightly under the influence of the falx.

### Sacrum

Influenced by dura, the sacral base moves posteriorly and the apex moves anteriorly about a transverse axis through the second sacral segment during the flexion phase. Although flexion and extension are the normal physiologic motions present, they may be restricted in one direction. The dysfunction may occur without other associated nonphysiologic dysfunction.

## General Findings and Observations

The general findings of a flexion or extension dysfunction are listed in Table 104-1.

## ■ TORSION

Cranial torsion is a rotation of the sphenobasilar symphysis along an anteroposterior axis (Fig. 104-3). The sphenoid and occiput rotate in opposite directions. The axis runs from nasion to opisthion. The torsion is named for the side of the high wing of the sphenoid (Figs. 104-4 and 104-5) (Table 104-2 lists the important findings).

The following relative changes take place in the other bones and the membranes.

1. **Temporal bone:** relative external rotation on the side of the torsion.
2. **Parietal bone:** relative external rotation on the side of the torsion.
3. **Mandible:** shifted toward the side of the torsion
4. **Orbit:** smaller on the side of the torsion.

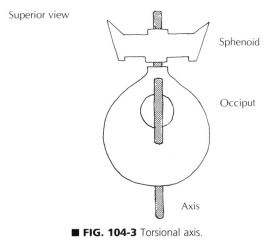

**■ FIG. 104-3** Torsional axis.

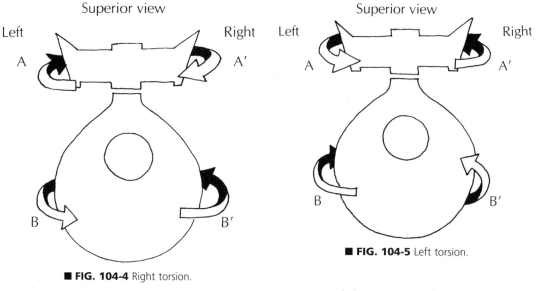

■ **FIG. 104-4** Right torsion.

■ **FIG. 104-5** Left torsion.

5. **Membranes:**
   a. Falx cerebri, also torsioned with the anterior end, twisting in the same direction the sphenoid rotates, and the posterior end twisting in the same direction the occiput rotates.
   b. Tentorium cerebelli: tentorium is side-bent in the same direction as the occiput rotates.

   c. Spinal dura: moves inferiorly on the side of the low occiput, allowing the sacral base on the side to move inferiorly.

■ **SIDE-BENDING AND ROTATION**

Side-bending and rotation are two separate motions of the sphenobasilar symphysis that occur simultaneously (Fig. 104-6). Side-bending occurs by rotation around two vertical axes, one through the center of the body of the sphenoid

**TABLE 104-2  FINDINGS IN TORSION DYSFUNCTION OF THE SPHENOBASILAR SYMPHYSIS**

| PARAMETER EVALUATED | SIDE OF HIGH SPHENOID WING | SIDE OF LOW SPHENOID WING |
|---|---|---|
| Frontal lateral angle | Anterior | Posterior |
| Orbit | Wide | Narrow |
| Frontozygomatic angle | Increased | Lessened |
| Eyeball | Protruded | Retruded |
| Zygomatic orbital rim | Everted and externally rotated | Inverted and internally rotated |
| Symphysis menti | To this side | Away from this side |
| Mastoid tip | Posteromedial | Anterolateral |
| Ear | Protruding | Close to head |

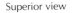
Superior view

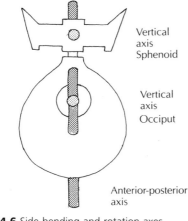

Vertical axis Sphenoid

Vertical axis Occiput

Anterior-posterior axis

■ **FIG. 104-6** Side-bending and rotation axes.

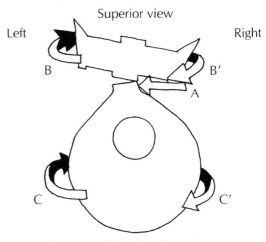

Superior view

Left                    Right

■ **FIG. 104-8** Left side-bending and rotation.

and the other through the center of the foramen magnum (Figs. 104-7 and 104-8). The sphenoid and occiput rotate in opposite directions on these axes, causing the side-bending.

Rotation occurs on the same axis as torsion; however, the sphenoid and occiput rotate in the same direction. Rotation occurs toward the side of the convexity, which is relatively inferior. Side-bending and rotation dysfunctions are named for the convexity of the side-bending motion.

The following relative motions occur in the other bones and membranes:

1. **Temporal bones:** externally rotated on the convex side.
2. **Parietal bones:** externally rotated on the convex side.

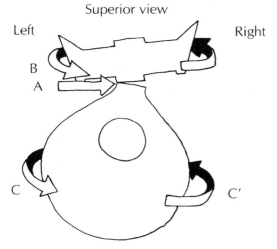

Superior view

Left                    Right

■ **FIG. 104-7** Right side-bending and rotation.

3. **Mandible:** shifted to the convex side.
4. **Frontal bone:** anterior on convex side.
5. **Orbit:** anterior on convex side.
6. **Membranes:**
   a. Falx cerebri, side-bent, following the convexity of the side-bending of the spheno-basilar symphysis.
   b. Tentorium: follows occipital motion.
   c. Spinal dura: inferior on the side of the convexity (interior occiput), dropping the sacral base inferiorly on that side.

## General Findings and Observations

In side-bending and rotation dysfunctions, one side of the head is relatively convex, the other relatively flat. Table 104-3 lists the important findings.

## Non-physiologic Motion Patterns

*Strains* are non-physiologic dysfunctions and are usually induced by trauma or systemic visceral disease. There are vertical and lateral strains, and a generalized compression strain. Dysfunctions of the facial bones, although relevant to complete cranial diagnosis and treatment, are beyond the scope of this chapter.

## ■ VERTICAL STRAINS

Vertical strains are named according to the position of the basishpenoid. It can move relatively superiorly or inferiorly, creating superior and inferior vertical strains.

## TABLE 104-3 FINDINGS IN SIDE-BENDING AND ROTATION DYSFUNCTIONS OF THE SPHENOBASILAR SYMPHYSIS

| LANDMARK | CONVEXITY | CONCAVITY |
|---|---|---|
| Lateral frontal angle | Posterior | Anterior |
| Orbit | Narrow | Wide |
| Frontozygomatic angle | Lessened | Increased |
| Eyeball | Retruded | Protruded |
| Zygomatic orbital rim | Prominent | Flat |
| Symphysis menti | To this side | Away from this side |
| Mastoid tip | Posteromedial | Anterolateral |
| Mastoid portion | Anterolateral | Posteromedial |
| Ear | Protruding | Close to head |

## General Findings and Observations

A vertical strain is flexion of the sphenoid accompanied by extension of the occiput, or extension of the sphenoid with flexion of the occiput. Side-to-side findings are symmetrical. Evidence of the anterior quadrants in external rotation would indicate a superior vertical strain (Fig. 104-9), if they are in internal rotation, there is inferior strain (Fig. 104-10).

## ■ LATERAL STRAIN

A lateral strain is a side-to-side shearing of the sphenobasilar symphysis (Fig. 104-11). It is usu-

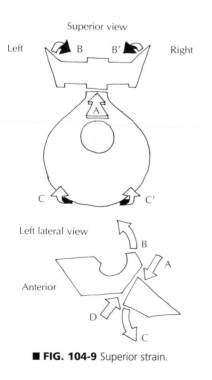

■ **FIG. 104-9** Superior strain.

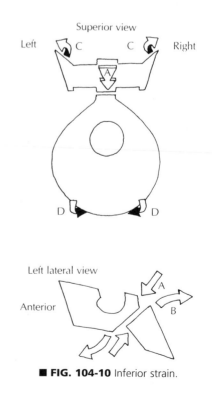

■ **FIG. 104-10** Inferior strain.

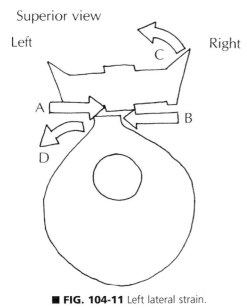

■ **FIG. 104-11** Left lateral strain.

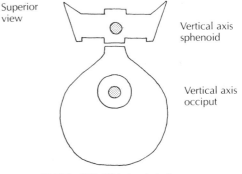

■ **FIG. 104-13** Lateral strain axes.

ally caused by trauma lateral to one side of the anterior cranium or the opposite posterior cranium (anterior or posterior to the sphenobasilar symphysis) (Fig. 104-11 and 104-12).

### General Findings and Observations

Both bones rotate on a vertical axis in the same direction (Fig. 104-13). The head may take on the appearance of a parallelogram (especially noticeable in infants). Regardless of age, side-to-side findings will not be symmetric.

### ■ COMPRESSION OF THE SPHENOBASILAR SYMPHYSIS

The dysfunction occurs as a result of pressure or trauma to the front of the head or face, to the back of the head, or to the entire periphery (i.e.,

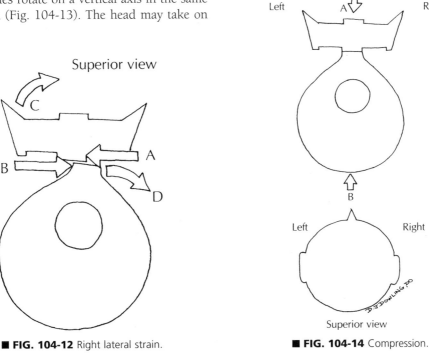

■ **FIG. 104-12** Right lateral strain.

■ **FIG. 104-14** Compression.

compression of the infant cranium during a difficult birth) (Fig. 104-14).

## General Findings and Observation

The dysfunction manifests as a restriction (mild, moderate, or severe) of all motions at the sphenobasilar symphysis. With severe compression, the cranium feels rigid.

### REFERENCES

Magoun HI. *Osteopathy in the Cranial Field, 3rd ed.* Kirksville, MO: The Journal Printing Co, 1976.
Sutherland WG. *Teachings in the Science of Osteopathy.* Cambridge, MA: Rudra Press, 1990.

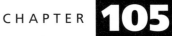

# Diagnosis and Treatment

*Hugh Ettlinger and Bonnie Gintis*

## ■ PRINCIPLES OF DIAGNOSIS

In his text, *Philosophy of Osteopathy,* Andrew Taylor Still stated, "To find health should be the object of the doctor. Anyone can find disease." How do we make sense of these words in the context of modern diagnosis and treatment? Any osteopathic diagnosis and treatment must use consideration of the whole patient in view of what maintains the individual's health, even in the presence of disease, injury, or dysfunction. The ability of the osteopathic physician to diagnose and treat patients using their health as a reference point and not their disease differentiates them from nonosteopathic physicians and adds a unique perspective to health care.

Making a diagnosis traditionally involves synthesizing information obtained from evaluation by history, observation, and physical examination. The osteopathic approach to these three aspects of diagnosis enhances the clinical information obtained by the traditional methods.

For the purpose of diagnosing cranial dysfunctions, the osteopathic physician must inquire about trauma and birth history. It is often surprising how widely varied symptoms are temporally associated with physical trauma and associated palpable tissue changes.

One must also consider the area, structure, and organ or system involved in the primary symptom, along with associated areas or systems, possible compensatory mechanisms, the anatomical "container" of the involved part or system, the associated connective tissue, fascial connections, the blood supply and lymphatics, the innervation, both somatic and autonomic, and hormonal or immune influences. Considerations must extend well beyond the musculoskeletal system and the cranium.

Visual cues provide information to further pursue in the physical examination. The patient's gait and general appearance reveal useful information. Asymmetry may represent a functionally normal anatomic variant, so function and dysfunctional asymmetries should be distinguished.

A light, gentle touch is required to receive information without altering the functioning of the tissue. Excessive pressure will obliterate the information being sought, just as an arterial pulse will be obliterated by heavy-handed compressive fingers.

The primary area of dysfunction, the site of original insult or injury, may exist in any area or system. A compensatory reaction may ensue anywhere in the body or not at all. Differing dysfunctions may create similar-appearing motion changes in the cranium but require significantly different treatment. For example, a side-bending rotation pattern in the cranial base may arise from a sprained ankle or a blow to the head, each requiring quite different treatment approaches.

Both observation and motion testing are used in the diagnostic process. When motion testing is used in the cranium, it must be performed with the utmost respect for the patient and with a consideration for the effect of the examiner's touch on the patient's response to that touch. The range of motion of the bone or membrane is tested within the context of the primary respiratory mechanism (PRM). Motion is simply initiated during the phase of the PRM that most closely resembles it, and then followed to the endpoint. Movement must not be forced beyond the range that occurs when the fluid carries on what you have initiated with gentle prompting.

Whenever possible, motion should be evaluated when the PRM begins the phase closest to the motion being tested. Motion is encouraged slowly and gently. When a response is observed, the operator simply follows the motion as the inherent forces carry it to its limit. If no response is observed, the motion being tested is not present and the examination should continue. The system should be allowed to return to its normal motion for several cycles before initiating another motion test. It is very easy to interfere with one's own diagnostic procedure if motion testing is performed too quickly or forcefully. Warning! The cranium can be very sensitive to the introduction of outside force and adverse reactions may ensue if excessive force is used.

## Methods

Two of the most common ways of contacting the cranium during diagnosis and treatment are the *vault hold* and the *fronto-occipital hold*. Each approach will give the operator a slightly different view of the system. The choice of which approach is most effective is one that the operator determines for each clinical situation.

1. **Vault hold:** The physician places his hands on either side of the head with the thumbs touching each other just above the sagittal suture (they should not be touching the patient's head). The index fingers contact the greater wings of the sphenoid, the little fingers contact the occiput, and the middle two fingers contact the temporal and parietal bones (one on each side of the ear). The finger pads, not the tips, are used. The entire finger and palm of the hand should contact the head.
2. **Fronto-occipital hold:** The physician places one hand under the patient's head, cupping the occipital squama. The other hand is placed across the forehead so that the thumb and index or middle finger of that hand contacts the grater wings laterally. The entire

hand, not just the finger pads, should contact the patient's head.

## ■ PRINCIPLES OF TREATMENT

Still made it very clear in his writing that osteopathic treatment is founded on the clinical applications of a set of principles and is not just a collection of techniques. There are many approaches to treatment that adhere to osteopathic principles.

William Sutherland designed his approach to treatment of the entire body based on what he observed. He designed many of his treatments using these principles of the power in the corrective forces within, direct action, exaggeration, which is now commonly referred to as "indirect," disengagement, molding, and opposite physiologic motion.

Molding and opposite physiologic motion are not described in this chapter.

1. **Indirect (exaggeration):** The dysfunction is guided in the direction toward the freedom of motion. It is the direction in which the point of balanced membranous tension is commonly found.
2. **Direct action:** The dysfunction is moved in the direction of the restriction to the motion barrier. Gentle encouragement is maintained against the restrictive barrier until release occurs. Matching treatment force and direction to the resistance felt in the tissues allows direct treatments to be performed from a point of balance and can enhance the treatment process.
3. **Disengagement:** The articulation is separated. Traction or compression may be necessary for disengagement, according to the anatomy of the articulation involved.

Other additional forces may be used to enhance the treatment, including:

1. **Directing the tide:** The force of the fluid fluctuation is used to achieve the changes necessary in the specific area requiring treatment. This approach is described in the next section.
2. **Respiratory assist:** Although the phases of the PRM are independent of the phases of breathing (Sutherland refers to this as *second-*

*ary respiration*), they do have the capacity to influence each other. Respiratory assistance can be used to enhance one phase of the PRM. Inhalation can be used to accentuate flexion and external rotation, and exhalation can be used to accentuate extension and internal rotation. The operator may ask the patient to coordinate his secondary respiration at a specific moment in the treatment to enhance a release or support a therapeutic motion.

## ■ BALANCED MEMBRANEOUS TENSION

Membranous articular strains may be treated using the principles of balanced membranous tension. This is a form of exaggeration where the cranium is guided in the direction of the pattern to the point of greatest ease. This may be performed using the vault, fronto-occipital, or temporal contact. The position is maintained until the inherent forces correct the dysfunction. Respiratory assist and/or directing the tide may be used to enhance the treatment. If more than one pattern is present, each pattern may be treated individually, or all patterns may be treated simultaneously, a process called *stacking*.

## ■ APPROACHES TO ALTERING THE PATTERN OF FLUID FLUCTUATION

### Compression of the Fourth Ventricle (CV-4)

This technique is commonly called the CV-4 technique because its effects are postulated to be caused by compression of the fluid in the fourth ventricle, which lies anterior to the occipital squama, and has a profound effect on the physiologic centers, located in the floor of the fourth ventricle. It is one of the most useful of all cranial techniques. Its relative contraindications include acute cerebral hemorrhage and increased intracranial pressure.

This technique has been used successfully to relieve headaches, reduce fever, assist in difficult labor, relieve congested sinuses and lungs, reduce edema, and generally promote the interchange of fluids throughout the body. It can also be used to reduce the effects of trauma, such as a whiplash injury. Administering a CV-4 may

also assist in the resolution of secondary somatic dysfunctions throughout the body.

One way to perform the CV-4 is for the operator to place her thenar eminences on the occipital squama, below the superior nuchal line. The hands must not be on the temporal bone or the occipitomastoid (OM) suture, because this will create dysfunctions. The OM suture should be located before the hands are placed to avoid its compression. Fingers may then be either overlapped or interlaced to cradle the occiput. It is crucial to remember that the intent of this technique is to affect the fluid of the fourth ventricle and not to compress the associated bones and meninges.

The operator begins by monitoring the primary respiratory mechanism through several cycles. The mechanism is then followed into the exhalation phase, with the operator gently resisting its motion toward the inhalation phase.

After a time, the fluid fluctuation will slow to a *still point*, during which no fluctuation will be palpable. At this point the operator may notice warmth in her palms or sweat on the patient's forehead, and the patient's breathing may change. To finish, the operator maintains her hand position, applying no pressure, until normal phasic fluid fluctuation returns. This may take from 15 seconds to several minutes. This signifies the end of the treatment. In cases of acute head trauma or tenderness, this approach may be applied to the sacrum with extension encouraged by directing the base anteriorly, resisting flexion.

### Venous Sinus Drainage

This relatively gentle technique may increase intracranial venous drainage. The hand contact on the bone of the external cranium exerts an influence on the dura that comprises the venous sinuses. Before treatment is initiated, the thoracic outlet, cervical, and occipitoatlantal joint dysfunctions must be mobilized to allow drainage from the venous sinuses, out the internal jugular vein and into the thoracic cavity.

**Step 1.** The physician places four fingers across the superior nuchal line, pointed directly anteriorly toward the patient's face. This position is maintained with slight pressure (usually the weight of the head will suffice) until release or an apparent softening of the bone is felt beneath the fingers. This release is followed to maintain balance of tension until both sides release (several minutes). This promotes drainage of the transverse sinus.

**Step 2.** To promote drainage of the confluence of sinuses, one finger is placed on the inion with the hands cradling the back of the head. The same procedure is followed until a "softening" response is felt.

**Step 3.** To promote the drainage of the occipital sinus, two or three fingers are lined up on either side of the midline from the inion down to the suboccipital tissues. Maintain this contact until softening is felt.

**Step 4.** To promote drainage of the superior sagittal sinus, the sagittal suture may be spread by moving superiorly and anteriorly from the lambda with two crossed thumbs on either side of the suture, disengaging the suture. After a local release is noted, treatment proceeds up the suture, one thumb at a time, toward the bregma. Continue anteriorly on the frontal bone with fingers lined up along both sides of the midline until a response is felt.

## V-Spread

V-spread is a combination of disengagement and directing the tide. The physician places two fingers of one hand on either side of the suture to be released and exerts gentle traction to disengage the suture. Simultaneously, one or two fingers are placed on the point of greatest distance from the suture on the contralateral side. The intention to direct the fluid with these fingers, combined with gentle pressure, if necessary, will send a fluid fluctuation toward that suture. This fluid fluctuation should be palpated by the V-spread fingers and will continue to manifest an effect between the two guiding and directing hands. The physician adjusts the directing fingers until a response is palpated between the two V-spread fingers. Release or an apparent softening of the tissues will occur.

## Lateral Fluctuation

Lateral fluctuation can be useful in calming patients after traumatic or other stressful situations in which a dysfunctional lateral fluctuation is persistent or in which no therapeutic motion is present. A lateral fluctuation may be initiated with a bilateral temporal hold, the thumbs over the anterior aspects of the mastoid processes and the fingers cupping the occipital squama. Motion is initiated by directing one temporal bone toward external rotation and the other toward internal rotation, shifting fluid toward the side of external rotation. Attention is placed on the shifting fluid, not the rotation of bone. Motion should be followed gently to its endpoint, and then initiated in the opposite direction, again focusing on the shift of the fluid. Repeat this process until the fluid shifts persist without assistance. At this point allow the fluctuation to continue, resisting each phase gently until a still point is reached. The treatment is complete when the PRM has resumed its normal phasic movement.

**REFERENCES**

Magoun HI. *Osteopathy in the Cranial Field, 3rd ed.* Kirksville, MO: The Journal Printing Co. 1976.

Still AT. *Philosophy of Osteopathy.* Kirksville, MO: Published by the author, 1889.

Sutherland WG. *Teachings in the Science of Osteopathy.* Cambridge, MA: Rudra Press, 1990.

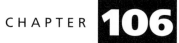

# CHAPTER 106

# Practical Applications of Cranial Osteopathy

*Sonia Rivera-Martinez*

T he osteopath reasons that order and health are inseparable and that when order in all part is found, disease cannot prevail. *Andrew Taylor Still*

Osteopathic physicians from the time of William G. Sutherland, DO, to the present date have recognized the cranial concept as a valuable therapeutic modality in clinical practice. Case histories describing the specific diagnosis and treatment of a large variety of disorders are widely documented in osteopathic literature. In this chapter, we discuss a few of these clinical applications.

## ■ ALLERGIC CONJUNCTIVITIS

Allergy to an airborne antigen is the typical cause of this type of conjunctivitis. It is acute in onset, recurrent, and commonly seasonal. In addition to bilateral conjunctivitis, ocular itching, and watery discharge, most patients will also report concomitant rhinitis. Diagnosis is made on a clinical basis. Avoidance of the inciting antigen, desensitization, and antihistamines are the mainstays of treatment. Structural dysfunctions tend to lower the resistance to allergens. Relieving restrictions of the facial bones, especially the zygoma, maxillae, and nasal bones, and also of the lacrimal ducts, postnasal circulation, and sphenopalatine ganglia may improve or relieve symptoms.

## ■ ASYMMETRY OF THE FACE

Stresses inflicted on the skull, whether by the birth process, use of forceps or vacuum extrac-tor, or by trauma, may result in asymmetry of the facial structures. In medical literature, such asymmetries have been documented with a broad array of implications, from simply cosmetic to clinically relevant. Whenever possible, these asymmetries should be treated in the postnatal period or soon after the trauma has occurred. Early correction can lessen the possibility of these becoming permanent; in infants and children, this may prevent these asymmetries from becoming incorporated into the pattern of growth.

## ■ FEEDING ABNORMALITIES IN AN INFANT

Structural abnormalities of the skull that interfere with the appropriate function of the muscles of mastication and nerves involved in the suckling and swallowing reflexes account for many difficulties infants experience in feeding. Breastfeeding is particularly affected by alterations to structures because it entails greater use of the suckling and swallowing mechanisms and requires strong muscles of mastication. Other considerations in the evaluation of an infant with suckling dysfunction are the assessment of the mother's breastfeeding technique and method of attachment. An infant's sucking reflex is strongest in the first half hour after birth, and successful breastfeeding largely depends on beginning during the neonatal period. Early postnatal treatment of cranial somatic dysfunctions may avert problems with latch-on and breastfeeding.

## ■ MIGRAINE HEADACHE

Somatic dysfunction of the sphenobasilar symphysis and temporal bone are common in migraine headache. In his observations, Magoun describes the greater wing of the sphenoid as usually being high on the side of the migraine pain. In this position, membranous tension would have a tendency to restrict the basilar region and vascular beds. Given that the cavernous sinuses are in the immediate vicinity, an anatomical alteration of the position of the sphenoid could potentially disrupt venous circulation. The resultant congestion and edema surrounding pain-sensitive structures may activate the cascade of events that produce migraine pain via the trigeminovascular system. Judicious and well-timed institution of manipulative treatment of cranial dysfunctions may terminate and even preempt a migraine attack.

## ■ STRABISMUS

Strabismus may result from paralysis or unequal tone of the ocular muscles. A lesion of the occulomotor nerve may cause the paralysis, and supranuclear abnormalities are the usual root of unequal tone. If strabismus is not corrected before the age of 4 to 6 years old, permanent vision loss may ensue. Medical treatment options include corrective lenses, orthoptic training, and surgery to correct the balance of the ocular muscles. Distortions of the orbit could produce a change in the origin and insertion of ocular muscles, and these can lose their inherent tonicity and become flaccid. Furthermore, cranial somatic dysfunctions may bring about deficient nerve trophism, affecting the cranial nerves that supply ocular muscles, thereby setting the stage for strabismus. Osteopathic treatment should focus on correcting these relationships.

## ■ TINNITUS

Tinnitus is a subjective experience characterized by a ringing, buzzing, roaring, whistling, or hissing sound in the ear. The perception of the noise occurs without an acoustic stimulus. The noise may occur intermittently, continuously, or in synchrony with the heartbeats. Hearing loss is usually present with this disorder. Almost all disorders of the ear may be associated with tinnitus.

Hearing aids and background music may help suppress the annoying noises. In the cranial direction, correcting dysfunctions of the temporal bones and releasing the cervical fascia may mitigate the tinnitus. This diminishing of symptoms may easily be explained because of the fact that temporal bone position affects the opening and closing of the cartilaginous portion of the Eustachian tube. High-pitch sounds occur with external rotation of the temporal bone in which the Eustachian tube is held open. A temporal bone in internal rotation will hold the tube closed and a low-pitch sound occurs.

## ■ VERTIGO

Lesions or disturbances of the inner ear, eighth cranial nerve, or vestibulocholear nuclei usually result in vertigo. The types of vertigo are the subjective type, in which the patient feels as if he or she is rotating, and the objective type, in which the environment appears to be rotating.

Therapeutic options include medications in the acute phase, and for the chronic state, vestibular and gait exercises may be effective. A common cranial dysfunction seen in patients with vertigo is one in which the temporal bone on one side is in external rotation while the other is in internal rotation. This dysfunctional arrangement may disrupt the orientation of the semicircular canals, producing vertigo. Balancing the temporals and the associated neck muscles may provide relief.

### Case 1

L.D. was a 12-hour-old girl with difficulty latching onto her mother's breast for feeding. This problem continued to persist even after the assistance of a lactation specialist on appropriate breastfeeding techniques and method of attachment. The baby's mother was frustrated because she had breastfed her two previous children with ease. According to the mother, the infant was not forming an adequate seal between the mouth and breast, and this caused poor sucking pressure. Most puzzling to the mother was that the infant was successful at feeding from a bottle.

At birth, the baby's anthropometrical measurements and APGAR scores were normal (weight 3702 g, length 53.2 cm, head circumference 33 cm; APGAR 10 and 9 at 1 and 5 minutes, respectively). She was born at 39 weeks via vaginal delivery with a vertex right occiput anterior presentation. Stage two of labor was 1 hour and 10 minutes, an episiotomy was performed, and vacuum extraction was used to assist the delivery secondary due to maternal exhaustion. In addition, no epidural anesthesia was administered throughout the birthing process. The pregnancy was uncomplicated without any maternal illnesses, and the only medication taken was prenatal vitamins. Presently, the mother reports the infant is feeding well on breast milk in a bottle and appears to have normal appetite, micturition, and bowel movements.

On physical examination L.D. was alert and active, freely moving all four limbs. Vital signs were stable, the anterior fontanelle was open and flat, a red reflex was noted bilaterally, the clavicles were intact, and Moro reflex was present. No cephalohematoma, subconjunctival hemorrhage, or caput succedaneum was noted. In addition, no facial nerve or brachial plexus-related palsies or other signs suggestive of obvious birth trauma were observed. However, oral examination revealed a weak suck reflex. Further, the infant had no observable facial congenital defects (i.e., cleft lip).

Findings observed on osteopathic examination were compression of the occipital condyles bilaterally (the left side greater than right), left parietal bone externally rotated, right medial pterygoid muscle spasm, and an anterior sacral base. No bossing of the frontal and parietal bones was noted and there was no overlapping of sutures present.

The osteopathic manipulative treatment of L.D. was performed while she was sleeping. Palpation for cranial motion and treatment with cranial techniques is difficult in an infant because they are, for the most part, continuously moving. For this reason, it is best to conduct a cranial examination and treatment as the infant is asleep or being fed. The dysfunctions found on the osteopathic examination of L.D. were addressed with balancing of membranous tension, decompression of the occipital condyles, and other cranial techniques, as well as sacral balancing. At the conclusion of the cranial treatment, L.D. was able to latch-on successfully to her mother's breast for the first time. She was discharged from the hospital 12 hours later with no further symptoms and instructions to follow-up in 1 week.

At the subsequent office visit, L.D. was found to have regained her birth weight and had continued to breastfeed without difficulties. Osteopathic examination revealed that the dysfunctions initially found had not recurred.

## ■ DISCUSSION

It is widely recognized that putting the infant to the maternal breast in the early postpartum period is important in facilitating mother–child bonding, successful breastfeeding, and enhances a mother's confidence that she can breastfeed. When possible, arrangements such as postponing the routine weighing and measurements of the infant can be postponed to allow the infant to root and latch on during the early prenatal hours. In addition, it is known that the baby's sucking reflex is strongest within a half hour of birth, and this timeframe coincides with when the baby is most alert.

Breastfeeding is a process that involves active participation of mother and infant. Evaluation of the baby's suckling reflex, the mother's breastfeeding technique, along with the method of attachment should be performed soon after delivery of the infant. To properly assess for suckling dysfunction in an infant, it is necessary to understand the mechanism of how babies are able to get milk into their bodies and the role of the anatomic structures involved in the process. For proper breastfeeding, the infant's lips and mouth must form a seal around the nipple, areola, and underlying breast tissue. With the suction that is created in the infant's mouth, the maternal breast tissues will elongate, forming a teat that will extend toward the soft palate. Then the baby's jaw and tongue compresses against the areola, causing maternal milk to move from the lactiferous sinuses into the infant's mouth. Next, the infant depresses and retracts the tongue in an undulating peristaltic motion to shift the milk to the back of the oral cavity where the receptors for the swallowing reflex are stimulated. Once the swallowing reflex is initiated, additional motions of the baby's tongue, soft palate, and larynx take place together with the closure of the nasal passages and trachea allows for milk to flow into the esophagus. In contrast, bottle-feeding is a more passive process. Milk from the bottle may flow easily without much suction or tongue/jaw motion by the infant.

This description of the breastfeeding and suckling mechanism in concert with the multitude of anatomical structures that are involved accentuate the significance of a properly functioning musculoskeletal system for an infant to feed successfully. Drs. Viola Frymann and Harold Magoun, among others, have described trauma to the skull that is sustained during labor and delivery as a possible source of feeding abnormalities in an infant. The use of forceps or vacuum extractor may be other causes of injury to the skull. As in the case of L.D., the most common presenting part is the occiput. As such, the occiput takes the greatest impact of the forces of labor. At birth the occiput is in four parts, namely the basiocciput, two lateral condylar parts, and the supraocciput. Lesions to the occiput that occur during labor mainly involve the condyles or lateral masses, which are driven into the superior articular facets of the atlas. The four parts of the occiput surround the foramen magnum and are in an intimate anatomic relationship with the hypoglossal nerve. This nerve supplies motor innervation to the tongue. As described, the tongue is a major player in the suckling reflex and has a significant role in the swallowing reflex. Other nerves involved in the swallowing process are the glossopharyngeal and vagus. Changes between the structural associations of the occiput may disturb these nerves, thereby causing suckling dysfunction. Decompressing the occipital condyles and addressing any dysfunctions of the muscles of mastication may result in relief of the suckling dysfunction, as was seen in the case of L.D. and the infants in the pilot study referenced later in this chapter.

In summary, it is essential that evaluation and treatment for suckling dysfunction take place in the early postpartum period. Timely intervention with appropriate osteopathic cranial techniques may aid in lactation success and in turn lead to a healthier infant.

## Case 2

W.R. was a 32-year-old white woman who presented to the office with a symptom of chronic migraine headaches since she was 15 years old. The headaches occured two to three times per week. However, when she was menstruating or was in a stressful period, the occurrence was daily. Her migraine headaches were described as throbbing, exacerbated with activity, eye movement, bright light, and loud noise. The episodes would usually last between 4 and 8 hours and were associated with nausea, dizziness, and sometimes vomiting. These attacks mainly affected the left side of her head, very rarely her right. W.R. stated she had no prodromal symptoms. Previous neuroimaging was negative. She had taken several different types of medications that initially provided relief but with time ceased to alleviate the pain. She further reported that she had been evaluated and treated by neurologists, acupuncturists, and many others in search of true relief. Over several months, her episodes had increased slightly in frequency and at times she had avoided her routine daily jogging because of the debilitating effect of the headaches. Moreover, the medications had become less effective in relieving the pain. With the exception of the small increase in occurrence, there had been no change in the signs or symptoms of her migraines and the pain did not awaken her from sleep. However, she found that the attacks were interfering more with her work and she was concerned about being dismissed from her job. At presentation her migraine pain was rated seven on a scale of ten, with ten being the worst and zero the least.

Her past medical and surgical history was remarkable for hypertension, which had been controlled with a beta-blocker, and a tonsillectomy when she was 5 years old. She worked as the head librarian for a large university and exercised regularly. She denied use of alcohol, caffeine, tobacco or illicit drugs, and history of trauma to the head. The family history was significant, because her mother and brother also have migraine headaches, but not as severe or frequent. Her medications included a beta-blocker daily for the hypertension and a selective serotonin agonist as needed for the migraine headache. W.R. had no known allergies.

The physical examination was unremarkable. Her vital signs were stable. Neurologic examination revealed that she was awake, alert, and oriented, the cranial nerves II to XII were grossly intact and no focal motor or sensory deficits were present. Deep tendon reflexes and motor strength for the upper and lower extremities were within normal limits.

On structural examination, there was a flattened cervical lordosis and an increased lumbar lordosis. A positive standing flexion test was noted on the left. Leg lengths were equal. There was inflare of the left ilia and a left-on-left sacral torsion, $OAFS_RR_L$, $AAR_L$, $C3ES_RR_R$, $T2FS_LR_L$, $L5FS_RR_R$, and Sibson fascia was strained bilaterally. The paravertebral muscles of the cervical and upper thoracic regions and the trapezius muscles were ropy and non-tender bilaterally. Cranial examination revealed tender points on the supraorbital notch, sphenoid, squamosal suture on the left; and posterior auricular on the right. In addition, the right occipitomastoid suture was compressed, the left temporal bone was internally rotated, and a left torsion pattern of the sphenobasilar synchondrosis (SBS) was present.

On the first visit, W.R. was treated using balanced ligamentous tension, myofascial release, muscle energy, counterstrain, progressive inhibition of neuromuscular structures (PINS) techniques, and cranial osteopathic techniques such as v-spread, distraction, and balancing. PINS was applied along the trigeminal distribution of the head and scalp. She responded well to the treatment reporting complete relief of her migraine pain. Stretching exercises were recommended for the cervical and upper thoracic spine. One week later, at the follow-up visit, W.R. reported that she had only one episode of migraine pain since the last visit and that it was less intense as compared to previous episodes requiring fewer doses of medication. During the structural examination it was noted that the tender points on the right side of skull had recurred. She was seen and treated on a monthly basis for 4 months. At the last scheduled visit, the frequency of her migraine headaches had decreased to less than once per month, the pain was readily relieved with a low dose of ibuprofen, and the tender points were no longer present. W.R. was discharged with instructions to continue the stretching exercises and to follow-up on an as-needed basis.

# ■ DISCUSSION

Migraine is the second most common type of headache in the United States. Approximately 10% to 20% of the U.S. population has migraine headaches. Migraine without aura is the most common type of migraine headache. The first migraine episode often occurs in childhood or during adolescence and is less likely to begin after age 50. The migraine without aura is defined as an idiopathic recurring headache disorder. An attack typically lasts between 4 and 72 hours and is characterized by unilateral location, throbbing quality, is aggravated by minor physical activity, intensity is either moderate or severe, and is associated with nausea, vomiting, photophobia, and phonophobia. The migraine with aura is also a recurring headache with similar syndrome characteristics, but the attacks are preceded by neurologic symptoms that last less than 60 minutes (the aura). A migraine attack can be severe and debilitating, often causing disruptions of lifestyle and job absenteeism. Typically a migraine attack is alleviated with sleep.

Several triggers to migraine attacks have been identified. Stress is the most common trigger. Both males and females report an increased frequency during stressful periods. In women, hormonal fluctuations, especially during menarche, pregnancy, breastfeeding, and menopause, are characteristically associated with a change in the frequency and severity of the attacks. Even oral contraceptive and estrogen replacement therapy may have similar effects on this pain syndrome. Other triggers are depression and anxiety.

The pathophysiology of migraine headaches is not fully understood. Vasoconstriction and vasodilation of the arterial blood flow of the brain and scalp occurs during a migraine event, yet it is unknown whether these are causative agents or effects of the migraine. Several phenomena occurring during a migraine attack seem to result from the activation of the trigeminovascular system. The trigeminovascular system acts as a sentinel system that causes pain to alert and protect the brain from insults such as ischemia and toxins. Migraine triggers, through direct or indirect means, cause the release of chemical activators such as prostaglandins, serotonin, and histamine. These mediators can stimulate the trigeminal nerve. Stimulation of trigeminovascular axons causes the release of vasoactive neuropeptides (substance P). Substance P acts on mast cells and platelets that lead to the release of histamine and serotonin, ultimately resulting in inflammation and local vasodilation. Furthermore, serotonin sensitizes pain receptors located in the blood vessels. This cascade of events provokes the prolongation of the pain and the hyperalgesia seen in migraine headaches.

In the evaluation of a patient with migraine headache, the physician may need to decide if neuroimaging is necessary. It is recommended that neuroimaging would be required if the patient exhibits an atypical headache pattern or if focal neurological symptoms are present. Other patients in whom neuroimaging may be indicated are patients who are awakened from sleep by the pain, those with a headache that is worsened with a Valsalva maneuver, those with rapid progressively worsening symptoms, and new onset in an older patient.

The goals of the treatment of migraine include headache prevention, reduction of severity, frequency and disability, restoration of patient ability to function, and improvement in the patient's quality of life among others. Management and treatment will depend on the duration and severity of the migraine, the associated symptoms, and response to initial treatment. The pharmacologic armamentarium consists of ergotamine and its derivatives, triptans, analgesics, and opiates. Overuse of some of these medications should be avoided because it may lead to rebound headaches. Preventive pharmacologic therapy is recommended in patients with more than two headaches per week. Complimentary therapies that may be considered and have been shown to help patient manage migraine attacks are biofeedback and cognitive behavioral therapies.

As with W.R, migraine patients may often present to an osteopathic physician after pharmacologic and other therapies have failed to give adequate pain relief. Osteopathy in the cranial field has much to offer a patient with migraine headache. Common areas of somatic dysfunc-

tions in migraine patients are the craniocervical junction, the upper cervical (C1–C3), and upper thoracic spine (T1–T4), temporal bones, and a torsion pattern of the SBS. Afferent pain stimuli from C1–C3 roots and cranial nerves V, VII, IX, and X converge on the trigeminal spinal tract and may be a factor in bringing about irritation of the trigeminovascular axons inciting the migraine cascade. It may follow that disturbances in the anatomic relationships (e.g., cranial bones, musculoskeletal) of these nerves could alter their function and activate the trigeminovascular axons. Sympathetic innervation of the head arises from T1–T4. Increased sympathetic tone triggers vasoconstriction leading to decreased blood flow, which in turn sets off the subsequent sequelae producing vasodilation and migraine. Appropriate manipulative treatment with emphasis to dysfunctions of the cranium, cervical, and upper thoracic spine may prove to have preventive and abortive effects in migraine therapy.

## REFERENCES

Atterberry OR. Migraine and its Treatment. *J Osteopathic Cranial Assoc* 1954;61–63.

Aukerman G, Knutson D, Miser WE. Management of the Acute Migraine Headache. *Am Fam Physician;* 2002;66: 2123–2130, 2140–2141.

Beers MH, Berkow R. *The Merck Manual.* Whitehouse Station, NJ: Merck Research Laboratories, 1999.

DiGiovanna EL, Schiowitz S. *An Osteopathic Approach to Diagnosis and Treatment, 2nd ed.* Philadelphia, PA: Lippincott-Raven, 1997.

Fraval MR. A pilot study: Osteopathic treatment of infants with a suckling dysfunction. *AAO Journal* 1998;2:25–33.

Frymann VM. The trauma of birth. *Osteopathic Annals* 1976; 5:197–205.

Kappler RE, Ramey KA. Head Diagnosis and Treatment. In: Ward RC, ed. *Foundations for Osteopathic Medicine.* Baltimore, MD: Williams & Wilkins 1997:535–536.

Magoun HI. The cranial concept in general practice. *Osteopathic Annals* 1976;5:32, 36–42.

Magoun HI. *Osteopathy in the Cranial Field, 3rd ed.* Biose, ID: Northwest Printing, 1976.

Magoun HI. *Practical Osteopathic Procedures.* Kirksville, MO: The Journal Printing Company, 1978.

Sinusas K, Gagliardi A. Initial Management of Breastfeeding. *Am Fam Physician* 2001;64:981–988, 991–992.

Ward RC. *Foundations for Osteopathic Medicine.* Baltimore, MD: Williams & Wilkins 1997:901–913.

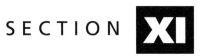

# Systemic Considerations

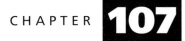

# Lymphatics

*Dennis J. Dowling*

## ■ THE IMMUNE SYSTEM

The immune system is actually not located in a single organ but is a multiorgan system that prevents damage from microorganisms and also maintains homeostasis. It includes first-line defenses that act as barriers and filtration mechanisms to reduce or eliminate incursion by particles and infectious agents. During the act of inhalation, air brought in through the nostrils is filtered through nasal follicles, humidified by mucus, and brought into the pharynx past the adenoidal and tonsilar lymphatic tissues. Offensive materials such as dust and bacteria are made soluble and subjected to the bacterostatic properties of mucus and saliva. If they manage to make it as far as the bronchi, an escalator-like action of the lining cilia brings some of these materials back up to the posterior pharynx, where they can be swallowed and subjected to the acids and enzymes of the stomach.

Scavenger cells called macrophages might consume other components that escape this process. If they still persist, the body may recognize them and send weapons known as antibodies to deal with recognized antigens.

The skin is a first line of defense for excluding bacterial and viral infection. Most often, it takes a breakdown in the skin's integrity to lead to infection via this route. Practically each of the body's fluids has some bacterostatic properties to reduce proliferation in anticipation of a more directed response. Perspiration contains lactic and fatty acids known to have this potential. Aberrant cell production, such as cancer, is also recognized and, for the most part, removed.

Thermostatic changes regulated by the central nervous system may actually be a basic attempt to reduce replication of microorganisms. Fever as a symptom shows evidence that there is invasion and response. Temperature gradients of a certain level inhibit protein synthesis. The problem in infection is not that there is a fever. The patient may suffer when it does not occur as it should, is dangerously high, occurs too rapidly, or remains elevated inappropriately after the infection has been adequately managed. Generally, the very old, the very young, or immune-impaired persons tend to show these difficulties. The use of antipyretic medications may be counterproductive to the defense process against microorganisms.

Modern medical pharmacological interventions have been very effective in facilitating the body's immune response. Medication augments the efficiency of the response but rarely replaces it. Most of the antibiotics and antiviral agents commonly used, especially on an outpatient basis, are bacterostatic in function (i.e., they inhibit further replication of the number of organisms, and thus allow the body to mount its own defenses to fight and destroy the invaders). When these defenses are absent or overwhelmed, more destructive and dangerous bacterocidal agents may prove helpful. In some cases, more harm comes from the side effects of these medications than the good accomplished.

When operating optimally, the body is an integrated machine capable of defending and repairing itself. These activities are dependent on each of the neurological, endocrinological, hematological, respiratory, urological, gastrointestinal, and vascular systems. The importance of the immune system in its more specific functions has implications for the constant health of the individual.

## ■ LYMPHATICS

### Functions

The two primary functions of the lymphatic system are filtering of particulate matter before it enters the vascular system and development and delivery of components to combat foreign substances. It is selective for particulate size and returns the nearly 200 grams of protein that leak out through capillary filtration every 24 hours.

### Components

Lymph, a clear, transparent, watery substance is produced primarily by the liver and gastrointestinal tract and contains fat, fatty acids, glycerol, amino acids, glucose, and other substances. These substances may give the lymph a more milk-like appearance. When produced by other regions, it is a filtrate of excess fluid drained away from the arterial ends of capillaries by lymph vessels. Normal lymphatic flow is approximately 2 liters per day for the entire body.

In combating foreign substances, the immune function of the lymphatic system relies on the phagocytic action of scavenger cells such as macrophages and competent cells such as the lymphocytes, which have varied functions. Some interact directly with foreign intrusions, whereas others, the *B-lymphocytes*, produce antibodies as a means of unlocking or weakening the invaders' defenses.

### Structure

The structure of the system consists of lymph nodes and channels. The lymph vessels usually traverse at least two nodes. Because not all of these are in use at any given time, there is a tremendous reserve capacity. Flow along these channels is unidirectional, controlled by a valvular system. Sections between the valves contract in sequential reaction to distension, further promoting one-way flow. Some of the larger vessels are also selective in the amount and size of the material they contain.

Both a deep and superficial system of vessels exist, with each servicing specific regions. The deep system (Fig. 107-1) drains the structures of the thorax, abdomen, pelvis, and perineum. The channels and their affiliated nodes surround major organs and vasculature and join into larger vessels until they unite with either the right lymphatic duct or the thoracic duct. The superficial lymphatic vessels (Fig. 107-2) drain the skin and other musculoskeletal structures and are located with their nodal components near veins and travel through the superficial fasciae. Again, the direction of flow is from the periphery to the core, with drainage symmetrically occurring toward the cervical, axillary, and inguinal regions, and thereafter to the deeper system. The thoracic duct, the largest of all lymphatic channels, is also under some direct neural influence from the sympathetic system.

### Lymphatic Flow

In the generally healthy individual, the abdominal lymphatics are responsible for most of lym-

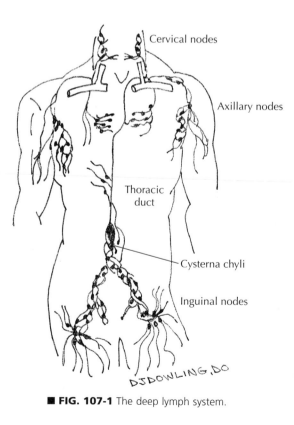

■ **FIG. 107-1** The deep lymph system.

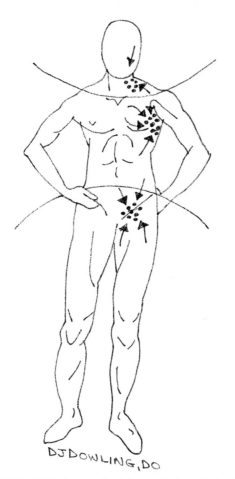

DJ DOWLING, DO

■ **FIG. 107-2** Symmetric drainage of the skin by the superficial lymph system.

phatic fluid production. Paradoxically, increased pressure on these vessels causes them to initially open rather than close. Intraluminal distension also creates some of the flow along with reactive contraction of the vessels. Intestinal motility, by direct pressure on the vessels and by increased production of the lymphatic fluid, produces flow.

## Diaphragm

The major pump of the lymphatic system is muscular activity, with the diaphragm acting as the primary engine. As the diaphragm descends into the abdominal cavity during inhalation, intra-abdominal pressure is increased, thereby creating increased pressure on the vessels and other lymphatic tissue such as the nodes. The contents

of the relatively large pleural lymphatic nodes are pressured by the expanding alveoli sacs to empty their contents. This causes the contents to be propelled along in a cephalad direction toward the subclavian veins. Elevation of the diaphragm during exhalation lowers the intra-abdominal pressure and creates a pressure gradient for more fluid to be drawn into the abdominal vessels. Increase in respiratory capacity therefore increases the function and efficiency of the system.

## Skeletal Muscle

Skeletal muscular activity is the other major pump of the lymphatic system. The intermittent action of contraction and relaxation during physical activity produces a change in interstitial pressure increasing flow by compression, especially against the influence of gravity, from the periphery toward the trunk. Even passive activity such as massage or manipulation alters the pressure on the smaller lymphatic vessels.

## Dysfunction

Impaired function of either of these muscular pumps, the diaphragm or skeletal muscle, leads to stasis of the lymphatic system. Restricted thoracic cage motion, as is often seen in chronic conditions such as asthma, emphysema, bronchitis, and acute respiratory illness, handicaps adequate function. This acts locally as well as systemically in the lungs. Peripheral edema is often seen in states of impaired musculoskeletal activity, especially when the other means of peripheral drainage, the venous system, is absent, blocked, stiff, damaged, or weakened. This is found most frequently in the lower extremities but can be observed in other gravity-dependent regions such as the sacrum and buttocks in a patient in a prolonged supine position.

## Pressures

As a system of tubes, the lymphatic vessels are closed endothelial tubes that are permeable to fluids and high molecular compounds. Four major pressures act to mobilize fluids into and out of the lymphatic capillary:

1. Capillary pressure moves fluids out through the capillary membranes.

2. Interstitial fluid pressure moves fluid inward when the pressure is positive and outward when negative.
3. The plasma colloid osmotic pressure causes osmosis of fluid inward through the membrane.
4. Osmosis outward through the membrane is caused by interstitial fluid colloid osmotic pressure.

## Lymph Nodes

Lymph nodes vary in size and are aggregates of lymphatic tissue. Kidney bean-shaped, each consists of a cortex containing germinal centers and an inner medulla. Reticuloendothelial cells are located along trabecular connective tissue and act as a filtration system for particulate matter. An efferent lymph vessel exits at the hilum, along with a vein, and is accompanied by an artery. An afferent lymph vessel enters on the convex side through the capsule.

## Spleen

The spleen is the largest of all lymphatic tissues and rests against the lower ribs (nine through eleven), the diaphragm, the stomach, and the left kidney in the left hypochondral region. A parenchyma of red and white pulp is surrounded by a capsule of fibrous connective tissue that contains efferent lymphatics, blood vessels, nerves, and some smooth muscle. The red pulp is a cordal and sinusoidal system concerned primarily with the production of blood products. The white pulp, which is lymphoid tissue, produces thymus-dependent *T lymphocytes* and *B lymphocytes* and *plasma cells*. The latter components produce the humeral antibody component of the immune system, and the T-lymphocytes are involved in the cell-mediated arm of the system. The vasculature consists of the splenic artery, the largest branch from the celiac trunk, and the splenic vein, which unites with the mesenteric vein to form the portal vein.

Five percent of the blood volume per minute enters the spleen. Normally, the spleen sequesters one third of the available platelet pool and approximately 40 to 50 mL of erythrocytes. These latter elements may be immature cells being readied for use, aged cells being prepared for retirement and recycling of their components, or abnormal red blood cells that have been removed from the pool. As a preparation site for newly produced cells, the surface area is increased by pitting the central portion of the cells in order that they are converted to normally functioning biconcave disks.

Embryologically, the spleen is responsible for the production of fetal hemoglobin and retains some potential for extramedullary hematopoiesis throughout life. Besides removing the effete, less functioning cells, the spleen also clears microorganisms and particulate matter. It produces jellylike substances called *opsonins*, which may cover certain particles or organisms. These amalgams are then more easily destroyed by the liver or macrophages. The spleen is more efficient than the liver at removing antigen/antibody complexes and poorly opsonized material.

Splenic activity can be influenced by several factors. A distended stomach or a full colon can compress the spleen. Several times per minute, the descent of the diaphragm pushes the spleen further inferiorly, and in intense activities such as exercise, it increases the rate and the extent of splenic compression. Sympathetic stimulation causes contraction of the capsule, which causes further expulsion of blood and other contents into the circulation. During times of injury, this can act as an auto-transfusion process, with the delivery of erythrocytes to compensate for loss and platelets to begin some of the bandaging process. The immunological components can be propelled to reach a site of active or potential infection.

## ■ INFECTION

In response to infection, the lymphatic tissue reacts much in the way a factory might to increased demand. Production of immunocompetent cells and destruction of the invading organisms or substances are increased. Lymphoid tissue that was previously non-palpable may hypertrophy. Upper respiratory infections frequently have findings of lymphadenopathy in the cervical chain lymph nodes. Inguinal lymph node adenopathy may be noted in cases of urinary or pelvic infection. Enlargement of the spleen, known as *splenomegaly*, occurs during diseases such as mononucleosis. Because it is normally covered by the stomach and the costal cartilage, a palpable spleen is a cardinal finding of this viral infection.

The spleen may also become enlarged when the marrow is unable to further undertake hematopoiesis. The primitive production of fetal hemoglobin can be reestablished and may help maintain the blood's oxygen-carrying capacity in spite of idiopathic anemia. The liver may increase in size from infection or other toxic influence. Hepatitis, or inflammation of the liver, frequently results in *hepatomegaly*. Subsequent to infection, it may be quite some time before the lymphatic tissue regresses to its previous size, if at all.

## ■ HISTORICAL PERSPECTIVE

> I have successfully treated many cases of pneumonia, both lobar and pleurotic, by convecting the ribs at their spinal articulations . . . I carefully adjust the misplaced ribs.
> Andrew Taylor Still, MD, DO

### Spanish Influenza

The Spanish flu pandemic of 1917 to 1919 has been called by some in the pre-HIV age as "the last great plague." The middle estimate of the worldwide death toll was approximately twenty million lives lost to the illness in that era. Perhaps as many as 500 million people had the illness commonly known as "grippe." Although other plagues had higher death rates, in terms of sheer numbers, the Spanish flu pandemic is credited as one of the worst, if not the worst. In the United States, one person in every four (approximately twenty million cases) became ill with the flu.

The symptoms were similar to that experienced with other influenza epidemics, but the especially virulent nature of the illness and the complication that ensued, especially the increased susceptibility to subsequent pneumonia, raised both the morbidity and mortality. One out of four American soldiers who died in the time of World War I actually died from this one–two combination of virus and bacteria. In the United States, close to 500,000 people are estimated to have finally died as a result of the disease or the post-flu pneumonia. Insurance companies estimated that 13% of the deaths were directly caused by influenza and 87% resulted from the combination with pneumonia. In some communities along the Atlantic seaboard, estimates were as high as a 50% risk of dying after pneumonia. A disease that had previously been called "the old man's friend" in quickly ending the suffering of the old and infirmed was indiscriminate in regards to the delivery of death, because most city morgues were grossly overwhelmed. There was no panic until it was almost over. Unlike the Black Plague, bodies were not collecting in the streets. Those who became ill took to their beds with the expectation that they would improve in a few days. The course of the illness was insidious, and after some time various cities and communities banned sports events and public gatherings and fined people for spitting, and the Red Cross manufactured 50,000 flu masks.

An infected individual would typically show the symptoms of flu, perhaps improve slightly, and then worsen dramatically as pneumonia set in. The Ute Native Americans in Utah were nearly decimated, and some families saw three-quarters or more of their members die as a result. There had been flu pandemics before, but none as deadly as this instance.

A survey conducted by the Journal of the American Osteopathic Association in 1919 revealed that 1,350 osteopathic physicians reported 43,500 well-defined cases. Of these, only 160 deaths were noted, with 10 of them attributed to pneumonia. A later survey of the era of 2,445 osteopaths resulted in an estimate that the mortality rate for DO-treated cases may have been as low as one-fortieth of that experienced by patients of MDs. Typically, the rate of cases of pneumonia after influenza was one out of sixteen cases, whereas insurance companies reported a rate as high as one out of two. At the mortality rate reported by osteopathic physicians, an estimate of potentially 73,500 American deaths would have occurred versus the 500,000 otherwise reported can be inferred. In other words, there was an apparent 2.5% mortality rate for allopathy compared to a 0.37% rate for osteopathy.

At least one distinguishing intervention was the attention of the osteopathic profession toward maximizing respiratory function, raising the ribs, mobilizing restricted spinal regions, and increasing vascular and lymphatic flow. Otherwise, descriptions of treatment by individual osteopathic physicians are not much different than those of their allopathic colleagues. It is possible that some potentially harmful interventions that were traditionally used by nonosteopathic physicians were also avoided by the DOs, but in the majority of cases, the pharmacological and other therapeutic approaches were similar.

# ■ OSTEOPATHIC RESEARCH

Other investigators over the years have studied the effect of osteopathic manipulation on the immune system. Castilio and Ferris-Swift studied the effect of manipulation in the splenic region on blood indices. They found an average increase of 2,000 in the leukocyte count in 80% of the cases with a right shift and an increase in the opsonic index in as many cases. The bacteriolytic power of the serum was found to be increased in 68% of the subjects, and a decrease in the erythrocyte count was found in 75% of the cases.

Watson and Percival examined pneumonia mortality rates in children at comparable inner-city hospitals. Children treated for bronchopneumonia with manipulation at Los Angeles County Osteopathic Hospital had a 10.66% mortality rate, versus 29.6% at an allopathic hospital. Lobar pneumonia had essentially the same mortality rate, with findings of 11.2% versus 10.8% for the respective hospitals. These were in the time before antibiotics.

Measel studied antibody response after manipulation twice daily for a week combined with administration of a polyvalent pneumococcal vaccine. The study subjects showed a significant increase in antibody response to many of the subserotypes when compared to matched control subjects. An unpublished study by this author found a trend toward increased white blood cell count in the majority of treated subjects as compared to controls within 1 hour after treatment. There was a significant increase in the lymphocyte absolute number and an insignificant decrease in hemoglobin as measured at an independent laboratory.

A limited study conducted at the Lake Erie College of Osteopathic Medicine published in 1998 saw significant basophilia in seven subjects treated with lymphatic pump techniques and no change in five similarly tested control subjects.

A study on immune response in hepatitis B-inoculated subjects at the West Virginia School of Osteopathic Medicine published that same year demonstrated that 50% of twenty subjects treated with lymphatic pump techniques showed immune level antibody response by the thirteenth week as compared to 16% of the control subjects. Such results should lead to a change in the practice of medicine in favor of using regular lymphatic manipulation in vaccinated patients to possibly bring about an earlier immune response than would be expected with vaccination alone.

Some of the effects attributed to the manipulative interventions have been discussed in the literature and attributed to the phenomenon of *demargination*. A significant percentage of hematological cells actually lie against inner vessel walls as a reserve. There is a great level of capacitance, but because many vessels, arterial, venous, and lymphatic, are in reserve, a large supply of cells is available. Activities such as exercise automatically lead to increased flow. It appears that these cells, the large majority of which are immunocompetent and mature, are then "knocked off" and delivered into the blood stream. Even if this were the only effect, it would still be an improvement over the stagnation that occurs in patients unable to move or exercise themselves. Manipulation may serve to mimic this natural process in the weak and debilitated.

# ■ TREATMENT

Much of the treatment performed historically within the osteopathic profession has been thoracic pumping. Other means of lymphatic pumping includes pectoral traction, rib raising, effleurage, Dalrymple pedal pumping, cervical lymphatic drainage, doming of the diaphragm and splenic and hepatic pumping. Air sinus drainage techniques performed about the face are used in conjunction with the other techniques to help promote the production and clearance of watery mucus from the upper respiratory region.

The most efficient approach is to first treat the central components, thereby freeing drainage into the larger lymphatic structures, and thereafter to work outward toward the periphery. Techniques directed at mobilizing the upper ribs, especially the first rib, assist in clearing the way for drainage to the subclavian veins. Working from proximal to distal makes the most sense as it allows for a more opened thoroughfare through which the congested fluid may flow. However, the real benefit of osteopathic manipulation may be in the restoration of more normal functioning and facilitating the patient's own innate restorative processes.

## Contraindications

Some of the techniques may be limited or inappropriate, depending on the patient's medical condition. Splenomegaly, hepatitis, pneumothorax, rib fracture, osteoporosis, pyelonephritis, thrombotic phenomenon, and recent surgery may preclude the use of thoracic manipulation for fear of further complications. Anemia, pregnancy, and a history of neoplastic processes are relative contraindications.

There has not been any proof that such manipulations promote metastasis of malignant cells by increasing circulation. In fact, an argument could be made that the presentation of neoplastic cells to bodily organs that can develop seek-and-destroy components for abnormal tissue may be beneficial. However, caution must be exercised in this regard. The same holds true if there is an abscess or other localized infection. Sometimes it is wiser to allow the body to wall off and deal with an invader than it is to break the compartment and allow further spread.

Cardiac and respiratory conditions most likely will benefit from this form of treatment. However, care must be taken to develop interventions that facilitate improvement without compromising other considerations. Thoracic pumping may increase respiratory capacity and fluid dynamics, but to one experiencing the sensation of extreme chest pressure, the benefits may be outweighed by the psychological considerations. As in all cases of manipulative or other interventions, decisions are best developed when a diagnosis is made and indications and contraindications are evaluated.

## Case 1

T.Z. was a 55-year-old woman with a long history of alcoholism who was admitted to the hospital for liver failure. She was icteric. The liver was four fingerbreadths below the right costal margin and palpated across the midline as well. On neurologicl examination, the patient demonstrated balance difficulties, some confabulation as well as asterixis. Her skin felt doughy and her lower extremities were edematous. Laboratory findings were consistent with the hepatitis, with SGPT, SGOT, AST, bilirubin, and LDH elevated several times greater than normal. Treatment was mostly supportive and there were dietary restrictions.

The patient refused to get out of bed and reported that her legs and feet hurt too much for her to do so. The girth of the ankles was 55 cm for the right leg and 50 cm for the left at the level of the malleoli. The osteopathic medical student requested permission from the attending physician and the patient to attempt incorporating osteopathic manipulative medicine into the treatment. This was agreed upon and the MD resident was present for the initial recording of the ankle diameters.

OMT consisted of pectoral traction, rib-raising, pedal pumping, effleurage, and passive range of motion of all extremities. This was performed twice in 1 day, separated by approximately 3 hours. At the conclusion of the second treatment, there was noticeable differences in the ankle circumferences and re-measurements were performed at the level of the pen marks that were still present on the patient's skin. The new diameters were approximately 30 cm each. The patient expressed that her ankles felt much better and she proceeded to get out of the hospital bed and walked around. She was quite enthusiastic and told physicians and other patients that she could walk because of the treatment. When she was examined the next day, there was some increase in edema and the circumferences were now approximately 35 cm but the patient was basically asymptomatic. She was again treated and they returned to 30 centimeters.

## Discussion

Obviously, treatment must be tailored to the patient. Compression of the chest and upper abdomen were contraindicated in this patient because of the hepatomegaly. The decreased fluid return was part of a vicious cycle of dysfunction. The probable portal vein hypertension restricted venous return from that route. Because of the discomfort, the patient did not move, and because of this more stasis occurred. The treatment with OMT lymphatic techniques allowed for greater return of fluid. Once this was accomplished and the compression was released, more normal circulation could occur. The patient, having fewer symptoms, was then able to move about and performed more of her own lymphatic pumping by ambulation.

## Case 2

V.S. was a 65-year-old man who presented for treatment for leg pain, swelling, and weakness. He was in his usual state of health 2 years previously when back pain suddenly developed. It was discovered that he had a 6-cm abdominal aortic aneurysm that was expanding and leaking. He underwent emergency surgery and received a graft to the aorta. While hospitalized, he reported chest pain and bilateral leg pain. It was discovered that he had ischemic changes of the cardiac muscle and of the lower extremities. More extensive surgery was performed, including a subclavian–femoral bypass with graft and a four-vessel coronary artery bypass with internal mammary arteries and greater saphenous vein grafts from the left leg. The patient did well and was able to be discharged from the hospital. He had persistent paresis and edema of both lower extremities. He underwent therapy but there was not much improvement in either of these two conditions.

The patient was directed by a family member to attempt osteopathic manipulative treatment. There was weakness of two out of five of the extensor hallucis muscles of both feet, and the left leg was dusky and had a +2 pitting edema extending to the tibial tuberosity. The patient had lost all of the hair from his legs below the patellae. Pulses were difficult to appreciate at times.

The OMT regimen for the lower extremities concentrated on fluid mobility. Pedal pumping and effleurage were applied after treatment to the pelvic diaphragm and inguinal region. The patient was instructed to perform home exercises, including tracing the alphabet with his feet while sitting or lying supine. He also performed exercises using an elastic band.

The patient underwent treatment with OMT on a weekly basis for 2 months, and then the interval was gradually increased to the more recent monthly treatments. The patient's strength increased to three out of five in the left foot and to four out of five in the right foot. The patient reported that the pain and swelling had decreased significantly. He also noted that the color had remained persistently normal in appearance. Also, he noted that the hair had begun to grow back on his legs.

## Discussion

The reason for the patient's lower extremity edema was primarily caused by the removal of the greater saphenous vein. Although in theory there was still the presence of lymphatic return, this system was probably overwhelmed. In addition, the surgical reaping of the saphenous vein most probably damaged the lymphatic vessels as well. The paresis was caused by a previously undiscovered spinal cord infarct.

The lymphatic treatment allowed for fluid return. This also contributed to improved arterial circulation to the extremities. The improved circulation from this and the frequent mobilization by the patient performing exercise facilitated the increase in strength and circulation. The hair growth demonstrated the effect of this treatment.

**REFERENCES**

Castilio Y, Ferris-Swift L. Effects of splemc stimulation in normal individuals on the actual and differential blood cell count and the opsonic index. *Kansas City College of Osteopathy and Surgery Bulletin* 1932;16:10–16.

Castilio Y, Ferris-Swift L. The effect of direct splenic stimulation on the cells and the antibody content of the blood stream in acute infectious diseases. *The College Journal, Kansas City College of Osteopathy and Surgery* 1934;18(7).

Chiles HL. Editorial: a new survey of public health. *J Am Osteopath Assoc* 1919;1:227–230.

Galewaler JE. Motion, the lymphatics and manipulation. *J Am Osteopath Assoc* 1969;69:247–254.

Guyton AC. *Textbook of Medical Physiology,* 7th ed. Philadelphia: W.B. Saunders, 1986.

Jackson, et al. Effect of lymphatic and splenic pump techniques on the antibody response to hepatitis B vaccine: a pilot study. *J Am Osteopath Assoc* 1998;98:155–160.

Kapandji IA. *The Physiology of the Joints*. Vol III, Edinburgh: Churchill Livingstone, 1974.

Kohn GC. *Encyclopedia of Plague and Pestilence*. New York: Facts on File, 1995.

Langley L, Telford IR, Christensen JB. *Dynamic Anatomy and Physiology, 5th ed.* New York: McGraw-Hill, 1980.

Measel JW. The effect of the lymphatic pump on the immune response: I. Preliminary studies on the antibody response to pneumococcal polysaccharide assayed by bacterial agglutination and passive hemaglutination. *J Am Osteopath Assoc* 1982;82:28–31.

Measel JW. Introduction: thoughts on osteopathic practice and infectious diseases. *Osteopath Ann* 1982;10:92–94.

Mesina J, Hampton D, Evans R, et al. Transient basophila following the application of lymphatic pump tech-

niques, a pilot study. *J Am Osteopath Assoc* 1998;98: 91–94.

Moore KL. *Clinically Oriented Anatomy, 2nd ed.* Baltimore: Williams & Wilkins, 1985.

Robbins SL. *Pathologic Basis of Disease, 3rd ed.* Philadelphia; W.B. Saunders, 1984.

Schiowitz S, DiGiovanna E, Ausman P. *An Ostecpathic Approach to Diagnosis and Treatment.* Old Westbury, NY: New York College of Osteopathic Medicine, 1983.

Smith RK. One hundred thousand cases of influenza with a death rate one-fortieth of that officially reported under conventional medical treatment *J Am Osteopath Assoc* 2000;100:320–323.

Tasker EE. Spanish influenza:what and why? *J Am Osteopath Assoc* 1919;2:270–273.

Watson JO, Percival EN. Pneumonia research in children at Los Angeles County Osteopathic Hospital. *J Am Osteopath Assoc* 1939;39:153–159.

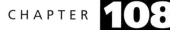

# CHAPTER 108

# Circulatory System

*Dennis J. Dowling*

Andrew Taylor Still stated, "The rule of the artery is supreme." Rather than elevate the artery above all other bodily components, Dr. Still was attempting to point out the importance of blood, its constituents, and its conduits. Without them, there would be no oxygen–carbon dioxide exchange, no nutrition, limited removal of waste products, and no life. The circulatory system serves the function of providing fuel, warmth, invader-fighting immune components, as well as returning any used or effete substances to the appropriate organs for recycling and elimination.

Blood moves and changes in a dynamic fashion and affects all structures. The absence of blood, *ischemia*, at best leads to reduced function and, at worst, tissue death. Stasis, or sluggish flow, can result in a lack of oxygenation of the affected structures. The signs and symptoms can include pallor in appearance and easy, persistent blanching after pressure. The skin can also appear smooth and hair that had previously been present can disappear. Occasionally, these are indications of single or regional somatic dysfunctions. Further impairment results in cyanosis. Skin demonstrates the blue tinge of deoxygenated blood and cell death can occur. Extending these phenomena to the other organs is reflected by atony and possible organ death. In cases of obstruction of coronary vessels, the cardiac muscle and the related intrinsic neural pacemaker control may be severely affected. If the blood supply is not quickly restored, myocardial infarction and death may occur. Constriction of renal vessels leads to hypertensive states and

progressive renal failure may result. Blood flow loss to the intestines can halt peristalsis and even lead to rupture. The effects to the central and peripheral nervous system include alterations of sensorium, consciousness, function, reflexes, and strength.

The body's innate capacities are capable of adapting to changes, to a limit. The use of collateral vessels and neovascularization are two of the mechanisms that reflect attempts to restore more normal functioning following persistent dysfunction. The adaptive response to acute decreased flow results in constriction of the blood vessels to relatively nonessential functions but even this is not as effective as resumed normal activity. The diameter of the arteries is under control of the sympathetic system and any event that brings about increased activity results in vasoconstriction. Therefore, decreased flow can be the result of local injury, shunting to another region, and/or persistent sympathetic stimulation. The final status depends on the ability of the terminal capillaries to deliver the blood to the target tissue.

There are two potential drainage routes for fluids in the body: the venous and lymphatic systems. When one is impaired, the other somewhat compensates. There are limits and even a temporary condition can set off a cascade of impaired function, compensation, and hopefully recovery. Too often, the compensation is inadequate

When noting circulation-related vital signs, such as heart rate and blood pressure, indicating alterations from normal, it is imperative that the reason for the condition be discerned. Aside from neural influences, circulation is affected by temperature and climate, endocrinological function, medications, and even food. The most obvious reason for decreased blood pressure and increased heart rate is blood loss. Hyperthyroidism will typically be associated with an increase in both heart rate and blood pressure, along with other signs and symptoms. Hypothyroidism will demonstrate the opposite. Many medications can cause subtle or severe alterations.

The body attempts to respond to excess heat, whether internally established such as in fever or because of the environment, by increasing perspiration and dilating surface vessels as a means of dissipating the heat. Fever is a natural process that serves at least a partial function of inhibiting microbial replication. Within normal parameters, it is best left alone. Except for the very young, very old, and those with some pre-existing conditions, a few hours of temperatures of 101 to 102 degrees Fahrenheit is tolerable. The archaic understanding of fever was that it was caused by excess in blood and the solution was to draw off the excess by phlebotomy. The result was a cooling that appeared to also quiet the agitated patient. Treating the symptom did not treat the cause of the disease, and it certainly was not focused on the patient. Such treatments were the mainstay of medical treatment, even into the twentieth century. It was only a few years ago that the method of treating fever was to rapidly cool the patient in ice blankets, by sponging the skin with alcohol, and even by infusion of cool fluids into the colon. Besides weakening the immune response, such treatments caused too rapid a shift and the dilated vessels may have led to greater permeability of the skin, increased absorption of isopropyl alcohol, and a lowered seizure threshold. The current approaches to fever, i.e., allowing tolerable temperatures to occur unchecked and slowly lowering those that exceed acceptable limits, are more consonant with osteopathic philosophy and practice. In response to cold, the vessels constrict as a means of maintaining core temperature. Contemporary treatment of hypothermia is a likewise slower process than had been previously used as the "standard of care." Slow warming leads to less tissue damage.

The blood delivers reparative and defensive substances. Platelets and vasoactive substances present to areas of damage to act as a temporary bandage. Subsequently, other components move into the clot area and promote healing. Both cell-mediated and humoral elements are drawn to areas of invasion in defense of the organism. Many of these wait along the inner walls of the vessels in a process known as margination. Injury and infection promote demargination and a more rapid blood flow may contribute along with chemotactic elements. When circulation is impaired, immune function is likewise affected. Besides serving an immune function, the spleen sequesters fifty or more milliliters of blood. Although much of this blood consists of aged red blood cells, they could still serve some function. When placed under stress or injury, the capsule of the spleen can contract and bring about a small amount of this autotransfusion.

If one were to take the heart as the starting point for circulation, blood enters the right atrium and is transferred to the same-side ventricle. The deoxygenated blood travels to the lungs by way of the pulmonary artery. The higher affinity of hemoglobin for oxygen as opposed to the carbon dioxide allows for easier transfer at the capillary level. The pulmonary veins conduct blood to the left atrium, through the mitral valve to the left ventricle, and then out of the heart through the aortic valve. Some blood is diverted for the heart's own use to the coronary vessels. The rest travels via the aorta to all parts of the body. Once at the target area, the blood exits temporarily by way of and reenters a capillary. Return to the heart begins in a venuole and through subsequent veins that increase in diameter. Alterations of intra-abdominal and intra-thoracic pressures, as caused by diaphragmatic movement, draws blood to the heart by way of the vena cavum. A subsidiary portal system specializes in blood return from the liver. Portal hypertension may show surface expression in a pattern of engorged blood vessels in the abdomen known as a "caput medusa." Valves within the veins prevent backflow. Harvey's original research hundreds of years ago established that flow within the veins was unidirectional and to the heart. Although both the arteries and veins both contain smooth muscle, the arteries' walls are thicker and these vessels are less compressible. When there is localized swelling, the veins are more likely to have their lumens narrowed and congestion ensues. Inflammation of the vessels can occur, both with and without clots.

The role of the osteopathic physician is to facilitate the normal processes, especially where flow to or away from a region is impaired. Using knowledge of structure and function, the removal of impediments to circulation needs to be addressed. Contraindications include circumstances where increased circulation could lead to increased blood loss, further damage, spread of infection, or dislodgement of a blood clot. Many of the techniques that can be used for the purpose of treating lymphatic difficulties can also be used.

## ■ CASE 1

S.B. was a 63-year-old man who was brought to the emergency department in an unconscious state. He had apparently taken an overdose of his prescribed anticoagulant medication, resulting in a bihemispheric bleed that caused compression of the brain parenchyma. Neurosurgeons and neurologists who were called to evaluate determined that his condition was inoperable.

Within hours of his admission, the patient demonstrated atrial fibrillation with a rapid ventricular rate (200 per minute), a blood pressure of 90/50 mm Hg, and he became hyperpyrexic at 106 degrees Fahrenheit. The patient was breathing on his own but occasionally demonstrated Cheyne–Stokes respiration. The patient frequently grimaced. Attempts at lowering the heart rate and raising blood pressure through pharmacological means were unsuccessful, as were attempts at performing carotid and ocular pressure. In fact, these did not affect the parameters in a positive way and the patient's blood pressure decreased.

There was some inconsistency in dealing with the family. On the one hand, they were being told that there was no hope; on the other hand, one of the attending physicians was giving more hopeful prognoses than were reasonable. The osteopathic intern received permission to treat the patient with manipulation.

The causes of the signs of the patient were from the compression of the cranial contents. The cardiac, respiratory, and temperature changes were all caused by this. There was a flexion pattern to the cranial motion and the amplitude was shallow and rapid. Treatment consisted of CV4 and indirect cranial techniques.

Within minutes of the onset of treatment, the patient's ventricular response lowered to approximately one-hundred fifteen beats per minute. The temperature lowered to 102 degrees Fahrenheit and the breathing became more regular. The blood pressure increased to 100/60 mm Hg. The patient ceased grimacing. These effects lasted 8 hours. The treatment was repeated with similar effects. A "do not resuscitate" order was obtained and the patient died the next day.

### Discussion

The reasons for the findings in this patient were caused by the effects on the relevant parts of the brain. The respiratory changes were most probably caused by compression of the pons. The stimulation from the brain was also responsible for the atrial fibrillation and rapid ventricular response. The rapid heart rate is directly related to the lowered blood pressure. Although there are other causes for the patient's grimaces, the abnormal cardiac rhythm does not allow for proper filling of the cardiac chambers and the coronary vessels may not receive adequate circulation. This is a frequent cause of chest pain in patients with cardiac dysrhythmias.

Although there should be some concern in performing cranial osteopathy in patients with intracranial bleeding, the extreme nature of this situation relatively lessened the contraindications. The bleeding was confined to a closed space and there was a tamponading process in effect. The decrease in blood pressure was not caused by the blood loss but was related to the cardiac arrhythmia. The compression of the brain parenchyma was responsible for the hyperpyrexia. Insufficient time and the suddenness in the increase in his temperature precluded the likelihood of an infectious cause.

The endpoint of treatment in this case was not so much improvement of the patient's condition but was to make the patient more comfortable. It is unknown whether he actually could appreciate pain or discomfort. However, the improvement of all signs appears to indicate this.

## ■ CASE 2

A 70-year-old woman presented with multiple symptoms of back and hip pain for 3 weeks. Although relevant somatic dysfunctions were noted to explain the chief symptom, examination of the lower extremities demonstrated +2 pitting edema. The patient stated that she had had swollen ankles for several years and was on diuretics and calcium channel-blocking medication for this and her hypertension. The edematous legs made it difficult for her to walk comfortably the distances to the stores in her immediate neighborhood. She denied any history of myocardial infarction or shortness of breath. Other than the chief symptom, hypertension, and peripheral edema, there were no other medical problems.

The chief finding in this patient was a posteriorly rotated ilium with a unilateral sacral shear. This was fairly simple to address and the patient felt that she returned to her previous level of functioning in this regard. The patient did accept treatment for the edema as well. The edematous legs also had an ashen appearance and the skin was flaky.

The treatment focused on increasing drainage from the lower extremities. Dalrymple pedal pumping, effleurage, and petrissage were used. She was shown how to pump her feet with the legs elevated at home. The patient returned 1 week later and reported that she had urinated more than usual the evening of the previous treatment and she felt that her ankles had decreased in size. Her ability to walk comfortably also increased. There was now a +1 pitting edema. Treatment continued over a period of 8 weeks at a weekly frequency. The patient's edema reduced significantly and the color and surface improved. There was some mild recurrence when she was returned 1 month later but still it was greatly improved over her initial appearance. The patient was followed-up for several years on a monthly to bimonthly basis. At one point she reported that she had to resume shaving her legs.

## Discussion

The evidence was present for a right-sided congestive heart failure as well as venous insufficiency. There is often a vicious loop that occurs with stasis—decreased function—increased stasis and so on. As the extremities become more edematous, the patients do not engage in as much activity. The pumping action that should occur to facilitate drainage is not performed. Diuretics have an effect of shifting fluids but the effect on the kidneys is to vasoconstrict the renal arteries. This can result in increased tolerance and the need for higher and higher doses to accomplish the same effect. There has also been some evidence for the involvement of calcium channel-blockers causing side effects of peripheral edema. The patient had been taking this medication for years without this apparently occurring.

The treatment had the effect of shifting the venous preload. More blood delivered to the right side of the heart increased the filling capacity, and more of it was then delivered to the kidneys. This accounts for the diuresis that the patient experienced on the night of the first treatment. With the decrease in edema, the patient was capable of walking to a greater extent and this combined with her home treatment allowed for greater more regular drainage. With improvement of venous drainage, arterial flow had less resistance to the tissue. The improved circulation had the unwanted, but fairly acceptable given the alternative, side effect of resumed hair growth.

### REFERENCES

Rogers FJ. An osteopathic perspective on cardiology. In: Ward RC, ed. *Foundations for Osteopathic Medicine, 2nd ed.* Philadelphia: Lippincott Williams & Wilkins, 2003: 345–369.

Sparks HV. Tissue respiration and circulation. In: Ward RC, ed. *Foundations for Osteopathic Medicine, 2nd ed.* Philadelphia: Lippincott Williams & Wilkins 2003:157–164.

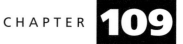

# Autonomic Nervous System

*Dennis Dowling*

The autonomic system is responsible for the moment-to-moment modification of practically all functions of the body. Although there are intrinsic plexi that promote normal activity, the sympathetic and parasympathetic systems enhance or retard function. Auerbach's and Meissner's plexi become activated by intraluminal distension and initiate peristalsis in an anterograde fashion. Increased parasympathetic activity, primarily from the vagus nerve in the cranial axis, increases gastrointestinal motility. The same can occur from microbial and chemical irritation of the inner walls. The effects are decreased transit time and decreased water absorption, among other effects. The person may also have other symptoms including discomfort, nausea, oating, and irritation.

The complementary activity of upgraded sympathetic activity has nearly the opposite effects, at least as far as the mechanical effects. Sphincters that would ordinarily be more likely to be open in effect close. Motility of the contents is radically reduced. All of this is expected, given that increased sympathetic activity is beneficial for fight or flight behaviors. Circulation to the locomotive components of the body, the arms and legs, becomes increased and is decreased to the viscera. Decreased bowel function, increased water absorption caused by increased transit time and inner surface contact, and a more solid production of fecal matter are effects. The patient may likewise have pain and discomfort from increased and trapped flatus. In some severe instances, dehiscence and rupture may occur.

The parasympathetic activity to all of the visceral organs has the unconscious result of increasing basically restorative and adaptive processes. Cardiac and respiratory functions slow, renal water conservation increases, and the senses dull. There are no parasympathetic fibers to the extremities. Sympathetic activity brings about increases in blood pressure, dilatation of some and constriction of other blood vessels, bronchodilation for increased surface area, and renal vessels constrict reducing flow to the kidneys. Pupils dilate to take in more of the surroundings and even hearing becomes more acute.

All of these are apparently for short durations under normal circumstances. They are examples of the adaptations affecting the structure and function of the body. However, dysfunction occurs when there is either persistence past the point of usefulness, inappropriate activation, a reflex loop pattern or any combination. The activation of any portion can be primary, secondary, or tertiary. The body responds to stress with vasoconstriction of all of the arteries as a means of shunting blood to the muscles. A normal reaction by the coronary vessels is to dilate, not because of an apparent paradoxical effect or receptor difference, but because the sympathetic stimulation increases the inotropic and chronotropic effects on the heart. The increased pressure, because of the rate and force of contraction, typically results in greater capacitance and perfusion of the heart itself. Partial or total occlusion by atherosclerosis or thromboembolic phenomena results in ischemia and possible infarction. The resultant pain and pressure contributes to even greater increase of sympathetic stimulation and worsening of the vessel narrowing.

In another instance, reflux esophagitis can affect the paraspinal musculature and vertebral facet joints from the middle thoracic vertebrae and upwards. Typically, the region will develop bilateral somatic dysfunctions and restriction of motion. Flattening of the region would be commonplace. Any incompetence of the gastroesophageal sphincter and acid reflux can decrease once the cause has disappeared. The somatic dysfunctions can spontaneously resolve or persist. Any persistence can then set up the reverse of the previous condition: a somatovisceral reflex as opposed to the initial viscerosomatic one. In other words, the dysfunctions, via the common innervation by the sympathetic fibers, can cause a recrudescence of the original effects in the absence of the original causes.

Some persistent conditions relate to either constant or intermittent irritation of the sympathetic nervous system. Reflex sympathetic dystrophy (RSD) is a difficult condition to treat. The precipitating injury can be significant or minor. Bone fractures of the extremities appear to be the most frequent causative element but sometimes apparently innocuous occurrences appear to be the preceding relevant event. The sensitivity of the system appears to be exquisitely set for any minor irritation. The affected person can show Raynaud syndrome and allodynia. Stimuli that should not elicit a reaction do so. The touch of clothing or a breeze touching the skin of the affected limb can show progressive reddening, blanching, and even subsequent cyanosis. The pain can be lancinating with all manner of sensory alterations.

The parasympathetic system is not without its own difficulties. Somatic dysfunctions of the suboccipital region can influence the region of the fourth ventricle and the underlying nucleus ambiguous. The stimulation of the vagus, especially if there is intermittent changes, result in such reactions as decreased blood pressure, alterations of thyroid and other endocrinological function, respiratory, cardiac blocks, gastrointestinal hyperactivity, and even pelvic changes. Cardiac effects, depending on the locus of the electrophysiological effect, can include slowing (the sinoatrial node in bradycardia) or absence

(atrioventricular nodal-mediated heart blocks) or other irregularity of heart rate and rhythm. There are many causes of diarrhea, but the wide traveling vagus is implicated in some persistence. This is evidenced by the choice of some pharmacological interventions typically used. The same can be said for some urological, gynecological, and even respiratory responses.

All of these considerations would be of no use to osteopathic physicians without the possibility of the application of the knowledge. The principle of rational treatment indicates that understanding the processes can be translated into treatment. This can involve the use of osteopathic manipulation in the integrative care of the patient. The goal, as usual, is to facilitate the normal, compensatory mechanisms of the individual's body.

Often, osteopathic physicians speak about decreasing or increasing some component. Although this is a theoretical perspective, probably the more accurate understanding is that the osteopathic physician acts to assist a resetting by removing the impedance to healthy functioning. Rather than work from a standard protocol, the development of a plan of treatment should hinge on understanding how the systems of the body interact in the discovery of the cause rather than focus on the effects, which are typically the patient's symptoms. This is sometimes difficult to accomplish, because the patient is often interested in the cessation of the symptoms. The focus must remain with determining the abnormal functions and structures and the means by which the inner health can be encouraged.

## ■ CASE 1

R.P. was a 66-year-old woman who presented with a new symptom of lower extremity pain and discomfort for 6 months. She had been seen previously in the clinic for back and neck pain and had not received osteopathic manipulation for at least one year. She had breast cancer and had undergone lumpectomy, radiation treatment, and chemotherapy. The patient had been doing well and then fell and fractured her fibula and tibia of the right leg. The fracture was caused by the trauma and was not felt to be related to any metastatic processes. She underwent surgery for the fracture and had open reduction and internal fixation of the tibial fracture. The approximation and eventual bony healing appeared to be adequate. However, the patient continued to report pain localized to the fracture site and to the whole lower extremity. These were also accompanied by sensations of burning and cold, flushing, blanching, and even times when the foot would turn blue. The patient noted that sometimes she was not able to tolerate the touch of clothing or bed sheets, and that the symptoms could drastically worsen even in response to a breeze blowing across it. The foot was often swollen. Another physician treated the patient with narcotic and non-narcotic analgesic medications. She had difficulty tolerating these and there was no improvement noted. She was begun on relatively high-dose oral steroids, which were then tapered. The symptoms improved slightly but then returned to the previous level when they were tapered. There was concern regarding the long-term side effects associated with corticosteroids.

On examination, the patient's vital signs were within normal limits with the exception of a slightly elevated blood pressure. The patient's x-rays were reviewed and there appeared to be satisfactory healing. The patient's leg was examined and had a $+1$ pitting edema and it was erythematous initially. As it was being palpated, the skin blanched and appeared mottled. There was restriction of motion of the fibular head in anterior glide, the talus was anterior, there was restriction in the popliteal region and tension and multiple tenderpoints along the iliotibial band. There was increased inversion of the right foot. The right ilium was anterior and there were single somatic dysfunction at L5, L1, and T12, among others.

The lower extremity was treated with progressive inhibition of neuromusculoskeletal structures, Myofascial release, counterstrain, muscle energy techniques, and high-velocity low-amplitude (HVLA) thrusting techniques. The latter two modalities addressed the iliac, fibular head and talus dysfunctions. The lumbar region was treated with fascial release and balanced ligamentous tension. Effleurage and lymphatic draining techniques were also applied. All treatments were selected and applied as the patient could tolerate. The patient had some initial

discomfort with all handling but the edema reduced, the patient had more mobility, and there was a change of color noted.

The patient returned the next week and noted that although the symptoms were not completely resolved, they had improved. She seemed to have greater tolerance for contact with the skin than previously. Treatment continued until the patient was able to tolerate wearing an ankle brace for support of apparently weaker talofibular ligaments. The patient was started on gabapentin as a means of addressing the neuropathic condition. The patient tolerated this.

## Discussion

Fractures are part of the cause in a majority of cases of *reflex sympathetic dystrophy* and limbs are affected in most. The symptoms can be unilateral or bilateral. There appears to be hypersensitivity of the sympathetic fibers. These accompany arteries and directly influence their diameters through increased stimulation. There appears to be a mix of both chronic and acute appearance to the condition. Prolonged constriction leads to ischemia and this can bring about inflammatory changes in the release of other vasoactive substances and increased reactivity, similar to migraine.

For this patient, treatment was directed at the more apparent region of symptoms as well as the origin of the sympathetic fibers to the lower extremity, the thoracolumbar region. Also addressed was the stasis that occurred. Not only is the arterial flow into the region impaired but also the venous and lymphatic return is also reduced.

Addressing the components of reflex sympathetic dystrophy appears to ameliorate the condition. However, given the nature of the condition, there may not be a full reversal or return to previous function. Improvement without resolution may be an acceptable goal. This also requires that the patient and the osteopathic physician come to an understanding regarding expectations.

## ■ CASE 2

A.D. was a 47-year-old woman who was referred by her gastroenterologist for back pain. The pain was nearly constant, graded as five out of ten, and described as "dull-to-sharp." There was limitation of motion. The pain was localized to the mid-thoracic region without any radiation. The patient had a history of gastroesophageal reflux and had been progressively placed on increasing doses of $H_2$ blockers and proton pump inhibitors. The abdominal symptoms that she had had previously abated but did not completely disappear. The patient had an endoscopic examination 2 weeks previously and was told that everything "looked good."

On physical examination, the patient's spine appeared to have no movement between the levels of T2 to T9, with multiple single somatic dysfunctions, and the paravertebral musculature was ropy in consistency. The patient was treated with myofascial techniques, muscle energy techniques, and HVLA thrusting techniques to the thoracic region. Exercises were added to increase mobility. She tolerated these interventions well and gradually felt improvement of her abdominalsymptoms. Over a period of 3 months, with the interval between treatments advanced to 3 weeks, the patient improved significantly. She did not have any continued symptoms of back pain. In addition, she no longer had any reflux symptoms. Her gastroenterologist agreed to reduction and then elimination of her medications. She returned 9 months later for a single visit for unrelated neck pain and reported that neither the back pain nor the abdominal discomfort had recurred.

## Discussion

The linkage between the gastrointestinal and musculoskeletal conditions is easily apparent when one considers the sympathetic innervation of the esophagus. In retrospect, it is difficult to determine whether there were viscerosomatic or somatovisceral reflexes. Whether the muscular and somatic dysfunctions occurred first and led to the gastrointestinal difficulty or if the opposite occurred is almost immaterial. What is more pertinent is that both dysfunctions, at some point, sustained the other. The pharmacological treatment only affected one aspect of the loop and in the absence of complete treatment, should be expected to be wholly or partially ineffective. By addressing both components, the condition was able to improve.

### REFERENCES

Kuchera ML, Kuchera WA. *Osteopathic Considerations in Systemic Dysfunction, 2nd ed.* Columbus, OH: Greyden Press, 1994.

Willard FH. Autonomic nervous system. In Ward RC, ed. *Foundation for Osteopathic Medicine, 2nd ed.* Philadelphia: Lippincott Williams & Wilkins, 2003:90–119.

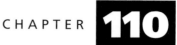

# Visceral Manipulation

*Eileen L. DiGiovanna and Dennis J. Dowling*

From the earliest days of osteopathy, direct manipulation of the viscera has been included in the armamentarium of the osteopathic physician. In his last book, *Osteopathy, Research and Practice,* Andrew T. Still, the founder of osteopathy, discussed the treatment of many disease entities and emphasized the treatment of "lesions" of the vertebrae and ribs as well as describing techniques applied directly to the viscera. His stated goal was always to improve the circulation of arterial and venous blood and lymphatic flow to and from the viscera, as well as assuring proper neural function. His preference in visceral treatment was to have the patient in a knee–chest position, from which he would lift the viscera being treated upward toward the diaphragm. He described using this type of technique in the treatment of dysentery and appendicitis. He used a technique for dyspepsia in which he placed the patient on his right side while he lifted the stomach toward to left.

The intestines are suspended in a sheath of fascia known as the mesentery. In quadrupeds, the intestines float in the abdominal cavity in coils and the chyme moves through the lumen unimpeded by gravity. In humans, peristalsis must overcome gravity as well as tensions created by the layers of intestines in a fairly narrow space. In addition, medications and some foods can have the effect of altering gastrointestinal function.

*Mesentery lift techniques* help to decongest the intestines and allow improvement in the arterial blood flow to them because their blood supply enters through the attached mesentery. These techniques also free the lymphatic channels from the intestines that lie in the tissues of the mesentery.

In her 1915 text, *Osteopathic Mechanics,* Edythe Ashmore, DO, describes three types of treatment of the liver:

1. Patient is supine, with knees flexed. The physician places one hand under the seventh to tenth ribs and one hand on top of the chondral junctions of the same ribs. The hands are compressed together and then released suddenly.

2. Patient lies on left side. The physician stands behind the patient and the patient is asked to reach his right arm behind the physician and grasp her shoulder. By leaning back the physician elevates the patient's ribs. The physician places her hands on the anterior and posterior rib cage as above. The patient inhales fully and as he exhales, the physician bends over and compresses the patient's lateral rib cage with her chest. The patient inhales fully and then at the end of exhalation the physician quickly released the compressive forces.

3. Patient in knee–chest position with the physician lifting upward if there is any visceral ptosis present.

Techniques, as described, are useful in decongesting the liver with the removal of toxic waste products. The liver possesses a rich bed of lymphatic channels and venous vessels in the portal system. It is a pressure-sensitive organ and these manipulative techniques, through pressure-gradient changes, assist in moving lymph through the channels.

Similar compressive techniques may be used for the spleen, also a pressure-sensitive organ. The spleen serves to store red and white blood cells and to remove damaged cells from circulation. It is an integral part of the immune system. Splenic pump techniques serve to assist patients who are in need of a heightened immune function, i.e., in the presence of systemic infections, and, in some anemic patients, to increase the numbers of red cells in circulation.

Both organs are fragile and care must be taken when performing these techniques. A splenic pump should not be performed on an enlarged spleen because of the danger of rupture. Compression of the rib cage in instances of hepatitis may cause damage to the liver.

Both Still and Ashmore urged use of the palmar surfaces of the fingers, not the tips of the fingers, when working with any of the abdominal contents to thus avoid injury to the internal organs.

In 1983, Jean-Pierre Barral and Pierre Mercier published a text in Paris on visceral manipulation entitled *Manipulations Vice'rales.* In 1988, this was translated into English as *Visceral Manipulation.* This text led to a renewed interest in direct treatment of the viscera.

Four types of visceral motion are described based on the system which influences or controls that motion:

1. Somatic nervous system
2. Autonomic nervous system
3. Craniosacral rhythm
4. Visceral motility

Motion of the neuromusculoskeletal system that occurs with activity such as walking, running, or movement of the trunk brings about passive motion of the viscera. The viscera need to be mobile for this motion to occur.

Motion under the control of the autonomic nervous system may be either direct or indirect. There are three major factors:

1. Diaphragmatic motion—this causes indirect motion of the contents of both the thoracic and abdominal cavities.
2. Cardiac motion—this directly affects the lungs, esophagus, mediastinum, and diaphragm.

3. Peristaltic motion—contractile waves of the hollow organs, lesser in effect than the others.

Craniosacral rhythm involves fluctuation of the cerebrospinal fluid, which bathes the brain and spinal cord. Its pressure changes, as well as variations in the pressures exerted by the arterial and venous systems affect the functioning of all systems.

Intrarectal and intravaginal techniques can be performed for the purpose of more direct manipulation of the pelvic viscera, as well as some musculoskeletal structures such as muscles and ligaments.

Visceral motility is described by Barral and Mercier as an "intrinsic, active motion." Each organ possesses this motion independent of extrinsic forces. This occurs in two phases, which Barral and Mercier name *"expir"* and *"inspir".* In "expir," the organs move toward the midline of the body, and during "inspir" they move away from the midline in a rotational manner. The rotations appear to occur around the axes of their embryologic origin. These motions may be related to the craniosacral rhythm.

Visceral osteopathic diagnosis, as with somatic diagnosis, is primarily palpatory. Each organ is evaluated for its motion characteristics. The mobility of the organs is assessed during inhalation and exhalation and by motion testing of the organ attachments. The inherent motility of each organ is assessed by palpation. Temperature changes over the organ are also noted.

The associated musculoskeletal structures are evaluated for evidence of dysfunctions. Viscerosomatic reflex findings and Chapman's points may be useful in diagnosis. Viscerovisceral reflexes, somatovisceral reflexes, and abnormal sympathetic or parasympathetic influences all affect viscera.

Osteopathic visceral manipulation is directed toward restoring normal mobility and motility of the involved organ, assuring normal lymph flow and circulation, establishing a normal cranial rhythmic impulse, and removing abnormal somatic or nervous influences on the viscera.

## ■ MESENTERIC LIFT

This technique is useful in treating patients with a wide variety of gastrointestinal problems with symptoms such as diarrhea, constipation, nausea, vomiting, and abdominal pain. Care must always be taken to assure a thorough examination to rule out more serious conditions of the abdomen.

1. **Patient position**: supine
2. **Physician position:** standing on the patient's left side initially
3. **Technique:**
   a. the physician reaches across the patient's abdomen and places the fingers on the right lower quadrant medial to the ASIS.
   b. The physician sinks the pads of his fingers into the abdomen until indirect contact is made with the cecum. The amount of resistance is noted.
   c. Traction is directed toward the umbilicus and maintained until there is a sense that there is potential additional movement of the structure.
   d. The physician then repositions his hands to the right side of the abdomen between the iliac crest and the lower ribs at approximately the mid-axillary line.
   e. The physician then uses the pads of his fingers to traction the ascending colon medially toward the umbilicus. The traction is maintained until there is a release noted. Occasionally, peristalsis may be noted.
   f. The physician then moves his fingers to the upper right abdominal quadrant and tractions the hepatic flexure of the colon medially and obliquely downward towards the umbilicus. The same end point is used prior to moving to the next region.
   g. The physician then places his right hand, oriented transversely, in the epigastric region. The ulnar edge of the hand is sunk into the region and can be assisted with the other hand in tractioning the transverse colon towards the umbilicus. The release should be noted prior to moving to the splenic flexure of the colon.
   h. The physician moves to the patient's right side.
   i. He then moves his fingers to the upper left abdominal quadrant and tractions the splenic flexure of the colon medially and obliquely downward toward the umbilicus until release is noted.
   j. The physician then uses the pads of his fingers to traction the descending colon medially toward the umbilicus. The traction is maintained until there is release noted.
   k. Then he reaches across the patient's abdomen and places the fingers on the left lower quadrant medial to the ASIS.
   l. The physician reaches across the abdomen and places the fingers on the left lower quadrant medial to the ASIS to traction on the sigmoid colon.
   m. The physician then places the pads of his fingers along a line oriented from the right ASIS to the left anterior axillary line where it crosses the rib cage. The fingers should be inferior and to either side of the umbilicus. Gentle pressure is gradually increased to introduce traction towards the right upper quadrant. This may be uncomfortable, so care must be taken.

## ■ ESOPHAGEAL RELEASE

1. **Patient position**: supine
2. **Physician position**: standing on either side of the patient at the level of the patient's chest
3. **Technique**:
   a. With his cephalad hand, the physician locates the tracheal cartilage just cephalad to the jugular notch.
   b. The thumb on the near side and the index finger on the far side are gently slid down either side of the trachea until contact is made with the esophagus. Asking the patient to swallow may assist in locating it.
   c. A gentle pinch is exerted and the esophagus is held.
   d. The thumb and forefinger of the caudad hand are spread 3 to 5 centimeters apart, with the thumb just lateral and inferior to the xiphoid process on the patient's left side. Both fingers are then directed posterior and inferior to the lower rib cage on that side.
   e. The physician exerts cephalad traction with the hand that is at the patient's neck and toward the patient's feet with the other hand.

f. The physician can translate either or both hands laterally and determines the relative freedom for each. The physician holds in the direction of freedom until there is a release noted.

Other techniques are beyond the purview of this text and can be obtained from books dedicated to this topic.

## ■ CASE STUDY

H.S. was a 25-year-old woman with a chief symptom of "irritable bowel syndrome." She had some of the classic symptoms of the condition, including episodes of pain and constipation, apparently alternating with watery loose stools that she described as diarrhea. She stated that these symptoms had been intermittent since she was 13.

A gastrointestinal workup, including radiological studies, failed to reveal any apparent cause. The patient had attempted use of various medications without any apparent success.

Examination revealed normoactive bowel sounds and tenderness to palpation in all four quadrants. There were type II somatic dysfunctions in the lower thoracic spine, with Chapman's points on the lateral right thigh. There was no abdominal rebound and the patient was afebrile.

Treatment began with inhibition to the paravertebral muscles in the thoracolumbar region as well as muscle energy and thrusting techniques to the somatic dysfunctions. A mesenteric lift was used with good release. The Chapman's reflex points were treated. The patient was encouraged to drink several glasses of water per day and to maintain a balanced diet.

Two weeks later she returned stating that she only had one episode of constipation that was not of the usual severity. She was again treated and followed-up in a month with marked improvement.

## Discussion

Irritable bowel syndrome (IBS) is a clinical condition that has not been related to a specific cause. The primary symptoms are constipation and abdominal discomfort and pain. Occasionally, it alternates with true diarrhea. Treatment with laxatives can lead to bloating, gas, and rebound constipation. Water and bulk are important for more normal stool movement. Sympathetic output from the thoracic region reduces peristalsis and increases sphincter tone.

Treatment of the thoracic spine is directed at reducing sympathetic outflow to the small and especially the large intestines. Chapman's reflexes are typically found in cases of gastrointestinal dysfunction.

The mesentery is a stretch sensitive organ and a cyclic loop of stretch-dysfunction-pain-sympathetic tone can occur. Pulling the mesentery in directions that bring it toward its attachments can reduce these stresses and assist in breaking the cycle.

### REFERENCES

Ashmore E. *Osteopathic Mechanics*. London: Tamor Pierston Publishers, 1915 (republished 1981).

Barral J-P, Mercier P. *Visceral Manipulation*. Seattle: Eastland Press, 1988.

Kuchera ML. Kuchera WA. *Osteopathic Considerations in Systemic Dysfunction*. Columbus, OH: Greydon Press, 1994.

Still AT. *Osteopathy, Research and Practice*. Seattle: Eastland Press, 1910 (republished 1992).

Ward RC. *Foundations for Osteopathic Medicine, 2nd ed.* Philadelphia: Lippincott Williams & Wilkins, 2003.

# CHAPTER 111

# HEENT Applications

*Eileen L. DiGiovanna, Donald E. Phykitt, and Mary-Theresa Ferris*

## ■ HEADACHES

Headache is a condition often seen by physicians. Most people suffer from headaches at some time during their lives and many people are significantly incapacitated by them. Millions of people treat themselves with over-the-counter medications such as acetaminophen or aspirin.

The causes of headache are many and varied. Some are life-threatening, such as intracranial aneurysms or bleeding, meningitis, or have the potential to be such as hypertension. Thus, the physician must keep these in mind when treating a patient with severe headaches. However, the majority of headaches are caused by muscle tension or migraine. A 28-year study at the Headache Unit of Montefiore Hospital found that 90% of headache patients had migraine, tension headaches, or a combination of the two.

## Pathogenesis

The brain itself is almost totally insensitive to pain. The scalp, arteries, muscles, mucous membranes of the sinuses, ear, and the teeth are all pain-sensitive structures. The crucial areas in the creation of headache are the suboccipital and upper cervical areas as well as the scalp. In the upper two cervical segments, the sensory fibers of the first three cervical segments are joined by the descending tracts of cranial nerves V, IX, and X. These three cranial nerves, along with the second cervical nerve, mediate the referral of excessive connective tissue tension in the cervical area as pain in the cranial vault or cephalgia.

Intracranially, only the dura, its arteries, the large arteries at the base of the skull, and the venous sinuses are sensitive to pain. Connective tissue stresses that cause tension or drag on the dura create an environment for the development of migraine headaches. This occurs through a reflex vasospasm mediated through a biochemical cascade with ensuing ischemia.

Some types of head or facial pain are mediated through three cranial nerves bearing sensory fibers—V, VI, and VII. Most notable among these are *trigeminal neuralgia* and *Bell's palsy*.

## Tension Headache

Tension headaches are probably the most common form of headache. These are generally of three types:

1. Emotional
   a. Stress and associated anxiety
   b. Depression
   c. Anger, particularly unresolved conflicts
2. Postural
   a. Occupational
   b. Postural imbalance
   c. Abnormal spinal curvatures
   d. Poor posture when seated or standing, especially when forward-bent
3. Muscle hypertonicity or fatigue
   a. Maintenance of a frown—affects the frontalis muscle
   b. Bruxism—affects temporalis and masseter muscles
   c. General fatigue—decreases proper muscle support of head and neck

Whe two or more components are involved, there are likely to be frequent, recurrent tension headaches.

Prolonged muscle contraction of scalp, face, and neck muscles is a major contributing factor in tension headache. This is often associated with reflex vasoconstriction of superficial vessels. The patient may experience a "band-like" pain around the head or pain in occipital region. The pain is usually bilateral and unaccompanied by nausea and vomiting. The upper cervical spine is often involved in head pain and must be evaluated in the headache patient.

## Migraine Headaches

Migraine headaches are a frequently seen type of headache; however, many patients diagnose their headaches themselves as migraine headaches, which are in reality tension headaches. Migraine headaches are usually recurrent, most often unilateral, throbbing, or pounding, and associated with nausea or vomiting. The patient may experience some prodromal warning such as visual auras, blind spots, or auditory changes.

One or more triggering factors, such as stress, certain foods, trauma, or hormone changes, usually initiate the onset of the migraine leading to vasoconstriction and subsequent vasodilatation of the adrenergically innervated blood vessels at the base of the brain and in the meninges.

## Osteopathic Considerations and Evaluation

The musculoskeletal system is intimately involved in tension and migraine headaches. The muscle involvement in tension headache is obvious and includes the muscles of the head and face, the cervical spine, and the upper thorax. Somatic dysfunction of the occipito-atlantal joint, the atlanto-axial joint, and C2 on C3 are frequent sources of headache. The levator scapula, with its attachments to the scapula and the cervical spine, and the trapezius must be considered. Facial muscles may be the major source of head pain. The patient must be evaluated for bruxism, teeth grinding, or jaw clenching, which affects the temporalis and masseter muscles. Bruxism may lead to dysfunction of temporal bone motion or to problems with the temporo-mandibular joint.

The patient with migraine headaches must be evaluated for a variety of cranial dysfunctions,

especially temporal bone motion and side-bending/rotation patterns. Dysfunctions of the upper thoracic spine may affect the sympathetic innervation to the blood vessels of the head. Somatic dysfunctions of the upper cervical spine are often related to migraine headaches. A combination of tension and migraine headache patterns is not uncommon.

## ■ THE TEMPORO-MANDIBULAR JOINT

### Anatomy

The temporo-mandibular joint (TMJ) is a synovial joint formed by the articulation of the condyle of the mandible with the mandibular (glenoid) fossa and the articular tubercle of the temporal bone. The joint is divided into superior and inferior compartments by a fibrocartilaginous disk. The major motions of the TMJ are depression of the mandible (opening the mouth) and elevation of the mandible (closing the mouth). These motions are achieved by rotation of the condyle in the mandibular fossa, accompanied by anterior or posterior glide on the articular tubercle, respectively. Furthermore, the joint allows protraction, retraction, and side-to-side glide of the mandible.

The mandibular fossa is an oval depression in the temporal bone just anterior to the external auditory meatus. It is bounded anteriorly by the articular tubercle, laterally by the zygomatic process, and posteriorly by the tympanic plate. The close proximity of the mandibular fossa to the external auditory meatus allows fingers placed in the meatus of each ear to palpate condylar motion as it rotates and glides in the fossa. Occasionally, a small ridge of bone (the postglenoid tubercle) forms a prominence at the posterior border of the fossa. The shape of the mandibular fossa does not exactly conform to the mandibular condyle. The articular disk molds the two surfaces together.

The articular disk is fibrous and is molded to the bony surfaces. It is variable in thickness, being thinnest centrally. Its margins merge with the joint capsule. The disk is more firmly attached to the mandible than to the temporal bone. Therefore, when the head of the mandible glides anteriorly on the articular tubercle (as when opening the mouth), the articular disk slides anteriorly against the tubercle.

The fibrous capsule of the TMJ is loose. It is attached to the margins of the articular area on the temporal bone and to the neck of the mandible. It is thickened laterally to form the *temporomandibular ligament*. This is a triangular ligament whose base attaches to the zygomatic process and the articular tubercle. Its apex is fixed to the lateral aspect of the neck of the mandible. The accessory ligaments of the TMJ are the *stylomandibular, sphenomandibular,* and *pterygomandibular ligaments*; none has any significant effect on joint movement.

The innervation of the joint is mainly supplied by the auriculotemporal branch of the mandibular division of the trigeminal nerve. Additional fibers are supplied by the masseteric branch of the mandibular nerve. The vascular supply is derived from the superficial artery and the deep auricular branch of the maxillary artery.

Movements of the TMJ result chiefly from the actions of the muscles of mastication—the *temporalis, masseter, medial pterygoid,* and *lateral pterygoid* muscles. The various movements of the TMJ result from the cooperative activity of several muscles, either bilaterally or unilaterally.

1. **Temporalis:** Extensive fan-shaped muscle covering the temporal region.
   Origin: Temporal fossa and temporal fascia.
   Insertion: Coronoid process and anterior border of the ramus of the mandible.
   Actions: Elevates the mandible (closes the mouth) and retracts the mandible after closure.
2. **Masseter:** A quadrangular muscle that covers the coronoid process and ramus of the mandible. It is easily palpated at the cheek when the teeth are clenched.
   Origin: Inferior margin and deep surface of the zygomatic arch.
   Insertion: Lateral surface of the ramus and corocoid process of the mandible.
   Actions: Elevates the mandible, clenches the teeth, and aids in protraction of the mandible.
3. **Lateral pterygoid:** A short, thick muscle with two heads of origin.
   Origin: Superior head—infratemporal surface of the greater wing of the sphenoid;

inferior head—lateral surface of the lateral pterygoid plate.
   Insertion: Neck of mandible and the articular disk.
   Actions: When contracted bilaterally, the lateral pterygoid muscles protract and depress the mandible. When contracted unilaterally they produce contralateral lateral glide of the mandible.
4. **Medial pterygoid:** A thick quadrilateral muscle located deep to the ramus of the mandible: it embraces the inferior head of the lateral pterygoid muscle.
   Origin: Deep head—medial surface of lateral pterygoid plate; superficial head—tuberosity of the maxilla.
   Insertion: Medial surface of mandible, near its angle.
   Actions: Contracting bilaterally, it assists in elevating and protracting the mandible; contracting unilaterally, it produces contralateral lateral glide of the mandible.

## Biomechanics

Mandibular movements may be classified as bilaterally symmetric or bilaterally asymmetric. Because the mandible is a single bone with two joints, movement through one joint cannot occur without a similar coordinating or dissimilar reactive movement in the other joint. Depression, elevation, protraction, and retraction of the mandible are bilaterally symmetric motions because they require similar motions in both joints. Lateral excursions (side-to-side movements) are bilaterally asymmetric, since there are dissimilar movements of the joints.

*Depression* is a hinge-like rotation of the mandibular condyle accompanied by simultaneous anterior glide of the condyles and articular disks on the articular tubercles. This is mainly produced by the lateral pterygoid muscles. Some assistance is gained from the suprahyoid and infrahyoid muscles. The axis of rotation is through the head of the mandible; the axis of glide is through the mandibular foramen.

*Elevation* is the opposite of depression. The motion is achieved mainly through the actions of the temporalis and medial pterygoid muscles, with assistance from the anterior fibers of the masseter.

*Protraction (protrusion)* is motion that involves anterior glide of both condyles and articular disks along the articular tubercles. It is achieved through bilateral contraction of the medial and lateral pterygoid muscles.

*Retraction* is a movement opposite that of protraction. It is produced by bilateral contraction of the horizontal fibers of the masseter muscles.

*Lateral excursion* is movement that involves lateral glide of the ipsilateral mandibular condyle, accompanied by slight medial rotation of the contralateral condyle about the medial, shifting axis. It is achieved by unilateral contraction of the contralateral medial and lateral pterygoid muscles.

## Evaluation and Treatment

TMJ dysfunction affects approximately 20% of the American population, with a 3:1 female-to-male preponderance. Pain associated with the temporo-mandibular joint was first described in the 1830s. The first treatment was an ostectomy.

The cause of TMJ dysfunction appears to be a combination of various factors, including malocclusion, trauma, psychological or emotional status, the neuromuscular apparatus, and the general health of a patient. Internal derangement is another etiologic factor, described as an abnormal relationship of the articular disk to the mandibular condyle, fossa, and articular eminence. Included in this category are perforation, fragmentation, and displacement of the disk.

Dental procedures such as forceful extractions can be considered traumatic, and bruxism (teeth grinding) is seen as repeated microtrauma to the TMJ. Muscular imbalance is another etiologic factor that may be a cause of or may be caused by malocclusion. Malocclusion may occur with the loss of a single tooth or several teeth, improper alignment of dentures, and other factors.

## Signs and Symptoms of Dysfunction

The most common signs of TMJ dysfunction are clicking or popping sounds in the joint, pre-auricular pain, limited jaw movements, and tenderness on palpation. Additional frequently en-countered symptoms include jaw, ear, and facial pain, headache, masticatory muscle pain, fatigue, and tightness. Although not as common, the following symptoms have also been reported: swallowing difficulties, tinnitus, backache, mouth dryness, nervousness, sleep disorders, snoring, loss of balance, and mental disorders.

## Evaluation

A thorough history is extremely important and must include trauma (not just to the head and neck), dental work, gum chewing, clenching or grinding of teeth, stress, psychological makeup, and postural habits. The TMJ stressor may be present for a long time before it manifests itself as a symptom.

A complete physical must be performed and any possible organic causes ruled out. Muscle spasms, scoliosis, leg length discrepancies, arches of the feet, craniosacral motion, and somatic dysfunctions must be evaluated. Asymmetries of any postural mechanisms can be reflected at the TMJ.

Examination of the TMJ should include the following:

1. Observation of facial symmetry or asymmetry.
2. Observation of a midline deviation of the mandible and palpation of the TMJ during opening and closing of the mouth.
3. Measurement of the jaw opening. The average adult opening is 40 mm.
4. Assessment of joint noises—when a click occurs with mandibular opening.
5. Palpation of the joint and surrounding areas for bony abnormalities and tenderness.
6. Assessment of musculature—spasms, imbalance, etc.
7. Evaluation of craniosacral motion, especially the temporal bones
8. Palpation of the TMJ through the external auditory meatus, noting tenderness or deviation with motion (Fig. 111-1).
9. It is fairly common to find dysfunctions of the occipitoatlantal joint, C2, and C3.

A dental examination is also essential for a complete evaluation of a TMJ dysfunction.

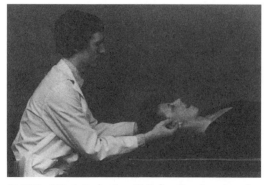

■ **FIG. 111-1** Evaluating TMJ function by observing tracking while palpating the joint through the auditory meatus.

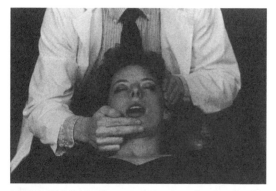

■ **FIG. 111-2** Muscle energy treatment for muscles that close the jaw.

The neck should be examined as it is fairly common to find dysfunctions of the occipitoatlantal joint, C2, and C3.

TMJ imaging may also be employed in the diagnostic evaluation. Magnetic resonance imaging is the procedure of choice for internal derangements and will demonstrate bony detail as well as soft tissues.

## Treatment

The treatment of TMJ dysfunction has three components:

1. Identifying and eliminating any treatable cause.
2. Osteopathic manipulative treatment.
3. Prescribing an exercise regimen for the patient to use at home.

Conservative treatment following these guidelines should be used before any consideration of surgical intervention.

Inter-occlusal stabilization devices, also known as splints or appliances, may be helpful. Repositioning is accomplished over several months and involves frequent readjustments as the muscles relax and the mandible shifts.

## Osteopathic Manipulative Techniques

### Muscle Energy Techniques

Muscle energy techniques are designed to treat and relax the various muscles of mastication—those that open and close the jaw, and those that move it from side to side.

1. **Patient position:** supine.
2. **Physician position:** seated at the head of the table.
3. **Technique:**
   a. To treat the muscles that close the jaw, ask the patient to open her mouth. Place two fingers on the patient's chin. Ask her to attempt to close her mouth against your resistance (Fig. 111-2). Repeat three times.
   b. To treat the muscles that open the jaw, ask the patient to close her mouth. Place two fingers on the patient's chin. Ask her to attempt to open her mouth against your resistance (Fig. 111-3). Repeat three times.
   c. To treat the muscles that move the jaw laterally, ask the patient to move her jaw away from the affected side. Place two fingers on the side of her jaw, and ask her

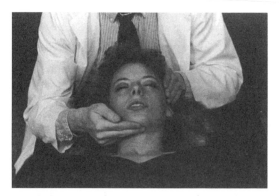

■ **FIG. 111-3** Muscle energy treatment for muscles that open the jaw.

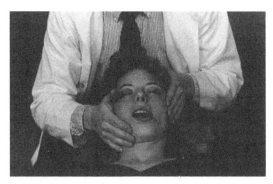

■ **FIG. 111-4** Muscle energy treatment for muscles that move the jaw laterally.

to move her jaw back against your fingers as you provide a resistance (Fig. 111-4). Repeat three times, attempting to move the jaw through its restriction.

### Counterstrain technique

1. **Patient position:** supine.
2. **Physician position:** seated at the head of the table.
3. **Technique:**
   a. One finger monitors the tender point in the muscle.
   b. The patient is asked to relax her jaw. With the other hand the physician moves the jaw toward the affected side until the point is no longer tender (Fig. 111-5).
   c. This position is held for 90 seconds. The jaw is then returned to the neutral position.

### Stretching the pterygoid muscles

In some cases of TMJ dysfunction, the pterygoid muscles are hypertonic. These muscles can be

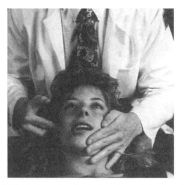

■ **FIG. 111-5** Counterstrain treatment for tender point in the right masseter muscle.

passively stretched by applying pressure with a gloved finger inside the mouth. The finger is gently slid along the muscle, massaging and stretching it. Inhibition of tender points in these muscles may also be used.

### Cranial treatment

Because the temporal bone is intimately involved in most TMJ cases, it must be evaluated and treated for any motion restriction found (see Section X, Cranial Osteopathy). Because the motion of the sacrum is closely related to motion of the cranium, evaluation and treatment of the sacrum may provide important help as well.

## ■ NASAL SINUSES

The nasal sinuses include four pairs of aerated cells in the bones of the skull, named after the four bones in which they are located: frontal, sphenoid, ethmoid, and maxillary. These sinuses are lined with epithelium similar to that of the nasal passages. This epithelium contains goblet cells that secrete mucus, which is normally moderately thin and clear, and ciliated cells whose purpose is to move the secretions out of the sinuses into the nasal passages, assisted by gravity.

The frontal sinuses drain primarily by gravity; the ethmoid, sphenoid, and maxillary sinuses rely heavily on the ciliated cells that line them to move mucus toward the nasal passages. The lining of the sinuses is subject to the same irritants, allergens, and infections that involve the upper respiratory mucosa.

Edema or tenacious mucus as well as slowing of ciliary movement, as is caused by tobacco smoking, may affect the discharge of secretions out of the sinuses. Secretory fluids build up, the passage of air is blocked, and unequal pressures result, leading to pain. This pain may be located over the sinuses in the forehead, the orbits, or the cheeks, and may be referred via reflexes to the occiput and neck, the teeth, the temples, or the ears.

Sympathetic innervation to the sinuses arises in the upper thoracic area and passes through the cervical ganglia. The upper thoracic and cervical areas should be evaluated for the presence of somatic dysfunction, and any dysfunction found should be treated. Probably the most consistent mechanical finding associated with sinusitis is occipitoatlantal dysfunction, which requires treatment for relief.

The osteopathic treatment of sinusitis has several goals: to relieve obstruction and pain; to improve venous and lymphatic flow from the area; to affect reflex changes; and to improve mucociliary clearance. Several manual techniques have been designed to aid in achieving these goals. Although only one set of sinuses may produce pain, the entire series of techniques should be performed to assist drainage of all the sinus areas.

## Treatment Techniques

The positions of patient and operator, described below, are identical for all the techniques:

1. **Patient position:** supine on the table, with her eyes closed, and relaxed.
2. **Physician position:** seated comfortably at the head of the table.

## Direct Pressure and "Milking"

Pressure may be applied directly with the thumbs over the frontal sinuses. The pressure is gradually increased and released in a gentle, rhythmic motion, never hard enough to cause severe pain. The cycle is repeated several times (Fig. 111-6).

The thumbs are then placed side by side in the center of the forehead and, with gentle pres-

sure downward, are moved laterally toward the temples. At the edge of the temporal fossae the thumbs are directed caudad to the zygoma. This cycle is repeated six or eight times.

For the *supraorbital notch,* gentle pressure may be applied over the supraorbital notch; then the thumbs are swept along the eyebrow ridge bilaterally (Fig. 111-7).

For the *maxillary sinuses,* the same technique can be applied to the maxillary sinuses. Pressure is applied over the sinuses with the thumbs. The nasal passages are "milked" by beginning with the thumb on each side of the nose and pressing down while sweeping the thumbs laterally along the maxilla (Fig. 111-8).

In the *temporal areas,* direct pressure may be applied over the temporal areas by gently placing the thenar eminences in the temporal fossae bilaterally and compressing these areas between the hands. Pressure is applied and released in gentle, rhythmic motions (Fig. 111-9).

## Indirect Pressure

The fingers of the operator's hands are interlaced and laid palm up on the table under the patient's head. The thenar eminence of each hand is placed against the patient's head laterally on the occiput. Gentle, rhythmic pressure is applied to the head by pressing the hands together and releasing them. A counterstrain technique is applied in the same manner. The pressure is main-

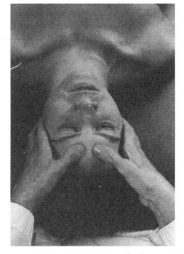

■ **FIG. 111-6** Direct pressure applied over the frontal sinuses.

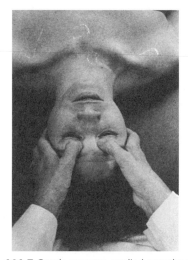

■ **FIG. 111-7** Gentle pressure applied over the supraorbital notch.

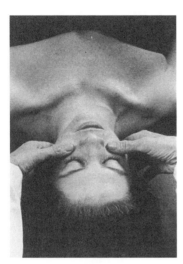

■ **FIG. 111-8** Pressure applied over the maxillary sinuses.

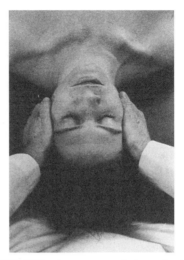

■ **FIG. 111-9** Direct pressure applied over the temporal areas.

tained for 90 seconds, then released very slowly. A similar technique involves cupping the occiput in one hand and placing the heel of the other hand in the center of the patient's forehead, compressing the head between the two hands in a gentle, rhythmic motion.

## Counterstrain Techniques:

In the m*axillary sinuses,* the tender points are over the infraorbital nerves. An effective counterstrain technique for the maxillary sinuses

is to interlace the fingers above the bridge of the nose with the thenar eminences resting on the lateral curve of the zygoma. Pressure through the thenar eminences, in a compressing and lifting motion, is maintained for 90 seconds, then released (Fig. 111-10).

*Supraorbital tender points* are located near the site of the supraorbital nerves. One arm rests on the patient's forehead, lightly pulling it superiorly, and, with fingers of the other hand pinching the bridge of the nose, the examiner distracts the nose caudad (Fig. 111-11).

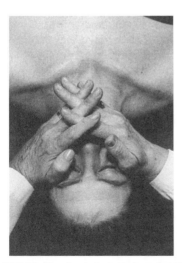

■ **FIG. 111-10** Counterstrain technique for the maxillary sinuses.

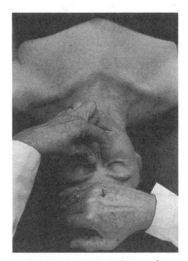

■ **FIG. 111-11** Counterstrain technique for supraorbital tender points.

## ■ NASAL PASSAGES

The nasal passages function as passageways for air to enter the respiratory system and for olfaction. The air is warmed, humidified, and filtered as it passes through them. A mucus blanket, secreted by goblet cells, covers the nasal mucosa, which is heavily ciliated. The mucosa requires a balanced autonomic nervous system in order to function properly. The blood vessels, which function to warm the air, rely on the sympathetic nervous system to create the necessary amount of dilation.

The nasal passages are subject to inflammation from irritants, viral and bacterial infection, and allergens. The inflammatory process initiates a production of thin, watery mucus leading to rhinorrhea. In some infectious processes, the mucus later becomes thick and tenacious, frequently colored green or yellow, especially in bacterial infections. The turbinates swell and block the nasal passages, making inhalation through the nose difficult.

Treatment of these inflammatory processes may include osteopathic manipulation. Lymphatic drainage of involved channels, especially the deep lymphatic chain, may be assisted through "milking" of the chains bilaterally. Because some of the lymph drains directly into the retropharyngeal area, treatment of the pharynx should be undertaken.

### Techniques for Drainage of the Nasal Passages

The nasal passages are milked by the examiner, who places the thumb of the right hand on the left side of the patient's nose and the left thumb on the right side of the nose, the thumbs crossing above the bridge of the nose. Pressure is applied alternately by each thumb, moving down the length of the nose (Fig. 111-12). This is performed several times, then the thumbs are reversed and a sweeping motion is made bilaterally down the sides of the nose and out over the maxillae.

## ■ THROAT/PHARYNX

The nasopharynx is the area above the soft palate and at the base of the nasal passages. The oro-

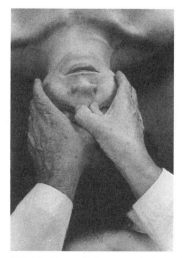

■ **FIG. 111-12** Sinus drainage technique for nasal congestion.

pharynx is the area posterior to the oral cavity from the soft palate down to the hyoid bone. Below the hyoid to the larynx is the laryngopharynx. The nasopharynx and laryngopharynx are lined with pseudostratified, ciliated epithelium while the oropharynx and the oral cavity are lined with stratified epithelium.

The palatine tonsils lie in fossae at the lateral edges of the soft palate. These are made up of lymphoid tissue. Adenoids are lymphoid tissue in the nasopharynx and on the posterior tongue. The tonsils and adenoids will enlarge in the presence of infectious processes as the immune system is called to combat the infection.

Infection, either viral or bacterial, is the most common of all pathological processes in the pharyngeal areas. While antibiotics are commonly used to fight bacterial infections, viral infections should not be treated with antibiotics. Osteopathic manipulation is helpful to assist in the treatment of both bacterial and viral pharyngeal infections.

### Techniques

Balancing the autonomic nervous system should be performed to assure proper circulation to the pharyngeal tissues. Both the upper cervical area and the upper thoracic area should be treated for any somatic dysfunctions found.

1. *Lymphatic drainage:* The anterior cervical chains should be assisted by "milking" the cervical chains from superior to inferior to move the lymph toward the large collection system in the thorax. One side should be treated at a time to assure that bilateral compression of the carotid sinus does not occur.
2. *Hyoid/tracheal motion:* The physician gently grasps the hyoid bone between the thumb and forefinger and moves it from side to side, gently stretching the muscles and fascia of the anterior throat. The physician moves the fingers from the hyoid to the trachea and continues the side to side motion. This is performed rhythmically up and down the anterior throat. This stimulates blood circulation, assists lymph circulation and free any tense tissues in the area for greater comfort.
3. Lymphatic drainage should not be attempted in the presence of very large cervical glands nor should it be used for *infectious mononucleosis* (Epstein-Barr viral infection).

## ■ MIDDLE EAR

The middle ear is separated from the external canal by the tympanic membrane. It contains the three tiny ossicles: the stapes, malleus, and incus. The cavity is air filled. Sound is transmitted through the middle ear to the cochlea of the inner ear and from there to the brain for interpretation. It is lined by the same ciliated epithelium as the respiratory system.

The middle ear is connected to the nasopharynx by the *Eustachian tube*, which lies partially in the temporal bone and is partially a cartilaginous tube. This tube only opens during swallowing or yawning and serves to maintain a balance between the air pressures in the middle ear and in the nasopharynx.

The most common pathology of the middle ear is *otitis media*. This may be of bacterial origin in which case the middle ear fills with infected fluid that is usually opaque. The level of this fluid may be seen behind the tympanum. The tympanum itself will be inflamed, swollen, and tense. The *cone of light* will not be present during the physical examination.

*Serous otitis media* occurs most frequently in children. In these cases, the middle ear is filled with serous secretions, again creating a fluid level seen behind the tympanum. The tympanum will be taut but generally not inflamed. This condition is often the result of restricted opening of the Eustachian tube so that secreted fluids are unable to drain from the middle ear.

Either type of otitis media has the potential risk of rupture of the tympanum, which may result in scarring and decrease or loss of hearing in the affected ear. To prevent the rupture, small tubes are often inserted through the tympanum of children to allow for fluid drainage. Antibiotics are necessary to clear the infectious process.

Osteopathic manipulation has proven effective in the treatment of otitis media to allow for a natural drainage of fluid through the Eustachian tubes.

## Galbreath Technique

The *Galbreath technique,* also known as the *jaw lift,* assists in the opening of the Eustachian tube. It is effective in otitis media and also in treating the stuffiness of the ear often experienced by airline passengers, especially if it persists despite swallowing and yawning.

1. **Patient position:** supine.
2. **Physician position:** standing at the patient's side opposite the affected ear.
3. **Technique:**
   a. The physician grasps the angle of the jaw on the contralateral side.
   b. The jaw is gently lifted toward the ceiling and pulled toward the physician.
   c. This position is held for several seconds and then the jaw is released. The patient may notice a popping sound in the ear as this is performed.
   d. This is repeated approximately six times.

## Temporal Bone

Because the medial third of the Eustachian tube lies in the temporal bone, it is important to free the motions of this bone. Osteopathy in the cranial field provides several techniques to assure that the motions of internal and external rotation of the temporal bone are free and symmetrical. Either direct or indirect techniques may be used.

## Muncie Technique

The Muncie technique is sometimes referred to as *finger surgery*. The physician's gloved fingers are inserted into the patient's mouth, with one finger being placed at the opening of the Eustachian tube. Structural adhesions may be broken up and/or tenacious mucus removed from the opening of the tube.

This technique is beneficial when other techniques have failed to provide relief from otitis media. It is also useful in patients with chronic symptoms of ear stuffiness, pain with altitude changes, vertigo or tinnitus.

## ■ INNER EAR

The structures of the inner ear lies within the temporal bone. They function both in hearing and in maintaining body balance. Any condition affecting the inner ear may result in hearing loss, hyperacusis, tinnitus, or vertigo.

Osteopathic treatment for any of the above relies heavily on treatment of the temporal bone. Normal circulation to the ear and normal lymphatic drainage of the ear must also be considered and treated.

## ■ CASE 1

J.J., a 2-year-old child, was seen in the clinic with a history of recurrent ear infections over the past year. There had been at least five episodes of ear pain with the child pulling at the affected ear, most often the right, but with two episodes in which both ears were infected. The child had been treated with antibiotics. Decongestants had been used for the past two episodes. The pediatrician was now recommending the insertion of tubes through the tympanum to prevent future ear infections and the danger of hearing loss. J.J. was on preventive antibiotics at the time of the visit, a course to be taken for 3 months. The parents did not want the surgery and were asking for some other form of treatment. Other than the ear infections, the child had been healthy except for one bout of bronchitis a year ago.

On physical examination, J.J. was a healthy-appearing child with all growth parameters within normal limits. The ear canal was clean; the tympanum was somewhat taut with a fluid level about a third of the way up the tympanum.

The nose and throat showed no inflammation, swelling of the turbinates, or enlargement of the tonsils. The heart and lungs were normal. Hearing did not appear to be affected—the child responded to his name when it was whispered behind him. On structural examination, he was found to have C2 $FS_RR_R$, $T4FS_LR_L$, an internally rotated temporal bone on the right, and external rotation of the left. There was mild condylar compression of the occiput.

The diagnosis was chronic serous otitis media. After a discussion with the parents, it was decided to try a series of osteopathic manipulative treatments before opting for the surgery.

The child was treated with the Galbreath technique bilaterally, myofascial release to the cervical spine, lymphatic pump to the thorax, and cranial treatment of the temporal bones and release of the condylar compression.

J.J. was treated weekly for 1 month and then every 2 weeks for 2 months, with follow-up examinations and treatment monthly for 3 months. During this time he completed his course of antibiotics. The fluid was reabsorbed by the fourth visit and did not return during the course of treatment. The mother called during the eighth month after institution of the osteopathic manipulative treatment to report that J.J. had not had any further occurrences of ear infections and was no longer on any medication for the otitis media.

## Discussion

Otitis media responds well to maintaining an open Eustachian tube, which can be facilitated by osteopathic manipulation. The Galbreath technique, or jaw lift, is useful in this regard. Because a portion of the Eustachian tube lies in the temporal bone, this bone must be kept functioning normally, i.e., internal and external rotation in conjunction with the normal cranial rhythmic impulse. The circulation to the ear and the normal flow of the lymphatics to and from the ear must be considered when formulating a treatment plan.

## ■ CASE 2

D.T., a 34-year-old secretary, presented with a symptom of nasal stuffiness, a sore throat, and pain in the left ear of 2 days' duration. She was requesting an antibiotic. She stated she had a similar condition 6 months previously that had been treated with erythromycin. Her medical history was pertinent for frontal headaches every spring with associated postnasal drip. She had a surgical history of appendectomy 3 years previously. She admitted to an allergy to penicillin and shellfish. She was on no medications other than a daily multivitamin and zinc lozenges for her throat taken the past 2 days.

Physical examination showed a healthy-appearing woman with hyperemic, swollen turbinates of her nose, a slight, clear nasal discharge, and mild redness of the throat. The ears showed no inflammation with a normal tympanic cone of light. Her lungs were clear to auscultation. On structural examination, a somatic dysfunction of the occipitoatlantal joint was diagnosed as $FS_LR_R$.

A common cold was diagnosed and it was explained to her why an antibiotic would not be helpful at this time because of the viral nature of a cold. She was instructed on the benefits of drinking sufficient fluids and getting plenty of rest. She was treated osteopathically with myofascial techniques to the cervical and upper thoracic spine and facilitated positional release to the OA somatic dysfunction. A lymphatic pump was used in conjunction with anterior cervical drainage to assure good movement of the lymph from the throat to the thoracic channels. Sinus drainage and nasal passage drainage were performed to relieve sinus and nasal congestion. The Galbreath technique was used to assure that the Eustachian tube would permit drainage from the middle ear and prevent congestion there.

## Discussion

Patients often request antibiotics to treat the common cold. They often assume a sore throat is a bacterial infection, when it is more often of viral origin. Osteopathic manipulation is ideal to make patients more comfortable as well as to assist their own immune system in fighting off the infection. The lymphatic system is a major part of the immune response and the movement of lymph is important. Fluids and rest assist the patient in the recovery process. Opening the nasal passages and assisting drainage from the sinuses make the patients more comfortable and prevent infected material being trapped in the sinuses. Ear pain is often caused by inflammation of the throat in the region of the opening of the Eustachian tube into the nasopharynx. Assisting the patient in opening the tube helps keep pressure balanced in the middle ear so that there is not an increased pressure leading to pain and stuffiness of the ear. Ideally, the patient should be treated in a day or two, especially if no improvement is noted.

### REFERENCES

Berkowitz BKB, Moxham BJ. *A Textbook of Head and Neck Anatomy.* Chicago: Yearbook Medical Publishers, 1988.

Blood SJ. The craniosacral mechanism and the temporomandibular joint. *J Am Osteopath Assoc* 1986;86:56–59.

DiGiovanna EL, Schiowitz S. *An Osteopathic Approach to Diagnosis and Treatment, 2nd ed.* Philadelphia: Lippincott-Raven, 1997.

Downs JR. Treating TMJ dysfunction. *Osteopath Phys,* 1976; 106–113.

Goulet JP, Clark PT. Clinical TMJ examination methods. *J Calif Dent Assoc* 1990;18:25–33.

Hasso AH, Christiansen EL, Alder ME. The temporomandibular joint. *Radiol Clin North Am* 1989;27:301–314.

Jones LH. *Strain and Counterstrain.* Indianapolis: American Academy of Osteopathy, 1981.

Kuchera ML, Kuchera WA. *Osteopathic Considerations in Systemic Dysfunction.* Columbus, OH: Greydon Press, 1994.

Royder JO. Structural influences in temporomandibular joint pain and dysfunction. *J Am Osteopath Assoc* 1981;80: 60–67.

Ward RC. *Foundations for Osteopathic Medicine, 2nd ed.* Philadelphia: Lippincott Williams & Wilkins, 2003.

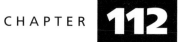

# Pulmonary Applications

*Eileen L. DiGiovanna and Sonia Rivera-Martinez*

The lower respiratory system includes the tracheobronchial tree, the lungs and their pleural covering, the pulmonary circulatory system, and the autonomic and visceral innervation to these structures. All of these visceral structures are enclosed in the bony thoracic cage—ribs, thoracic spine, clavicles, sternum—with their fascia and muscles and the muscular diaphragm separating the upper thoracic cavity from the lower abdominal one.

Osteopathic manipulation adds a markedly different and significantly effective dimension to the treatment of the pulmonary patient. Treatment of chronic pulmonary disease can be particularly challenging to the physician. The ability to assist respiration through manual contact with the musculoskeletal structures of the thoracic cage is an important adjunct to the osteopathic physician in treating acute and chronic conditions of the pulmonary system.

The process of breathing consists of two phases: inhalation and exhalation. Inhalation brings oxygenated air from the outside into the upper and then the lower respiratory tract. The air is cleansed of particulate matter and warmed in the upper respiratory tract. The air passes through the trachea, the bronchopulmonary tree, and into the alveoli of the lungs. Oxygen passes through the alveoli into the pulmonary circulation where, via erythrocytes, it is carried throughout the body. Also in the lungs, carbon dioxide in particular is removed from the blood and passes out of the body during the exhalation phase. This entire process is respiration.

Respiration uses not only the upper and lower respiratory tracts but also a large segment of the body's musculoskeletal system including the ribs, sternum, clavicles, thoracic (and to a lesser extent the lumbar) spine, the multiple muscles attached to these skeletal structures, the thoracic diaphragm, connected fasciae, ligaments and tendons. Osteopathic manipulation plays a significant role in the maintenance of these structures for optimum function in the work of respiration.

## ■ SOMATIC DIAGNOSIS OF PULMONARY DISEASES

Osteopathic somatic dysfunction diagnosis may be a valuable tool in identifying the presence of pulmonary pathology. Numerous studies have been performed over the years to find the best somatic predictors of respiratory disease. Myron Beal reviewed many previous studies and also reported one of his own. The most consistent findings were at T2–T7, with significant representation at C2–C3. Beal found somatic dysfunction of two or more adjacent vertebrae in this region, deep muscle splinting, and resistance to compressive springing of the involved area. These areas represent viscerosomatic reflexes from the lung to the soma and are useful as diagnostic findings by the osteopathic physician. It is in these areas that autonomic innervation to the lower respiratory tract passes from the spinal cord through the musculoskeletal structures or lies in associated ganglia. When the findings noted here are resistant to treatment, the physician must be suspicious of pulmonary pathology.

The presence of myofascial tender points, known as Chapman's points, may also assist in the diagnosis of pulmonary disease. The Chapman's points for the lungs are found near the sternum in the fourth and fifth intercostal spaces.

# ■ EVALUATION

When evaluating the pulmonary patient, it is also important to evaluate all components involved in respiration, including rib motion, ability of the spine to straighten during inhalation and curve with exhalation, diaphragmatic motion, and accessory muscles of respiration such as the scalenes, sternocleidomastoids, and abdominal muscles.

The thoracic diaphragm must be properly domed to allow for its maximum excursion. An increase in the workload of the diaphragm may strain the attachments on the ribs and the thoracolumbar junction. From the tension, the lumbar lordosis is increased and the diaphragm is flattened and spastic. Because the diaphragm is responsible for moving air into and out of the lungs, a decrease in its excursion prevents optimum exchange of essential gases.

Besides the proper functioning of the muscles and bony structures, other components necessary for healthy tissues include:

1. Good arterial supply
2. Motor and sensory innervation
3. Adequate biochemical environment
4. Free venous and lymphatic return

# ■ BRONCHITIS AND PNEUMONIA

The benefits of osteopathic manipulation in viral influenza was demonstrated in 1918 when, for the first time, statistical records were kept of patients who received osteopathic treatment as opposed to those who received standard medical care of the time. A severe outbreak of Spanish influenza occurred that year. Antibiotics were not available to treat the bacterial pneumonia that was a common complication of the viral condition. Kuchera and Kuchera note in *Osteopathic Considerations in Systemic Dysfunctions* that of the more than 100,000 persons who received osteopathic manipulation while being treated for the influenza, there was only a 0.25% mortality rate. This is quite significantly lower than the estimated 5% overall mortality rate for those receiving only standard medical care at the time. Of persons in whom pneumonia developed as a complication, the mortality rate of those medically treated was between 30% and 60%; for those who received osteopathic care, it was 10%.

Both bronchitis and pneumonia are generally infectious in nature, either bacterial or viral. In bronchitis, the bronchial tree is the structure affected, and in pneumonia, the infection is in the parenchyma of the lungs. Although the exact cause and the manifestations may differ, the goals of treatment are relatively the same in any of these conditions:

1. To improve venous and lymphatic flow
2. To improve arterial circulation to carry immune system products to the lungs
3. To ease removal of accumulated bronchial secretions and phlegm.
4. To decrease the workload of breathing

Osteopathic manipulation should address these goals to assist the body's fight against infection.

Various forms of lymphatic pump or thoracic pump will aid in improving venous and lymphatic flow as well as favorably affecting arterial circulation. Rib-raising techniques may be used to free bronchial secretions so they may be more easily expectorated and to normalize sympathetic innervation to the lung. The workload of breathing may be decreased by improving the compliance of the thorax—that is by freeing the ribs, vertebrae, clavicles, and sternum to restore the intrinsic elastic forces in the thorax.

The thoracic diaphragm may be re-domed by standing behind the seated patient, reaching around the chest, and curling the finger pads under the anterior inferior border of the rib cage. The patient is asked to exhale slightly as the fingers are gently pressed into the soft tissues. He is then asked to inhale deeply as the physician resists descent of the diaphragm. As the patient exhales again, the finger pads are pressed more deeply under the border of the rib cage and inhalation repeated. This is performed several times, moving the finger pads from medial to lateral slightly with each exhalation.

# ■ BRONCHIAL ASTHMA

Bronchial asthma represents a group of symptoms of various causes. The lungs of asthmatics are highly sensitized and react to such varied stimuli as allergens, irritants such as strong odors or fumes, emotion, and exercise. Whatever the trigger, the asthmatic attack is manifested through an inflammatory response, including spasm of the bronchioles, edema of the mucous membrane, and increased production of thick, tenacious mucus. These three incidences create difficulty in emptying air out of the alveoli, with resultant dyspnea and a wheezing sound, or crackles throughout the lung fields, on exhalation. The patient generally will brace himself with his arms and use the accessory muscles of respiration to assist his breathing. In severe cases, hypoxia occurs and the patient may exhibit cyanosis of the lips.

In treating an acute attack of asthma, it is essential to address the patient's immediate needs. Indicated medications should be given first and a nebulizer used as needed. Hydration is very important, because there is a great loss of fluids due to the rapid respiration. As respiration quiets, the osteopathic treatment can begin with seated rib raising techniques or some myofascial to the thoracic region, both useful in assisting the patient's respiratory efforts and loosening mucous plugs. Balanced ligamentous tension techniques are suitable for use during the acute phase.

Between acute attacks, it is important to treat all components of the respiratory system. In particular, all viscerosomatic reflex areas should be treated to prevent possible abnormal autonomic feedback to the lungs. Freeing the occipitoatlantal joint may treat possible increased vagal involvement.

Because of the emotional involvement in asthma as an etiologic factor and the fear elicited by the dyspnea, the very act of placing the hands on the patient will have beneficial effects and serve to calm him as you treat. This alone can be a significant therapeutic factor.

# ■ CHRONIC OBSTRUCTIVE PULMONARY DISEASE

As a result of cigarette smoking and air pollution, chronic obstructive pulmonary disease (COPD) has become a major cause of pulmonary illness in the world today. It is of insidious onset and is devastating to its victims. Dyspnea may become quite significant and require frequent to constant use of an oxygen tank. As dyspnea increases, physical activity is curtailed. Chronic bronchitis produces large amounts of thick mucus, and emphysema produces lesser amounts.

Musculoskeletal changes occur during the course of the disease. The chest assumes a barrel shape in which the anteroposterior (AP) diameter equals the transverse diameter. The accessory muscles of respiration gradually hypertrophy. Hypertrophic scalene muscles may impinge on neurovascular structures passing between or near them. Rib motion is markedly restricted and eventually contributes to the dyspnea. The thoracic spine becomes kyphotic and immobile. Motion of the diaphragm is restricted.

Osteopathic manipulation contributes to the overall well-being of the patient, even though the basic pathophysiology may not be reversible. The thoracic spine is treated to restore mobility and to address the viscerosomatic reflex changes in the upper thoracic spine. Rib motion may be improved with muscle energy or counterstrain techniques as well as myofascial techniques to relax hypertonic thoracic muscles. Fascial release and re-doming of the diaphragm should be performed. Thoracic pumping will improve lymphatic flow and the expectoration of tenacious mucus.

It is best not to use thrusting techniques on these patients. Many COPD patients have been on heavy doses of corticosteroids, which predisposes them to having osteoporosis. Caution should be observed in performing the thoracic pump and in directing pressure onto the sternum rather than the ribs.

The cervical spine should be treated, with attention given to the accessory respiratory muscles. The clavicles should be freed and any sternal restrictions, including the angle of Louis, treated. Upper extremity motion restriction may be found in chronic lung disease. Spencer techniques free the upper extremity range of motion

After osteopathic manipulation, COPD patients frequently report subjective increase in their sense of well-being and sleep better at night. They experience less effort breathing and improved physical functioning.

## ■ CASE 1

A.L. was a 78-year-old man with a history of long-term heavy smoking who presented to the clinic with symptoms of shortness of breath, often without exertion, but limiting even slow walking. He was required to sleep in an almost upright position on multiple pillows. The patient was specifically requesting osteopathic manipulation, which he had heard might help him. A pulmonologist already diagnosed moderately severe chronic obstructive lung disease in A.L. as a result of his earlier smoking habit. He sometimes was forced to use an oxygen tank when the weather was hot or when he wanted to travel more than a short distance. Bouts of coughing would be productive of thick mucus.

On physical examination, he appeared moderately distressed with a rapid respiratory rate. A.L.'s thorax was "barrel-chested," with the anteroposterior diameter of his chest equal to the transverse diameter. His lungs exhibited scattered crackles throughout the lung fields bilaterally. The heart rhythm was regular, with a rate of eighty. Otherwise his physical examination was within normal limits for a person his age.

The structural examination revealed marked restriction of all ribs. The first ribs were elevated bilaterally. The thoracic spine was kyphotic with restricted motion of the vertebrae. The scalene and sternocleidomastoid muscles were hypertrophied and tense. The trapezius and other scapular muscles were hypertonic. Shoulder motion was restricted bilaterally in flexion and abduction. The sternum was rigid with no flexibility at the angle of Louis. Cervical motion was restricted in all directions. The lumbar spine was flattened with hypertonic paraspinal muscles.

A.L. was treated with general myofascial techniques to the entire spine; passive and active were used. Spencer techniques were used to improve shoulder motion. Muscle energy was used to treat the cervical muscles and the lumbar muscles, as well as the trapezius. Fascial release was performed on the sternum and both scapulae. The first ribs were treated with counterstrain.

At the second visit, he reported that he had been sore for a while after the treatment but that he had noticed greater ease in breathing for approximately a day and a half after the treatment.

Most of the same structural findings were present at the second visit and were treated in a similar manner adding some rib raising techniques.

He was treated weekly for 6 weeks and then every 2 weeks. He continued to show some improvement. Most of the changes for him were quality of life issues. He experienced an ease of breathing for several days after a treatment. His shoulders showed improved range of motion that allowed greater use of his arms. The best improvement in his opinion was the increased sense of well-being that he experienced with treatment.

He died of complications of his conditions and pneumonia one year after he discontinued treatment with osteopathic manipulation.

### Discussion

Chronic obstructive lung disease causes great limitation of function. The lifestyle effects are devastating to most people, including the caregivers. Although the condition itself will not be cured by osteopathic manipulation, the ability to breathe with greater ease and the ability to move more freely are greatly appreciated by the patient.

There is less work to breathing when the ribs are able to move more freely and when the spine is made more flexible, because deep inhalation and exhalation require flexion and extension of the spinal segments. Loosening the cervical structures gives comfort to the patient who is dependent on the accessory muscles of respiration.

One can consider the major goals of osteopathic treatment in these cases to be improvement of quality of life.

## ■ CASE 2

R.B. was a 36-year-old Hispanic man who presented to the emergency room with symptoms of acute-onset shortness of breath, wheezing, cough, and a tight feeling in his chest. The patient reported that his symptoms started immediately after being exposed to a very cold blast of wind while walking toward his car. He felt out of breath and was gasping for air. In a short period of time, he began to cough and wheeze. R.B. denied contact with sick persons, fever, nasal congestion, ear pain, and sputum production. During childhood he had similar "asthma attacks" and frequent visits to the emergency room for flare-ups; however, he never underwent intubation. The last exacerbation occurred in his early teens.

R.B.'s past medical history was remarkable for hypertension, which was well-controlled with an angiotensin-converting enzyme (ACE) inhibitor. He denied allergies to animals, insects, dust, food, and medications. The patient reported a 20 pack-year tobacco use, occasional consumption of alcohol, and denied use of illicit drugs. R.B. jogged 3 miles every morning, frequently played soccer, and worked for the sanitation department. His mother and two brothers had a history of asthma and his father had atopic dermatitis as a child.

On physical examination the patient appeared anxious, had difficulty speaking, was mildly diaphoretic, and exhibited labored breathing while sitting bent in a forward position. He was afebrile, had a heart rate of 120 beats per minute, and a respiratory rate of 30 breaths per minute. His chest excursion was diminished with rapid short breaths and he was using accessory muscles of respiration. Suprasternal retractions and nasal flaring were noted. The lung examination revealed diffuse inspiratory and expiratory wheezing bilaterally and hyper-resonance to percussion of the chest.

The osteopathic structural examination was remarkable for severe exhalation restrictions of ribs three to ten with rigid intercostal muscles bilaterally. In addition, there was markedly decreased diaphragmatic, thoracic inlet/outlet, sternal, and clavicular motion. Somatic dysfunctions included $OAES_RR_L$, $C2ES_RR_R$, and $T2$-$T6NS_LR_R$ with increased tonicity of the intrascapular paravertebral muscles.

In the emergency department, R.B. was given a beta2 agonist and an anticholinergic medication via nebulizer, intravenous steroids, and oxygen. As he was receiving the nebulized medications, his ribs and intercostal muscles were treated with balanced ligamentous tension techniques and respiratory augmentation techniques bilaterally with the patient in a seated position. There was a notable increase in his ribcage excursion and motion of the intercostal muscles

throughout the application of the osteopathic manipulative techniques. In addition, the patient felt less anxious, which aided in diminishing the work of breathing. Once the acute symptoms subsided and the patient felt comfortable lying supine, additional manipulative treatment, including a variety of techniques, was instituted to address the motion restrictions to the occipitoatlantal joint, cervical and thoracic spine, paraspinal muscles, sternum, clavicles, thoracic inlet/outlet, and thoracoabdominal diaphragm. R.B.'s symptoms improved significantly and he was discharged in stable condition from the emergency room with instructions to avoid exposure to exacerbating factors such as a cold environment. A prescription for beta 2 agonist and steroid inhalers, a peak flow meter, and a follow-up appointment with the family care center were then given.

## Discussion

Asthma is a common chronic inflammatory disorder that affects the airway passages of the lungs. Primarily, asthma is characterized by reversible, episodic narrowing of the airway's smooth muscle secondary to hypersecretion of mucus, hyper-reactivity, and mucosal edema. The narrowing may be of sudden or prolonged onset, which accounts for the varying degrees of airway obstruction seen in this disease. The hallmark of airway obstruction is a reduction in the forced expiratory volume in 1 second ($FEV_1$) and the ratio of $FEV_1$ to the forced vital capacity (FVC).

Asthma exacerbations may be precipitated by inhaled allergens such as perfumes or pollens, irritants, exercise, cold air, airway infection, smoking, or emotional stress. Typical symptoms are wheezing, which is most notable on expiration, breathlessness, anxiety, hypoxia, chest tightness, and paroxysmal cough.

The autonomic nervous system through homeostatic mechanisms adjusts airway size to meet the body's demands. An imbalance of these mechanisms may increase the work of breathing throughout an asthmatic attack. During relaxed situations when there is a decreased demand for airflow, parasympathetic stimulation promotes broncho-constriction leading to increased airway resistance. In contrast, during increased demand for oxygen consumption sympathetic domination takes place, causing bronchodilation to occur, which ensures minimal resistance to airflow.

The goal of treatment of the asthmatic patient is the control of symptoms and thereby the control of the condition. Decreasing airway resistance is essential in the treatment of the patient with asthma as this will diminish the effort to breath. Limited mechanical motion of the ribcage and adjacent anatomical structures may contribute to poor respiratory excursion and patient distress. The osteopathic physician may easily incorporate manipulative treatment, in addition to medications and avoidance of exacerbating factors into the management of the asthmatic patient. The goal is to maximize the patient's potential for health. In the acute state, patients with severe asthma symptoms may not be able to lie supine as breathing is more difficult in this position. Seated techniques such as gentle rib release are suitable for these cases. Treatment emphasis should be placed on any rib dysfunctions in both the acute and chronic settings. Mobilization of the ribs not only improves respiratory excursions but also may stimulate sympathetically mediated airway bronchodilation.

In severe asthmatic attacks, it may be necessary to repeat treatment at half-hour intervals to obtain significant relief of symptoms. The amount of treatment should be gauged so the patient can tolerate the treatment. As was seen in R.B.'s case, manipulative treatment does not interfere with the delivery of medications and can be instituted concomitantly. It is important to note that during an acute asthma attack, stimulatory treatment of the upper cervicals (OA, C1–C2) should be avoided because vagal stimulation may further exacerbate bronchospasm.

After the acute asthma symptoms have abated, or in between exacerbations, manipulative treatment may include direct or indirect (including articulatory) techniques to treat motion restrictions of the clavicles, cervical and thoracic spine, ribs, thoracic inlet, sternum, and thoracoabdominal diaphragm. Treatment of these areas may improve chest wall motion, thereby diminishing the work of breathing ultimately to the benefit of the asthmatic patient.

## REFERENCES

Ali J, Summer WR, Levitzky MG. *Obstructive Airway Disease in Pulmonary Pathophysiology.* New York, NY: McGraw-Hill, 1992;97–102.

Beal M, Morlock J. Somatic dysfunction associated with pulmonary disease *J Am Osteopath Assoc* 1984;84: 179–183.

DiGiovanna EL, Schiowitz S. *An Osteopathic Approach to Diagnosis and Treatment, 2nd ed.* Philadelphia: Lippincott-Raven Publishers, 1997:466–467.

D'Alonzo GE, Krachman SL. Respiratory System. In: Ward RC, Ed. *Foundations for Osteopathic Medicine.* Baltimore, MD: Williams & Wilkins, 1997:441–458.

Greenman P. Manipulative therapy for the thoracic cage. *Osteopath Ann* 1977;3:140–149.

Hoag JM, Cole WV, Bradford SG. *Osteopathic Medicine.* New York: McGraw-Hill Book Company, 1969:693–697.

Howell RK, Allen TW, Kappler RE. The influence of osteopathic manipulative therapy in the management of patients with chronic obstructive lung disease. *J Am Osteopath Assoc* 1975;74:757–760.

Kuchera ML, Kuchera WA. *Osteopathic Considerations in Systemic Dysfunction.* Columbus, OH: Greyden Press, 1994: 33–52.

Paul FA, Buser BR. Osteopathic manipulative treatment applications for the emergency department patient. *J Am Osteopath Assoc* 1996;96:403–407.

Stiles E. Manipulative management of chronic lung disease. *Osteopath Ann* 1981;9:300–304.

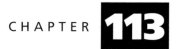

# Cardiac Applications

*Charles J. Smutney III, Eileen L. DiGiovanna, Sonia Rivera-Martinez*

The heart provides the pumping action for arterial circulation throughout the entire body. Its proper functioning is required for life itself. Understanding its significance and its interactions with the neuromusculoskeletal system is key to the osteopathic approach to manipulative intervention in a variety of cardiac conditions.

Andrew Taylor Still, founder of osteopathy, pointed out the significance of proper functioning of the heart and the arterial system when he stated, "The osteopath's foundation is that all the blood must move all the time in all parts to and from all organs."

Edward Stiles, DO has shown that osteopathic manipulative treatment significantly decreased morbidity and mortality of patients with a number of cardiovascular diseases. Felix Rogers, DO reported that osteopathic manipulation used in the treatment of patients with coronary artery disease was of significant value to some of these patients.

## ■ ANATOMY

The heart lies in the thorax, generally to the left, surrounded by the pericardium. It consists of striated muscle that is very similar in structure to that of the musculoskeletal system with the exception that cardiac muscle functions as a *syncytium,* that is, whenever a stimulus is applied to any one part of the muscle, the entire muscle contracts. The heart has an intricate electrical system that controls the rate and rhythm of the contractions, which serve to pump the arterial blood between the pulmonary system and the rest of the body.

The heart has four chambers for the collection and distribution of blood as it moves through the body. The left and right sides are separated by septae. The upper and lower chambers, the atria (above) and the ventricles (below), are also separated by septae, but the blood flows from the atria to the ventricles through valves that assure a unidirectional flow of the blood. These act as two pumps in series: one through the pulmonary system and the other through the rest of the body. Contraction of the ventricles is known as *systole* and relaxation of the ventricles, with elastic recoil of the walls of the larger arteries, propelling the blood is called *diastole.*

The innervation of the heart is significant to the ability of the osteopathic physician to diagnose and treat heart disease. The sympathetic innervation arises from the T1 to T6 region. The fibers from the right side of the cord pass to the deep cardiac plexus and serve the sinoatrial (SA) node and right side of the heart. On the left they innervate the atrioventricular (AV) node and left cardiac plexus. Parasympathetic innervation arises mainly from the vagus with the right vagus going to the SA node and the left to the AV nodes. The upper thoracic region and the occipitoatlantal, atlantoaxial, and C2 are all areas where the physician can find tissue changes and somatic dysfunction associated with heart disease.

## ■ MYOCARDIAL INFARCTION

The heart, itself, is supplied with blood through the coronary arteries and their small branches. Blockage, partial or complete, of a coronary artery leads to tissue damage or death known as *myocardial infarction*. The occlusion of an artery is most commonly caused by *arteriosclerotic plaque* formed on the lining of the inner surface of the arteries. Calcification of these plaques may occur. Blood clots tend to form on the plaques, especially if there is a tear or breakage of the plaque. The occlusion of the artery is the result of the narrowing of the channel by the plaque with a clot breaking loose and becoming caught in a narrowed artery, preventing the free flow of blood to the heart muscle.

The usual symptoms are chest pain, which may be crushing in nature, radiation of the pain to the left arm, jaw, or epigastric area, diaphoresis, and a heightened sense of anxiety.

## Cardiac Nociception

The fundamentals of osteopathic philosophy are clearly expressed in the cardiac patient with chest pain. The most easily understood osteopathic concepts are expressed here with examples of the structure–function relationship evidenced in viscerosomatic pain.

Nociceptive (pain) fibers from the visceral walls of the myocardium, the myocardial vasculature, and the pericardium return to the dorsal horn of the spinal column in the thoracic segments from T1 to T6 with the heaviest concentration at T4. The nerve pathway travels from the cardiac structures via a cardiac plexus and synapses with nerves in the superior, middle, and inferior cervical ganglia near the levels of C2, C5, and C7, respectively. Information is passed from these points along the spinal chain ganglia downward to the dorsal horn levels of T1 to T6. Here they synapse with wide dynamic array interneurons. These interneurons connect multiple sensory axons coming into zone one through zone seven in the dorsal horn. They function (in this case) as summation units that interconnect with nociceptive (pain) fibers from other areas of the body including the left upper extremity, epigastric region, left ribs, thorax, upper back, and the left jaw. Because of this wiring pattern, the brain often interprets visceral pain as somatic pain. Thus, the pain of myocardial infarction may be referred to the typical sites mentioned.

Facilitation from any of the inputs at these segments increases the likelihood of a response with additional input anywhere else in the circuit. Interestingly, muscular contraction, exhibited as a fusiform paraspinal muscle contraction, edema, erythema, and diaphoresis within the segmental region, continues to appear even in the absence of perceived pain. Conscious awareness of this facilitated response may be interpreted as pain, discomfort, and weakness in the musculoskeletal system or not at all.

In the presence of certain metabolic neuropathies, as an example diabetic neuropathy, nociceptive fibers may not signal pain. This leads to the potential for a silent myocardial infarction (MI). On physical examination, the restriction in movement and other up-regulated sympathetic findings will continue to be noticeable to the trained eye and hand. This simplified system of pain reporting for the viscera has a backup system with certain key organ structures.

The cardiac system also has vagus afferent sensory nerves that duplicate the transmission of nociceptive information but it bypasses the gating mechanism in the spinal cord. This feedback circuit carries information directly to vagal motor neurons that regulate sinoatrial and atrioventricular nodal firing rates. This can functionally override the inherent cardiac rhythm generators. It is clear that there is a complex interaction between the sympathetic and parasympathetic nervous system.

> The great vessels on the superior aspect of the heart are surrounded by a mixed plexus of parasympathetic vagal fibers and sympathetic fibers from the cardiac nerves. Embedded in the plexus are parasympathetic ganglia that receive the vagal preganglionic fibers. The plexus supplies postganglionic fibers to the sinoatrial and atrioventricular nodes, cardiac muscle itself and to the coronary vasculature of the heart. Stimulation of the sympathetic fibers accelerates cardiac output and can be arrhythmogenic, especially left-sided stimulation of the sympathetic pathways . . . Stimulation of the parasympathetic vagal fibers stabilizes the heart rate. Thus the balance between the sympathetic and parasympathetic pathways is crucial to cardiac function.
> —Willard and Carriero, 1994.

Distant mechanoreceptors and chemoreceptors, including the pressure-sensitive structures within the hypothalamus, the carotid bodies, the arch of the aorta, and the kidney near the mesangial complex, further duplicate nociceptive feedback, although these receptors may not trigger conscious awareness. In addition, there is evidence that cells of the neuroendocrine immune system can also directly and indirectly regulate heart rate via neuropeptide or hormonal secretion. As an example, consider how many mechanisms exist that release epinephrine from the adrenal glands. Nociception (pain) plays a large role in visceral function and dysfunction. Still said, "Drive a single nail through one toe. Would you be surprised if the heart made seventy-five (beats per minute)? Or even 125 beats per minute?"

Additional nociceptive information is often provided by chemoreceptors that detect oxygen deprivation. These chemoreceptors also report back to the segmental interneurons along the spine as well as to the vagal nuclei, further enhancing the capacity for balancing the parasympathetic and sympathetic systems. In a healthy system, this feedback circuitry maintains balance, but when a healthy system has become compromised, this protective balance may not function to the patient's advantage. As an example, in advanced cardiovascular disease, exertion can often be an initiating event. Exertion creates an increase for oxygen demand. When demand is high enough and supply is insufficient, immediately chemoreceptors begin to signal increasing levels of pain. As the demands continue to exceed supply, recruitment of ever wider areas of influence signal the familiar advancing of chest pain to include the left arm and then jaw pain. This process leads to increases in heart rate, stroke volume, cardiac output, coronary blood flow, systolic blood pressure, pulmonary blood pressure, cerebral blood flow, muscle blood flow, oxygen consumption, lactic acid production, respiration, and alertness. This is accompanied by a decrease in total peripheral resistance at the epidermis, increased subcutaneous and renal blood flow creating the familiar clammy, diaphoretic skin, and transient increased urine output. This can precipitate a feed-forward effect for the increasing oxygen demands that can quickly outstrip the ability of the compromised heart to adapt. The resulting electrochemical environment signals significant pain of between five and ten on a visual analog scale and, if left unabated, may lead to tissue damage (MI). Prolonged tissue damage without repair or large areas of tissue damage precede the evolution of congestive heart failure (CHF).

## Viscerosomatic Reflexes

The somatic effects of cardiac disease are probably better documented than for any other visceral pathology. The pain patterns of myocardial infarction are well known: left arm, left side of the jaw, epigastric region, and the anterior left chest wall. Somatic dysfunction and tissue changes are also common and consistent with cardiac disease. A number of studies have shown that the most frequent findings occur at T2 and T3 on the left. Also relatively frequent are findings at T1 and T4 on the left and T1 and T2 on the right. More than 70% of all somatic dysfunctions occur between T1 and T5 on the left. The changes include tissue texture changes of the intercostal muscles on the left and somatic dysfunction at any of the aforementioned thoracic vertebrae. Chapman's points are also fairly consistent in the presence of cardiac problems. The anterior point is located in the second intercostal space near the sternum. Changes also are found in the upper cervical region, especially with posterior or inferior wall infarction.

## Considerations in Osteopathic Treatment

Treatment of the patient in the earliest stages of MI is preferable. In any case, treatment must follow standard of care and address issues that are potentially life-threatening first. Use of oxygen, morphine, nitrates, recanalization of the vessels with clot-reduction medications or mechanical means, and aspirin or antiplatelet aggregation agents underscores some of the most basic pharmacologic approaches. Issues of hypertension must be addressed pharmacologically.

Once these interventions have begun, further decreasing oxygen demand is clearly prudent. Manipulative procedures that decrease facilitation at segments T1 to T4 as well as in the cervical spine should further decrease oxygen and energy demands. Issues of hypertension may have musculoskeletal influences that must be addressed. A high percentage of hypertension patients in a pilot study show a consistent somatic dysfunction pattern of C6, T2, and T6, as reported by William Johnston, DO.

At the segmental level of C2, the location of the superior cervical ganglia, there is an influence from the vagus and the sympathetic chain ganglia that can decrease the propensity for arrhythmias as well as decrease heart rate. In addition treatment of the structural elements that influence excursion and the work of breathing may further increase oxygen supply. With increasing excursion, the lymphatic system and the venous system will drain more functionally further decreasing peripheral and central chemotactic load stress.

## ■ ARRHYTHMIAS AND PALPITATIONS

The electrical system of the heart is disrupted by a number of factors, most commonly tissue damage, involving electrical nodes or pathways, from MI. Congenital factors, such as septal defects, may play a role. Some are of unknown cause.

The rhythm changes may be either an increase or a decrease in cardiac rate, or an irregularity of rhythm. Slow irregularities are known as *bradyarrythmias* and rapid rates are known as *tachyarrhythmias*. Some involve the atria and others the ventricles.

Significant for the patient in regards to arrhythmias is the fact that most pharmacologic agents used to treat them have numerous side effects, some potentially serious and even life-threatening.

The patient feels some of the arrhythmias as *palpitations*. Palpitations are felt as "skipped beats," thumping or pounding in the chest, rapid heart rate, or irregular beating of the heart. This is uncomfortable and frightening for the patient. Palpitations may be symptomatic of serious cardiac problems or the result of anxiety and benign with no cardiac dysfunction. MI establishes the potential for either type of palpitation.

It is typical to find somatic dysfunction in the upper thoracic region, both of the vertebrae and their ribs. Upper cervical somatic dysfunction is often present. A fairly common finding is that of a trigger point in the left pectoralis major muscle.

### Osteopathic Treatment

In come cases of arrhythmia, medications may be essential or use of a pacemaker or implanted defibrillator may be required. Even in these cases, use of manipulative care may be used adjunctively. If the arrhythmia is not life-threatening or if the palpitations are not of cardiac origin, osteopathic manipulation may be all that is required to prevent or decrease the frequently of palpitations.

All somatic dysfunctions of the T1–T6 vertebrae must be treated. Rib somatic dysfunctions may be secondary to the vertebral dysfunctions or may be the primary dysfunction requiring treatment. Rib-raising may address the excessive sympathetic nervous system tone and assist lymphatic movement. Chapman's points for the heart should be treated and if a pectoralis trigger point is found, it also should be treated to prevent feedback to the heart.

## ■ CONGESTIVE HEART FAILURE

The heart may begin to enlarge as a result of excessive stresses placed on it: chronic high blood pressure with an increase in cardiac workload, congenital heart abnormalities such as septal defects, valvular defects, infectious cardiomyopathies, or loss of significant heart muscle caused by infarction. The heart muscle becomes less effective in pumping blood and fluids begin to accumulate in the various parts of the body. If the major failure involves the right side of the heart, the dependent parts of the body are the first to manifest edema: feet, ankles, legs, and sacral region. In left-sided failure, the lungs are the first to demonstrate the backup of fluids as *pulmonary edema* in which the patient experiences cough and difficulty breathing.

### Osteopathic Treatment

Pharmacological intervention is necessary to relieve resistance to cardiac output and to remove excess fluids from the lungs and other body parts. The basic cause must be addressed if possible, such as treating hypertension.

Osteopathic intervention should address the autonomic nervous system and the lymphatics. The sympathetic and parasympathetic systems must be balanced. Lymphatic techniques are important but should be used with caution so that an overload of fluid from the extremities is not dumped back into the inefficient cardiovascular system.

Physical exertion taxes the heart when it is already in failure. It therefore becomes important that all dysfunctions are corrected to prevent unnecessary work in the use of the extremities and postural muscles.

## ■ OTHER CARDIAC DYSFUNCTIONS

Knowledge of specific structural findings that are consistent with unique disease processes may assist in the diagnosis of and refine the osteopathic treatment chosen for these conditions. One description of structural findings that are frequently associated with certain cardiovascular conditions is:

1. Coarctation of the aorta: greater muscular development of the upper extremities than the lower extremities.
2. Ventricular septal defect: in children there may be bilateral prominence of the anterior part of the chest with bulging of the upper two-thirds of the sternum.
3. Ventricular septal defect: in the adult there may be a unilateral bulge at the fourth and fifth intercostal spaces at the left lower sternal border.
4. Atrial septal defect: bulging in the area of the second and third intercostal spaces at the left sternal border.

Hurst's *The Heart*, ninth edition and Braunwald's *Heart Disease* sixth edition describe flattening of the thoracic spine with evolving MI and progressive narrowing of the anterior posterior (AP) diameter in advancing mitral valve prolapse.

Distinguishing between cardiac and noncardiac causes of pain and dysfunction is somewhat simplified when using osteopathic approach. Structuring a treatment plan that includes the standard of care and the addition of intelligently applied osteopathic treatment may reduce the severity and frequency of cardiac disease and decrease the length of hospital stay.

## ■ CASE 1

K.S. was a 64-year-old Hispanic woman who came to the clinic stating, "I have heart failure."

In January 1998, she had dilated cardiomyopathy diagnosed secondary to longstanding hypertension and underlying coronary artery disease. In the past 3 years she had been hospitalized sixteen times for heart failure complications.

K.S. stated that she was unable to walk more than 50 feet without fatigue, shortness of breath, weakness, and palpitations. Occasionally she awoke at night, coughing and out of breath. She constantly has lower extremity edema, has gained 32 pounds, and laments not being able to play with her only granddaughter.

The past medical history was remarkable for hypothyroidism, hyperlipidemia, an appendectomy, tonsillectomy, and 30 pack-years of tobacco use. The echocardiogram of November 2000 showed an ejection fraction of 20%.

Her medications included levothyroxine, an angiotensin-converting enzyme (ACE) inhibitor, an alpha beta-blocker, two diuretics, a nitrate, a lipid-lowering agent, and aspirin.

The physical examination was remarkable for jugular venous distention, a holosystolic murmur, a point of maximum impulse displaced to the left, and pedal edema.

An osteopathic structural examination revealed the following somatic findings: the most severe restrictions to motion were found at the facilitated segments of T2 to T4 on the left, occipitoatlantal joint, thoracic inlet, thoraco-abdominal and pelvic diaphragms, and the lower ribcage. These findings may place an extra workload on an already compromised cardiac pump.

At every treatment session, the autonomic nervous system and lymphatics were addressed in addition to other osteopathic findings. The goal of the treatment plan was to support the cardiovascular homeostatic mechanisms and enable the patient to lose weight.

With osteopathic treatment, the patient's condition began to improve. She was then challenged with an exercise program of daily walking.

Table 113-1 illustrates the changes that took place after 9 months of osteopathic treatment. The ejection fraction increased to 45%. She was able to walk 2.5 miles daily without shortness of breath, had not had any hospitalizations, the dosage of all her cardiac medications had been reduced, and one diuretic was removed from her

**TABLE 113-1 CASE 1: CHANGES AFTER 9 MONTHS OF OSTEOPATHIC TREATMENT**

| INDICATORS | FEB. 2001 (BEFORE) | NOV. 2001 (AFTER) |
| --- | --- | --- |
| Ejection Fraction | 20 % | 45% |
| Exercise Capacity | < 50 feet | 2.5 miles |
| Hospitalizations | 4–6/year | None/11 months |
| Medications | ↑ dosage | ↓ dosage |
| Weight Gain/Loss | 32 lbs gain | 38 lbs loss |

regimen. She lost 38 pounds, seldom had lower extremity edema, and her hypertension came under control.

Most important to the patient was her ability to again play with her granddaughter.

## Discussion

Heart failure is a clinical syndrome of which a diseased heart is the centerpiece. It is characterized by the inability of the heart to meet metabolic demands. One may look at the preload, afterload, and contractility components associated with cardiac function in health and disease being affected by this syndrome. Congestive heart failure may be caused by a deficit of cardiac contractility or an increased workload.

Heart failure in patients with dilated cardiomyopathy is mainly caused by systolic dysfunction in which there is a diminished capacity to eject blood against the afterload. Therefore, afterload reduction becomes an essential component of the treatment plan.

Afterload may be reduced by a decrease in vasoconstriction and weight loss. The lymphatic and autonomic nervous systems play a key role in hemodynamics and thereby in afterload reduction.

Research published in the *Mayo Clinical Proceedings* has demonstrated that a chronic increase in sympathetic tone is a potent risk factor for cardiovascular events, especially in patients with heart failure. Normalizing the sympathetic nervous system tone decreases vasoconstriction and increases venous capacity. These lead to a decrease in the afterload.

Compensatory mechanisms in heart failure tend to increase the heart rate, further diminish-

ing cardiac output. Normalizing the parasympathetic nervous system may reduce the heart rate to normal allowing for an increase in output.

Heart failure is associated with an elevated venous pressure. Treating the lymphatics increases lymphatic return and reduces the central venous pressure. Proper motion of the ribcage and the many diaphragms of the body are important in maintaining the pressure gradients for lymphatic and venous return.

Fascia envelops every organ in the body. It forms the pathways for all nerves, blood vessels, and lymphatics. Releasing fascial restrictions reduces tissue congestion, enables normal motion of the organ systems, and increases circulation.

## ■ CASE 2

N.S. was a 68-year-old woman with a chief symptom of pounding in her chest on occasions. She had a history of an atrial septal defect that was diagnosed 45 years previously, for which she underwent surgical repair. Several years after the surgery, an irregular heart beat developed, for which she eventually had a pacemaker implanted. She was well for a while, but an arrhythmia developed again, which was not controlled by the pacemaker. This time the ventricle had become involved and, after physiologic testing, required an implanted combined pacemaker/defibrillator. She was also placed on anti-arrhythmic medication. As a result of the bouts of arrhythmia, gradual weakening of the cardiac muscle occurred, resulting in congestive heart failure. She reported that when under stress, on exertion, or sometimes for no apparent reason, her heart would pound or she would hear her heartbeat in her ears. She found this very uncomfortable and disconcerting.

Her medications included digoxin, a diuretic, and a beta-blocker.

On physical examination she was normotensive. The heart rate was eighty-six and the rhythm at the time was regular. No murmur was evident. The point of maximum impulse was shifted to the left. There was jugular venous distension and mild ankle edema. She had scars of the neck, anterior chest—midline and left pectoral area, relative to previous surgeries. The protrusion of a mechanical device was evident in her abdominal wall.

Osteopathic structural examination revealed marked tenderness in the upper left thoracic area with somatic dysfunction of T2, T3, T4, and the third rib. The first ribs were elevated bilaterally and there was marked tension and tenderness in the trapezius bilaterally. Cervical somatic dysfunctions were also found: OA F $S_LR_R$, C2 F $S_LR_L$, and C3 F $S_RR_R$.

Osteopathic manipulation was added to her treatment plan. The muscle hypertonicity was treated with passive myofascial techniques and facilitated positional release. The somatic dysfunctions were treated with muscle energy, facilitated positional release, and balanced ligamentous tension. Rib-raising was used to induce adequate lymphatic drainage and normalize sympathetic tone.

She responded well to the treatments and, in addition to feeling more comfortable, she had fewer episodes of palpitations, and some episodes that were present were stopped with treatment.

## Discussion

Cardiac arrhythmias are very complex to treat because of multiple causes and because of problems with the treatments available. Medications for this condition have many side effects, some quite serious, and the medications and pacemak-ers have a significant failure rate. Palpitations are frightening and the added stress of the fear tends to aggravate the frequency and severity, so that a vicious cycle is formed. The somatic problems that result from the cardiac condition can become quite uncomfortable to even painful in nature, further complicating the patient's life.

Osteopathic manipulation is aimed at the autonomic nervous system, particularly seeking to balance the sympathetic and parasympathetic arms. Removal of somatic problems makes the patient more comfortable and thus more able to cope with the other issues in life.

### REFERENCES

Beal MC, Kleiber GE. Somatic dysfunction as a predictor of coronary artery disease. *J Am Osteopath Assoc* 1985;85: 302–307.

Curtis BM, O'Keefe JH. Autonomic Tone as a Cardiovascular Risk Factor: The Dangers of Chronic Fight or Flight. *Mayo Clin Proc* 2002;77:45–54.

DiGiovanna EL, Schiowitz S. *An Osteopathic Approach to Diagnosis and Treatment, 2nd ed.* Philadelphia: Lippincott-Raven, 1997.

Fuster V, Alexander RW, O'Rourke RA. *Hurst's The Heart, 10th ed.* New York: McGraw-Hill, 2002.

Goldman L, Braunwald E. *Primary Cardiology*. Philadelphia: W.B. Saunders Company, 1998.

Johnston W. Palpatory findings in the cervicothoracic region: Variations in normotensive and hypertensive subjects, A preliminary report. *J Am Osteopath Assoc* 1980;79: 300–308.

Kuchera ML, Kuchera WA. *Osteopathic Considerations in Systemic Dysfunction, 2nd ed.* Columbus, OH: Greyden Press, 1994.

Rogers FJ. Cardiology. In: Ward RC, ed. *Foundations for Osteopathic Medicine*. Baltimore, MD: William and Wilkins, 1997.

Shamsham F, Mitchell J. Essentials of the Diagnosis of Heart Failure. *Am Fam Physician* 2002;61:1319–1328.

Thomas PH. *Congestive Heart Failure.* In: Hoag JM, ed. *Osteopathic Medicine*. New York:. McGraw-Hill Book Company, 1969.

Wallace E, et al. Lymphatic System. In: Ward RC, ed. *Foundations for Osteopathic Medicine*. Baltimore, MD: William and Wilkins, 1997.

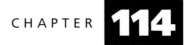

# Gastrointestinal Applications

*Dennis J. Dowling and Michael F. Oliverio*

## ■ STRUCTURE AND FUNCTION

The gastrointestinal system is a series of structures that mechanically process food, contribute to the process by means of chemicals and hormones, or both. It literally begins at the lips and ends with the anus. As a tube, it contains the openings at the two ends with various doors or sphincters acting as valves checking retrograde movement. Food enters the mouth and is subjected to mechanical and chemical digestive processes almost immediately. Hunger begins with signals received in the central nervous system as to glucose level, the status of stomach filling, odors, and even visual cues. Increased production of saliva can begin with a thought of food but is enhanced by other stimuli.

Foods are made soluble in the mouth through chewing and salivation and create vapors that stimulate the fibers of the olfactory nerve. The olfactory nerve (cranial nerve I) passes through the cribiform plate of the ethmoid. Whether the nerve is injured or compressed, decreased ability to smell can impair the ability to taste and reduce the enjoyment of food.

Mastication is innervated by the trigeminal nerve (cranial nerve V), which activates all of the muscles of mastication. Taste of the anterior tongue is conducted by sensory fibers from the facial nerve (cranial nerve VII), and from the posterior aspect and sides by the glossopharyngeal nerve (cranial nerve IX), while swallowing is innervated by the hypoglossal nerve (cranial nerve XII) and, to a lesser extent, the vagus nerve (cranial nerve X). The glossopharyngeal also mobilizes the tongue and food is pushed to the teeth and posterior pharynx.

Impairment of any or all of these components, especially in the absence of known cause, requires understanding of the course of each of the nerves and the possible constrictions and impediments that may occur as they pass through and around other structures. The courses of the maxillary and mandibular divisions of the trigeminal nerve pass through the foramina ovalle and rotundum. *Problems of chewing* may result in pain and discomfort. The facial nerve courses through a common opening in the temporal bone and is sometimes compressed along with a branch of the vestibulocochlear nerve in the auditory canal. The hypoglossal and vagus, as well as the spinal accessory nerve (cranial nerve XI), arise from the nucleus ambiguous in the medulla and upper cervical region (CN XI) and then descend through the jugular foramen. The hypoglossal nerves exit through the same-named foramen medial to the occipital condyles. *Difficulties in swallowing* may be related to cranial dysfunctions of the occiput, temporal, and sphenoid bones in particular and involve the upper cervical spine.

The next aspect concerned with processing involves gravity to a slight extent and intrinsic neural processes. The epiglottis shields the larynx and trachea during swallowing as a means of preventing aspiration of food contents into the respiratory system. Food, as it enters the esophagus, causes distension of the tube. Lubricated with saliva and facilitated by expansion, the food is pushed along by smooth muscle contractions. A gastroesophageal sphincter marks the entrance in the stomach. It lies just inferior

**631**

to and is reinforced by the muscular diaphragm. *Reflux esophagitis or gastroesophageal reflux disease (GERD)* most often results from incomplete closure, increased acid production, and most probably both. Variations in contour of the stomach serve the function of permitting expansion for meals and providing greater surface area for the further breakdown of the chyme, or products of digestion.

Increased acid production, already cued by the notion and oral processing of the food, lowers the pH of the environment, contributing to both the chemical breakdown of the food and the facilitation of other enzymes capable of breaking protein, fat, and starch molecular bonds. Although there has been positive identification for the involvement of *Helicobacter pylori* in the development of peptic ulcers, there must be an opportunity for it to exert its influences. The pharmacological approach to treatment combines antibiotics and proton pump inhibitors as a means of making the environment less hospitable by raising the pH. Alterations in the environment probably allow the microorganism to take root and flourish.

The lining of the stomach wall is protected by prostaglandin-mediated mucous production. This is impaired by the use of steroids, non-steroidal anti-inflammatory drugs (NSAIDS), and other medications. An individual's mental condition can also impair the ordinary protective elements of all systems. *Prolonged sympathetic activity* does not so much increase acid production as it does reduce the integrity of the mucoid lining. Other structures, such as the liver, spleen, gallbladder, and pancreas, are embryologically related to the intestines and connected, for the most part, by ducts. There are also sympathetic and parasympathetic influences on these structures. The splenic and hepatic capsules contract slightly in response and the process alters some of the functions. As with other sphincters, the ducts leading to and from the gall bladder react.

The combination of acid, food products, and other juices are released from the pylorus of the stomach and through a sphincter into the proximal small intestine of the duodenum. Without the buffering provided by bicarbonate products produced in the liver, concentrated in the gall bladder, and delivered by small ducts, the walls would be eroded. Glucose is processed to glycogen and stored in the liver, insulin from the pancreas drives glucose into cells, and fats, protein, and water are further processed. Some commensurate enteric microorganisms assist in the breakdown of substances and help to maintain the internal milieu. This balance may be upset by the nonspecific action of antibiotics.

Peristalsis, the rhythmic contraction of the gastrointestinal system that reacts to local expansion and pushes the contents in an anterograde manner, is a localized process that does not require cognitive intervention but is modified by it and the autonomic nervous system. The intrinsic plexi manage the function of stimulating the smooth muscle as a response to intraluminal stretching. Vagal influences affect the gastrointestinal system all the way until very nearly the distal portion and upgrade the process. Other functions, including locomotion and mentation, are reduced as the organism goes through the restorative processes mediated by the parasympathetic system. Increased peristalsis and faster processing times result from increased parasympathetic influences. There is a disadvantage in this being maintained for a prolonged time: the decreased absorption of nutrient components and water. When this is prolonged, the stool produced is watery and loose. These results are usually termed *diarrhea,* even though the correct definition includes a critical amount of approximately a liter or more. At times this may be an advantage, as when infective agents invade the gastrointestinal system. Toxic and other waste components irritate the inner wall lining and accelerate peristalsis. Although there is discomfort from the filling of the intestines and more frequent bowel movements, the faster transit time reduces the opportunity for the organisms to reproduce and invade. The irritation of the gastric walls of the stomach and the lining of the intestines may result in the reflex contraction of the smooth muscle and retrograde expulsion from the stomach by the process of emesis. Mucous production may also be increased. There can also be severe nutritional and health consequences in that the individual's health may be endangered and impaired by malnutrition and dehydration because of the limited absorption allowed in these circumstances.

The complementary component of the parasympathetic system in the autonomic nervous system, the sympathetic system, also can modify the gastrointestinal system function. Nerve fibers arise from all thoracic and the uppermost lumbar spinal segments and accompany the arteries to the various organs. Increased sympathetic activity results in the opposite effects to that of the parasympathetic. Activation results in decreased peristalsis, contraction of the sphincters, and slowed or even shut-down of gastrointestinal activity. A relatively mild, benign, and usually self-limited form occurs with *constipation*. When appropriate, such activity delays the relatively unnecessary restorative processes while preparing the individual to escape ("flight") or defend ("fight") by redirecting the efforts to the skeletal muscle. Physiologically, it is also of direct benefit to the gastrointestinal system.

Whether by trauma or by surgical intervention, the gastrointestinal system nearly stops functioning when the abdominal cavity is entered. Sometimes this occurs without trauma, as when a rupture occurs in the intestines and the contents cause an inflammatory process known as *peritonitis*. Disturbance of the peritoneum results in a rigid response of the more superficial abdominal muscles as well. These responses reduce the amount of blood loss by way of sympathetically constricted arteries as well as limiting the amount of intraluminal contents spilling into the cavity. Again, this is useful in temporary situations but interferes with normal functioning when it persists past the point of usefulness.

Prolonged sympathetic activity, as occurs in a *postoperative ileus*, results in increased absorption of water, greater energy requirements, and disorganization of some of the normal processes. The stool may become hard and difficult to mobilize. Fissures may develop in the stool and proximal fluids may leak around, creating the impression of loose stools when the opposite is the truth.

Some conditions, such as *irritable bowel syndrome* (IBS), appear to involve alternating patterns of upgraded parasympathetic and sympathetic activity rather than what would be considered normal. Sufferers appear to experience bouts of diarrhea with intervening episodes of constipation. Rarely do they have periods of prolonged comfort. Although psychological factors cannot be solely to blame in such conditions, they are often implicated and some pharmacological interventions focus on reducing elements of anxiety, depression, and other feelings, there may also be a commonality with some of the involved neurotransmitters.

Although the obvious treatment for *appendicitis* is surgical, the clinical presentation presents with some typical findings and pattern. The appendix exists as a blind pouch in the pocket of the cecum. The T10 spinal level innervates the region. The initial symptom in appendicitis is the referred pain and cramping to the umbilical region. When the muscles become tight and rigid, a viscerosomatic reflex occurs. At T10 or thereabouts, acute somatic dysfunction may also arise. Later, if the appendix touches the anterior peritoneum, the localized right lower abdominal quadrant becomes more symptomatic. If the appendix is retrocecal, the psoas becomes irritated and may even go into spasm and shortening. A Chapman's point is located at the tip of the right twelfth rib and is helpful in the diagnosis of appendicitis.

The structure and function of the gastrointestinal system is primarily visceral. The aforementioned muscles of mastication comprise skeletal muscle. The diaphragm bridges the thoracic and abdominal cavities and acts as more than as a septum or wall. The descent of the diaphragm during respiratory inhalation results in mechanical compression of the liver, stomach, and intestines. This is made more intense by the closing of the glottis and addition of the contraction of other abdominal muscles as when a *Valsalva* maneuver is performed. In some cases, this may trigger a vasovagal reaction by way of a *viscerovisceral somatic reflex*.

Other skeletal muscle contributions include the contraction of the muscles of the pelvic floor. The sling of the puborectalis and other levator ani muscles are responsible for maintaining fecal continence along with a trained sympathetic reflex. Relaxation of these muscles and the rectal sphincter is under voluntary control and is facilitated by diaphragmatic contraction when necessary. The diaphragm is also involved in a type of mechanical irritation of the diaphragm and referral to other parts. Whether from free air under the diaphragm, spastic contractions of the stomach, an inflamed gall bladder, or other structure, irritation of the diaphragm results in radiation of pain to the ipsilateral shoulder, neck, and scapula.

*Hiccups or hiccoughs* can also involve a soma-tosomatovisceral response, and attention should be directed not only to the immediate region but also to the origins of the phrenic nerve at the C3, C4, and C5 levels.

The parasympathetic influences to the lowest region of the gastrointestinal system arise not from the cranial-originating vagus but from the second, third, and fourth sacral nerves. The free mobility of the pelvic components, the sacrum, innominate, and even the coccyx, is necessary for proper functioning. Likewise, somatic dys-functions of the region can be related to *hemor-rhoids, diverticular disease, abscesses,* or other dis-eases. The dural core-link from the foramen magnum through the spinal column and with attachment to the second sacral segment con-nects the cranial mechanism to its inferior sacral component. Local restrictions, especially of the sacrum, can affect the sigmoid colon, rectum, and anus mechanically and neurologically as well as restrict optimum cranial functioning. The inverse is also true.

## ■ CASE ONE

Mrs. A.M. was a 49–year-old obese woman who had a history of chronic cholecystis. She had three episodes that occurred within the past year before elective hospitalization for a cholecystec-tomy. Each event appeared to be precipitated by eating a meal with a relatively high fat content. She reported nausea, vomiting, and severe right upper abdominal pain with radiation of the pain to the shoulder and scapula. Treatment con-sisted of narcotic analgesia and she was dis-charged from the emergency department with-out being hospitalized after each event. Murphy's sign was positive. Pulse, temperature, and blood pressure were all mildly increased. Plain x-ray, ultrasound, and MRI confirmed the diagnosis of cholecystis. The walls of the com-mon cystic duct and those of the gall bladder are thickened. There were also radiolucent

stones and sludge noted. Mrs. M. had no other significant medical problems. Rather than undergo another attack, the patient had elected to undergo surgery.

Mrs. M. wanted the procedure to be per-formed laparoscopically. Although the surgeon had agreed to attempt to do so, he advised the patient that an open procedure would probably need to be performed given her obesity and the inflammation of her gall bladder. After attempt-ing the laparoscopic procedure, the surgeon al-tered the process to the open procedure because of the difficulty of access and surgical accuracy that he encountered during the surgery.

The gall bladder was removed successfully. She was medicated for pain with a narcotic com-bined with an antihistamine administered intra-muscularly by injection, was given intravenous fluids, and was allowed sips of water. She was not to eat until allowed to do so by the surgeon. Within the next 6 hours, the surgeon, her pri-mary care physician, the nurse, and the intern examined her. There were no bowel sounds aus-cultated, she did not pass flatus, and her abdom-inal girth increased. Percussion of her abdomen revealed tympanitic sounds. The surgeon or-dered a nasogastric tube to be placed by the in-tern for the purpose of decompressing the gas production of the gastrointestinal system. There was also some discussion as to the possible need for a rectal suction tube to be placed. Concern was expressed that further increase in abdominal girth could precipitate dehiscence of the abdom-inal sutures. The intern requested permission and orders to perform osteopathic manipulation as an adjunct to treatment for the postoperative ileus.

The intern examined the patient further and found rigid paravertebral musculature as well as somatic dysfunctions in the region of T5 to T9 on both sides. The most significant of these was a T7 E $S_R$ $R_R$. The patient was advised of the situation and she expressed preference for the osteopathic manipulation over the insertion of the rectal tube. The intern sat with his arms rest-ing on the mattress on the patient's right side, with the palms of his hands under the patient and the fingers curled upwards. The pads of the fingers of both hands contacted the hypertonic paravertebral muscles as a means of applying inhibitory pressure. This was maintained for more than 2 minutes, with the endpoint being the resultant relaxation of the muscles. The muscles, which had also been tender to palpation previously, were no longer so. The procedure was repeated in other areas of the thoracic and lumbar spine on the same and opposite sides with similar results. The single somatic dysfunction was addressed by balanced ligamentous technique (BLT). The spinous process of T7 was pushed toward the left side while the spinous processes of T6 and T8 were drawn toward the right. This was maintained until there was a release and an exaggeration was felt. Motion was then introduced toward the barrier directions. The other posterior transverse processes, reflecting the less rigid vertebral dysfunctions, were gently sprung anteriorly.

Finally, the patient's abdomen was also treated. The intern stood on the patient's left side and reached over the patient and placed the pads of his fingers against the lateral aspect of the abdominal muscles in the posterior axillary line between the tenth rib and the iliac crest. The patient tolerated this and it was maintained for approximately a minute until the musculature relaxed. The same was repeated with the intern on the patient's right side and addressing the patient's left side. Lastly, the intern placed the edge of his hand on the edge of the abdominal bandage below and parallel to the surgical incision. Gentle pressure was exerted obliquely toward the incision for approximately 30 seconds. The patient tolerated all manipulations well and the whole treatment took a little more than 10 minutes.

Two hours later the patient expressed that she was in less pain and reluctantly offered that she had passed flatus. Auscultation of the abdomen revealed fairly normal bowel sounds in all four quadrants. The patient was able to resume eating the next day and was discharged 2 days after that. No rectal or oral tubes were necessary.

## Discussion

The process of postoperative ileus is one involving both mechanical and autonomic nerve-mediated processes. Even though the surgery barely affected the intestines, there was a need to physi-

cally manipulate them as a means of allowing greater exposure for the operative field. In response, the process of peristalsis slows and even shuts down. The other factor is the irritation and apparent up-regulation of the sympathetic nervous system. This further maintains sphincter closing and reduced peristalsis. This is reflected and maintained by the increased spinal rigidity, the viscerosomatic reflex. The pain from the incision and the stress from the procedure further served to maintain the skeletal rigidity and sympathetic activity. Some of the effect could also be attributed to the side effects of the operative anesthesia. Narcotics also have the effect of reducing peristalsis, which calls to mind considerations of benefit versus risks. With sphincter closure, decreased motility, increased stasis, and unimpaired enteric activity, the production of gases continues with no easy escape.

The common intervention is to try to decompress the buildup of gas while awaiting the return of the patient's own inherent functions. This does not always happen spontaneously and approximately 7% to 8% of patients undergoing abdominal surgery can be expected to have a postoperative ileus. Hermann (1963) performed a study in which the subjects were assigned for treatment with osteopathic manipulation after surgery. Of the 317 patients who were treated, only one had a postoperative ileus (0.3%). The next 92 patients went untreated and seven of them had ileus. The seven were treated and only one case remained unresolved and required other interventions. The treatment, paravertebral inhibition, was similar to what was applied in this case.

## ■ CASE TWO

Ms. T.C. was a 25–year-old woman who presented with a chief symptom of alternating diarrhea and constipation. She stated that each would last a few days and she rarely had periods when she felt "normal." The constipation she described as consisting of, at most, one bowel movement per day, which required straining, and it was accompanied by abdominal bloating and cramping. She would take laxatives to try to relieve these symptoms. When she had diarrhea, she would have several loose-formed bowel movements per day. She would often finish one bowel movement and would feel that she needed to again return to the bathroom approximately an hour later. Although she did not have the same level of abdominal discomfort, she found the diarrhea almost as disconcerting because the frequent movements would also lead to her hemorrhoids becoming inflamed and painful. She would try to increase her dietary intake of fiber when these symptoms developed and used topical agents on her hemorrhoids. Other than the chief symptom, the patient had no other medical problems.

She had attempted dietary changes, including subtraction diets, to try to eliminate problematic foods and has undergone testing for food allergies. None of these avenues demonstrated any usefulness. There was no apparent correlation with her menses, because she had attempted to track its influence previously. She was unmarried, was not in a relationship, and was employed as a first grade teacher. She expressed that she enjoyed her work but sometimes found it stressful.

On physical examination, the patient was afebrile and had normal vital signs. There were no remarkable findings other than some slight abdominal discomfort on palpation of the left quadrants. Bowel sounds were relatively normal and present throughout. Somatic dysfunctions were noted as being an occipito-atlantal compression and OA $ES_LR_R$, C3 $ES_LR_L$, C4 $ES_LR_L$, C7 $FS_LR_L$, T3 $ES_RR_R$, T7 $FS_RR_R$, T9 $ES_LR_L$, T10 $ES_RR_R$, L5 $ES_RR_R$, and L-on-L sacral torsion. There was a mild right torsion cranial dysfunction and paravertebral muscle spasm in a noncompensatory pattern. Besides the tenderness of the left half of the abdomen, the underlying structures felt full and resistant.

The patient was treated for her somatic dysfunctions on the first visit with a combination of techniques including, muscle energy, facilitated positional release, high-velocity low-amplitude (HVLA), and cranial osteopathy. In addition, ventral visceral techniques were used. The left hemi-diaphragm was discovered to be restricted as well and a diaphragmatic release was used. Beginning in the left lower quadrant, the physician scooped the abdomen toward the umbilicus and held until the structures released. This was directed at supporting the mesentery and the sig-

moid colon. The procedure was repeated for the descending, splenic flexure, transverse, hepatic flexure, ascending, and cecal portions of the large intestines in sequence. The direction of traction was toward the umbilicus for each of the efforts. A direct posterior pressure was used to treat the central region into the locations of the mesenteric ganglia. This was moderately uncomfortable for the patient. The sacral and occipital portions were treated with a rocking maneuver and CV4, respectively.

The patient was directed to discontinue her use of the over-the-counter and prescriptive medications that she had been using. She could use a bulk-forming agent if necessary for either diarrhea or constipation. She was also advised to exercise by walking and look into other such activities that would possibly interest her. She was also directed to increase her daily intake of water and limit her intake of caffeine-containing beverages and foods. Ingestion of vegetables with some limitations was recommended. Some consideration was given to possible behavioral counseling to manage the stress but this was deferred for the next visit.

The patient returned two weeks later and reported that she felt improved and no longer a "prisoner of the bathroom." She was having one to two normal bowel movements per day. She did express that she had abdominal aches for 24 hours after the treatment and had two large bowel movements the evening of her first treatment. Some of her somatic dysfunctions noted on the first visit were present but were in a more compensatory pattern. The abdominal examination was unremarkable and there were no apparent restrictions. The patient was again treated with similar methods to the first visit. She called before her next scheduled visit and cancelled her appointment with the statement that she felt that she "was cured."

## Discussion

The condition of irritable bowel syndrome (IBS) is just that, a "syndrome." It is not truly a diagnosis. It is a set of symptoms and signs indicating some commonality. The most likely cause concerns the effects of the autonomic system. The sympathetic and parasympathetic systems are not adversarial but are complementary. The former is for modifying preparedness and interaction with one's environment. The latter adjusts the visceral components in their function of repair, energy storage, and rebuilding. One cannot function without the other. The most probable sequence of occurrences in IBS is an upgrading of sympathetic efferent modification of the gastrointestinal system. In effect, the processes are shut down. This leads to increased absorption of fluid, the production of a more compact and difficult to mobilize stool, and finally discomfort. The stoppage results in a backup of contents prior. Sometimes the dense stool fractures and the relatively non-absorbed stool leaks around and may appear to be diarrhea. A parasympathetic rebound may also be possible and transit time may accelerate as a means of trying to reestablish equilibrium. There may in fact be an overcompensation. The original instigating precipitant may be a physical injury, anxiety, fear, anger, or some other event or thought. The cascade of events can repeat indefinitely. The musculoskeletal system acts as a mirror, refractor, and anchor. The appearance of viscerosomatic reflexes marks the underlying elements and may act as part of a reverberating circuit to maintain the existence of the visceral end. Manipulation of the available findings allows the osteopathic physician entrance into breaking the circuit, reducing magnification, and reestablishing harmony.

The patient may have contributed to the alternating pattern by her use of anti-diarrheal medications. Many are irritating to the lining of the gastrointestinal system. Somatovisceral and viscerosomatic reflexes occur in patterns related to the structures being innervated by the same segmental levels. Their persistence may maintain dysfunctions longer than the original condition would have. The effect of osteopathic manipulative medicine may not be so much an upgrading of the sympathetics or parasympathetics as it is in removing impediments and reflex patterns to allow a resetting of the system towards health.

## ■ CASES THREE AND FOUR

C.B. and B.C. were two infants, both female, who were brought to the osteopathic physician by their respective parents with symptoms of "colic." They both were inconsolable at almost all times, fussy, and difficult to manage. Both were 6 months old and had been through the gamut of attempts at changing formulas. None of the pharmacological interventions appeared to work and for the parents the frustration was that their first babies were not the "bundles of joy" that they had expected. The babies ate, gained weight, had bowel movements, and slept fitfully. All touching and activities, especially feeding and defecation, seemed to aggravate their condition. The birth histories were unremarkable and both were delivered full-term by normal spontaneous vaginal delivery.

C.B. was the first child presented. She never smiled and she struggled whether touched or left alone. On examination, the occipito-atlantal joint had relatively free motion. The key element was a spastic diaphragm. There was also a posterior protrusion at approximately the level of the sixth rib on the left. The baby was held and treated. Gentle pressure was placed anteriorly, a fingerbreadth below the left sided ribs. The baby fussed and cried for minutes and then fell asleep. This was almost coincident with the release of the diaphragm. A slight anterior pressure placed on the posterior rib resulted in an audible and palpable movement of the rib. The parents were a bit disconcerted by the process but accepted the sleeping baby.

A call was received the next day. The first statement was, "What did you do to our baby?" She had slept all of the way home in the car, awoke and had a meal, was relatively quiet and then slept through the night. These were all first occurrences. A follow-up that occurred several days later revealed that this had become the more consistent behavior. The parents noted that she smiled and seemed to interact with them, which she had not done to any extent previously.

C.B.'s parents referred B.C.'s parents a few weeks later. On the surface, her clinical history was almost identical. However, there were different findings. B.C. had a compressed OA joint and a free diaphragm. The treatment was directed at the dysfunction. There was some slight improvement after OA decompression. It actually took a total of three successive weekly treatments before the same results as were obtained with C.B. could be obtained with B.C. Although initially disappointed, the parents were quite happy with the ultimate outcome.

There were some clinical clues as to the differences between the two babies. C.B. would practically take in full meals and then regurgitate much of it. B.C. could make a good seal around the bottle nipple but demonstrated difficulty in swallowing, and half, if not more, of what she took in her mouth would not be swallowed. Both babies had a great deal of gas and flatus and were apparently uncomfortable for much of the day. They slept little, cried a great deal, and did not smile or seem to react well to being held. C.B.'s difficulty stemmed from a spastic diaphragm whereas B.C.'s was related to OA compression affecting the hypoglossal nerves where they exited medially from the occipital condyles.

## Discussion

Colic is a fairly common condition. Approximately 10% to 30% of babies experience it. The main symptom is continuous crying for long periods of time, usually worsening in the evening. Beyond sometimes apparent endless periods of crying, a baby with colic may also look uncomfortable and appear to be in pain. Babies may lift their head or legs, become red in the face, pass wind, refuse to eat, or become fussy soon after eating. Disturbed sleep is another common symptom. Babies do continue to eat and gain weight. The parents also have disturbed sleep and experience heightened stress and anxiety. The usual treatment is dietary change, even though less than 5% of the babies with diagnosed colic have a discernible food allergy. If the mother is breast-feeding, then she also must change her diet. All in all, this may be more of a temporizing effect in that most children will outgrow it, after 3 or 4 months.

Unrecognized are the mechanical causes. A birth history, although useful, may not give much information. The findings of the osteopathic structural examination may reveal cranial, cervical, thoracic, rib, diaphragmatic, lumbar, or pelvic findings. All significant findings should be treated with osteopathic manipulation. Generally, infants are fairly plastic and the forces necessary are minimal.

### REFERENCES

Adams RD, Victor M. *Principles of Neurology, 5th ed.* New York: McGraw-Hill Inc, 2001.

Barral J-P, Mercier P. *Visceral Manipulation.* Seattle, Washington: Eastland Press, 1988:67–183.

Carreiro J. *An Osteopathic Approach to Children.* New York: Churchill-Livingstone, 2003:85–103.

Educational Council on Osteopathic Principles. *Clinical Osteopathically Integrated Learning Scenarios.* American Association of Colleges of Osteopathic Medicine, 2001: 87–92.

Finet G, Williame C. *Treating Visceral Dysfunction,* Portland, OR: Stillness Press, 2000.

Hermann E. *The D.O.* 1965;Oct: L163–L164.

Kuchera ML, Kuchera WA. *Osteopathic Considerations in Systemic Dysfunction, 2nd ed.* Columbus, OH: Greyden Press, 1994;79–122.

Magoun, HI Sr. The dental search for a common denominator in craniocervical pain and dysfunction. *J Am Osteopath Assoc* 1979;78:810–815.

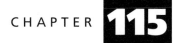

# Renal and Urological Considerations

*Stanley Schiowitz*

The renal system serves as a filtration system to remove waste products from the circulatory system, passing them out of the body through the urine. The urological system serves two purposes:

1. It provides the ducts through which the urine is moved from the kidneys and out of the body via the ureters, bladder, and urethra.
2. The male urological system is intimately bound to the male reproductive organs. These two separate systems are generally considered as one.

## ■ BENIGN PROSTATIC HYPERTROPHY

Benign prostatic hypertrophy (BPH) is an enlargement of the prostate that creates lower urinary tract obstruction accompanied by urinary tract symptoms. It is a condition that will likely occur in almost all males, if they live long enough. Autopsy studies show that microscopic evidence was found in 90% of men older than age 80, but it was also found in as many as 25% of 40-year-old men.

### Etiology

Aging and androgens are the only presently established factors in the development of BPH. Estrogen, growth factors, such as basic fibroblast growth factor, and stromal epithelial interactions are known to play a part in the growth of the prostate. Diets that are high in butter, margarine, seed oils, and low in fruit content and zinc may predispose to the development of symptoms.

### Signs and Symptoms

Obstructive symptoms are seen related to bladder outlet obstruction. These include changes in the force and stream of the urine, polyuria, nocturia, urinary dribbling, urgency, and urge incontinence. There is usually a palpable enlargement of the prostate, when examined digitally through the rectum, but the size may have no relationship to the degree of symptoms presented. Over a period of time, secondary bladder changes can develop consisting of bladder wall thickening, trabeculation, and the formation of calculi. The intensity of lower urinary tract syndrome signs and symptoms generally progress over time. However, spontaneous improvement can occur in the untreated patient.

Treatment is usually conservative in nature, primarily dedicated to relief of the symptom complex and improvement of the quality of life. There are a number of newer pharmaceutical agents that are presently being employed that have varied effects on these symptoms.

Indications for surgical intervention usually include azotemia, recurring hematuria, bladder calculi, recurrent large amounts of residual urine, recurrent infections, and incontinence.

### Osteopathic Concepts

The prostate is innervated from the prostatic plexus of the autonomic nervous system. It arises

**639**

from the inferior hypogastric plexus. These nerves are distributed to the prostate, seminal vesicles, prostatic urethra, ejaculatory ducts, corpora cavernosa, corpus spongiosum, membranous and penile parts of the urethra, and the bulbo-urethral glands. The preganglionic efferent sympathetic fibers of this plexus are derived from the lowest three thoracic segments and the upper two lumbar segments of the spinal cord. The parasympathetic preganglionic fibers originate in the second, third, and fourth sacral segments of the spinal cord.

Chronic somatic dysfunctions are commonly found at the eleventh and twelfth thoracic and the first lumbar segments. Chapman's points for the prostate, as well as restrictions of the cranial-sacral mechanism, can be present. All of these, when present, should be treated as a means of resolving many of the presenting symptoms. It is also important to treat any structural deficits, such as a short leg or thoraco-lumbar scoliosis, as a means of lessening the effects created by the stimulation of the autonomic nervous system involved.

## ■ NEPHROLITHIASIS

There are sixteen to twenty-four cases of nephrolithiasis per 10,000 persons reported in the United States yearly. Males have a three-fold to four-fold increased risk of the development of renal calculi over females. Uric acid and calcium stones are the most prevalent types of calculi found in men, whereas infectious stones are more common in females.

The composition of these calculi can be any of the following: calcium, phosphate, mixed calcium and phosphate, magnesium ammonium or phosphate, uric acid, cystine and some are of miscellaneous minerals. Of these, the calcium, phosphate, and uric acid stones are most prevalent in this order.

## Cause of the Specific Types of Calculi

Calcium oxalate stones develop in an acidic urine, whereas calcium phosphate stones develop in an alkaline urine. In addition to the pH of the urine, the cause of the hypercalcemia that may be present should be identified. Among the

conditions that can be present to create a hypercalcemia are: hyperparathyroidism, hypervitaminosis, Paget disease, multiple myeloma, other malignancies that metastasize to bone, such as lung, breast, kidney, head, and neck, as well as immobilization.

Uric acid stones are a product of purine metabolism and a diagnosis of gout should be considered. Chronic renal infections and urinary retention syndromes are other major causes. It is easy to see the importance of obtaining a comprehensive history and the chemical definition of any stone that is passed. Dietary advice and strenuous treatment of infections can prevent reoccurrence of the calculi.

## Signs and Symptoms

Pain is the most common symptom presented. It can be mild or extremely intense and require hospitalization. Renal colic is a result of the obstruction caused by the stone. The condition can be asymptomatic when obstruction is absent. The pain usually starts suddenly in the early morning and rapidly becomes more intense as the stone moves down the ureter. A history of relative dehydration can precede the onset of an attack. The location of the pain will depend on the position of the stone. Upper ureteral and pelvic obstruction will cause flank pain with costovertebral tenderness and may radiate into the abdomen. A positive Lloyd's sign is usually present. Lower ureteral obstruction can cause pain that radiates into the groin, testicle, or labia. Nausea and vomiting may develop and a differentiation from an acute appendicitis must be made. A low-grade fever may develop. If the stone is passed, the patient will have relief of symptoms. Failure to pass the stone, with maintenance of obstruction, will require therapeutic intervention. The following methodologies for treatment of the calculi are presently available. Extra-corporeal shockwave, lithotripsy, pericutaneous nephrostilithiotomy, rigid and flexible uteroscopy, or open surgical approaches.

## Osteopathic Concepts

One of the most important of the osteopathic concepts is prevention. The emphasis must be placed on hydration, a dietary prescription, and the prevention of recurring urinary infection by immediate and intensive treatment of an acute urinary infection, as well as the treatment of all underlying pathology.

The renal and ureteric plexuses of the autonomic nervous system innervate the kidneys and ureters. The renal plexus is formed by filaments from the celiac ganglion, celiac plexus, aorticorenal ganglion, the lowest thoracic splanchnic nerve, the first lumbar nerve, and the aortic plexus. The ureteral plexus is derived from the renal and aortic plexuses, the superior hypogastric plexus, the hypogastric nerve, and the inferior hypogastric plexus. The efferent fibers of the autonomic nervous system related to the kidney and ureter are derived from the vagus nerve and the first, second, and third lumbar segment of the spinal cord.

Somatic dysfunctions are commonly found at the twelfth thoracic, and first two lumbar segments. Chapman's points for the kidney, as well as the cranio-sacral mechanism, must be evaluated. Any dysfunctions found should receive osteopathic manipulative treatment at the time of the acute incident, with a follow-up evaluation and treatment as necessary when the symptom complex has subsided.

## ■ PYELONEPHRITIS

Acute pyelonephritis is an acute infection of the renal parenchyma and collecting system of the upper urinary tract. Chronic pyelonephritis follows repeated attacks of acute pyelonephritis leading to changes characterized by progressive renal scarring, usually asymmetric and irregular, involving both the cortex and the pelviocalyceal system.

Acute pyelonephritis is commonly caused by a bacterial agent. *Escherichia coli* and other enterobacteria account for 90% of these infections. Chronic recurrences of acute episodes are usually caused by predisposing factors such as functional abnormalities including indwelling catheters, anatomic abnormalities of the urinary tract that cause stasis or obstruction, urolithiasis, malignancy, neurogenic bladder, and foreign bodies. Other risk factors include diabetes mellitus, age, and the presence of immune deficiency. Females are more prone to urinary tract infection because of the relative position of the urethra in close approximation to the rectum.

## Signs and Symptoms

Patients usually present with fever, chills, and flank pain with or without radiation to the groin. Additionally, depending on the severity of the condition, they may show other signs of sepsis, including malaise, nausea, and vomiting. Lower tract symptoms such as dysuria, increased urinary frequency, and urgency may be present. Examination will show the presence of tenderness of the costovertebral angle of the involved side. A urinalysis will show pyuria, bacturia, and gross or microscopic blood. A complete blood count will report a leucocytosis with predominance of neutrophils. Urine cultures are diagnostic and a sensitivity study will identify the appropriate antibiotic therapy.

A patient with a history of recurrent attacks must be evaluated for any predisposing factors that may be present. The elimination of these findings must be vigorously pursued. In the pediatric female patient, simple instructions on the proper wiping of the anus and urethra from front to back can eliminate the reoccurrence of acute cystitis and the danger of its being the cause for the creation of pyelonephritis.

## Osteopathic Concepts

The innervation of the kidneys and related organs has been reviewed in the previous topic of nephrolithiasis. This included common sites of the development of somatic dysfunctions.

Cole reported that the animal research he had performed in 1951 showed that "in the kidneys some of the glomeruli were swollen, as were the cells of the collecting tublules of the cortex." In his summary he states that "it may be stated that spinal fixation in experimental animals resulted in cellular and vascular alterations in visceral structures reflexly (sympathetically associated)."

Frymann, in the 1950 yearbook of the Academy of Applied Osteopathy, reviewed research previously reported by Davis, McConnell, and Burns. She noted that in addition to the expected sites for the finding of somatic dysfunctions secondary to renal pathology, involved somatic dysfunctions were found in the cervical region.

In the same yearbook, Zirul states in the conclusion of his article that "the osteopathic lesion, especially of the sixth cervical to the first lumbar spinal segments, causes aberrant neural impulses to the kidneys."

Nelson, in the 1951 yearbook of the Academy of Applied Osteopathy, found that "pyelonephritis, in concomitant urethral spasm and structure, has its spinal lesion counterparts at the level of the fourth and fifth lumbar segments, with emphasis on the fourth."

These all are different sites than had been discussed in the previous topic of nephrolithiasis. It emphasizes the fact that structural diagnosis must be all-inclusive and osteopathic manipulative treatment must be applied to try to resolve all structural abnormal findings.

## Case One

A 38-year-old man was seen in the emergency room of the local hospital. He had called at four o'clock that morning with the symptom of severe pain in the right side of his back. The pain awakened him from his sleep at three o'clock in the morning and had been gradually worsening. He was told to proceed to the emergency room. At that time he noted that his pain was still very severe and seemed to have traveled down into his right groin. In addition, he had urgency and dysuria, as well as some nausea. He denied any previous history of back pain or renal difficulties. He stated that he had given up smoking a year previously but did consume three to four cans of beer daily. His appetite was usually very good and he admitted to having gained approximately 25 pounds in the past few years. He had no food restrictions and noted that he was "a meat and potatoes guy."

Further questioning elicited a history of multiple joint pains of recent onset, with most of the discomfort in his left ankle and foot, especially his left big toe. He had taken an over-the-counter anti-inflammatory medication that gave him relief of the symptoms. His occupation was accounting and he was not restricted from physical activity and was able to perform all of his duties.

Physical examination revealed a well-developed, overweight male who was in obvious pain. Lloyd's sign was positive on the right. The ab-

dominal examination did not reveal any guarding, mass or organ enlargement. All other systems were found to be within normal limits. His temperature, orally, was 99 degrees.

A structural examination revealed severe hypertonicity of his right back, from his upper thoracic region down to his sacrum. In addition there was a somatic dysfunction present at T8–T9, and a reduction of cranial-sacral rhythm.

A urinalysis was performed and the microscopic examination was positive for erythrocytes and an acidic pH. A flat plate x-ray of the abdomen showed some gas in the large colon, but there was no evidence of renal calculi.

A tentative diagnosis of a right renal uric acid calculus was made. The patient was placed on intravenous fluids and parenteral analgesics. A CAT scan was performed, which showed a translucent calculus present in the lower right ureter close to its insertion into the urinary bladder. A serum uric acid was completed and was reported as above normal. His urine was continually monitored to note total output as well as to attempt to obtain the stone should it be passed.

The patient noted within the next four hours that his pain was completely alleviated. All analgesics were discontinued, but observation of his urine was maintained.

He received osteopathic manipulative treatment (OMT) to relieve the muscle hypertonicity, the somatic dysfunction, and to increase the cranial-sacral motion. In addition, he was given allopurinol and K-citrate to assist in reducing his uric acid as well as to create alkaline urine.

A few hours later a stone was recovered from his urine and was sent to the pathologist for further evaluation. It was later confirmed that it was a uric acid calculus.

The patient was discharged later that day and was instructed on his further care at home. He was placed on a low purine diet and was told to continue taking allopurinol and potassium citrate.

The patient returned to work within the next 48 hours and was next seen in the office 30 days later. At that time he had no symptoms. He had no urinary symptoms and his joint pains were no longer present. A repeat of his serum uric acid was reported as within normal values. He had lost 5 pounds and was maintaining his diet. The somatic findings were no longer present. He was told to continue on the present course of treatment and to return for further testing in 3 months time.

## Discussion

This patient presented with a very typical history and symptom complex for a uric acid calculus. This is a condition that usually occurs in males, and there usually is a familial history. In addition, his diet contributed to the condition. He was in some ways very fortunate that the urinary problem developed at an early stage in his development of gout. His maintenance of a proper diet and medication should prevent him from pathological changes developing that would have occurred in his joints, because the condition was diagnosed before the onset of bony changes with joint destruction.

He will have to continue on a restricted diet, medication, as well as making sure that his urine remains slightly alkaline.

T8–T9 somatic dysfunction is usually found with renal disease. It assists in the diagnosis of a renal problem and should be treated to assure that there is no negative autonomic feedback to the kidney from the soma and to relieve some of the somatic pain associated with the kidney stone.

## Case Two

A 66-year-old man was seen in the clinic with a chief symptom of nocturia. He was a patient at the clinic for the previous 5 years and was being seen for the management of his hypertensive vascular disease. He was being seen semi-annually and was under good control. He was taking a beta-adrenergic blocking agent, atenolol 50-mg. daily.

He had no history of angina, dyspnea, swelling of his ankles, or other indications of water retention. All of his past medical history was non-contributory. On further questioning, he noted that he had had nocturia over the past 3 years. He was awakened on the average of two times every night by the need to urinate. In the past 6 months, he noted that he was being awakened on the average of four to five times during a night. In addition, during the day, he had increased urgency and experienced the need to rush to the bathroom and then had trouble starting the flow. The strength of the flow was diminished and he "dribbled" out the balance of his urine. The entire process was taking much longer than had been necessary previously.

Physical examination revealed a slightly obese male, with no obvious deformities. His blood pressure was 128/78 mmHg; he had a regular sinus rhythm; no murmurs were noted. He chest sounds were clear. There were no abdominal masses or organomegaly noted. There was no evidence of swelling of his lower extremities.

A structural examination revealed somatic dysfunction present at T12–L1 and L1–L2. In addition, the cranial–sacral rhythm was diminished.

A rectal examination revealed that he had a slightly enlarged prostate gland that was mildly boggy to palpation. There were no nodules or firm masses palpable. In comparing these findings to previous years, it was noted that there was a small increase in size and bogginess.

A urinalysis was performed that was negative for any signs of infection, albumin, blood cells, or sediment. A PSA test was performed, and it was normal with no change from those performed in previous years. A routine blood chemistry profile showed an increase in his cholesterol level (200 mg/dL), with a low-density lipoprotein of 160 mg/dL and high-density lipoprotein of 45 mg/dL.

A diagnosis of benign prostatic hypertrophy was made, as well as obesity and hyperlipidemia. The patient was placed on a weight reduction regimen that included exercise. The urinary problem was fully discussed with the patient and it was agreed that he would start taking finasteride orally for at least the next 6 months and see if it had any effect on his condition. The use of other medications to reduce his immediate symptoms of urgency and nocturia was discussed as well, and it was agreed that should his symptoms worsen, then he would receive the necessary prescription.

He received OMT to relieve the dysfunctions that had been found, and he was told to return for further evaluation in 6 months. His lipid profile would be re-evaluated after the period of diet control.

## Discussion

The aforementioned describes a typical case of benign prostatic hypertrophy. The physician must be aware of the possibility of carcinoma of the prostate as well as the development of urinary retention. Either one of these conditions will require more intensive evaluation and possible surgical intervention. A large percentage of these patients will have their symptoms resolve with no therapy given at all. It is important to discuss the entire condition, as well as possible outcomes and all alternate approaches to therapy with the patient, because using a pharmaceutical agent, such as finasteride, can entail a lifetime commitment to the taking of the drug.

The finding of somatic dysfunction at the T12–L1 region is common in the presence of prostate disease. Dysfunctions of the pubic symphysis and congestion of the ischiorectal fossa should be explored. These should be treated to relieve or prevent discomfort in this area.

## Case Three

A 38-year-old woman was seen as an emergency patient in the clinic. She reported fever, chills, and pain in her back, as well as urinary frequency. This had developed over the previous 24 hours. She did not recall any previous incidents that were similar. Her past history was positive for multiple incidents of cystitis as a child and occasional bouts of dysuria and frequency of urination over the past 3 to 4 years. She had seen her physician for these and was placed on antibiotics for relief. She often medicated herself for these symptoms. She had no other major illnesses or surgery and had two pregnancies that were uneventful. She stated that her menstrual cycles were regular and that she did not take oral contraceptives.

Examination revealed a well-developed female in apparent distress. Her temperature, orally, was 101°F. Her pulse was 94 beats per minute; her respirations were normal. Her blood pressure was 110/75 mm Hg, and she had normal cardiac and breath sounds. Her abdomen was generally tender throughout without rigidity being present and she had pain on palpation of the right back at the costovertebral region. A structural examination revealed a somatic dys-

function at L3–L4, and a reduction of the normal cranial-sacral rhythm.

A sterile sample of urine was obtained and an immediate urinalysis was performed. It revealed, on microscopic examination, the presence of bacteria, red blood cells, and debris. There was no evidence of the presence of albumin or glucose. The urine was submitted to the laboratory for culture and sensitivity tests and blood was sent for complete blood count and blood chemistries.

A tentative diagnosis of pyelonephritis was made and the patient was sent home for bed rest. In addition, she was given a prescription for an antibiotic to be started at once. It was felt that E. coli caused the majority of these types of infections and the antibiotic was chosen to treat this organism, pending the results of the culture and sensitivity tests. She was to increase her fluid intake and told she could take acetaminophen as needed. She was to call within 24 hours and daily for 4 days to monitor her progress and was to return for a follow-up visit to the clinic in 1 week.

Daily improvement of all of her signs and symptoms was noted. The antibiotic, previously prescribed, was shown to be effective for the treatment of her infection, which was caused by E. coli as predicted.

When seen a week later, the patient felt well. She had no signs or symptoms, except for a general feeling of fatigue. Her microscopic urine examination no longer revealed bacteria or blood cells. The pain in her back was no longer present. The previously seen somatic dysfunctions had returned and were treated once more.

It was recommended that she continue on the antibiotic for the next week, when the culture would be repeated.

A discussion was had with the patient regarding her previous history of cystitis and her self-medication for it. It was explained that she had been using her medication improperly and not taking the drug until the infection had been completely resolved. This led to repeated incidents and the present condition, and could lead to her developing severe renal damage. She was instructed on the care that she had to take when wiping herself after defecation or urination. In addition, it was felt that once the urine culture was reported as negative, she should be placed on a long-term medication to maintain an aseptic urinary tract for at least 3 months.

## Discussion

This case is typical of pyelonephritis as seen by the primary care physician. The patient is usually female and has had a previous history of urinary tract infections. It is seen in patients who, as children, had multiple incidents of cystitis. In addition, patients are prone to self-medication, underusing the amount of the pharmaceutical needed to completely treat the infection. This leaves them prone to repeated infections and gradual development of renal pathology. Among factors to be aware of is the tendency for having multiple sexual partners with the development of chronic gynecologic infections of which they are not aware. If they are aware of the gynecologic infection, they often feel that the urinary condition is a symptom of vaginal infection and treat it locally, allowing the infection to ascend from a cystitis up the ureters and to the kidneys into pyelonephritis.

Somatic dysfunctions in the lower thoracic and upper lumbar regions are often found in association with renal and urological conditions. Pubic and other pelvic somatic dysfunctions may occur due to regional inflammation or as viscerosomatic reflexes. These need to be treated to relieve discomfort and to remove viscerosomatic and somatovisceral reflexes from creating cyclical feedback conditions.

### SELECTED READINGS

Cole WV. Somaticovisceral Reflexes. *J Am Osteopath Assoc* 1951;50:309–314

Cole WV. *Somaticovisceral Reflexes (Part two)*. The Cole Book. Newark, OH: American Academy of Osteopathy.

Frymann VM. *The Role of the Osteopathic Lesion in Functional and Organic Renal Pathology,* Year Book. Colorado Springs: Academy of Applied Osteopathy, 1950.

Hanno PM, Malkowicz SB, Wein AJ. *Clinical Manual of Urology,* third ed. New York: McGraw Hill, 2001.

Isselbacher KJ, Braunwald E, Wilson JD, et al. *Harrisons's Principles of Internal Medicine,* 13th ed. New York: McGraw-Hill, Inc, 1994.

Kuchera M, Kuchera WA. *Osteopathic Considerations in Systemic Dysfunction,* 2nd ed. Kirksville: Kirksville College of Osteopathic Medicine, 1994.

Nelson CR. *Structural Diagnosis and Treatment of Urological Problems.* Colorado Springs: Year Book, Academy of Applied Osteopathy, 1954.

Resnick MI, Novick AC. *Urology Secrets,* 3rd ed. Philadelphia: Hanley and Belfus, Inc, 2002.

Teichman JMH. *Urology.* New York: McGraw-Hill, 2000.

Warwick R, Williams PL. *Gray's Anatomy, 35th British ed.* Philadelphia: W.B. Saunders Company, 1973.

Zirul EE. *The Role of the Osteopathic Lesion in Functional and Organic Renal Pathology.* Colorado Springs: Year Book, Academy of Applied Osteopathy, 1950.

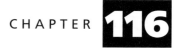

# Gynecologic Considerations

*Charles J. Smutny III, Mary E. Hitchcock, and Sonia Rivera-Martinez*

## ■ DYSMENORRHEA AND PREMENSTRUAL SYNDROME

Two of the most frequent ailments of females of reproductive age are dysmenorrhea and premenstrual syndrome. Dysmenorrhea can be subdivided into two distinct forms, primary and secondary. Although all three can be found in the same patient, premenstrual syndrome, primary dysmenorrhea, and secondary dysmenorrhea are often discussed separately.

## Definitions

1. **Primary dysmenorrhea (functional dysmenorrhea):** painful menses in the absence of discrete organic disease. (This is to be distinguished from premenstrual syndrome in that symptoms persist after the onset of menses or initiate earlier than 14 days before menses).
2. **Secondary dysmenorrhea (acquired dysmenorrhea):** painful menses associated with definable pathology.

   Pain is a highly subjective part of history taking. Alone, it is not sufficient to make a diagnosis. Symptoms must alter the patient's activities of daily living (ADL) and persist for more than several hours. The symptoms may last as long as several days in acute situations. In the case of secondary dysmenorrhea, weeks to months may pass with major ADL changes before the patient seeks attention.

3. Premenstrual syndrome (PMS): an interrelated constellation of physical, metabolic, hormonal, and psychological imbalances, variable in nature, and beginning an average of 7 to 10 days (with a range of 2 to 14 days) before menses. Symptoms include headache, bloating or abdominal swelling, irritability, tiredness, and food cravings such as sweets and/or salt. Hormonal imbalances may predispose a woman to anxiety, depression, and even open hostility. Symptom complexes often potentiate mood swings. Symptoms and imbalances decrease rapidly with the onset of menses.

(All three entities may be associated with vasovagal effects and their associated nausea.)

a. **Premenstrual dysphoric disorder (PMDD):** a severe form of PMS. The symptoms of PMDD are similar to those of PMS but are severe enough to interfere with work, social activities, and relationships.

Dysmenorrhea and PMS tend to be diagnoses made in women in their teens and twenties.

Thinking osteopathically requires a clear understanding of normal and pathological anatomy and physiology (structure and function) and educated hands with palpatory experience. Combined with the knowledge of a range of osteopathic techniques for both diagnosis and treatment, one can separate these three entities and treat them efficiently and cost-effectively.

## Premenstrual Syndrome (PMS)

The cause of PMS is complex and not well understood. Some theories propose progesterone deficiency, endogenous opiate peptide excess, or pyridoxine deficiency as potential causes. Blood serum studies clearly show that there are some transported elements that can trigger symptoms. Decreased calcium and magnesium have been clearly shown to increase the severity of PMS. Borderline thyroid function with thyroid stimulating hormone in the middle to high range and active T-3 in the low normal to below normal range have been associated with increased PMS symptoms. Inappropriate production of follicle-stimulating hormone and/or luteinizing hormone has also been associated with increased symptoms. Balancing estrogens and progesterones has further indicated that hormones play a significant role in PMS. Prostaglandins and arachidonic acid rank highly in the suspected pain causing agents secondary to their known characteristics of influencing the release of substance P. Studies of a variety of pharmacologic agents used to treat PMS show as high as 30% to 40% of patients responding to placebo. The placebo side of the equation is very poorly studied, although there may be much to be gained by a thorough investigation of placebo. This is evidenced by the substantial amount of money dedicated to the study of placebo by the National Institutes of Health (NIH).

The preponderance of inconclusive studies has led some practitioners to ascribe a psychological diagnosis to PMS without giving consideration to other factors. The psychological aspects of the patient are more clearly understood when looking at the psyche's impact on the limbic system. This is especially so when considering how well placebos have worked in some studies. Treatment of limbic system influences is more clearly defined in the psychiatric literature with respect to the anxiety and depression symptoms that are commonly associated with PMS.

From the perspective of hormonal influences on brain and systemic function via the influence on all three legs of the neuroendocrine immune system, alterations in somatic function become more easily understood. This relationship is best expressed via the autonomic systems structural influence and can be detected as increases in muscle tone, diaphoresis, hypervigilance, hyperesthesia, increased heart rate, and the increased frequency and severity of mood swings (up-regulated sympathetic drive).

Somatic dysfunctions that are commonly associated with PMS and dysmenorrhea include organ-specific segmental dysfunctions from T10 through L2 in the sympathetic distribution to the primary organs of reproduction, occipital atlantal junction dysfunction, and C2 dysfunction influenced by the sympathetic facilitation of the superior cervical chain ganglia. C2 is also associated with parasympathetic influence from the vagus nuclei, further impacting on cervical and visceral muscle tone. The sacral and pelvic region has direct influence from inflammation and muscle spasm in the pelvic bowl and may show parasympathetic response in the hypogastric plexus secondary to the influence of sacral restrictions and lymphatic retention.

## Dysmenorrhea

*Primary dysmenorrhea* is a diagnosis by exclusion that may be considered after secondary dysmenorrhea has been effectively ruled out. The physiology of menses and the mechanism of uterine contracture, in particular, are significant in understanding primary dysmenorrhea. Physical deconditioning and gravitational strain can constitute a formidable problem for many women, especially when they are postpartum. This can negatively influence the essential function of contraction for the expulsion of endometrial products as well as increased ligamentous strain. Both processes can produce significant pain.

Pain secondary to endometrial product retention is largely regulated by the hormonally controlled production of specific prostaglandins (PGs). The PGs are produced as a result of the disintegration of the endometrial lining and subsequent breakdown of the cellular fats into arachidonic acid byproducts. The frequency and severity of subsequent cramping is increased in direct proportion to the concentration of PG and/or the pooling of natural fluids during menses. This triggers a severe contracture of the uterine musculature and increases potential for ischemia secondary to the muscle contracture. A common descriptor for this type of pain is "it feels like I am in labor." This pain may be localized to the abdomen or extend into the back and the thighs and may last from hours to days. It most commonly presents as an annoyance, but at its worst, it has the potential to be totally incapacitating. Since the symptoms are often the result of prostaglandin influence, and the drugs of choice have become nonsteroidal anti-inflammatories (NSAIDs) because of their mechanism of action as prostaglandin inhibitors.

*Secondary dysmenorrhea* includes pathology such as, but not limited to, endometriosis, entrapped or irritating intrauterine devices, uterine polyps, fibroids (especially submucous fibroids, which may cause ball valve effects or fluid pooling of breakdown products), anovulatory menorrhagia, pelvic congestion syndrome (associated with a retroverted uterus, venous stasis, and lymphatic stasis), strictures, pelvic inflammatory disease, ovarian cysts, adenomyosis, hydrosalpinx, ectopic pregnancy (a surgical emergency), and retention of endometrial fragments that act as foreign bodies. An anteroflexed uterus, hyperplasia or fibrosis, and estrogen-progesterone imbalances may play significant roles. Poor physical conditioning, multiparous uterus, and/or weakness or damage to the suspensory ligaments must also be considered as potential factors.

Practiced palpatory skills applied to physical diagnosis and a good history combined with appropriately selected diagnostic laboratory and radiologic examinations should separate secondary dysmenorrhea from both primary dysmenorrhea and PMS.

## Treatment

Osteopathic treatment can begin with the initial physical examination and should include treatment of the primary somatic dysfunctions. Treatment of the uterus and pelvic floor during bimanual examination is most appropriate.

Treatment should include the upper thoracic and upper cervical regions especially when sympathetic tone is elevated. This can have an influence on the adenohypophysis output via the sympathetic fibers branching off from the carotid complex following the blood supply to the secretory structures. It may also decrease fluid retention in the upper thoracic region, increase lymphatic drainage both locally and systemically, and may reduce breast tenderness commonly associated with dysmenorrhea. Additional treatment of the thoracic and pelvic diaphragm along with segmental dysfunctions of the thoracolumbar junction and sacral pelvic regions can further enhance resolution or remediation of the physical expression of these conditions. Increasing range of motion in all these areas reduces venous and lymphatic stasis that is a known contributor to increased pain.

Lymphatic techniques completed after segmental and localized somatic dysfunction correction, reinitiates normal lymphatic flow. This can reduce the degree of water retention commonly associated with PMS and dysmenorrhea.

Treatment techniques should be chosen according to the tissue responses at each area. Effort should be made to use indirect treatments when possible to reduce the chance of the upregulating nociceptive (painful) stimulation. Counterstrain and facilitated positional release are uniquely apropos in this patient population because they tend to reduce pain rapidly. In addition, they can be readily taught to the patient for self-administration.

A simple yet helpful technique is the use of inhibitory pressure on the sacrum to quiet uterine contractions. The patient is prone as the physician maintains a deep, steady pressure on the sacrum until the contractions cease (Fig. 116-1). At home, the patient may perform a similar maneuver by using a book to create the pressure as she lies supine with the book under the sacrum (Fig. 116-2). Flexing the knees while in this position increases the pressure on the sacrum (Fig. 116-3).

A similar technique may be used anteriorly, applying the pressure over the symphysis pubis (Fig. 116-4).

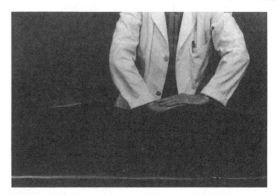

■ **FIG. 116-1** Sacral pressure for the relief of dysmenorrhea.

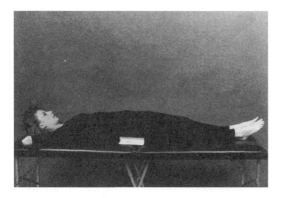

**■ FIG. 116-2** Self-treatment by sacral pressure using a book.

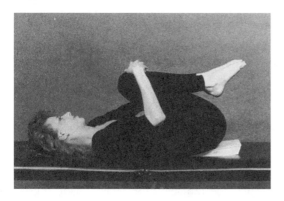

**■ FIG. 116-3** Increasing sacral pressure by flexing legs on trunk.

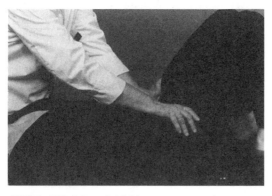

**■ FIG. 116-4** Deep inhibiting pressure on tissues overlying the pubic symphysis.

Failure of the patient to respond to treatment is a strong indicator for potential visceral disease as the underlying cause. This would warrant further examination and special diagnostic testing.

The standard of care in evaluation and treatment of these patients must include nutritional, electrolyte, hormone, and structural considerations that should be properly balanced, while social and family history, familial support structures, and secondary gain issues should be investigated. Nutritional supplements, replacement hormone therapy, and surgical interventions should be considered as a matter of course in an appropriate sequence dictated by standard of care.

Medications including serotonin reuptake inhibitors have been shown to be helpful and should be considered in patients that are resistant or not responsive to osteopathic treatment. Adjunctive therapy combining medication and osteopathic manipulative techniques is often more effective in severe cases than either is independently. Use of outside resources including support groups, social services, and psychological interventions may also need to be considered.

## ■ CASE 1

S.S. was a 28-year-old woman who was first evaluated for symptoms of abdominal pain, bloating, mood changes, and headaches associated with the impending onset of menses within 2 to 3 days before the start of her flow. Pain eased within 1 to 2 days after the onset of menses. Visual analogue scale of pain is variable from three to seven out of ten during this part of her cycle. Some cycles were described as worse than others. Pain scales less then five out of ten represent days when she was not capable of going to work or completing activities of daily living at home beyond toileting and bathing. She had an established history of premenstrual syndrome by diagnosis since age 15. She has seen her physician regularly twice per year and has had negative Pap smears yearly since the onset of sexual activity at age 21. The onset of menses was at age 12. She has had a regular cycle of 28 to 29 days, followed by a period of 3 to 5 days of flow that regularly had a heavy onset (seven to nine heavy-duty pads per day) lasting 1 to 2 days and a slow tapering decrease. She has had four sexual partners in her lifetime and denied ever having had a sexually transmitted disease. She had never been pregnant. She stated that she had "always used barrier contraception and had never, ever been without protection." She knew that her period was about to begin within a few days after the onset of headache, followed in 24 hours by the onset of abdominal cramping, bloating, and mood swings that range from crying to anger. She was reluctant to use oral contraceptives secondary to a family history of breast cancer. She has used multiple analgesics, nonsteroidal anti-inflammatories, opioid narcotics, and herbal remedies for pain control without significant success. She also stated that she did not like to use medication in general.

Socially, she never imbibed alcohol or smoked anything. Her family history included breast cancer in her mother and her older sister. Both sustained multiple "lumpectomies" and the mother had had a single modified radical mastectomy on the right. Both were without persistent sequela for more than 5 years. Both mother and sister had experienced significant problems with premenstrual syndrome

She had arrived 2 days after the most recent headache began and was weepy. She was approaching her calendar date for the onset of menses in 2 days. Her abdomen was visibly distended. Evaluation of the head, eyes, ears, nose throat, chest, and heart was normal. The abdomen was soft and tender in the left and right lower quadrants in the suprapubic region. There was a mild increase in temperature medial to the right ASIS. There was edematous accumulation of fluids in the inferior aspect of the small panniculus with widespread edema in the four extremities easily noted. There was mild to moderate pitting in the pretibial region down over the dorsum of the foot bilaterally.

The occipital atlantal junction was restricted in flexion and extension but symmetric and side-bending in rotation. There was tenderness along the superior nuchal line bilaterally. There was a mild thoracic and lumbar flattening with a decreased excursion of the diaphragm and rib structures on inhalation. The left first rib was restricted with the rib in the elevated position. The thoracolumbar junction was tender to palpation in the midline and bilaterally across the

surfaces of the erector spinae, paraspinals, and quadratus lumborum muscles. There were anterior tender points in the L1, L2, and L3 distributions with the right greater than the left. Sacral motion was restricted both in inhalation and exhalation. Seated flexion was positive on the right with a negative spring test, right sacral base anterior, and left inferior lateral angle posterior and superior. L5 was rotated to the right. There was a minor restriction in hip extension bilaterally with the right greater than the left during gait. Speculum examination was within normal limits and the bimanual examination did not identify any masses. The pelvic floor was elevated and demonstrated poor excursion with respiration. The right ovary was more tender to touch than the left. The uterus appeared normal in contour and texture.

During pelvic bimanual examination the pelvic floor was treated with respiratory assisted muscle energy bilaterally. Occipital atlantal decompression was used to decrease cervicogenic headache muscle tension and to rebalance sympathetic and parasympathetic tone. Facilitated positional release to the first rib on the left was followed by rib-raising bilaterally and redoming the diaphragm. The purpose of this set of procedures was to increase potential for drainage through the thoracic duct of lymphatic fluids and to improve the excursion of the diaphragm which pumps that fluid. This was followed by counterstrain to the anterior tender points sequentially from L1 through L3. The patient then rolled to the prone position and respiratory-assisted muscle energy was applied to the sacrum to restore symmetrical motion during respiration. Soft tissue and myofascial release was used in the thoracolumbar region and the patient was returned to the supine position. Bilateral pedal pump was administered to initiate movement of lymphatic fluid into the now-open lymphatic channels, with both the pelvic and abdominal diaphragms assisting in the movement of fluid with respiration.

On reassessment, somatic dysfunctions and tenderness had been reduced, rotations normalized, and range of motion had become more symmetric during gait. She stated that her headache had resolved. She showed mood improvement with a smile on her face and an appropriate sense of humor.

She was instructed on how to self-administer a counterstrain treatment and a standing bilateral pedal pump. She was asked to return in 4 days, or sooner if the pain returns, for follow-up treatment and to review her self-treatment program.

## Discussion

The sequence of somatic dysfunctions that were treated is significant in that the osteopathic thought process should include an attempt to restore normal function on a systemic basis as well as treating the local area of dysfunctions (treat the whole patient). With edema in all four extremities, lymphatic techniques become more prominent in the treatment plan. The headache symptom associated with increased cervicocranial junction muscle tone is indicative of an increase of sympathetic tone, probably secondary to nociceptive (pain) input. Balanced ligamentous tension, counterstrain, and cranial techniques are indirect techniques that can achieve reductions in muscle tone and reduce facilitation in the nervous system restoring a more normal balance.

Restoring sacral function and pelvic diaphragmatic motion is central to the movement of localized lymphatic fluid from the pelvic bowl up into the abdominal cavity. There, the lymphatic fluids and debris can be moved via visceral peristaltic movements and diaphragmatic excursion through the cysterna chyle into the thoracic duct and upward toward the left subclavian vein for return to the intravascular space. Movement of the accumulated interstitial fluids into the terminal lymphatic ducts using a pedal pump initiates fluid movement into a now open system that had facilitated to maintain normal function. This reduces the accumulation of proteinaceous fluids in the pelvis and the subsequent accumulation of substance P and other pain-generating chemicals. Using osteopathic techniques with an understanding of normal physiologic function as a background, the practitioner can address physiologic dysfunctions via the direct influence of the somatic system on the physiologic environment.

## ■ OSTEOPATHIC CONSIDERATIONS IN THE OBSTETRIC PATIENT

Osteopathic care throughout pregnancy provides a woman with the special benefit of adjusting the functions of her body to the demands of a progressing pregnancy. Seemingly minor problems, especially those involving the back, may be the beginning of a lifetime of musculoskeletal difficulties. Childbearing women without other clear traumatic or visceral causes of back pain can often trace part of their own history to a difficult labor and/or postpartum onset.

An exercise program begun in the early prenatal period, or, ideally, before conception, may strongly reduce the potential for developing low back dysfunctions. If manipulation and an exercise regimen are developed and continued postpartum, the patient may return to normal function much more rapidly.

In a discussion of obstetric back pain, the pelvis may serve as a starting point. It is the foundation on which the entire spinal column is balanced. Forward tilting of the pelvis occurs during pregnancy, with a resulting increased lumbar lordosis as a counterbalance. Often this increase in spinal curves may extend as far as the cranial base and may induce cranio-sacral strains. This may lead to acute and, if uncorrected, chronic backache and a host of other symptoms. Lordosis is commonly more marked in women than in men. Obesity and/or a growing fetus compound the stresses, exaggerating the curve (Fig. 116-5). Alterations in posture shift the stresses from their normally ligamentous and disk-oriented balance to a strenuous muscle-controlled balance. As the pregnancy continues to develop, distension of the abdomen further reduces the muscular capacity to counterbalance. This is a living example of the physiological principle of the length–tension relationship in which muscles can be stretched beyond their capacity to contract efficiently.

Anatomically, the body is designed to resist gravity through one primary and two subsidiary centers of transition (Fig, 116-6). These transition zones at the C7–T1, T12–L1, and L5–S1 junctions serve as fulcrums for the transmission of force upward and downward through the column. They serve as balance points for the ante-

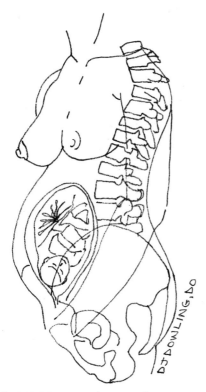

■ **FIG. 116-5** Pregnancy increases the curvature of the spine, especially the lumbar lordosis.

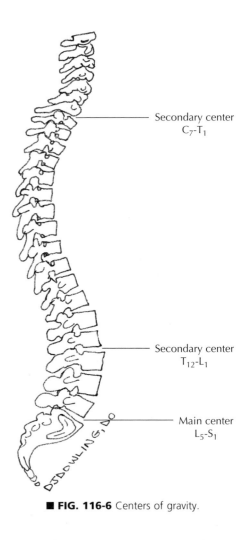

■ **FIG. 116-6** Centers of gravity.

rior–posterior (A-P) curve and may serve as proprioceptive references to the longitudinal center of gravity. The compound functions at these points subject them to higher stresses than at other spinal areas. This adaptation is to human advantage, however, because this arrangement can resist ten times that of a straight column. With an engineer's eye, the spinal column can be viewed as the mast of a ship with a series of muscular and ligamentous stays placed for balance and control through a range of motion. A good example is the trapezius and its wedge-shaped form from spinous process to scapular spine. A-P curve changes in the column result in an increase of the thoracic A-P diameter and transverse diameter and a shortening of the longitudinal axis. This reduces the efficiency of the "stay and mast" system.

The iliopsoas muscle is often considered the "mainstay" in the column support system. It therefore has the potential for a significant role in the back pain of pregnancy and in back pain

in general. Crossing the critical area of the L5–S1 junction, it can help distribute forces from the large range of motion above through to the relatively limited movement of the sacrum. Equally important is its capacity to help distribute forces from below upward. Its origins at the inferior borders of the transverse processes of L1–L5, the anterolateral surfaces of the vertebral bodies of T12–L5, and the intervertebral disks between them give this muscle a unique range of functions similar in some respects to the sternocleidomastoid. As a result, its structure and function require complex innervation, great recruitment capacity, and significant power capacity. The iliopsoas may be involved in respiratory function as an anchoring mechanism for the crura of the diaphragm. It is involved in the stabilization of the lumbar spine in standing, sitting, and loco-motion. It supports the viscera and forms a major part of the posterior and lateral bowl of the faux pelvis. It may also support the growing fetus, keeping the body of the uterus in the faux pelvis and the abdomen until descent at term begins.

One key may be in understanding the iliop-soas' role in nutation and counternutation (phys-iologic A-P rocking of the sacrum). The psoas muscle acts as a prime mover of the lumbosacral junction and may strongly influence sacral me-chanics. This becomes focal in studying the me-chanics of gait, respiration, and the sequence of engagement, flexion, descent, and internal rota-tion of the fetus. The muscularly controlled counternutation of delivery is assisted by proges-terone and relaxin, which induces ligamentous laxity. This facilitates the opening of the true pelvic inlet, which must occur for engagement to begin.

During delivery, the hip, pelvic, and abdomi-nal musculature undergoes maximum physical strain, with resulting stress on the back and the pelvic and sacroiliac ligaments. The lithotomy position further exacerbates stress because grav-ity cannot assist in the process (as opposed to squatting which is the most natural position).

The sympathetic innervation to the female pelvic structures is derived from nerves at the spinal levels of T10–T12 and L1–L2. Nocicep-tive fibers also follow these tracts and share in-terneurons with musculoskeletal nociceptive fibers at the same levels. Parasympathetic: inner-vation arises from S2–S4 through the pelvic splanchnic nerve (Fig. 116-7). Changes in A-P curves can facilitate segments and lower pain thresholds. This information becomes more use-ful diagnostically when one is attempting to sep-arate out other visceral problems that may occur during pregnancy. As the curves progress, there may be an increase in the tortuosity of viscera as they traverse the pelvic brim. This may lead to compression of some of the structures that are normally suspended freely. The mass and size of the uterus and the fetus may further com-

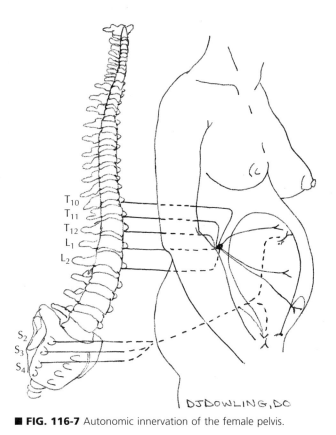

■ **FIG. 116-7** Autonomic innervation of the female pelvis.

pound these restrictions. Respiratory and circulatory function may be altered leading to commonly found constipation, edema, and backache. Urinary frequency, susceptibility to infection, leg cramps, varicosities, acrodyesthesia (tingling and numbness of the hands), breast soreness, and joint pains are also common complaints. Each of these has structural strain as a component to be considered.

Although lumbar and sacral backaches are the most common musculoskeletal symptoms of pregnancy, symptoms from the apex of the skull to the plantar surface of the feet may frequently be encountered. Secondary to large postural changes, muscle fatigue and discomfort initiate many symptoms. Increasing breast mass may exaggerate this. Rib dysfunctions and thoracic and cervical pain may increase in frequency and duration. Muscle tension headache may occur more frequently as these dysfunctions accumulate. Postural changes may alter the weight-bearing distribution of the seated patient toward the coccyx, predisposing to coccygodynia. These manifestations might herald subsequent hypertension, edema, altered glucose balance, preeclampsia, and other symptoms that define a pregnancy in difficulty. Non-osteopathic medicine relies upon frequent checkups for early intervention, nutritional supplements, and dietary advice as the tools to prevent these conditions. Their true battle with these entities only begins once they have occurred. Medications may appear to be the only avenue for holding the symptoms at bay until delivery or termination.

The osteopathic approach provides greater opportunity for treatment, quite literally at the practitioner's fingertips. "Traditionally, osteopathic manipulative management of the obstetric patient has been limited to soft tissue relaxation especially to the lumbar region and, occasionally, to making corrections of the isolated somatic dysfunctions" (Zink, 1977). This is often effective in improving the comfort of the patient but does not directly address: (1) gravitational strains; (2) optimization of external or pulmonary respiration; or (3) facilitation of drainage of the venous and lymphatic systems. It certainly does not address optimization of the primary respiratory mechanism.

To treat the patient as a unit, the osteopathic physician must consider the neurologic model,

the respiratory–circulatory model, the energy model, the fluid model, and osteopathy in the cranial field in an integrated manner. It may also be important to consider other models of function. The key is to integrate the information into the understanding of the patient as a unique, interrelated unit of function.

Osteopathic medicine utilizes observation, palpation, motion testing, and special testing as a matter of course. These skills may take on refined meaning here. Alterations in normal respiratory mechanics can often yield signs of other problems beginning. The mechanics of pulmonary respiration is often a good place to begin the diagnostic and therapeutic process of assisting the patient back toward health.

Normal breathing is dependent, both anatomically and physiologically, on a level pelvis and a straight spine (in which the movement of all segments is unhindered). This allows the thoracic cage, which is suspended from the spine, to function properly, thereby ensuring maximum external respiration. When proper external respiration occurs, there is an effective negative pressure in the thorax that guarantees the continuous return of blood from the central nervous system. This, in turn, allows the cerebrospinal fluid to move more freely. At the same time, an effective negative pressure in the thorax draws the venous blood from the rest of the body as well as promoting terminal lymphatic drainage (Zink, 1977).

Tettambel stated:

> A well-tuned engine or balanced musculoskeletal system is capable of good performance. It's prepared to accommodate the traveling fetus by regulating its own contractions and assisting the muscles to cooperate with the flexion, extension, and rotations of the fetal skull . . . . By maintaining the body fluid homeostasis and re-evaluating the ever changing pregnant posture and gait, the obstetrician helps the kidneys to maintain their efficiency and regulate their filtration system and the heart to maintain a healthy beat, keeping the pumping station running without being on overload. Therefore, edema and late breaking preeclampsia may be kept at bay.

Treatment programs must be designed to address all of these issues, from prenatal planning and treatment to postpartum follow-up. It must be emphasized that the treatment protocol will evolve from a good medical, surgical, gynecological, social, nutritional, psychological, and trauma history combined with a thorough diag-

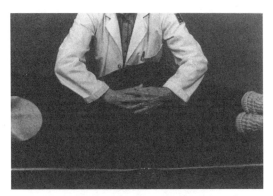

■ **FIG. 116-8** Sacral rocking on obstetric patient.

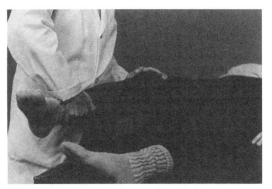

■ **FIG. 116-10** Adduction, internal rotation, and extension of the hips.

nostic and structural examination. This will elucidate a fair portion of the balances and imbalances as they affect the intricate workings of the patient's inherent mechanisms.

Some additional treatment techniques and exercises included here may add to the battery of tools to assist the patient in seeking and maintaining a healthy pregnancy and delivery. Still stated:

> The knee chest position will place the abdomen in the proper form for unloading the pelvis and any impacted condition. Then place the hands low down on the abdomen and draw the contents of the pelvis forward toward the umbilicus and up from the pelvis, to give free passage of blood and other fluids circulating in the lower part of the abdomen.

Sacral rocking may be used to release sacral restrictions, both before delivery and during early delivery (Fig. 116-8). After delivery, the woman's legs are removed from the stirrups and her hips are put through adduction and internal rotation while still flexed, followed by extension (Figs. 116-9 and 116-10). This reduces the po-

tential for sacroiliac dysfunction, which may result from the increased elasticity of pelvic ligaments combined with the intense ligamentous strain of delivery.

In breech presentations, an external cephalic version may be attempted. This has a success rate as high as 75%. The major risk of this procedure is abruptio placentae. Risk of occurrence is greatly increased with the presence of placenta previa and only somewhat increased with leiomyoma. It may be prudent to attempt this with delicate hands and gentle forces over a period of time because heavy handedness may result in a different outcome (cesarean section).

Manipulation may also be used immediately postpartum and minimally as early as 4 or 5 hours after a cesarean section, and then up to three times per day, to alleviate hyperextension of the lumbar spine.

Within minutes to a few hours after delivery, simple in-bed exercises may begin. The patient may be instructed to approximate the scapulae while sitting (Fig. 116-11). This encourages motion of the chest and shoulder girdle and may reduce some of the muscular stress accumulated during delivery. Within hours on the same day, the woman may lie in bed with her knees bent and raise the buttocks approximately an inch. By pressing the lumbar area against the bed, she can tilt the pelvis (Fig. 116-12). This may begin the abdominal and low back rehabilitation process. Walking, even for short distances, should be encouraged early.

As tolerated, she may stand with legs apart about shoulder width and twist the trunk from right to left and back slowly (Fig. 116-13). Em-

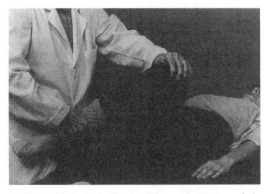

■ **FIG. 116-9** Adduction and internal rotation of the hips.

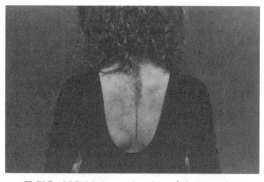

■ **FIG. 116-11** Approximation of the scapulae.

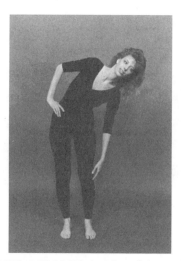

■ **FIG. 116-14** Side-bending of the trunk.

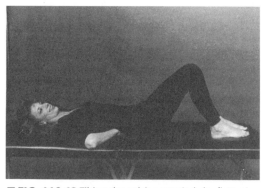

■ **FIG. 116-12** Tilting the pelvis posteriorly by flattening the lumbar lordosis.

phasis should be placed on slow motion and maximal range of motion without incurring pain. There is no place for a "no pain, no gain" mentality. In the same position, she may bend the trunk sideways and forward (Figs. 116-14 and 116-15). This may help strengthen and stretch both internal and external obliques, restoring more normal abdominal muscle function. The woman may continue adding exercises as tolerated.

When possible, to lying on the floor with her legs straight and arms out to the sides, the patients reaches with one knee to the opposite arm,

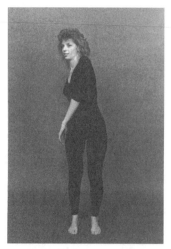

■ **FIG. 116-13** Trunk twists.

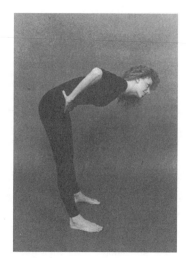

■ **FIG. 116-15** Forward bending of the trunk.

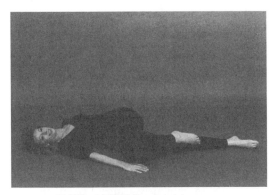

**■ FIG. 116-16** Trunk twists prone.

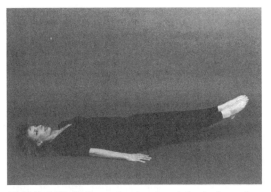

**■ FIG. 116-18** Strengthening the abdominal muscles.

returns, and does the same with the other arm and knee (Fig. 116-16).

When the iliopsoas is severely contracted, a stretching exercise is suggested. While standing, the unaffected leg is placed at a height of 2 to 2.5 feet from the floor, on a chair or stool. The affected leg is stretched approximately 3 feet behind in an anterior rotation position. With continuous gentle stretch, the foot of the affected leg is gradually rotated internally. The woman then applies pressure over the buttock on the affected side, adding full body weight to the stretch at the level of the compromised hip (Fig. 116-17).

A passive stretch may be accomplished by lying supine on a rolled-up towel that has been placed at the thoracolumbar junction. This should relieve some of the flexion stress accumulated during the day. Leg-raising with the legs not more than 6 inches from the floor will strengthen abdominal muscles (Fig. 116-18). If the legs are raised higher than this, the psoas muscle becomes involved in flexion, which is not desirable in some low back problems.

All exercises should be repeated ten times without pain. Mild to moderate discomfort is to be expected. Patients should strive to work up to ten repetitions and then, as tolerated, work toward exercising two to three times per day. Gentle passive stretching should follow each exercise period. Moving on to more strenuous aerobic and anaerobic exercises gradually may speed the return toward normal with reduced risk of injury. High-impact aerobics may cause more trouble than good because of increased risk of injury.

Studies by Myers, Muller-Tyl and Wimmer-Puchinger, Ringrose, and Copper each point out that psychological stress and emotional turmoil may manifest themselves via the hypothalamic–autonomic axis as the physical phenomena of obstetric complications.

### Contraindications to Manipulation Are of Great Importance

1. *Stimulatory treatments should not be used during premature labor.* Stimulation of spinal nerves may be sufficient to promote a labor that might otherwise have been halted by complete rest.
2. *Stimulatory treatment should not be used in the presence of abruptio placentae.* Abruption is

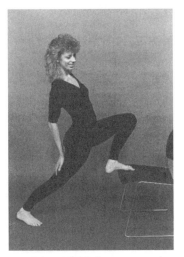

**■ FIG. 116-17** Iliopsoas stretch.

considered a medical urgency or emergency and may require an emergency cesarean section. Abruptio placentae occurs after the twentieth week of gestation and most commonly in the last ten weeks of pregnancy. Any detachment earlier in pregnancy is regarded as spontaneous abortion. Where symptoms of shock or changes in fetal activity and heart sounds occur, placenta previa should be suspected.

3. *Treat with extreme caution if membranes rupture without labor.* Without amniotic fluid protection, the fetus is more vulnerable to outside trauma. External cephalic version is more difficult in the absence of amniotic fluid. The use of fetal movements in response to gentle sustained pressure may be effective but may take time.

4. *Treatment should be avoided in cases of an incompetent cervix.* There is a higher incidence of premature labor, spontaneous abortion, and oligohydramnios.

5. *Eclampsia requires rapid medical treatment.* The malignant hypertension and seizures require protect measures and probably rapid delivery.

6. *An ectopic pregnancy requires emergent surgery.*

The list of absolute contraindications is short, itself giving some hint to the extensive applications of osteopathic philosophy and practice to the obstetric patient. "Osteopathic obstetrics can be a reality. Integration of structure, function, and palpatory skills can expand the diagnostic acumen that cannot be appreciated through technology or textbook" (Tettambel, 1997).

### ■ CASE TWO

This case reports on the use of osteopathic manipulation as an alternative to vacuum-assisted delivery.

X.R. is a 36-year-old Hispanic female gravida 1 para 0. Mrs. R. presented at 39 weeks with symptoms of spontaneous rupture of membranes, contractions every 3 to 4 minutes, and mid to low back muscular pain. She reported active fetal movements and sparse vaginal bleeding. During this pregnancy, she had no complications and gained 32 pounds. Mrs. R. had no significant medical history and her only medication was prenatal vitamins.

On admission her vital signs were stable. Fetal heart rate was 150 beats per minute and reactive. Uterine contractions were irregular. The estimated fetal weight was 3,500 grams. Pelvic examination found no active bleeding and no external lesions. The cervix was dilated 7 cm, 80% effaced, station was−1, with a right occiput anterior vertex presentation, and tested positive for spontaneous rupture of membranes.

Because this patient was in active labor, the focus of the osteopathic structural examination was on the sacrum, pelvis, lumbosacral junction, and lumbar spine. Notable on the osteopathic examination were the restriction of the psoas and sacroiliac joint bilaterally.

Mrs. R. was admitted to labor and delivery and a normal spontaneous vaginal delivery was anticipated. Her first stage of labor was uneventful. She refused epidural anesthesia and reached full dilatation 4 hours after admission. During this phase of labor, her muscular back pain was treated with gentle myofascial stretching techniques. In general, obstetric patients in active labor tolerate these types of soft tissue techniques. However, as labor pain intensifies, patients may be unable to bear any manipulative treatment. This patient expressed relief of her muscular back pain but was unable to endure treatment of the sacrum and iliopsoas because of labor pain.

After 2.5 hours of strenuous bearing down throughout the second stage of labor, her expulsive efforts became poor because of fatigue. Mrs. R. was taken to an operating room to assist the delivery with vacuum extraction.

Considering the osteopathic structural findings in this case, the risks involved with vacuum extraction, the patient's wishes for a natural birth, and the absence of fetal distress at the time, consent was obtained for a trial with osteopathic manipulation before attempting delivery with the assistance of a vacuum extractor.

The osteopathic treatment selected for this patient was balanced ligamentous tension technique to the sacrum, inhibition of the psoas muscle, pelvic diaphragm release, and lateral spread of the vaginal walls.

Osteopathic treatment was successful. Baby R. was delivered without the assistance of the vacuum extractor. Her APGAR scores were 9 after 1 and 5 minutes. Furthermore, Mrs. R. did not sustain any tearing and/or lacerations of the cervical or vaginal tissues during delivery. Mother and infant were discharged 24 hours after delivery in stable condition.

## Discussion

As demonstrated in this case, the tension of the iliopsoas and restrictions found at the sacroiliac articulations may impede descent of the fetal head. Prolongation of this stage may very well result in maternal fatigue and the inability to deliver the child by usual means. If normal vaginal delivery is unfeasible, assistance with instrumentation, such as forceps or a vacuum extractor, may be attempted. The indications for vacuum assisted delivery include maternal exhaustion and inadequate expulsive efforts. Suction forces used with vacuum extraction range from 12 to 18 pounds per square inch. Further, vacuum extraction carries a risk of complication three times greater than normal vaginal delivery.

Dr. Melicien Tettambel states that restriction of sacral motion may interfere with rotation of the head, which could lead to cessation of fetal descent .This was the case with Mrs. R. Her sacrum was locked in counternutation, hindering further fetal descent. The physiologic motions of the sacroiliac joint during fetal descent are counternutation and nutation. In counternutation the sacral base moves posteriorly and the apex moves anteriorly. The iliac crests are separated and the ischial tuberosities move together. These motions result in widening of the pelvic inlet and narrowing of the pelvic outlet. The motions occurring with nutation are opposite to those of counternutation and result in widening of the pelvic outlet. Counternutation of the sacrum must occur for entry of the fetus into the true pelvis and for engagement to begin. Sacroiliac nutation assists fetal descent through the pelvic outlet .Throughout pregnancy the iliopsoas supports and maintains the fetus in the false pelvis. Relaxation of the psoas muscle permits fetal engagement in the true pelvis. Release of the pelvic diaphragm and lateral spread of the vaginal walls relax the superficial and deep muscles of the pelvic floor, thus aiding in final descent.

As seen in this case, osteopathic manipulation may be a useful treatment modality to assist normal vaginal delivery before using forceps or a vacuum extractor, thus potentially preventing complications to mother, child, or both.

### REFERENCES

Buster JE. Dysmenorrhea and premenstrual syndrome. In: Hacker N, Moore JC, eds. *Essentials of Obstetrics and Gynecology.* Philadelphia: W.B. Saunders, 1986.

Copper AJ. Psychosomatic aspects of pre-eclamptic toxemia. *J Psychosom Res* 1958:2.

Dalton K. *Premenstrual Syndrome and Progesterone Therapy.* London: Heinemann, 1977.

DiGiovanna EL, Schiowitz S. *An Osteopathic Approach to Diagnosis and Treatment, 2nd ed.* Philadelphia: Lippincott-Raven, 1997:459–465.

Golay J, Vedam S, Sorger L. The squatting position for the second stage of labor: effects on labor and on maternal and fetal well-being. *Birth* 1993;20:73–78.

Kapanji IA. *The Physiology of the Joints, 2nd ed.* Edinburgh, UK: Churchill Livingstone, 1974:64–66.

Kuchera ML, Kuchera WA. *Osteopathic Considerations in Systemic Dysfunction, 2nd ed.* Columbus, OH: Greyden Press, 1994:216–217, 229.

Michele AA. *Iliopsoas.* Springfield, MO: Charles C. Thomas Publisher, 1962:187–189.

Moore KL. *Clinically oriented anatomy. The Abdomen.* Baltimore: Williams & Wilkins, 1985:275–276.

Muller-Tyl E, Wimmer-Puchinger B. Psychosomatic aspects of toxemia of pregnancy. *J Psychosom Obstet Gynecol* 1(3–4).

Myers R. Maternal anxiety and fetal death: In: Zichella and Pancheri, eds. *Psychoneuroendocrinology and Reproduction.* New York: Elsevier, 1979.

Northrup C. *Women's Bodies, Women's Minds.* New York: Bantam, 1994.

Putta LV, Spencer JP. Assisted vaginal delivery using the vacuum extractor. *Am Fam Physician* 2000;62:1316–1320.

Plauche WC, Morrison JC, O'Sullivan MJ. *Surgical Obstetrics.* Philadelphia: W.B. Saunders Company, 1992:288–289.

Ringrose CA. Psychosomatic influences in the genesis of toxemia of pregnancy. *Can Med Assoc J* 1961:84:905–907.

Still AT. *The Philosophy and Mechanical Principles of Osteopathy.* Kirksville, MO: Hudson, 1902.

Tettambel MA. An Interview: structural focus: key to osteopathic obstetrics concept. *Pharma* 1994.

Tettambel MA. Obstetrics. In: Ward RC, ed. *Foundations for Osteopathic Medicine.* Baltimore, MD: William and Wilkins, 1997.

Towner D, Castro MA, Eby-Wilkens E, Gilbert WM. Effect of mode of delivery in nulliparous women on neonatal intracranial injury. *N Engl J Med* 1999;341:1709–1714.

Zink JG. Respiratory and circulatory care: the conceptual model. *Osteopath Ann* 1977;3:108–112.

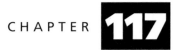

# Neurological Considerations

*Eileen L. DiGiovanna and Michael Rowane*

The human nervous system is extremely complex and has an effect on and is affected by the entire body. The central nervous system consists of the brain, including the cerebral cortex, the cerebellum, basal ganglia, and the brain stem, along with the spinal cord. From the brain arise the twelve cranial nerves and from the spinal cord arise the peripheral nerves:

1. Motor
2. Sensory
3. Autonomic
   a. Sympathetic
   b. Parasympathetic

## ■ BRAIN

The cerebral cortex is the center of conscious activity of the brain. Initiation of motor function begins here at the conscious level. Sensory input to the brain is processed and interpreted here. Speech, visual processing, and memory all have their centers in the brain. It is only in the human brain that rational thought and emotions are capable of being used at an advanced level.

The basal ganglia are structures that act as control centers between the sensory and motor systems. They control automatic movements and inhibit segmental reflexes. When dysfunctional, tremor, rigidity of muscles, or postural disorders may result.

The cerebellum has a proprioceptive function that controls posture, balance, and smoothness of muscle functioning. When this function is disturbed, symptoms such as dysfunctional movement, muscle tremor, loss of balance, or ataxia may be manifested.

The brain stem is the main connection between the superior parts of the central nervous system (CNS) and the spinal cord. All nervous impulses ascending from the cord to the CNS or descending from the CNS to the cord pass through the brain stem. Within the brain stem are the nuclei of the cranial nerves and the autonomic centers. Significant damage to the brain stem is inconsistent with the continuation of life.

Motor pathways in the brain consist of an *upper motor neuron* and a *lower motor neuron*. The upper motor neuron is located in the cerebral cortex and the lower motor neuron in the brain stem. A lesion of the upper motor neuron will result in muscle weakness or paralysis, with no muscle atrophy early and a disuse atrophy developing after a period of time. If a body part is bilaterally represented in the cortex, this would not be as noticeable. Increased muscle tone may be present along with increased tendon reflexes. The lower motor neuron is located in the brain stem. A lesion of the lower motor neuron is generally manifested as muscle weakness, flaccid paralysis, loss of reflexes, and an atrophy of the muscles.

### Cranial Nerves

There are twelve cranial nerves arising from the central nervous system. They arise from the brain as opposed to the spinal cord. They supply innervation, both motor and sensory, to the head and neck. There are three types of motor and three of sensory innervation from the cranial nerves:

I. Motor
  A. Somatic—to muscles developed from somites.
  B. Branchial—to muscles developed from the branchial arches
  C. Visceral—to muscles of the viscera, including smooth muscles and glands
II. Sensory
  A. General—pain, pressure, temperature, touch
  B. Special—vision, hearing, balance, smell, and taste
  C. Visceral—input from the viscera

Somatic motor fibers are carried in three cranial nerves to the muscles of the eye, the occulomotor (III), trochlear (IV), and abducens (VI), and in one to the tongue, hypoglossal (XII). Branchial motor fibers are carried by the trigeminal (V) to the temporalis and masseter muscles, by the facial (VII) to the muscles of expression of the face, by the glossopharyngeal (IX) and vagus (X) to the muscles of the pharynx and larynx, and the accessory nerve (XI) to the sternocleidomastoid and trapezius.

Visceral motor fibers are carried in the occulomotor nerve (III) to the muscles of the pupil of the eye. They are carried in the facial nerve (VII) to the glands of the head other than the parotid, which is innervated by the glossopharyngeal nerve (IX). The vagus (X) innervates all thoracic viscera and abdominal viscera to the splenic flexure of the colon.

Cranial nerves carrying special sensory input are:

1. Olfactory (I)
2. Vision (II)
3. Taste (VII, IX)
4. Balance (VIII)
5. Hearing (VIII)

The trigeminal nerve (V) is the only cranial nerve carrying general sensory fibers. It innervates the head, neck, meninges, and sinuses. The glossopharyngeal nerve (IX) and the vagus (X) carry visceral afferents, sensory input from the viscera such as nausea, but not pain.

It is important that the osteopathic physician understand the course and function of each cranial nerve. Dysfunction of a nerve may result from numerous factors including trauma, infection, or tumor. Assistance may be given to the healing process by discovering and treating any somatic components of the dysfunction with osteopathic manipulation. Improving circulation to the area, removing edema fluid and freeing compression of the nerve by bone or muscle are some ways in which the physician can assist.

## Spinal Cord

The spinal cord extends from the brain stem to the second lumbar vertebra at which level it becomes the *cauda equina,* separating into individual nerve bundles. The cord is segmented with nerve roots exiting each segment. Within the cord are the anterior horn cells from which arise the peripheral motor nerves and the dorsal horns into which the sensory nerves enter.

## Autonomic Nervous System

The autonomic nervous system provides access to most of the viscera of the body through either the sympathetic or parasympathetic systems, or by balancing the two systems. The autonomic nervous system is discussed in detail in Chapter 109.

## Impingement Neuropathies

Impingement neuropathies occur when surrounding tissues entrap a nerve, causing mechanical irritation or injury to the nerve. The most common ones occur to nerves of the upper or lower extremity and are discussed in those sections of this book.

## ■ BELL'S PALSY

Bell's palsy is a result of dysfunction of the facial nerve (VII), the cause of which is not known for certain, but may be related to cold, viral infection, or trauma resulting in an inflammation of the nerve. It is a lower motor neuron lesion, with all muscles being paralyzed to various degrees on the side of the lesion. There is generally a marked facial asymmetry with drooping of the corner of the mouth and the eyebrow, loss of nasolabial fold, and creases in the forehead. Typically, because of crossed fibers, there is sparing of the frontalis muscles. The eyelids do not close firmly and blinking is difficult so that the tears are lost, or the lacrimal gland fails to produce tears so that the eye dries out. It must be kept lubricated until normal tear production returns. Food tends to become lodged in the cheek or is lost from the corner of the mouth. Perception of sound is increased causing discomfort and taste may be lost. There may be significant pain in the jaw and around the ear.

The osteopathic physician will frequently find tenderness to palpation of the facial and cervical muscles, including the sternocleidomastoid and scalene muscles, on the ipsilateral side. There is often a somatic dysfunction at the level of C3. There may be occipitomastoid compression with an internally rotated temporal bone on the involved side.

Myofascial soft tissue treatment with counterstrain and muscle energy techniques may relieve the facial pain associated with Bell's palsy. The occipitomastoid compression should be released and the temporal bone assisted into normal internal/external rotation. Normal lymphatic flow should be assured by correcting dysfunctions of the cervical spine, cranial motion, and sacrum. C3 should always be evaluated and any dysfunction corrected.

## Parkinson's Disease

Parkinson's disease is a degenerative neurologic disease in which dopaminergic synapses in the *corpus striatum* deteriorate leading to tremor, bradykinesis, and muscular rigidity. Neurons, high in dopamine, are gradually lost from the *substancia nigra*. The patient loses voluntary control of muscles and will often "freeze" and be unable to initiate motion or will be unable to stop motion until some obstacle is met, e.g., walking into a wall. Many medications available for the treatment of the disease lead to dyskinesias, so medications must be carefully balanced.

Parkinson's patients begin to adopt a flexed posture, with the head tilted forward and an increased kyphosis of the thoracic spine. The gait is slow and shuffling. Flexion of hips, knees, and ankles is decreased, so tripping and falling occurs frequently causing multiple injuries. Occasionally an extension of the head and neck occurs, making it difficult for the individual to see where they are walking. The quality of life deteriorates for both the patient and the caregiver.

Generally, patients with Parkinson's disease are disabled beyond that caused by the disease itself. This is probably caused by the fact that they tend to decrease their activities with resultant loss of muscle strength and muscle tightness is increased by inactivity and prolonged flexed postures, i.e., sitting. Osteopathic manipulation has been shown to improve several facets of the Parkinson's disease complex, including the quality of life. A combination of manipulation, physical therapy, and strength training can, especially in the earlier phases, accomplish several things for the patient:

1. Improve head and body posture
2. Increase stride length
3. Increase hip, knee and ankle flexion with increased elevation of the foot from the floor
4. Decrease number of falls
5. Improve quality of life with decreased depression

Muscle energy techniques seem to be especially helpful in treating these patients.

Stretching of tight, hypertonic muscles increases range of motion of joints and aids in decreasing flexion deformities. Areas of somatic dysfunction may be treated with muscle energy, counterstrain, or facilitated positional release. Thrusting techniques are not as useful because of the muscle rigidity that often prevents movement through a barrier. Patients should be given a structured exercise program to perform at home, including muscle strengthening of the extremities. They and their caregivers need to be taught how to make their home safer from tripping and loss of balance, such as removing throw rugs, covering or removing wires from the floor, and installing safety bars in tubs and beside toilets.

## Reflex Sympathetic Dystrophy

Reflex sympathetic dystrophy (RSD) manifests unstable vasomotor activity in the distal extremities. Although it is most common in the upper extremity (hand), it can occur in the lower (foot) as well. The cause is poorly understood, but RSD seems often to follow a painful condition involving the extremity that has caused the extremity to be immobilized for a time. Myocardial infarction with pain in the left arm has preceded some cases. Injury to an extremity or stroke involving the extremity may be precipitating causes.

It appears that an abnormal stimulation of the sympathetic nervous system occurs, with symptoms manifesting weeks to months after the precipitating event. Initially, there is redness, edema, and burning pain of the extremity. The sympathetic fibers of the autonomic system travel with the arteries. Hypersympathetic activity results in vasoconstriction, inflammatory changes, and release of vasoactive substances. The pain may be so severe as to prevent use of the extremity. Often in the upper extremity, the shoulder of the involved arm is painful as well as the hand, known as *shoulder/hand syndrome*. Later the skin becomes atrophic with pallor or cyanosis of the digits, much as a Raynaud's phenomenon. If not resolved soon, irreversible changes occur, including contracture of extremity muscles and osteoporosis.

Prevention, if possible, is key. Patients who have had a stroke or myocardial infarction should be mobilized early. It is important to search for and treat any somatic dysfunctions related to the sympathetic system innervating the involved extremity; cervical, upper rib, and upper thoracic for the upper extremity, and lower thoracic or lumbar for the lower extremity. Pain must be controlled so that exercises may be prescribed and performed on a regular basis. Sympathetic nerve block may be required.

## ■ CASE ONE

R. B. was a 68-year-old white man with a history including cervical spinal fusion, 14 years of Parkinson's disease, and 8 years of neck tightness, with his head chronically in a forward bent position. He has had difficulty with ambulation in the past, in which he seems to cross one leg in front of the other and fall. The patient's family has used a private physical therapist to assist him, several times per week, with exercise and provide soft tissue massage to decrease the muscular tension in the cervical spine and improve his ability to raise his head.

The physical examination revealed the patient in a wheelchair with his body curled forward and his head in a flexed-forward position. The patient was able to communicate, but his speech varied in clarity of articulation. A neurological examination revealed his cranial nerves to be grossly intact. He had a slight action tremor, especially of extremities. His muscle strength was four out of five bilaterally; the deep tendon reflexes were decreased one-and-one-half out of four bilaterally; and sensation appeared to be equal bilaterally.

Key findings of the patient's structural examination involved a significant increase in the kyphotic curve of the thoracic spine and associated flattening of the lordotic curves of the cervical and lumbar regions. There was a decrease in range of flexibility of the right piriformis and left psoas muscles, as well as a pelvic asymmetry of the innominate bones being anterior/inferior on the right and posterior/superior on the left. There was mid- to upper thoracic paravertebral restriction on the right, especially at T3 and T6. The cervical spine examination revealed a marked decrease in range of motion with the head flexed forward and greater rotational motion to the left. There was an upper cervical somatic dysfunction at C2. There was obvious poor tone and laxity of the posterior cervical musculature, whereas there was tension and contraction of the anterior cervical muscles.

The primary focus of the initial treatment was to perform a full evaluation for primary and secondary sites of somatic dysfunction. Although the primary concern of the patient was the cervical region, it was important to correct any structural problems affecting the other parts of the body. Soft tissue and muscle energy techniques were complemented with moderate velocity–low amplitude (MVLA) techniques except for the cervical spine, where myofascial release techniques were the primary modality used. Trapezius inhibition techniques were performed with a compression myofascial technique to the right trapezius.

A series of specific exercises to stretch the cervical spine and rehabilitate it were given to the patient and his caretaker. Other modalities to aid in rehabilitation included the use of heat, attention to improving posture, and activity alteration.

Mr. B. was seen over the next few months on a monthly basis with some gradual improvement. He had a history of chronic anterior cervical tightness leading to forward bending. His wife noticed that during periods of fatigue, he would return to this position. In further treatment sessions, the goals were to increase range of motion, loosen the anterior cervical musculature and to encourage strengthening of the posterior cervical musculature. These had been distorted because of the prolonged flexed state of the patient's cervical spine. The patient found that after a few treatments he was able to hold his head up better and stopped falling. There was a long discussion with the patient on the need for a long-term rehabilitation program, in light of the progressive nature of Parkinson's disease. A time span of 4 weeks between treatments seemed to be optimum for the patient to maintain head control and avoid falling. The family was committed to performing all measures to help improve the status of the patient.

## Discussion

Parkinson's disease is a frustrating condition with a serious progressive decline of motor capabilities leading to complete disability. Any modality that can help enhance quality of life should be explored. There have been studies from the New York College of Osteopathic Medicine demonstrating the benefits of osteopathic manipulation, including one by Wells et al. A simple protocol had been used on ten patients with Parkinson's to evaluate the effect on gait. What is interesting is that a single session of OMT protocol had an immediate impact on the typical Parkinson's gait. A few other studies support the integration of a multidisciplinary team with physical therapy, proprioceptive and strength training, along with osteopathic manipulative treatment, especially one by Smutny et al. All of the 35 Parkinson's patients with 193 patient encounters had measurable improvements in one or more elements of gait analysis, whereas 71% had measurable improvements in every aspect of gait analysis.

Osteopathy in the cranial field (OCF) appears to be another area that may offer benefits to Parkinson's patients. Rivera-Martinez et al demonstrated that strain patterns involving bilateral occipitoatlantal and occipitomastoid compression were reduced significantly with OCF.

There is a body of literature developing on osteopathic manipulation for Parkinson's patients. The benefits of osteopathic manipulation do warrant further exploration as to specific manipulative protocols. This could encourage widespread use by primary care physicians to administer osteopathic manipulation in a time efficient manner. The benefits of osteopathic manipulation were tremendous for this patient and his activities of daily living. The patient had the number of falls reduced and was able to maintain head control if he received OMT at least every 4 weeks. This is one of the most dramatic benefits to a specific population that osteopathic manipulation can offer.

### REFERENCES

Berne RM, Levy MN. *Physiology*. Mosby, St. Louis, 1998.

Lehman SK, Wells MR, Smutny C, et al. Development of "The NYCOM osteopathic physical treatment program for patient's with Parkinson's disease." *J Am Osteopathic Assoc* 1998;98:390.

Rivera-Martinez S, Wells MR, Capobianco JD. A retrospective study of cranial strain patterns in patients with idiopathic Parkinson's disease. *J Am Osteopathic Assoc* 2002; 102:417–422.

Smutny CJ, Wells MR, Bosak A. Osteopathic considerations in Parkinson's disease. *J Am Osteopathic Assoc* 1998;98: 389.

Ward RC ed. *Foundations for Osteopathic Medicine, 2nd ed.* Philadelphia: Lippincott Williams & Wilkins, 2003.

Wells MR, Giantinoto S, D'Agate MS, et al. Osteopathic manipulative treatment acutely improves functional gait performance in patients with Parkinson's disease. *J Am Osteopathic Assoc* 1999;99:92–98.

Wilson-Pauwels L, Akesson EJ, Stewart PA. *Sandoz Course, Cranial Nerves, Anatomy and Clinical Comments*. Toronto: BC Decker Inc., 1988.

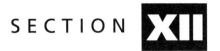

# OSTEOPATHIC MANAGEMENT

# CHAPTER 118

# The Manipulative Prescription

*Eileen L. DiGiovanna*

The osteopathic physician has the opportunity and responsibility to apply osteopathic principles in the management of all patients. Osteopathic manipulation should play a prominent role in the care of patients when appropriate. This chapter describes how osteopathic manipulation fits into the plan of management along with the information given in the practical applications chapters throughout this text. This plan is often called the "osteopathic prescription." As the physician would prescribe surgery or medications, the osteopathic physician will provide the additional prescription of manipulative care.

## ■ PATIENT EVALUATION

In no area of medicine is any treatment begun without benefit of a careful history and physical examination. From these follow a *differential diagnosis* list, which should include all possible causes of the patient's chief symptom. In the problem-solving process, the physician must determine whether further evaluative testing is needed to narrow the differential diagnosis to a *working diagnosis*. The information gathered from the history, physical examination, and additional testing is used to "rule in" or "rule out" conditions from the differential diagnostic list. In all cases, life-threatening illness must be excluded first.

An important part of the physical examination for the osteopathic physician is the *structural examination*. This not only provides information regarding the patient's neuromusculoskeletal system but also provides clues to visceral problems as well through viscerosomatic reflex findings and Chapman's reflex points.

In determining which adjunctive testing to use, the physician may use a variety of guidelines:

1. Know exactly what information you are seeking when you order adjunctive testing. The performance of indiscriminate testing is not a replacement for clinical insight. Differential diagnosis should form the basis of decision-making as to adjunctive testing.
2. Know which tests will provide the most information with the least risk to the patient and which are most cost-effective. Tests that will not confirm or alter the course of treatment should be avoided. The timing of some examinations may need to be taken into consideration (i.e., electrophysiological testing generally requires a 6-week latency before it is useful, certain radiological changes may only become apparent at certain intervals).
3. Plan the order in which the testing should be performed to assure that the most serious illnesses or injuries are addressed first. Generally, a sequence of least to most invasive is followed.
4. Inform the patient as to why the test is being ordered and what information it will provide. The patient is more likely to cooperate in obtaining the test if he understands the reason for it.

### Adjunctive Testing

1. Blood tests: These should be performed when looking for infectious processes, metabolic problems, specific visceral involvement in a disease process, autoimmune diseases, hema-

tologic problems, and other disease entities that may be identified through the blood.

2. Radiographic studies: x-rays of the musculoskeletal system should be taken under the following conditions:
   a. Suspicion of fracture or dislocation
   b. Suspicion of significant arthritis
   c. Significant musculoskeletal trauma occurred
   d. Anyone older than age 50 with bone or joint pain
   e. When a patient has been injured in a manner that has legal implications
   f. When there is a significant risk of a medical malpractice suit
   g. To diagnose and monitor the progress of structural scoliosis
   h. To measure leg length discrepancies and pelvic tilt

3. Magnetic resonance imaging (MRI): MRI is useful in identifying soft tissue injury or herniation of an intervertebral disc. It need not be performed for every suspected disc herniation unless the finding of such will change the treatment plan for the patient.

   Certain bony pathologies found on x-ray may be investigated in more detail with MRI.

4. Bone scan: A bone scan is particularly useful in a search for cancerous metastatic disease and should be used when there is a suspicion of this. Occult fractures may also be detected.

5. Bone density studies: Bone density studies are helpful in determining the presence and extent of bone mass loss in such conditions as osteopenia and osteoporosis. This is often a valuable screening test for women who have entered the menopause or for persons using long-term steroid medication.

6. Electromyographic/Nerve Conduction Studies (EMG/NCS): EMG/NCS are useful to identify specific nerve and muscle involvement, both which nerve is involved and the extent of the involvement. While the results may be helpful, it is not entirely accurate in all cases.

7. Positron emission test (PET): PET scanning may be useful in the determination of actual brain or other tissue functioning.

# ■ DEVELOPING A MANAGEMENT PLAN

The next step is to develop a management plan for the patient. Some considerations are:

1. Relief of pain
2. Control of any infectious process or metabolic disorder with appropriate medications
3. Improving patient mobility and quality of life
4. Necessary lifestyle changes
   a. Smoking cessation
   b. Good nutrition plan that will meet any special needs the patient may have
   c. Appropriate exercise regimen
   d. Assessment of risk factors with appropriate changes including preventive measures against future injury or illness

# ■ OSTEOPATHIC PRINCIPLES

Osteopathic principles should be an integral part of the overall evaluation and management of every patient.

1. **The body is a unit:** As the physician approaches the diagnosis of the patient's condition, the unity of the body should be kept in mind. It is never a good practice to isolate the focus of the examination to a single body part, even though the symptom seems related to only one area. A clear example is shoulder pain; pain in the shoulder may be caused by a cervical problem, shoulder joint or shoulder girdle involvement, an elbow or wrist problem, temporomandibular dysfunction, cardiac ischemia, irritation of the diaphragm, gall bladder disease, or even a postural imbalance that has caused compensation from the sacrum to the cervical region. Visceral problems may manifest in the soma and vice versa. Trigger points may refer pain some distance from the point itself. The physician must consider all facets of interrelatedness of the body.

   The concept of body unity includes consideration of the mental health and spiritual health of the patient as well as their physical status. Development of and recovery from illness is powerfully affected by depression, anxiety, fear, anger, guilt, feelings of helplessness and hopelessness, family relationships, and spiritual support systems.

2. **Structure and function are interrelated:** The physician must recognize that an abnormal structure is likely to result in abnormal functioning of that body part. Likewise, long-standing abnormal function will eventually

affect the structure involved by creating a compensatory position or motion pattern, changes in the structure itself, or stresses on the structure that will result in a breakdown of tissue. A treatment plan must focus on improving the structure and function of the patient to the nearest normal possible for that patient, even when those found do not seem to be related to the problem at hand.

The musculoskeletal system is the osteopathic physician's gateway to the treatment of many conditions both of that system and other systems connected to it by the nervous and the circulatory systems.

3. **The body is self-regulating and self-healing:** The wise physician will use the body's ability to repair and maintain itself. It then is the role of the physician to know when and where to intervene to assist the body in its healing process. Osteopathic considerations in doing so include:
   a. Maintaining good circulation to involved body parts.
   b. Maintaining good lymphatic flow to assure the best functioning of the immune system.
   c. Preventing facilitation of spinal segments that may send inappropriate feedback to involved structures through the nervous system, motor, sensory, or autonomic.
   d. Removing any sources of pain or discomfort that are treatable manually.
   e. Treating all somatic dysfunctions that interfere with motion of any body part or mobility of the patient in general.

## ■ OSTEOPATHIC MANIPULATIVE TREATMENT PRESCRIPTION

Once the physician has determined the working diagnosis and developed a plan for the management of the patient, it is necessary to decide on a plan for the use of osteopathic manipulative treatment (OMT). In making a decision as to which techniques to use, it is helpful to determine the goals of this treatment:

1. Relieve musculoskeletal pain or discomfort
2. Improve motion of specific joints
3. Improve arterial and/or venous circulation
4. Improve lymphatic flow

5. Affect nervous system involvement
   a. Autonomic input
   b. Nerve impingement
      (1) Peripheral nerve
      (2) Nerve root
      (3) Nerve plexus
   c. Spinal cord facilitation
   d. Reflexes
      (1) Viscerosomatic
      (2) Somatovisceral
      (3) Somatosomatic
      (4) Chapman's points
      (5) Trigger points
6. Affect patient's mental state
   a. Assist relaxation
   b. Relieve anxiety
   c. Improve patient's sense of well-being

Every physician and every patient must understand at the beginning of any course of treatment that not every condition is fully "curable." Many times the goal must be improvement and, even then, not every condition and not every patient will respond favorably to manipulative management. Goals need to be reassessed periodically to assure that they are still proper and reasonable.

## Models of Manipulative Treatment

As part of the determination as to the type of manipulative treatment to be selected, Greenman has proposed some manipulative models to assist in this selection. The models focus on specific goals for the treatment. In some patients it may be necessary to consider several goals and, therefore, more than one model may be used.

1. **Biomechanical model:** This model focuses on the postural and structural aspects of the patient's condition. This model is useful in treating patients with musculoskeletal pain and dysfunction, postural imbalances, joint injury or dysfunction, muscular and tendinous injury or imbalances, ligamentous injuries, gait abnormalities, and motion dysfunctions.

   The goals of this model are pain relief, quality of joint motion, joint function, toning of muscles, and overall health of the musculoskeletal system.

2. **Neurological model**: This model is indicated for influencing the nervous system through osteopathic manipulation. This model includes direct effects on the nervous system such as relieving a nerve impingement, as in carpal tunnel syndrome, or on viscera through the autonomic nervous system or treatment of viscerosomatic reflexes or Chapman's points. It can be for the relief of neurologically maintained pain or for improving quality of life for persons disabled by chronic neurologic disease processes.

3. **Respiratory/circulatory model**: The goals of this model include use of musculoskeletal system function in the maintenance of good arterial and, especially, venous circulation as well as assistance in the normal flow of lymph throughout the body. It includes maintaining proper functioning of the thoracic diaphragm, assuring proper motion of the thoracic cage, use of lymphatic pumps and effleurage, removing obstructions to the flow of blood or lymph, and assuring flow of all fluids in the body, including removal of tissue edema fluid and sinus drainage.

   Viscerosomatic reflexes from the heart and lungs will be treated as a combination of the two models of respiratory/circulatory and neurological when this is determined to be useful.

4. **Bioenergy model**: The bioenergy model focuses primarily on the inherent energies of the body and assuring a free flow of these energies, which the body uses in its regulatory and reparative efforts. An example of this is the cranial rhythmic impulse, the normal inherent force of the central nervous system, which may be accessed through osteopathy in the cranial field. Some thermal energies of the body may be used diagnostically by those trained in this method. The *percussion hammer*, as used and taught by Robert Fulford, DO, affects and normalizes vibratory energies in the body.

5. **Psychobehavioral model**: The effects of osteopathic manipulative medicine can be powerful in the realm of the patient's mental health. Touch has long been documented as a strong bond between individuals and is a physical demonstration of caring and concern. Stress is a known contributor to illness, pain, mental suffering and maintenance of conditions within the body which allow illness and injury to occur. A hands-on approach to treatment not only reassures the patient, but relaxes the muscles affected by stress and improves the sense of well-being. As pain decreases, so do anxiety and feelings of helplessness and hopelessness.

   Many patients experience an emotional release during an osteopathic manipulative treatment. They may laugh or cry, sometimes almost uncontrollably. A physician who is able to deal with these episodes can do much to relieve the patient's mental distress.

   While treating a patient with OMT, an excellent opportunity is provided for exploring the patient's concerns, fears, social problems, and other aspects of the patient's life that may be affecting his or her health.

## Choosing Techniques

Once a treatment model or models have been selected, the physician will need to determine the type of techniques she will use. The type of technique(s) will depend on a number of factors:

1. Patient's physical condition and stamina
2. Patient's age
3. Acuteness or chronicity of problem
4. Ability of patient to move into certain positions
5. Location of dysfunction or injury
6. Physician's knowledge and skill with various techniques
7. Physician's age, strength, and body habitus
8. Environmental factors
   a. Availability of treatment table
   b. In hospital, home, or office setting
9. Effectiveness of previous osteopathic treatments
10. Contraindications to certain techniques in specific patients
11. Risk/benefit considerations

The osteopathic physician will be well served to add as many techniques to his armamentarium as possible, including both direct and indirect types. This allows a wider choice of techniques. He should understand the principles of technique application and have a good knowledge of anatomy. He will then be able to modify techniques to the patient's advantage and comfort.

## Frequency of Treatment

Because each patient is unique, the frequency of treatment may vary from patient to patient, even for a condition that seems the same in both. A general rule that may be used is that a weekly treatment is generally sufficient for a subacute condition or in the early treatment of more chronic conditions. Some acute conditions necessitate more frequent treatment, perhaps even daily in the early stages.

However, it is important to remember that the patient requires time to allow the body to accommodate to the changes instituted during treatment and for the body to proceed with its own healing processes. Too frequent treatments can be more detrimental than helpful. Being aware of the changes that have occurred since the previous treatment assists the physician in determining the time between visits which is most productive of improvement.

## Duration of Treatment

There are two aspects to duration of treatment:

1. Length of treatment at one visit
2. Length of total treatment for any given condition

The duration of the treatment may vary from several minutes to an hour depending on the type of techniques being used and the amount of time available to the physician for the performance of the treatment. It is important to continually assess the tissues to assure that not too much is being done to them. It is also important to understand that it is not always possible to deliver a head-to-toe treatment to every patient. The patient will not tolerate it or may even be harmed by it. Finding the main source of the problem and addressing that first may relieve the physician of the necessity of treating many compensatory findings that will resolve when the central dysfunction is no longer present. Techniques such as cranial treatment may require more time caused by the sometimes slow and delicate nature of motion and responses.

The length of the total treatment plan will vary depending on the response of the patient to the treatment. Most acute conditions should respond within a reasonably short period of time, perhaps one treatment or perhaps after four to six treatments. After that amount of time, most dysfunctions will resolve or become subacute, although due to individual unique response, it could take a longer time or more treatments. Once the acute phase has passed, many patients will respond best to treatments administered every 2 to 3 weeks. Their bodies continue the healing process with less outside assistance.

Treatment of chronic conditions is much more variable and in some conditions become a matter of maintenance treatments in specific time frames. Often a monthly or bimonthly treatment is sufficient, while others may only require treatment every 3 to 6 months. The patient and physician will be able to determine the time span the responses to treatment will last based on the return of symptoms to their former state.

## Risk–Benefit Considerations

Although osteopathic manipulation is a highly effective and safe treatment for many conditions and a useful adjunct in the treatment of others, certain precautions, contraindications, and side effects must be taken into consideration when formulating a treatment plan. Because of the wide variety of techniques available to osteopathic physicians, there is no absolute contraindication to at least some form of manipulation in any given patient or condition as long as the patient's condition is stable and motion is permitted.

Because manipulation is practiced not only by osteopathic physicians but also by many nonosteopathic medical doctors, chiropractors, physical therapists, and others involved in manual medicine, it is obvious that millions of such treatments are given annually to patients with but few complications reported in the literature. It is generally reported that the incidence of untoward events occurring as a result of manipulative treatment is in the range of 1:400,000 to 1:3,000,000 cases. Few other medical interventions have this degree of safety.

It is important to differentiate between side effects and complications. For example, it is common for patients to experience some soreness after techniques such as counterstrain. This is not a complication, but a side effect of placing the patient in a position that stretches one group of muscles while shortening others. Cranial osteopathy may cause a sense of lethargy or fatigue in some cases, but this is not a complication, rather it is a side effect.

Many incidences considered as complications, such as vertigo, are often the result of something other than the treatment. Vertigo, for example, may be the result of the patient's head being turned and the inner ear may be the cause of the vertigo rather than the technique itself.

Some patients have a fear of certain techniques, notably the thrusting forms, and it may be best to hold off on doing these until the patient is more comfortable and trusting with the physician.

### Thrusting Techniques

Most of the severe iatrogenic complications reported as a result of manipulation are related to thrusting techniques. According to reports in the literature, most have involved the upper cervical spine. Complications include neurovascular accidents, some resulting from insult to the vertebrobasilar artery, aggravation of disk syndromes, and fractures. Missed diagnoses contributed significantly to complications, emphasizing the need for careful patient evaluation.

Physician-related problems include lack of skill, diagnostic error, and the use of inappropriate force. Patient-related problems include abnormal bony structure, pathologic entities, intolerance of head motion leading to vertigo, and psychological intolerance of this type of manipulation.

Perhaps the most significant complication reported is vertebrobasilar accident with rotary cervical manipulation, such as reported by Gittinger. In some persons, rotation and extension of the cervical spine cause narrowing of the vertebral artery on the side opposite the rotation. Pre-existent compromise of cranial collaterals, such as the carotids, must be considered. Occipital infarction may result, with various neurologic sequelae. Some considerations when using cervical high-velocity, low-amplitude (HVLA) techniques include preventing extreme extension, assuring there is no carrying of the head and neck out of the midline, and using minimal to no rotation. Many other techniques are available for the cervical spine so the risk versus the benefit of performing a thrusting technique, especially to the upper cervical region, must be considered.

Testing the patient's tolerance by extending and rotating the patient's head for 30 seconds while watching for nystagmus, nausea, or dizziness has sometimes been recommended. However, this screening test, known as the *DeKleyn test*, may actually incite an incident and frequently yields no accurate information.

One of the more common side effects of cervical HVLA appears to be vertigo. Although this may indicate impending vascular problems, in most cases it is of positional origin. True contraindications to thrusting techniques likely include the acute phase of rheumatoid arthritis, osteoporosis, bone cancers, fractures, known atherosclerotic plaques, and cervical spondylosis with vertebral artery ischemia. Care should be exercised in treating patients with radicular pain from herniated disks, pregnant women, or patients with acute whiplash, Scheuermann's disease, and postsurgical conditions. Patients on anticoagulant therapy or who have used bone matrix depleting medications should be treated with great caution.

### Muscle Energy Treatment

Muscle energy treatment is quite safe. Occasionally, some muscle stiffness and soreness occur after the treatment. If the area being treated is not localized well or if too much contractive force is used, pain may be increased.

Sometimes the patient is in too much pain to contract a muscle or for some reason is unable to cooperate with the physician's instructions or positioning. In such instances, muscle energy treatment may be difficult to apply.

Some complications reported as a result of muscle energy treatment include aggravation of herniated disk syndrome and increased pain. When the technique is performed properly, these are unlikely to occur.

## Counterstrain Techniques

Counterstrain is one of the safest of the techniques because it is purely positional and the patient or physician generates no force. Patients do need to be warned that they may feel sore after a treatment, because this is a common side effect. It can be expected that any resultant soreness should be gone within 24 to 48 hours, followed by relief of the original symptom.

The major problem with counterstrain is the patient's inability to assume certain positions because of pre-existing conditions that prevent them.

## Facilitated Positional Release (FPR)

Although FPR is a positional technique, some facilitating force is used. FPR with a compressive force should not be used in radiculopathy of the cervical spine; a traction force may be substituted.

## Myofascial Release, BLT, and LAS

Perhaps the gentlest of all the techniques when performed in an indirect manner, this still has some complications and side effects to be aware of. Aggravation of disc symptoms and muscle spasm are perhaps the most common, although even these are rare. Headaches, increased pain, and costochondral separation have been reported, none of which should happen when the technique is performed in a skillful manner.

## Cranial Treatment

These techniques are generally gentle; however, they may have the farthest-reaching effects when complications and side effects do occur.

Fatigue and lethargy are the most common side effects. Nausea, vomiting, headache, dizziness, and loss of appetite are seen. The most serious complication the author has heard of is hypopituitarism, after an intra-oral technique, which was a reversible problem. Emotional release, which may occur with any type of manipulation, most commonly occurs with cranial treatment, and the physician needs to be prepared to deal with this situation.

## Inhibition Techniques

While these may initially be painful in their application, they seldom have any side effects or complications. The most common would be a mild bruising in some patients at the site of the applied pressure.

# Eclectic Manipulation

Mastery of the multiple techniques of manipulative treatment will help the clinician determine and apply the most appropriate treatment in each patient. An analogy can be drawn with prescribing drugs: the more one knows about medications, their interactions, and their effects, the better one can tailor treatment to the individual case. Similarly, the more manipulative techniques the clinician knows, the more safely and effectively he or she can choose and use them. Each patient and each physician is different from any other. The manipulative procedures used should reflect these differences.

## REFERENCES

Bourdillon JF. *Spinal Manipulation, 3rd ed.* Norwalk, CT: Appleton-Century-Crofts, 1982.

Brownson RJ, et al. Sudden sensorineural hearing loss following manipulation of the cervical spine. *Laryngoscope* 1986;96:166–170.

DiGiovanna EL, Banihashem M, et al. *1996 Survey of American Academy of Osteopathy.* unpublished.

DiGiovanna EL, Schiowitz A. *An Osteopathic Approach to Diagnosis and Treatment, 2nd ed.* Philadelphia: Lippincott-Raven, 1997.

Gittinger JW. Occipital infarction following chiropractic cervical manipulation. *J Clin Neuroophthalmol* 1986;6:11–13.

Grayson MF. Horner's syndrome after manipulation of the neck. *Br Med J* 1987;295:1381–1382.

Greenman PE. *Principles of Manual Medicine, 2nd ed.* Baltimore: Williams & Wilkins, 1996.

Laughlin TM. Complications of spinal manipulation: a literature review 1975–1984. *Osteopath Ann* 1987;14:21–23.

Maitland GD. *Vertebral Manipulation, 4th ed.* Stoneham, MA: Butterworths, 1977.

# Index

Pages with *f* indicate figures; pages with *t* indicate tables.